HORMONES AND BRAIN FUNCTION

HORMONES AND BRAIN FUNCTION

Edited by

K. LISSÁK

Member of the Hungarian Academy of Sciences
Professor of Physiology
University Medical School
Pécs, Hungary

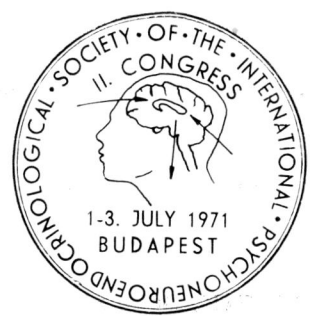

PLENUM PRESS • NEW YORK

Proceedings of the Second Congress of the International Society of Psychoneuroendocrinology held in Budapest (Hungary) from July 1 to 3, 1971

Published in the U.S.A. by

PLENUM PRESS

a division of

PLENUM PUBLISHING CORPORATION

227 West 17th Street, New York, N.Y. 10011

A copublication of Plenum Press, New York and Akadémiai Kiadó, Budapest

Library of Congress Catalog Card Number 72-87943
ISBN 0-306-30712-X

© Akadémiai Kiadó, Budapest, Hungary 1973

Printed in Hungary

CONTENTS

List of contributors	9
Preface	13
Ford, D. H.: Opening address	15
Brambilla, F.: Max Reiss memorial lecture	17

Section I

Neonatal and ontogenetic aspects of neuroendocrinology

Chairman: B. Flerkó

Gorski, R. A.: Mechanisms of androgen induced masculine differentiation of the rat brain	27
Dörner, G.: Sex hormone-dependent differentiation of the hypothalamus and sexuality	47
Kovács, S.: The role of thyroid and adrenocortical hormones in the biochemical maturation of the rat brain	53
Tsujimura, R., Kariyama, N. and Hatotani, N.: Disturbances of myelination in neonatally thyroidectomized rat brains	69
Vernadakis, A.: RNA synthesis in embryonic cerebellar explants cultured with estradiol	79
Nyakas, Cs.: Influence of corticosterone and ACTH on the postnatal development of learning and memory functions	83

Section II

Control, biosynthesis and release of pituitary hormones

Chairman: C. Fortier

Fortier, C.: Interrelationships in the control of ACTH and TSH secretion	93
Dupont, A., Bastarache, E., Bernatchez-Lemaire, I., Endrőczi, E. and Fortier, C.: Relationship of active avoidance learning to the pituitary–thyroid and pituitary–adrenocortical responses to cold exposure in the rat	105

Telegdy Gy.: Foetal steroidogenesis — 109

Halász, B. and Lengvári, I.: On the location of the neural structures involved in the reserpine induced hypersecretion of ACTH — 117

Martini, L.: Hypothalamic mechanisms controlling anterior pituitary functions — 123

Schreiber, V.: Thyroxine binding to anterior pituitary proteins in vitro: correlation with anterior pituitary growth — 143

Labrie, F., Pelletier, G., Lemay, A., Lemaire, S., Poirier, G., Barden, N., Béraud, G., Boucher, R., Gauthier, M. and Deléan, A.: Hypophysiotropic hormones, cyclic AMP and anterior pituitary protein synthesis and release — 157

Hilliard, J. and Sawyer, Ch. H.: Psychoneuroendocrine interactions in a reflex ovulator — 183

Shiotani, Y., Sakagami, M., Fujimoto, K. and Ban, T.: Influence of synthetic TRF administration and hypothalamic stimulation upon the ultrastructure of thyrotrophs — 195

Tallián, F.: The effect of oestradiol on pituitary–adrenal function in intact and thyroidectomized rats — 203

Halmy, L.: Studies on the regulation of pituitary–adrenal–thyroid and gonadal functions in rats with hypothalamic lesions — 207

Steiner, H., Piva, F., Motta, M., Gavazzi, G., Collu, R. and Martini, L.: Effect of synthetic TSH-releasing factor (TRF) and of some TRF analogues on pituitary function — 213

Motta, M., Collu, R. and Martini, L.: Effect of hypothalamic deafferentations on puberty in the male rat — 219

Fraschini, F., Collu, R. and Müller, E. E.: Mechanisms controlling pituitary gonadotropin secretion in prepuberal rats — 225

Piva, F., Schiaffini, O., Motta, M. and Martini, L.: The role of pineal principles in the control of ACTH secretion — 231

Debreczeni, L.: Effect of dehydrobenzperidol on pituitary–adrenal function — 237

Section III

Psychopharmacological and neurochemical bases of drug actions

Chairman: S. V. Anichkov

Anichkov, S. V. and Ryzhenkov, V. E.: Action of neurotropic drugs on the tropic functions of the pituitary — 243

Bekhtereva, E. P.: Action of central cholinolytics and oestrogens on gonadotropic release after the destruction of amygdala in rats — 253

Pfeifer, A. K. and Unyi, G.: The role of brain monoamines in the susceptibility to seizures brought about by chemical and electrical stimulations — 259

Kelemen, K.: Analgesia, tolerance and drug dependence — 273

Ryzhenkov, V. E.: Brain monoaminergic mechanisms and hypothalamic–pituitary–adrenal activity — 285

Sapronov, N. S.: Influence of some neurotropic drugs on the hypothalamo–pituitary–adrenal system after dexamethasone blockade — 287

Kuriyama, K. and Israel, M. A.: Effect of chronic ethanol administration on adenyl cyclase and cyclic 3',5'-nucleotide phosphodiesterase activities of mouse brain — 293

Hyyppä, M., Lehtinen, P. and Rinne, U. K.: L-dopa: its action on sexual behaviour and brain monoamines of the rat   297

Lehtinen, P., Hyyppä, M., Lampinen, P. and Rinne, U. K.: Sexual behaviour after neonatal reserpine and pCPA treatment with comment about hypothalamic indole amines in the rat   305

Mislow, J. F. and Friedhoff, A. J.: A comparison of chlorpromazine-induced extrapyramidal syndrome in male and female rats   315

Section IV

Hormonal influences on brain functions

Chairman: D. H. Ford

Ford, D. H. and Rhines, R. K.: Accumulation of ^{3}H-lysine in limbic and brainstem structures   329

Taleisnik, S. and Carrer, H. F.: Facilitatory and inhibitory mesencephalic influence on gonadotropin release   335

Kawakami, M., Terasawa, E., Kimura, F. and Kubo, K.: Correlated changes in gonadotropin release and electrical activity of the hypothalamus induced by electrical stimulation of the hippocampus in immature and mature rats   347

Schadé, J. P. and Wilgenburg, H. van: Steroid sensitivity of the nervous system   375

MacLean, P. D.: An evolutionary approach to the investigation of psychoneuroendocrine functions   379

Wied, D. de: The role of the posterior pituitary and its peptides on the maintenance of conditioned avoidance behaviour   391

Endrőczi, E. and Fekete, T.: Correlations between the pituitary–adrenal function and the exploratory activity, learning behaviour and limbic functions   399

Fuxe, K., Hökfelt, T., Jonsson, G. and Lidbrink, P.: Brain—endocrine interaction: are some effects of ACTH and adrenocortical hormones on neuroendocrine regulation and behaviour mediated via central catecholamine neurons?   409

Korányi, L. and Guzmán-Flores, C.: Pituitary–adrenocortical hormone influences on multiple units in the brainstem and forebrain structures   427

Murgaš, K. and Kvetňanský, R.: Effect of septal lesions on adrenal cortical and medullary activity during stress   437

Meyerson, B. J. and Lindström, L.: Sexual motivation in the neonatally androgen-treated female rat   443

Záborszky, L., Lénárth, Cs., Marton, J. and Palkovits, M.: Afferent brainstem pathways to hypothalamus and to limbic system in the rat   449

Peterfy, G. and Pinter, E. J.: Some physiologic aspects of emotional stress   459

Section V

Recent developments in clinical neuroendocrinology

Chairman: N. Hatotani

Hatotani, N.: Endocrinological studies on periodic psychoses	477
Wakoh, T. and Hatotani, N.: Endocrinological treatment of psychoses	491
Takahashi, S. and Gjessing, L. R.: Longitudinal study of catecholamine metabolism in periodic catatonia	499
Julesz, M.: Metabolism of androgenic steroids in human skin	507
Rubin, R. T., Kales, A. and Odell, W.: Secretion of LH and FSH during sleep in man	521
Legros, J. J., Palem, M., Servais, J., Margoulies, M. and Franchimont, P.: Basal pituitary–gonadal function in impotency evaluated by blood testosterone and LH assays	527

LIST OF CONTRIBUTORS

Anichkov, S. V. Institute of Experimental Medicine, U.S.S.R. Academy of Medical Sciences, Leningrad, U.S.S.R.
Ban, T. Department of Anatomy, Osaka University Medical School, Osaka, Japan.
Barden, N. Department of Physiology, Medical Faculty of Laval University, Quebec, Canada.
Bastarache, E. Department of Physiology, Medical Faculty of Laval University, Quebec, Canada.
Bekhtereva, E. P. Institute of Experimental Medicine, U.S.S.R. Academy of Medical Sciences, Leningrad, U.S.S.R.
Béraud, G. Department of Physiology, Medical Faculty of Laval University, Quebec, Canada.
Bernatchez-Lemaire, I. Department of Physiology, Medical Faculty of Laval University, Quebec, Canada.
Boucher, R. Department of Physiology, Medical Faculty of Laval University, Quebec, Canada.
Brambilla, F. Ospedale Psichiatrico Paolo Pini, Milan, Italy.
Carrer, H. F. Instituto de Investigación Médica Mercedes y Martín Ferreyra, Córdoba, Argentina.
Collu, R. Department of Pharmacology, University of Milan, Milan, Italy.
Debreceni, L. Mohács Hospital, Mohács, Hungary.
DeLéan, A. Department of Physiology, Medical Faculty of Laval University, Quebec, Canada.
Dörner, G. Institute of Experimental Endocrinology, Humboldt University (Charité), Berlin, G.D.R.
Dupont, A. Department of Physiology, Medical Faculty of Laval University, Quebec, Canada.
Endrőczi, E. Central Research Division, Postgraduate Medical School, Budapest, Hungary.
Fekete, T. Department of Neurology and Psychiatry, University Medical School, Pécs, Hungary.
Flerkó, B. Department of Anatomy, University Medical School, Pécs, Hungary.
Ford, D. H. Department of Anatomy, State University of New York, Downstate Medical Center, Brooklyn, N. Y., U.S.A.
Fortier, C. Department of Physiology, Medical Faculty of Laval University, Quebec, Canada.
Franchimont, P. Département de Clinique et de Pathologie Médicales, Université de Liège, Liège, Belgique.
Fraschini, F. Department of Pharmacology, University of Milan, Milan, Italy.
Friedhoff, A. J. Department of Psychiatry and Neurology, New York University Medical Center, School of Medicine, New York, N.Y., U.S.A.
Fujimoto, K. Department of Anatomy, Osaka University Medical School, Osaka, Japan.

Fuxe, K. Department of Histology, Karolinska Institutet, Stockholm, Sweden.
Gauthier, M. Department of Physiology, Medical Faculty of Laval University, Quebec, Canada.
Gavazzi, G. Department of Pharmacology, University of Milan, Milan, Italy.
Gjessing, L. R. Central Laboratory, Dikemark Hospital, Solberg, Norway.
Gorski, R. A. Department of Anatomy and Brain Research Institute, UCLA School of Medicine, Los Angeles, Cal., U.S.A.
Guzmán-Flores, C. Insituto de Investigaciones Biomédicas, Universidad Nacional Autónoma de México, Mexico City, Mexico.
Halász, B. Department of Anatomy, University Medical School, Pécs, Hungary.
Halmy, L. 4th Department of Internal Medicine, Postgraduate Medical School, Budapest, Hungary.
Hatotani, N. Department of Psychiatry, Mie Prefectural University School of Medicine, Tsu, Japan.
Hilliard, J. Medical Research Programs, Long Beach VA Hospital, Long Beach, Cal. U.S.A
Hökfelt, T. Department of Histology, Karolinska Institutet, Stockholm, Sweden.
Hyyppä, M. Department of Anatomy, University of Turku, Turku, Finland.
Israel, A. M. Department of Psychiatry, State University of New York, Downstate Medical Center, Brooklyn, N.Y., U.S.A.
Jonsson, G. Department of Histology, Karolinska Institutet, Stockholm, Sweden.
Julesz, M. 1st Department of Medicine, University Medical School, Szeged, Hungary.
Kales, A. Department of Medicine, Harbor General Hospital, Torrance, Cal., U.S.A.
Kariyama, N. Department of Psychiatry, Mie Prefectural University School of Medicine, Tsu, Japan.
Kawakami, M. 2nd Department of Physiology, Yokohama City University School of Medicine, Yokohama, Japan.
Kelemen, K. Department of Pharmacology, Semmelweis Medical University, Budapest, Hungary.
Kimura, F. 2nd Department of Physiology, Yokohama City University School of Medicine, Yokohama, Japan.
Korányi, L. Department of Physiology, University Medical School, Pécs, Hungary.
Kovács, S. Department of Physiology, University Medical School, Pécs, Hungary.
Kubo, K. 2nd Department of Physiology, Yokohama City University School of Medicine, Yokohama, Japan.
Kuriyama, K. Department of Psychiatry, State University of New York, Downstate Medical Center, Brooklyn, N.Y., U.S.A.
Kvetňanský, R. Institute of Experimental Endocrinology, Slovak Academy of Sciences, Bratislava, Czechoslovakia.
Labrie, F. Department of Physiology, Medical Faculty of Laval University, Quebec, Canada.
Lampinen, P. Department of Neurology, University of Turku, Turku, Finland.
Legros, J. J. Département de Clinique et de Pathologie Médicales, Université de Liège, Liège, Belgique.
Lehtinen, P. Department of Psychology, University of Turku, Turku, Finland.
Lemaire, S. Department of Physiology, Medical Faculty of Laval University, Quebec, Canada.
Lemay, A. Department of Physiology, Medical Faculty of Laval University, Quebec, Canada.
Lengvári, I. Department of Anatomy, University Medical School, Pécs, Hungary.
Léránth, Cs. 1st Department of Anatomy, Semmelweis Medical University, Budapest, Hungary.
Lidbrink, P. Department of Histology, Karolinska Institutet, Stockholm, Sweden.
Lindström, L. Department of Pharmacology, University of Uppsala, Uppsala, Sweden.
Lissák, K. Department of Physiology, University Medical School, Pécs, Hungary.
MacLean, P. D. National Institute of Mental Health, Poolesville, Md., U.S.A.
Margoulies, M. Département de Clinique et de Pathologie Médicales, Université de Liège, Liège, Belgique.
Martini, L. Department of Pharmacology, University of Milan, Milan, Italy.
Marton, J. 1st Department of Anatomy, Semmelweis Medical University, Budapest, Hungary.

Meyerson, B. J. Department of Pharmacology, University of Uppsala, Uppsala, Sweden.
Mislow, J. F. Department of Anatomy, Rutgers Medical School, New Brunswick, New Jersey, U.S.A.
Motta, M. Department of Pharmacology, University of Milan, Milan, Italy.
Müller, E. E. Department of Pharmacology, University of Milan, Milan, Italy.
Murgaš, K. Institute of Experimental Endocrinology, Slovak Academy of Sciences, Bratislava, Czechoslovakia.
Nyakas, Cs. Central Research Division, Postgraduate Medical School, Budapest, Hungary.
Odell, W. Department of Physiology, Medical Faculty of Laval University, Quebec, Canada.
Palem, M. Département de Clinique et de Pathologie Médicales, Université de Liège, Liège, Belgique.
Palkovits, M. Institute of Experimental Medicine, Hungarian Academy of Sciences, Budapest, Hungary.
Pelletier, G. Department of Physiology, Medical Faculty of Laval University, Quebec, Canada.
Peterfy, G. Department of Psychiatry, Reddy Memorial Hospital, Montreal, Canada.
Pfeifer, A. K. Institute of Experimental Medicine, Hungarian Academy of Sciences, Budapest, Hungary.
Pinter, E. J. Department of Medicine, Reddy Memorial Hospital, Montreal, Canada.
Piva, F. Department of Pharmacology, University of Milan, Milan, Italy.
Poirier, G. Department of Physiology, Medical Faculty of Laval University, Quebec, Canada.
Rhines, K. R. Department of Anatomy, State University of New York, Downstate Medical Center, Brooklyn, N.Y., U.S.A.
Rinne, U. K. Department of Neurology, University of Turku, Turku, Finland.
Rubin, R. T. Department of Psychiatry, Milton S. Hershey Medical Center, Hershey, Pennsylvania, U.S.A.
Ryzhenkov, V. E. Institute of Experimental Medicine, U.S.S.R. Academy of Medical Sciences, Leningrad, U.S.S.R.
Sakagami, M. Department of Anatomy, Osaka University Medical School, Osaka, Japan.
Sapronov, N. S. Institute of Experimental Medicine, U.S.S.R. Academy of Medical Sciences, Leningrad, U.S.S.R.
Sawyer, C. H. Department of Anatomy, UCLA School of Medicine, Los Angeles, Cal., U.S.A.
Schadé, J. P. Netherlands Central Institute for Brain Research, Amsterdam, The Netherlands.
Schiaffini, O. Department of Pharmacology, University of Milan, Milan, Italy.
Schreiber, V. IIIrd Medical Clinic, Faculty of General Medicine, Charles University, Prague, Czechoslovakia.
Servais, J. Département de Clinique et de Pathologie Médicales, Université de Liège, Liège, Belgique.
Shiotani, Y. Department of Anatomy, Osaka University Medical School, Osaka, Japan.
Steiner, H. Department of Pharmacology, University of Milan, Milan, Italy.
Takahashi, S. Central Laboratory, Dikemark Hospital, Solberg, Norway.
Taleisnik, S. Instituto de Investigación Médica Mercedes y Martín Ferreyra, Córdoba, Argentina.
Tallián, F. Department of Gynaecology and Obstetrics, Postgraduate Medical School, Budapest, Hungary.
Telegdy, Gy. Department of Physiology, University Medical School, Pécs, Hungary.
Terasawa, E. 2nd Department of Physiology, Yokohama City University School of Medicine, Yokohama, Japan.
Tsujimura, R. Department of Psychiatry, Mie Prefectural University School of Medicine, Tsu, Japan.
Unyi, G. Institute of Experimental Medicine, Hungarian Academy of Sciences, Budapest, Hungary.

Vernadakis, A. Department of Psychiatry, University of Colorado Medical Center, Denver, Col., U.S.A.
Wakoh, T. Mie Prefectural Hospital Takachaya, Tsu, Japan.
Wied, D. de Medical Faculty of University of Utrecht, Utrecht, The Netherlands.
Wilgenburg, H. van Netherlands Central Institute for Brain Research, Amsterdam, The Netherlands.
Záborszky, L. 1st Department of Anatomy, Semmelweis Medical University, Budapest, Hungary.

PREFACE

The International Society of Psychoneuroendocrinology organized its second congress in Budapest between 1 and 3 July, 1971. The sudden death on the 27th of July, 1970, of Professor Max Reiss, the President of the Society, nearly caused a break in the preparation of the Congress, but with the invaluable help of Professor Donald H. Ford, Treasurer and Acting President, and Professor Francesca Brambilla, Secretary of the Society, the Organizing Committee surmounted the difficulties. The Organizing Committee of the Congress set out five main topics discussed in five sections by invited lecturers and collective papers by registered discussants.

Technically, the Congress was organized by the Hungarian Physiological Society in cooperation with the Federation of Hungarian Medical Societies in the building of the Hungarian Academy of Sciences. Thanks to the generosity of the Medical Section of the Hungarian Academy of Sciences we are able to publish the Proceedings of the Congress by the Publishing House of the Hungarian Academy of Sciences jointly with Plenum Press, New York.

The Congress was sponsored by the International Society of Psychoneuroendocrinology, the Hungarian Academy of Sciences, the Hungarian Pharmaceutical Industry, the Factory of Electronic Measuring Instruments, the Upjohn Co., Kalamzoo, Michigan and the Wellcome Research Laboratory, Langley Court, Backenhom, Kent, England. On behalf of the Organizing Committee may I express our grateful thanks for their generous assistance which, despite many difficulties, made the successful organization of an international congress possible.

This volume contains the papers presented at the five sections of the Congress.

K. Lissák
President of the Congress

OPENING ADDRESS

D. H. FORD

Department of Anatomy
State University of New York
Downstate Medical Center
Brooklyn, N.Y., U.S.A.

Members of the International Society of Psychoneuroendocrinology, members of the Hungarian Academy of Sciences and friends, it is a great pleasure to be here today at the opening of the second international meeting of our Society.

May I thank our hosts, Dr. Lissák and his associates for planning what I am sure will be a most enjoyable conference. I know from my own experiences that they have worked long and hard to prepare an unforgettable educational and cultural experience for us. We all owe them a debt of gratitude for their labors.

As most of you know, ours is a very young society, being only two years old and I think its members are to be congratulated in supporting two international meetings within its first two years of life. I sincerely trust that this signifies the vigor with which the society will attempt to fulfil its mission of bringing psychiatry and neuroendocrinology together to effect an improved approach to our treatment of mentally disturbed patients. Hopefully, this will be paralleled by increasing cooperation between the clinical and preclinical branches of medicine to facilitate our research endeavors. While I am sure it is too early to point to great steps in this direction, the mere fact of our meeting together here to share our research experiences in a variety of fields points toward a future of continuing shared experiences. To this end, I hope that I will see many of you again next year at the workshop on the Neurobiology of Maturation and Aging in Brooklyn, N.Y. and at our annual meeting, which will be in London.

Hormones and Brain Function, Budapest 1971, pp. 17–23 (1973)

MAX REISS MEMORIAL LECTURE

F. BRAMBILLA

Ospedale Psichiatrico Paolo Pini
Milan, Italy

I have been asked to come here today to honour, together with all of you, the memory of Prof. Max Reiss, the founder and first president of the International Society of Psychoneuroendocrinology.

Max Reiss died 12 months ago, but I believe that he is still here with us, to see his ideals and his work to continue through our work and our faith in his basic principles, strive for knowledge, for truth, for honest work; not sterile research, done in order to obtain fame and honours, but the need to help human beings to understand the physiology and pathology of body and mind, and therefore to help other human beings to recover from their suffering.

I hesitated to accept the undeserved honour to talk about Max Reiss to outstanding researchers like you, who much better than me can understand and appreciate the value of his work and his message. But I am here only to express the feelings that we all share.

And because I believe that, in spite of the extremely relevant researches that he did and results that he obtained, the most important message coming from him is that we are only here to search for knowledge, and the one who possesses it is only a messenger to transmit knowledge to the others. So, here I am nothing else than the representative of those people who are trying to receive the message, to understand it, and to achieve it. Because, if Max Reiss worked and talked to people like you, who shared with him the possibility and ability to study and discover what is lying under the mistery of physical and mental phenomena, he worked and talked also to people like me, who long for knowledge and ask for help from all of you.

Very frequently in his lectures Max Reiss mentioned the "ivory tower" of science, only to condemn it and try to remove the remoteness of it. That is why the death of Max Reiss is for us something more than the loss of an outstanding researcher; and it is important that all of you, and the people like you, understand that what we expect and need from you is to carry on what he has started.

To talk about the scientific life of Max Reiss is not easy: the amount of work that he did, and the quality of it, could only be described as unbelievable from a single human being.

He started in 1922, at Prague University as assistant of the famous Prof. Biedl, and then Associate Professor of the Endocrine Department of the Institute for

General and Experimental Pathology, until 1938. The papers and books published in this period cover the most extensive and impressive field of hormonal research; physiology and pathology of endocrine glands, peripheral metabolic effects of hormones, methodological developments for hormonal assays, hormone extractions from animal glands, each research is a basic step in the field which was a mistery at that time.

We can only mention briefly his work: studies on the metabolic effects of insulin and epinephrine; on the adrenals, thyroid, gonad secretions and their general biochemical influence; on the multiple stimulatory activities of the pituitary. It seems to me, however, that the most relevant point in his research is that, already in those early days, he was trying to demonstrate and assess the existence of the peculiar interrelationship existing among all the different glands, their secretions and their general metabolic effects. He examined and demonstrated the now well-known phenomenon of the central regulatory function of the pituitary, and the peripheral activities of the thyreotrophic, corticotrophic, follicle-stimulating, luteinizing and somatotrophic substances, as stimulators of trophism and secretions of the target glands, and as regulators of a multitude of general metabolic mechanisms.

One of his most interesting fields of research was on the relationship between hormones and tumours, examined both as regards the cause–effect phenomena, and the possible therapeutic approach to the disease, a field, which has been later so largely developed by other scientists, and from which so many extremely important informations as to the mechanism of tumour growth, their biochemistry, and therapies have resulted. In 1938 in Brussels, Prof. Reiss, won the Cancer Society's prize for these researches. In 1938 Max Reiss emigrated to England to work with Prof. Golla in Maudsley Hospital, London, and then to become director of the Endocrine Department of the Burden Neurological Institute of Bristol, until 1946. From 1946 to 1957 he was research director of the Bristol Mental Hospital, honorary consultant of the S. Ebba's Hospital in Epsom, consultant in Mental Health of the South Western Regional Hospital Board under the Ministry of Health. At this time Max Reiss, even though continuing his basic research on the multiple pituitary functions, starts to confront the problem of mental health and to establish the basis of his main course of future research. I could say that he starts to think, believe and assess the necessity of the work that we are doing here today. His approach to the problem of the relationship between physiology and pathology of the brain and mentality is certainly the most audacious, modern, polymorphous and at the same time conclusive among all those that have been proposed up to now. The first experiments are the results of extremely significant researches on the effects of hormones on basic brain metabolism including extensive study of the relevant literature. For years psychiatrists and biochemists had been trying to establish the hormonal patterns of various mental diseases, divided according to the usual nosological definitions. The results obtained were contradictory, and, what is worse, the hormone therapies mostly failed. Max Reiss controlled first a large series of patients, according to the usual transversal method, and it was evident soon to him that the method itself was incorrect. First, the nosological division in big groups included patients too heterogeneous from the psychopathological and physical point of view. Second, the transversal method was inconclusive, due to the day-to-day spontaneous variations in the hormonal patterns. Third, the examination of a single gland activity did not give information about the complete biochemical profile of the patients, considering that the metabolic homeostasis of the human body is the consequence of a coordinate correlation between a multitude of hormonal and enzymatic processes. That is why his first experiments on thyroid and adrenal secretions were discouraging. Apparently in the same group of patients, considered erroneously homogeneous, a peculiar hormonal impairment typical of a peculiar mental disease did not seem to exist. Hypo-, hyper- and eusecretion of the thyroid and adrenals were present, changing from day to day, sometimes spontaneously, sometimes after therapy. This wide variability was the consequence of a methodological error. Either we can make really homogeneous groups of patients, classified according to the presence of peculiar psychopathological and physical phenomena and not according to the usual nosological divisions, or else we must study each patient with a longitudinal method, through months and years of psychiatric and biochemical observations. Each patient is an entity with a peculiar mental and hormonal profile, and therefore with the need of a specific personal therapy.

To understand why psychoses and neuroses develop in patients in connection with certain physical conditions, why the same mental disease proceeds according to different patterns in an apparently homogeneous group of patients, why the same therapeutic approach ends up in positive or negative results, we must keep in mind the fundamental theory of the vicious cycle proposed by Max Reiss.

In the appearance and development of a mental disease the following factors are fundamental:

1. Premorbid personality, often genetically determined, the quality of which decides the outcome of the future mental disturbance.
2. Lability in the endocrine equilibrium, which determines the individual adaptability to normal surroundings, to arising emergencies, to external or internal stimuli, to stress.
3. External precipitating cause (like mental and physical strains, increased environmental demands for adaptation, etc.).

The importance of a premorbid personality in relation to mental diseases is well known by the psychiatrists. But the importance of the individual biochemical, or better endocrine substrates cannot be ignored. The adaptation of the human body to different psychophysical situations depends at least in part on a well-balanced hormonal system. The endocrine glands receive stimuli from the environment through the afferent nervous connections, through the cells of central nervous system neurotransmitters, neurohormones. In turn, the variations in the hormonal patterns act on the structures and functions of brain cells, behaviour, psychological adaptability and reactivity to the surroundings, in one word on mentality, closing therefore a vicious cycle which most of the time cannot be spontaneously interrupted. And if the premorbid personality of the subject is determinant for the appearance of peculiar psychopathological symptoms, it seems decisive, too, for the direction in which the neuroendocrine vicious cycle develops. The fundamental point once established, that each patient presents a specific premorbid personality and a peculiar endocrine lability responsible for the development of psychopathological phenomena, it is easy to understand the kind of diagnostic and therapeutic approach of Max Reiss.

Especially significant were his experiments on schizophrenia. First, from the longitudinal observations of the patients he could demonstrate a frequent deficiency in the pituitary–gonadal axis, a relatively low percentage of thyroid impairment, in the sense of both hyper- and hypothyroidism, a wider range of variations from day to day of the adrenal secretions with an impaired hypothalamo–pituitary–adrenal axis, a rather frequently abnormal adrenal circadian rhythm. All these alterations seemed to correlate with the development and prognosis of the mental disease. Either in untreated patients, or in subjects under different psychiatric or hormone therapies, the improvement of the endocrine substrate was constantly connected with a psychiatric improvement. And more important again, the patients who maintained the newly acquired endocrine homeostasis did not relapse into the previous psychopathological disorders. The biochemical effects of different psychiatric therapies were examined. Electroshock treatment, insulin coma, leucotomy, general hospital care, hormone therapies, psychotropic drugs, when successful for the mental disorders, seemed to induce an analogous biochemical improvement. Especially interesting was the observation that both hypo- and hyperfunctions of the different glands seemed to improve after the same therapy. According to Prof. Reiss all these therapies do not induce a stimulation or an inhibition of a single endocrine axis, but re-establish a new equilibrium of the neurotransmitters and neurohormones, acting through different pathways. Electroshock therapy influences directly the brain biochemistry; insulin coma interferes with the basic metabolism of the nervous cells, through its specific action on the carbohydrate levels; leucotomy modifies the supraoptic–hypothalamic connections; general hospital care acts at the level of higher brain centres, due to the change in the environment and emotional involvements; psychotropic drugs seem to influence the neurotransmitters; hormone therapy, through the now well-known positive and negative feedback mechanisms, has an effect on the hypothalamic centres and probably on suprahypothalamic specific areas. The same results occur in the field of manic–depressive psychoses. However, certain endocrine impairments seem to occur with a relatively more constant frequency. In the depressive phase a hypersecretion of thyroid and adrenals is often present, together with a reduced pituitary–gonadal function. The opposite endocrine patterns are present in the manic phase. However, as in schizophrenia, it is difficult to assess the existence of a specific endocrine impairment related to a phase of the disease, due to the overlapping results in both groups. Here again the therapeutic approach, if successive, seems to influence both the psychopathological and biochemical aspects of the syndrome.

In 1958 the publication of the book on Psychoendocrinology was the first tentative to establish a new branch of scientific research, a precursor of the work that we are doing today in our Society.

In 1957 Max Reiss left England for the United States, and became the director of the Neuroendocrine Research Unit at Willowbrook State School, Staten Island, N.Y., an outstanding Institute for mentally retarded patients.

He started here to approach the problem of mental deficiency which was to be his field of research until his death.

Again the first problem which arises is the definition of mental deficiency, from the point of view of the causes and of the interfering factors. Mental deficiency is too wide a classification, which includes the most disparate psychophysical syndromes. Sometimes it is just a diagnosis which defines the end-result of an unknown disease.

The importance of certain endocrinopathies as the cause of mental deficiency is well known. But the pathogenesis of dysmetabolic mental deficiencies, of mongolism, of the so-called socio-familiar syndrome, is still under discussion. In too many cases the endocrine system seems unbalanced, either from the point of view of clinical symptoms such as delayed growth, physical and sexual retardation, or in the laboratory findings. Here again the theory of the interrelationship between the genetically determined metabolic constitution, the psychological influence of the surroundings, the severe childhood diseases, as combined causes of most of the syndromes, could represent the answer to the problem. All these different factors act on brain development and maturation, and in the meantime influence, via the hypothalamo–pituitary axis, endocrine secretions.

We know that most of the hormones interfere with the adequate development and function of brain cells in general and in specific areas of the central nervous system. That is why, here again, the theory of the vicious cycle is extremely relevant. Genotypical and phenotypical alterations of the brain cells induce a hypothalamo–pituitary target gland impairment: the hormonal imbalance, through multiple biochemical alterations, determines a secondary aggravation of damaged brain metabolism.

The studies on mongolism and dysmetabolic mental deficiencies, carried out by Prof. Reiss, reveal a multitude of minor hormonal disturbances. They are often not fully developed endocrine diseases; but pituitary–thyroid–adrenal and gonadal deficiencies seem present in many cases, either as a combination of errors, or as a single endocrine imbalance. In the mongoloids, the thyroid hypofunction reported by previous investigators, was not confirmed, except for a small percentage of the subjects. However, the examination of different parameters (such as BMR, PBI, ^{131}I uptake, red blood cell uptake of ^{131}I triiodothyronine, TSH stimulation test) pointed out discrepancies from one test to another, suggesting the possibility of metabolic impairments along the axis pituitary–thyroid–peripheral tissues. The adrenal and gonadal secretions, too, revealed frequently a mild deficiency.

We all know that the cause of the disease is chromosomal; but we do not know what is the basis of the chromosomal error. The hypothesis of an endocrine impairment of the placenta, as a cause of the foetal chromosomal alterations, proposed by Prof. Reiss, is certainly interesting. It is based on an extensive study of the literature on the effect of triiodothyronine (Tata and Widnell 1964), cortisol (Sekeris and Lang 1964) and androgens (Freemann et al. 1964) on the DNA–RNA relationship, and on personal experiments on the effect of testosterone, progesterone and hypophysectomy on mitotic index and liver cell content in RNA–DNA. Among the different syndromes of dysmetabolic mental deficiencies, phenylketonuria has been chosen and extensively studied by Prof. Reiss as a model for similar mental impairments related to different biochemical alterations. This disease seems related to an enzymatic deficiency, or probably to multiple enzymatic deficiencies, interfering with the metabolism of phenylalanine.

Phenylketonuric patients present a poor physical and sexual development and maturation, either in untreated cases or in subjects following specific phenylalanine poor diet. Hormone examinations reveal defective thyroid, adrenal and gonadal secretions, with a well preserved answer to stimulation tests, demonstrating therefore an impairment related to a hypothalamo–pituitary hypofunction. In the experimental animals Reiss demonstrated that a phenylalanine overload leads to a decrease in phenylalanine–hydroxylase levels. Therefore, the enzymatic defect of phenylalanine hydroxylase could be the result of the disease and not the initial cause. Hormone treatments, with growth hormone, chorionic gonadotrophin, anabolic steroids, both in animals and humans, reduce the high values of phenylalanine, and in children, precautiously treated, seems to induce also a significant mental improvement. It seems therefore that a more extensive study of the disease, taking into consideration an endocrine nosographic and therapeutic approach, should be worthwhile.

The wider group of the so-called socio-familiar mental retardation, where the environmental factors seem to represent the cause of the disease, shows also signs of multiple hormone disturbance. It must be mentioned that probably the group itself is not homogeneous. However, he stated, as in the case of endocrine disturbances of the psychoses, that in this case, too, a congenital mental and physical impairment exists, aggravated by the phenotypical factor of a negative socio-familiar influence. Extremely relevant are the results obtained by Prof. Reiss with hormone therapies, selected specifically after extensive metabolic studies of each patient. Growth hormone, anabolic steroids, thyroid extracts, probably through their specific influence on the development and maturation of brain cells, sexual hormones and chorionic gonadotrophin, through their effect on the maturation of specific brain areas, sensibly improve the mental deficiency, the accessibility, cooperation and learning ability of the patients, resulting in a better possibility for psychotherapy, specialized school instruction and vocational training.

A very interesting phenomenon, demonstrated by Prof. Reiss, is the presence of substances inhibiting luteinizing hormone, serotonin action and spontaneous activity in the blood and urine of mentally deficient subjects. This factor is present usually in a small quantity in normal children and adults, it is a substance which shows striking similarity to pineal extracts, both in the biochemical characteristics and peripheral effects, such as inhibition of serotonin and oxytocin actions, of TSH, ACTH and gonadotrophin secretions.

The physiological activity of the pineal gland itself has been extensively studied by Prof. Reiss: from the experiments with pinealectomized animals and after treatment with pineal extracts, it seems that this gland possesses both a stimulatory and an inhibitory effect on the pituitary and peripheral glands, together with a very impressive secretion of serotonin and its metabolites. It seems therefore an area where regulation of brain function and endocrine secretions occurs simultaneously. The possible meaning of such a strict relationship is impressive.

We could continue for hours to report and discuss the experiments and the results obtained by Max Reiss. But the conclusions that we can draw from his work are more important. The first one is that body and mind are a single unit, which cannot be examined separately if we want to understand and improve their functions. But it is more important for us that the work of a single group of scientists, examining a peculiar physical or psychological area, with a specific methodological approach, cannot lead to conclusive results. Only a combined effort of anatomists, physiologists, biochemists, neurologists, psychologists and psychiatrists can give the answer to the problem of normal and pathological psychophysical structures of the human being. And that is why Max Reiss made great efforts for the creation of our Society and the success of a group, which is the first one to represent a tentative of combined work toward the same goal. If our team will be successful, if we make even a small step toward the knowledge of human mental and physical entity, the exhaustive life-work of Max Reiss will not have been in vain. That is what he longed for, that is the heredity which he has left to us, that is what we must fight for. It is a difficult task but also the most generous gift we could receive. And I know that I can say for all of us that we understand his message and we will try to accomplish it.

REFERENCES

FREEMANN, J. J., HOLF, R., IOVINO, A. J. and MICHEL, I. (1964): Effects of steroids upon weight, protein and nucleic acid concentration of the preputial gland of the female rat. *Endocrinology* **74,** 990.

SEKERIS, C. E. and LANG, N. (1964): Stimulation of messenger RNA synthesis in rat liver by cortisol. *Life Sci.* **3,** 169.

TATA, J. R. and WIDNELL, C. C. (1964): Nucleic acid synthesis during the early action of thyroid hormones. *Biochem. J.* **92,** 26.

SECTION I

NEONATAL AND ONTOGENETIC ASPECTS OF NEUROENDOCRINOLOGY

Chairman: B. FLERKÓ

MECHANISMS OF ANDROGEN INDUCED MASCULINE DIFFERENTIATION OF THE RAT BRAIN*

R. A. GORSKI

Department of Anatomy and Brain Research Institute
UCLA School of Medicine
Los Angeles, Cal., U.S.A.

In order to put our more recent work in proper perspective, I would like first to review briefly the concept of sexual differentiation of the rat brain (for a more complete review see Gorski 1971a, b). Reproductive activity of the intact male rat is markedly different from that of the female. The adult male secretes androgen and forms mature spermatozoa essentially continuously. In addition, the male rat will display sexual behavior whenever presented with a receptive female. Although male sexual behavior is inhibited by a novel environment, once the experienced male adapts to the new environment of the testing cage, he will mate with the receptive female.

In contrast, reproductive activity of the female rat is cyclic. Mature ova are released only at ovulation which occurs spontaneously every four or five days. Ovulation in turn, is produced by a cyclic surge of gonadotrophin (GTH) release from the pituitary. In contrast to the relatively stable production of androgen by the testes, the ovaries of the female rat secrete markedly different amounts of estrogen and progesterone throughout the reproductive cycle. Cyclic ovarian activity is responsible for the characteristic four- or five-day vaginal cycle, and for the display of sexual receptivity only on the evening of vaginal proestrus.

Ovulation, which is the key to the estrous cycle of the female, is brought about by the neural activation of the pituitary gland in response to circulating levels of ovarian estrogen. Because of the dependence of this brain function upon estrogen, one might assume that the sex difference in reproductive activity is due to the presence of a functional ovary in the female and its absence in the male. However, when an ovarian graft is transplanted into the castrated male rat, ovulation does not occur. Even in the presence of ovarian steroids the brain of the male rat cannot bring about ovulation. The pituitary gland itself is not the factor which determines the reproductive pattern since pituitary transplants from the male will permit the resumption of ovulatory estrous cycles in the hypophysectomized female. With respect to the pattern of pituitary activity, the ability of the brain of the female rat to regulate the cyclic surge of GTH responsible for ovulation is the fundamental sex difference. The concept of sexual differentiation states that

---

* Original research by the author supported by Grant HD-01182 from the National Institute of Health and by the Ford Foundation.

this fundamental sex difference in brain function is not established directly by neuronal genetic expression. On the contrary, the production by the neonatal testes of a substance, presumably androgen, is the factor which determines the course of development of the brain.

THE NEURAL REGULATION OF OVULATION

An important aspect of the possible mechanism of action of androgen neonatally would be its probable focus of action. Since the neural regulation of ovulation is the key to the sex difference in pituitary activity, the elucidation of this system is critical to our topic. On the basis of much experimental evidence (Flerkó 1966, Everett 1969, Gorski 1971a) it is now generally accepted that the neural control of GTH secretion can be divided into several distinct levels (Fig. 1). The lowest level of control can be represented by the medial basal hypothalamus, perhaps the arcuate nucleus in particular. Neurons within this region regulate the basal level of pituitary activity responsible for follicular growth and estrogen secretion, but cannot independently bring about ovulation. In the male rat this region is sufficient to maintain near normal testicular activity without afferent neural input (Halász 1969).

In the female, ovulation is regulated by a higher level of control. In Fig. 1 we have indicated that this control system may involve the preoptic-anterior hypothalamus, a concept which is in good agreement with deafferentation studies (Halász and Gorski 1967, Köves and Halász 1970), and with studies which indicate that this region has special affinity for labeled estrogen (Pfaff 1968, Anderson and Greenwald 1969, Stumpf 1970, Zigmond and McEwen 1970). The figure also indicates, however, that extrahypothalamic circuits may modify ovulatory function.

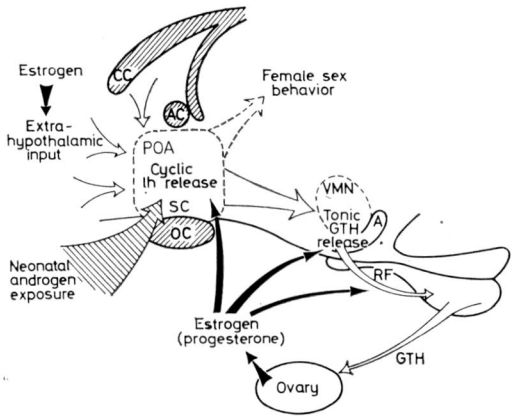

Fig. 1. Localization on a schematic parasagittal diagram of the brain of the neural control of hypophyseal secretion. Solid arrows indicate ovarian steroid feedback. The preoptic-anterior hypothalamic area (POA) is important both for the regulation of ovulation and female sexual behavior, and may be the focus of the permanent neonatal action of androgen. Abbreviations: A, arcuate nucleus: AC, anterior commissure; CC, corpus callosum; OC, optic chiasm; RF, releasing factors; SC, suprachiasmatic nucleus; and VMN, ventromedial nucleus. (Reprinted from Gorski 1970)

In this scheme I have not attempted to distinguish between the regulation of follicle stimulating hormone (FSH) and luteinizing hormone (LH) since both are released in the ovulatory surge. Flerkó (1966) has established a specific role for the anterior hypothalamus in the regulation of FSH release. Although Kordon (1967) has suggested that the premamillary region may also regulate FSH secretion, his observation that lesions of this region will restore ovulatory cycles in rats made anovulatory by suprachiasmatic lesions has not been confirmed by Illei-Donhoffer et al. (1970). Moreover, in response to a similar observation by Taleisnik (1966), we placed mamillary lesions in anovulatory androgenized females. Although ovulation occurred, presumably in response to the stimulatory component of the lesioning procedure, ovulatory cycles were not induced (Hagino et al. 1964). Although certainly not complete in detail, Fig. 1 does represent an adequate working model for the neural control of ovulation in the rat.

SEXUAL DIFFERENTIATION OF THE CONTROL OF OVULATION

The preceding figure indicates that neonatal androgen may act at the level of the preoptic-anterior hypothalamic control system to block ovulation irreversibly. Evidence for this hypothesis is gradually accumulating. Barraclough and Gorski (1961) demonstrated that this region is refractory to electrical stimuli in the androgenized rat. Several studies have demonstrated that the direct application of testosterone propionate (TP) to this general region in the neonatal female will induce anovulatory persistent estrus (Wagner et al. 1966, Nadler 1968, Lobl and Gorski 1969, Sutherland and Gorski 1970). The latter study showed that intrahypothalamic infusion of estradiol benzoate (EB) produces a similar effect. Very

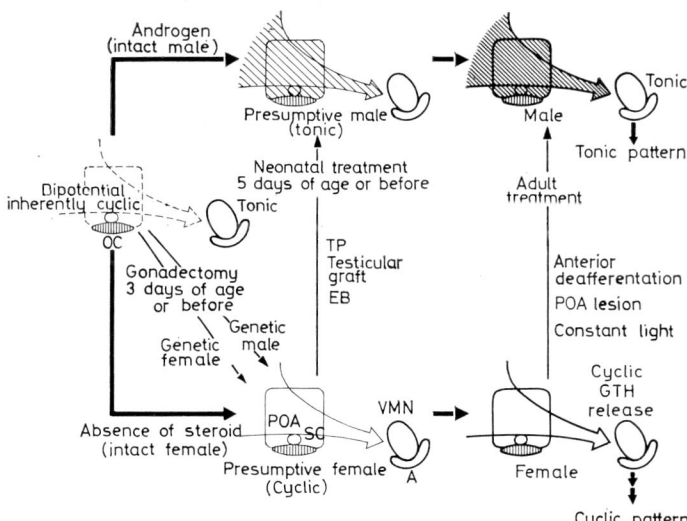

Fig. 2. Summary of the data which support the concept of the sexual differentiation of the neural control of GTH secretion in the rat. Please refer to text for discussion. (Based on experiments reviewed by Gorski 1971a, b)

recently, Field and Raisman (1971) have reported a sex difference in the ultrastructural anatomy of this region, while Dörner and Staudt (1969) have reported the existence of sex differences in neuronal nuclear size in this region of the brain.

The present status of the concept of sexual differentiation of the neural control of the pituitary gland is summarized in Fig. 2 and in Gorski's study (1971b). The preoptic-anterior hypothalamic area is considered to be undifferentiated at birth in the rat, or inherently cyclic. In the absence of gonadal steroids, e.g., the normal or ovariectomized female or the neonatally castrated male, this region develops its full potential for the cyclic regulation of GTH secretion. If the hypothalamus develops in the presence of gonadal steroids, the male pattern of GTH secretion develops. Although the physiological examples of this process would be the intact male, exogenous TP, and EB as well, when administered to the female or castrated male within the first few days of life, will masculinize the brain. The fact that the neural substrate for the cyclic release of GTH is comparable in the genetic male and female is indicated by the observation that anterior deafferentation, suprachiasmatic lesions, or exposure to constant light will block ovulation in both the adult female and the adult male subjected to neonatal castration.

SEXUAL DIFFERENTIATION OF THE NEURAL CONTROL OF SEXUAL BEHAVIOR

The concept of sexual differentiation also applies to the regulation of sexual behavior, or more specifically, of female sexual behavior. Although the normal female rat will show lordosis behavior after ovariectomy and priming with EB and progesterone, lordosis behavior in the androgenized female is suppressed as indicated in Fig. 3 (Clemens et al. 1969, 1970). Moreover, although the male castrated as an adult will not display lordosis behavior upon priming with ovarian hormones, the neonatally castrated male obtains a lordosis quotient (LQ; number of lordoses × 100/number of mounts) not different from that of the female (Grady et al. 1965). A possible role of perinatal exposure to androgen in the development of male sexual behavior is difficult to establish because the penis, which is necessary for normal male behavior, is itself dependent upon early androgen exposure (Whalen 1968).

Our previous studies on the differentiation of sexual behavior have revealed several important points:

1. The behavioral system appears to be less sensitive to TP and/or it appears to differentiate somewhat later than the GTH-regulating system.

2. Androgenization of sexual behavior may be due to a decrease in neural sensitivity to progesterone.

3. Since progesterone may facilitate sexual behavior by acting on the mesencephalic reticular formation, it is possible that androgen has an important influence on the development of extrahypothalamic circuits.

4. The evaluation of the influence of neonatal androgen exposure on sexual behavior depends critically on the method of testing.

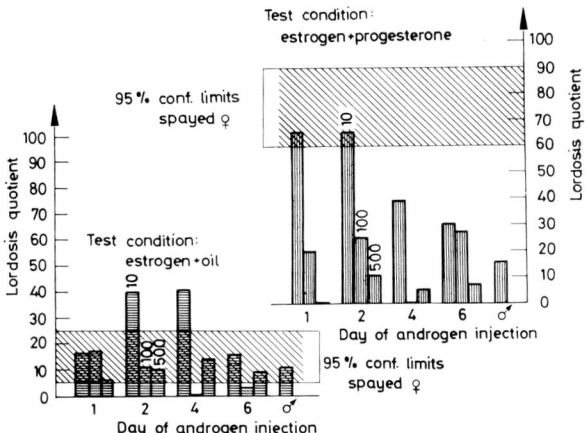

Fig. 3. Influence of 10, 100, or 500 μg TP, administered to female rats of 1, 2, 4, or 6 days of age, on their adult display of the lordosis response to the mounting male, subsequent to ovariectomy and replacement treatment with estradiol benzoate and progesterone (solid bars) or with estradiol benzoate alone (shaded bars). The mean response of the male rat orchidectomized as an adult, as well as the 95% confidence limits for the response of normal ovariectomized females similarly primed with ovarian hormones is also indicated. Lordosis quotients are based on a 10-mount test. (Reprinted from Gorski 1971a)

Evidence for the first two points is illustrated in Fig. 3. When as little as 10 μg TP is administered to the one- or two-day-old female, ovulation is prevented (Gorski 1968), but when such females are tested for lordosis behavior after ovariectomy and replacement therapy, with both EB and progesterone, they display normal levels of female behavior (Clemens et al. 1969). As one increases the dose of TP injected neonatally, however, lordosis behavior is suppressed (Clemens et al. 1970). Although these observations suggest that the behavioral system is less sensitive to TP, further analysis of the data suggests that there may also be a difference in the temporal pattern of the differentiation of GTH and sexual behavior control. Note that an injection of 10 μg TP given on day 6 is equally effective as 100 μg TP in suppressing lordosis behavior. However, by the sixth day of age the GTH controlling system is only minimally sensitive to systemic TP. This suggests that the behavioral system is most sensitive to the organizing action of TP between days 4–6, or several days after the period of maximal sensitivity of the GTH controlling system.

When lordosis behavior is analysed after ovariectomy and priming with both EB and progesterone, the male and androgenized female display an obvious deficit in female behavior. However, when the lordosis quotient was obtained in these same animals after priming with ES alone, we could detect no difference between males, females, or androgenized females (Clemens et al. 1970; Fig. 3). In fact, we established that females androgenized by the injection of 10 μg TP on day 1, 2 or 4 displayed a significantly higher LQ following EB treatment than control females (Fig. 4). This observation of possible increased sensitivity to EB

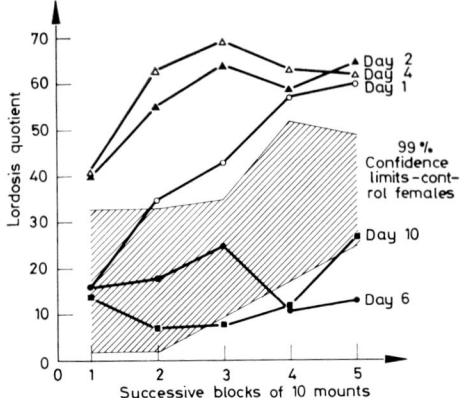

Fig. 4. Changes in the mean lordosis quotient over 5 consecutive blocks of 10 mounts for groups of androgenized females ovariectomized and primed only with estradiol benzoate for behavioral testing. The age at which 10 µg TP was administered is indicated in the Figure. The 99% confidence limits were derived from females which were not treated neonatally. (Reprinted from Gorski 1971b)

does not parallel the demonstration that estradiol uptake by the hypothalamus of the androgenized rat is decreased (Flerkó and Mess 1968, McGuire and Lisk 1969, but *see* Green et al. 1969). Although the dose of TP used to androgenize the rats may be one key to an understanding of this discrepancy between behavioral and chemical observations, the dose of EB used to induce lordosis behavior may be important as well. Davidson (1969) and Whalen et al. (1971) have clearly shown that there *is* a sex difference in the ability of exogenous EB to induce high levels of female sex behavior. The physiological significance of sexual behavior induced by the inundation of the brain by massive amounts of EB is unknown.

Ross et al. (1971) have recently demonstrated that progesterone will rapidly facilitate lordosis behavior in EB primed ovariectomized normal female rats when implanted in the mesencephalic reticular formation (MRF; Fig. 5). If the androgenized female is insensitive to progesterone, does the observation that progesterone acts in the MRF indicate that androgen also modifies the development of the MRF in the neonatal rat? This question, which would challenge the concept that androgenization is limited to the preoptic-anterior hypothalamus, must be studied further.

Finally, the precise method of testing lordosis behavior can significantly alter the results, particularly in the androgenized female rat. Figure 4 demonstrates that the LQ is not a stable parameter, and that it is dependent upon immediate previous experience, i.e. with increased numbers of mounts the probability that the next mount will be accompanied by a lordosis response is increased. Thus the number of mounts which constitute a behavioral test, or the number of mounts occurring within the time period of a test, may influence the results of that test. In addition, lordosis behavior is restored to the level of the normal female when the apparently androgenized female is permitted to adapt to the testing arena prior to the introduction of the experienced male (Fig. 6). Thus, when attempting

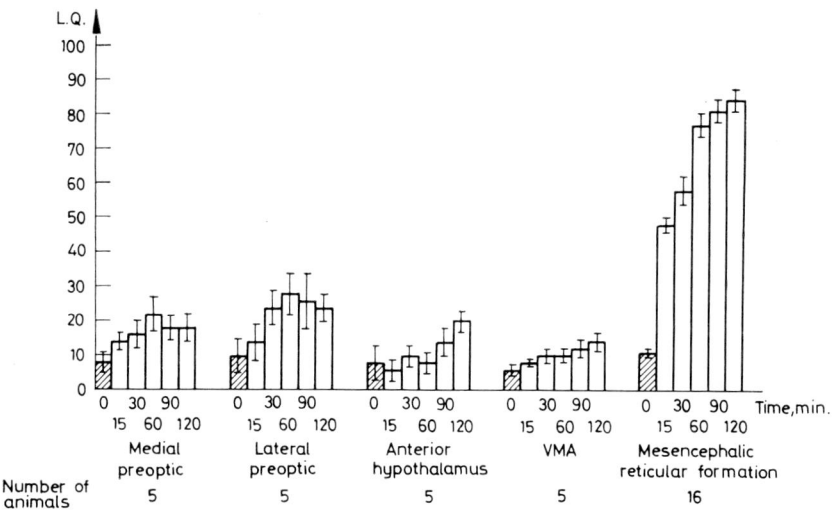

Fig. 5. Lordosis quotient (LQ) in estradiol benzoate-primed females at indicated intervals following unilateral intracerebral implantation of progesterone in the designated areas. Shaded bars (time 0) represent the pre-test scores after estrogen priming alone. Vertical lines indicate standard error of the mean. (Reprinted from Ross et al. 1971)

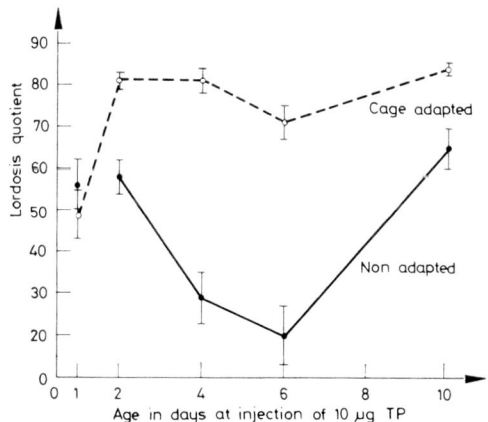

Fig. 6. Facilitation of the lordosis quotient (LQ), based on a 10-mount test, of adult female rats injected on day 1, 2, 4, 6, or 10 of life with 10 µg TP induced by a two-hour "adaptation" to the testing arena. The closed circles indicate the mean LQ of these same females when not allowed the pre-test adaptation period. All behavioral tests were performed after ovariectomy and replacement with estradiol benzoate and progesterone. (Reprinted from Gorski 1971b)

to compare the results of behavioral studies in one laboratory to those of another, the dose of TP, the age at injection, probably the age at testing, the hormonal replacement, and the conditions under which the tests are conducted are critical factors which must be taken into account.

THE MECHANISM OF ANDROGEN INDUCED ANOVULATORY STERILITY

Our studies of the possible mechanism of androgen induced masculine differentiation of the brain have been restricted to the regulation of GTH secretion, and to the action of exogenous TP in the female. Although differentiation could be considered a physiological process only in the male, little is known about the dynamics of neonatal testicular activity. However, in the female the amount of androgen and the time it is administered are under experimental control. The fact that androgenization is dependent upon the dose of TP is well known, but equally important is the age of the rat both at injection and at observation. Thus, 10 μg TP given to the 6-day-old female is much less effective in inducing anovulatory persistent estrus than the same dose given on day 4, when the animals are laparotomized shortly after puberty (Fig. 7). However, when these same rats were autopsied at approximately 100 days of age, almost all were anovulatory. Although 10 μg TP given on day 6 was very effective in inducing the anovulatory state, there was a marked delay in its appearance. The mechanism of this delayed anovulation syndrome (DAS) as we have called it (Gorski 1968) appears to involve postpubertal feedback of ovarian steroids (Kikuyama and Kawashima 1966, Arai 1971).

Thus limited by choice to the study of the development of ovulatory capacity in the female, our approach to the possible mechanism of androgenization has been twofold: (i) to identify and characterize those agents which can attenuate

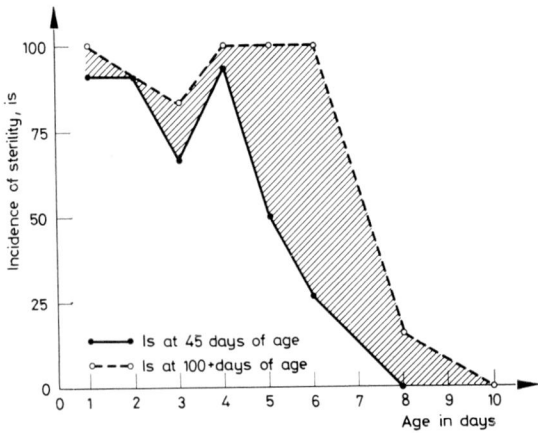

Fig. 7. Influence of animal age, at injection of 10 μg TP and at observation, on the incidence of sterility. The shaded area reflects those animals which exhibited the delayed anovulation syndrome. (Reprinted from Gorski 1968)

androgenization; and (ii) to elucidate the temporal characteristics of androgenization. Although we have confirmed in previous reports that reserpine, chlorpromazine, and progesterone can attenuate androgen action (Arai and Gorski 1968a), we focused our attention on the barbiturates phenobarbital (PhB) and pentobarbital (PB), and the anti-androgen cyproterone-acetate (CA). As illustrated in Fig. 8 the simultaneous injection of PhB, PB or CA with 30 µg TP to the 5-day-old female significantly reduces the incidence of sterility (IS) at both 45 and 90 days of age. With this knowledge we attempted to determine the critical exposure period necessary for androgenization of GTH regulation by timed injections of these agents (Arai and Gorski 1968b, c).

As indicated in Fig. 8, if one allows TP to be in the rat for as little as 3–6 hours, PhB and CA no longer significantly lower the IS to TP. PB injection as late as 6 hours after TP is still effective in reducing the IS at 45 days of age, but because of the DAS this group of animals at 90 days of age was no different from control rats injected with TP alone. These experiments demonstrate that there is an early and relatively brief period during which the process of androgenization is highly labile to barbiturate. It should be stressed that this observation does not necessarily contradict the suggestion of Ladosky et al. (1970) that steps important in sexual differentiation of the brain occur as late as day 12 of life. It is possible that androgen initiates changes which eventually culminate in anovulatory persistent-estrus. Although the entire process could last many days, we have focused our attention on the initial events.

One criticism of the concept that barbiturates inhibit androgenization at the level of the brain is the well-known ability of barbiturate treatment to induce liver enzymes capable of inactivating plasma steroids. Sutherland and Gorski (1970) studied this possibility by injecting neonatal females with PB for several days

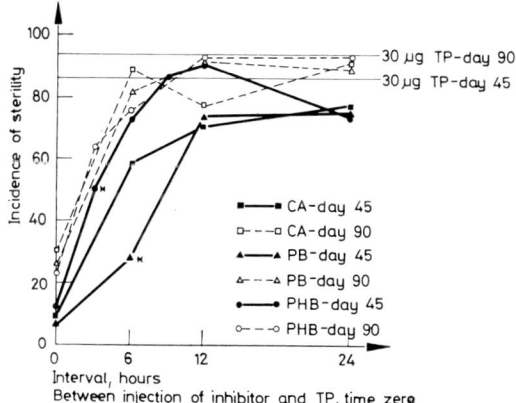

Fig. 8. Incidence of sterility (IS) at 45 and 90 days of age following the injection of 30 µg TP alone, simultaneously with, or at various times prior to the injection of cyproterone acetate (CA), pentobarbital (PB), or phenobarbital (PhB) to the 5-day-old female rat. Asterisk indicates a significantly decreased IS in comparison to the injection of TP only. Although not indicated by an asterisk, all three agents significantly reduced the IS both at 45 and 90 days of age when administered simultaneously with TP. (Reprinted from Gorski 1971b)

prior to the administration of TP. As seen in Table 1, an injection of 0.03 mg/g PB on days 2, 3 and 4 did not inhibit the action of TP given on day 5. However, when a fourth injection of PB was given on day 5, the IS was significantly reduced, even though TP was injected on day 5 after the rats had apparently recovered from the anesthetic effects of PB. The fact that multiple injections of PB were required argues against a role of the liver in the inhibition of androgenization by a single simultaneous injection of PB with TP.

TABLE 1

Influence of daily pentobarbital (PB) priming on effect of neonatal androgen injection (Sutherland and Gorski 1970)

Treatment	Incidence of sterility			
	No. anovulatory at 45 days of age	%	No. injected at 90 days of age	%
30 µg TP on day 5	12/24	50	23/24	95
0.2 mg PB on days 2, 3, 4; 30 µg TP on day 5	9/22	40	20/22	90
0.2 mg PB on days 2, 3, 4, 5; 30 µg TP on day 5*	10/23	43	16/23	69**

* Administered after recovery from anesthetic effect of PB.
** $p < 0.03$, X^2 analysis.

Sutherland and Gorski (1970) attempted to document a neural focus for the interaction between TP and PB by infusing the latter drug into the hypothalamus at the time TP was given systemically. Unfortunately these experiments were essentially negative, an observation which forced us to reinvestigate the ability of PB to block androgenization. These experiments were performed several years after the initial observation (Arai and Gorski 1968a) and yielded different results. The initial studies had indicated that a single injection of 0.05 mg/g PhB or two injections of PB (0.03 mg/g) approximately 4 hours apart would markedly inhibit androgenization. We were unable to confirm our previous observations (Table 2). Because many rats died following the second injection of PB, we attempted to increase survival by injecting PB only at the time TP was injected. With this regime we were able to confirm the observation that PB can attenuate androgen action (Table 2).

During these experiments we determined that the rate of absorption of androgen is a critical factor. We observed that a dose of 30 µg TP given on day 5 was significantly less effective when given in a volume of 0.02 ml rather than 0.05 ml (Table 2). Moreover, the intraperitoneal injection of 30 µg TP in 0.05 ml oil was totally ineffective. In order to interfere with androgenization an agent would have to be given in an adequate dose and at a time which would correspond to the action of androgen. A small change in the temporal pattern of androgen absorption might be a significant variable in those experiments designed to interfere with androgenization, and indeed, in androgenization itself.

Since we were able to repeat the inhibition of androgenization by PB, we considered the possible mechanism of action, if any, which might be common for the various inhibitors including tranquilizers, progesterone, and PB. One possibility is that any perturbation in brain function during androgen action could inhibit androgenization. However, refrigeration for 4 hours beginning with TP injection or the injection of a dose of Metrazol which was just below that which caused fatal convulsions, did not interfere with androgenization. We have tentatively

TABLE 2

Influence of phenobarbital (PhB), pentobarbital (PB), volume of vehicle, refrigeration, and Metrazol on the effect of neonatal injection of androgen

Group	Injection on day 5	Incidence of sterility			
		No. anovulatory at 45 days of age	%	No. injected at 90 days of age	%
1	30 μg TP in 0.05 ml oil only	29/37	78	34/37	92
2	+ 0.05 mg/g PhB	8/9	89	9/9	100
3	+ 0.03 mg/g PB, twice	6/9	67	8/9	89
4	+ 0.03 mg/g PB, once	3/14[a]	21	7/14[a]	50
5	30 μg TP in 0.02 ml oil only	15/30[b]	50	23/30	77
6	+ 0.03 mg/g PB, once	0/8[c]	0	3/8[d]	38
7	30 μg TP in 0.05 ml oil + 4 hours refrigeration	4/5	80	5/5	100
8	+ 0.5 mg Metrazol	5/6	83	5/6	83
9	given intraperitoneally	0/5[a]	0	0/5[a]	0

[a] Significantly different from Group 1, $p < 0.005$.
[b] Significantly different from Group 1, $p < 0.02$.
[c] Significantly different from Group 5, $p < 0.02$.
[d] Significantly different from Group 5, $p = 0.05$.

concluded that the inhibition of neural function at the time androgen exerts its initial effect may be an important factor in blocking androgenization, but suppression of what neural function?

Since the effect of neonatal androgen exposure is permanent we argued that TP might alter genomic expression within the brain. Barbiturate injection has been shown to depress DNA, RNA, and protein metabolism in certain non-neural tissues (Baserga and Weiss 1967). Could the suppression of these fundamental processes in the brain prevent androgenization? Although our initial experiments indicated that the injection of 1 μg actinomycin-D, a DNA-dependent RNA synthesis inhibitor, or 10 μg puromycin, a protein synthesis inhibitor, could attenuate androgenization (Kobayashi and Gorski 1970), the fact that both the antibiotic and the TP were administered subcutaneously did not confirm or deny the possibility of a specific interaction of these two agents at the level of the brain. In an attempt to provide more conclusive evidence for this possibility, we have implanted various antibiotics directly into the suprachiasmatic region of the hypothalamus, the area thought to be the site of androgen suppression of ovulation.

This experiment raised a fundamental question which has not been studied to date. Although it is well established that the newborn rat of either sex has the potential to develop the cyclic pattern of GTH regulation, what processes are required for that potential to become manifest in the sexually mature rat? The answer to this question is critical to an understanding of the action of androgen. Does androgen merely prevent the maturation or development of the fully functional cyclic regulatory system, or does it induce changes which actually masculinize the brain? Ladosky and Gaziri (1970) have reported that brain levels of serotonin increase significantly at 12 days of age in the female. If this observation proves to be functionally significant, it would be important to know if testicular androgen secretion in the male prevents development of a serotonergic system, or induces the development of another system, which is antagonistic to the serotonergic system.

Considering the former possibility, perhaps neuronal genetic expression is necessary to establish this serotonergic system. Androgen might act by *inhibiting* these genomic processes. If this were true, one would expect that antibiotics placed in this region of the brain at this critical period might mimic androgen action and induce anovulatory sterility. Although we implanted various antibiotics including the DNA synthesis inhibitor sarkomycin (12 µg), the RNA synthesis inhibitors actinomycin-D (0.2 µg) and rifampicin (15 µg), and the protein synthesis inhibitors chloramphenicol (16 µg), puromycin (1.4 µg), streptomycin sulfate (15 µg) and cycloheximide (0.7 or 14 µg), none of these agents interrupted the development of normal ovarian activity (Fig. 9).

If androgen masculinizes the brain by *stimulating* genomic expression at some level, then these antibiotics might be expected to inhibit androgenization in

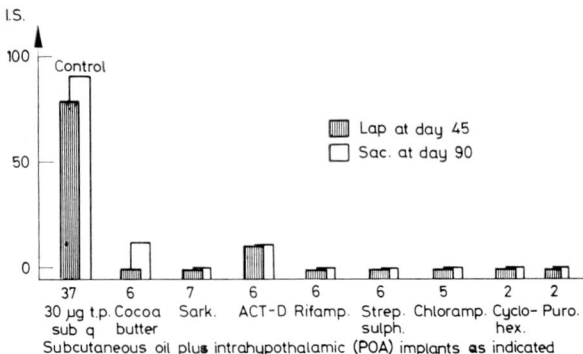

Fig. 9. Incidence of sterility (IS) following intrahypothalamic implantation of various antibiotics in the 5-day-old female. Androgen was not given to these females. For control purposes, 5-day-old females were given 30 µg TP SC. Numbers at the base of each column indicate the number of rats which reached autopsy. (From Gorski and Shryne 1971)

response to 30 μg TP. As indicated in Fig. 10, intracerebral cycloheximide did significantly attenuate androgenization. Implantation of identical pellets of cycloheximide subcutaneously did not interfere with androgenization (Gorski and Shryne 1971).

Although I have used the development of a serotonergic system purely as an example, these data support the view that androgen alters fundamental neurochemical processes, perhaps protein synthesis, within the suprachiasmatic region

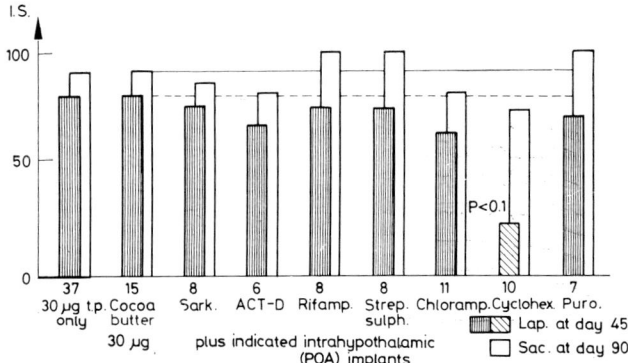

Fig. 10. Incidence of sterility (IS) following intrahypothalamic implantation of various antibiotics in the 5-day-old female rat simultaneously injected SC with 30 μg TP. Control groups included females injected with TP alone, and females which received an intrahypothalamic implant of cocoa butter, the excipient for the antibiotics. Numbers at the base of each column indicate the number of rats which reached autopsy. (From Gorski and Shryne 1971)

and that this in some way prevents the cyclic release of GTH in the adult. Two published experiments are consistent with this general concept. Shimada and Gorbman (1970) reported that the forebrain of the androgenized female rat contains a unique species of RNA, and Clayton et al. (1970) have reported that three hours after testosterone injection RNA synthesis throughout the brain of the two-day-old female is significantly decreased except in the medial preoptic area, and the amygdala. Although our studies were performed with a respectable number of female rats (95 animals survived intracerebral implantation of antibiotics), they must be considered preliminary. In experiments of this type the appropriate antibiotic, at an adequate dose, must be present at the site of androgen action and at the proper time within the temporal sequence of both androgen action and cerebral development. Nevertheless, these studies do support the view that androgen may masculinize the brain by an action at a very fundamental level of neuronal activity.

THE REGULATION OF NEONATAL TESTICULAR ACTIVITY

Although our preceding discussion has been limited to the possible mechanism of action of exogenous androgen on the female hypothalamus, we hold the view that elucidation of this system will also explain the action of endogenous androgen on the developing brain in the intact male rat. Recently B.D. Goldman and I have turned our attention to the male; what regulates the critical activity of the testes (presumably androgen secretion) which is responsible for physiological differentiation in the male?

Goldman and Mahesh (1970) stimulated interest in this question by demonstrating that the injection of antibodies to GTH (anti-GTH) on days 1, 3 and 5 of life reduced fertility in the male rat. This important observation was based on the analysis of vaginal smear records in female rats housed with experimental and control (injected with normal rabbit serum, NRS) males. We decided to repeat their basic experiment but to include direct behavioral observations. Antibodies to GTH (NIH-LH-SI2) were prepared as before (Goldman and Mahesh 1970) and injected (0.1 ml/injection) on days 1, 3 or 5 of life. All tests were performed on the same animals according to the following schedule. At approximately 90 days of age anti-GTH and NRS treated males were housed individually with a single female for 2–3 estrous cycles. In confirmation of the previous study, only one of 16 anti-GTH males was able to impregnate the female, while 13 of 14 RNS males mated successfully. At about 110 days of age the males were tested for male sexual behavior for 30 minutes with EB-progesterone primed spayed females. Because sexual experience is an important factor in male behavior, all males at 120 days of age were housed overnight with sexually receptive spayed females. A second male behavior test was performed at 150 days of age. At 180 days of age all males were castrated and the testes weighed and studied histologically. Approximately 50 days after castration the male rats were themselves primed with EB and progesterone and tested for their ability to display lordosis behavior with experienced stud males. Two months later the males were given a subcutaneous transplant of immature ovarian tissue. The ovarian grafts were removed after one month and studied histologically. At approximately 340 days of age, and after two weeks of daily injection of TP, these males were given a third 30 minute test for male behavior and then autopsied.

Figure 11 illustrates the results of the three tests for male sexual behavior. It is clear that the anti-GTH treated males did not show normal male behavior. They achieved intromission into the vagina significantly fewer times, and rarely ejaculated. It is very likely, therefore, that the decreased fertility originally observed by Goldman and Mahesh (1970) was due to this deficit in male sexual behavior.

Figure 12 illustrates the deficit in male behavior in another way (percent intromission, i.e. number of intromissions plus ejaculations $\times$ 100/total number of mounts) and as well illustrates the results of the additional experiments. Although the percent intromission was significantly reduced in the anti-GTH males on the first and second test, is this due to inadequate testicular function? Two observations argue against this. First, there was no difference in testicular weight at autopsy, nor were any histological differences detected. Second, when male behavior was retested after exogenous TP, the anti-GTH treated males

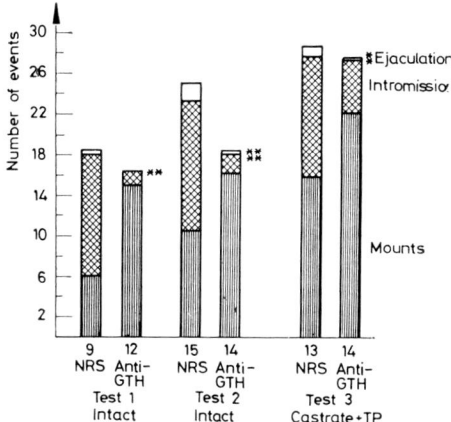

Fig. 11. Influence of neonatal treatment with GTH antiserum (anti-GTH) on parameters of male sexual behavior (number of mounts, intromissions, and ejaculations) in intact or castrate rats. Statistical analysis by the Mann-Whitney U test; ** $p < 0.001$. (From Goldman, B. D., Quadagno, D. M. and Gorski, R. A., unpublished observations)

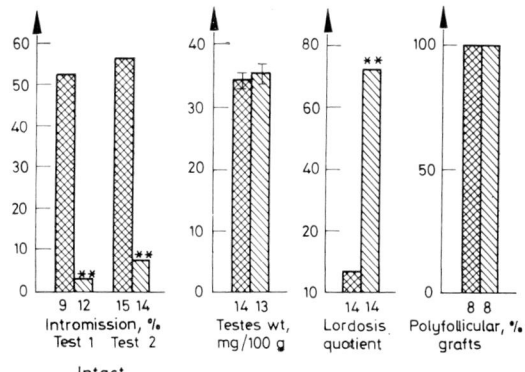

Fig. 12. The influence of neonatal treatment with GTH antiserum (anti-GTH) on sexual differentiation of the regulation of pituitary secretion, and sexual behavior, and on the development of the penis. All tests were performed on the same animals in the sequence as indicated. See text for experimental procedures. Statistical analysis of behavioral data by the Mann-Whitney U test, autopsy data by the Student's t test; ** $p < 0.001$. (From Goldman, B. D., Quadagno, D. M. and Gorski, R. A., unpublished observations)

still displayed significantly poorer male behavior. Thus male sexual behavior was significantly reduced after anti-GTH treatment, apparently independent of the level of adult testicular activity. However, this cannot be taken to indicate that anti-GTH treatment necessarily prevented an action of androgen on the brain. As illustrated in Fig. 13, the weight and length of the penis, and the number of penile spines, were significantly reduced in the experimental males. Since normal penile development is essential for male sexual behavior as measured in this study (Whalen 1968) it is impossible to attribute the present results to a central or peripheral mechanism. However, since Beach and Holz (1946) have shown that the responsiveness of the penis to androgen is permanently suppressed if it is not exposed to androgen neonatally, these results do suggest that neonatal treatment with anti-GTH had prevented or reduced androgen secretion.

Moreover, this study does provide evidence that anti-GTH prevented a central effect of androgen. As I indicated earlier the male rat castrated as an adult does not display lordosis behavior; however, the anti-GTH treated males exhibited female levels of lordosis behavior. Goldman and Mahesh (1970) reported that anti-GTH treatment did not prevent masculinization of the neural regulation of GTH secretion. This observation is confirmed by the present study since none of the ovarian grafts developed corpora lutea. All ovarian grafts which survived transplantation contained follicles in various stages of development.

Earlier in this discussion I indicated that in the female rat the neural system which regulates lordosis behavior is less sensitive to androgen, or differentiates later than the GTH-controlling system. Anti-GTH treatment of the neonatal male suggests that this observation applies to the genetic male as well. Anti-GTH treatment as performed in this study appears to reduce, but not to eliminate endogenous androgen. A sufficient amount of androgen is released to masculinize the GTH controlling system, but not enough to suppress lordosis behavior. In addition, sufficient anti-GTH was injected to prevent normal development of the penis. Perhaps solely as a consequence of this, male sexual behavior is markedly disturbed.

In summary, sexual differentiation of the female rat under the influence of exogenous TP may involve a permanent change in neuronal genomic activity. In the intact male, the secretion of androgen during this critical period in development appears to be at least partially dependent upon the pituitary gland. The

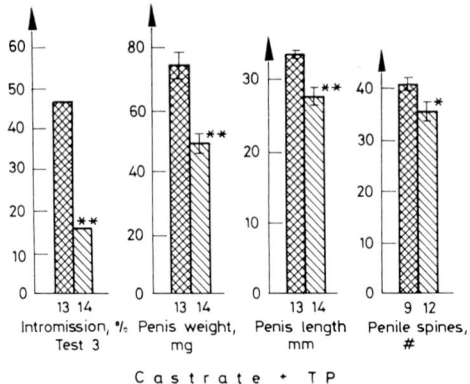

Fig. 13. Subcutaneous ovarian graft removed one month after transplantation to a male treated on day 1, 3, and 5 with GTH antiserum. When primed with estradiol benzoate and progesterone prior to ovarian grafting, this male developed a lordosis quotient of 93.3 over a 30 mount test. Statistical analysis of behavioral data by the Mann–Whitney U test, autopsy data by Student's t test; * $p < 0.025$, ** $p < 0.001$. (From Goldman, B. D., Quadagno, D. M. and Gorski, R. A., unpublished observations)

fact that testicular grafts in the female also induce masculine differentiation of the brain, suggests that the key to this process may be the genetically determined capacity of the male gonad to respond to GTH. Nevertheless, it is interesting to ponder this fundamental question: Is androgen induced differentiation of the hypothalamus dependent upon hypothalamic activity? Or perhaps more clearly, which came first, the chicken or the egg?

REFERENCES

ANDERSON, C. H. and GREENWALD, G. S. (1969): Autoradiographic analysis of estradiol uptake in the brain and pituitary of the female rat. *Endocrinology* **85**, 1160—1165.

ARAI, Y. (1971): Some aspects of the mechanisms involved in steroid-induced sterility. In: *Steroid Hormones and Brain Function*. Ed. by C. H. Sawyer and R. A. Gorski. University of California Press, Los Angeles.

ARAI, Y. and GORSKI, R. A. (1968a): Protection against the neural organizing effect of exogenous androgen in the neonatal female rat. *Endocrinology* **82**, 1005—1009.

ARAI, Y. and GORSKI, R. A. (1968b): The critical exposure time for androgenization of the developing hypothalamus in the female rat. *Endocrinology* **82**, 1010—1014.

ARAI, Y. and GORSKI, R. A. (1968c): Critical exposure time for androgenization of the rat hypothalamus determined by anti-androgen injection. *Proc. Soc. exp. Biol. (N.Y.)* **127**, 590—593.

BARRACLOUGH, C. A. and GORSKI, R. A. (1961): Evidence that the hypothalamus is responsible for androgen-induced sterility in the female rat. *Endocrinology* **68**, 68—79.

BASERGA, R. and WEISS, L. (1967): Inhibition of deoxyribonucleic acid synthesis by pentobarbital. *Biochim. biophys. Acta (Amst.)* **145**, 361—367.

BEACH, F. A. and HOLZ, A. M. (1946): Mating behavior in male rats castrated at various ages and injected with androgen. *J. exp. Zool.* **101**, 91—142.

CLAYTON, R. B., KOGURA, J. and KRAEMER, H. C. (1970): Sexual differentiation of the brain: effects of testosterone on brain RNA metabolism in newborn female rats. *Nature (London)* **226**, 810—812.

CLEMENS, L. G., HIROI, M. and GORSKI, R. A. (1969): Induction and facilitation of female mating behavior in rats treated neonatally with low doses of testosterone propionate. *Endocrinology* **84**, 1430—1438.

CLEMENS, L. G., SHRYNE, J. and GORSKI, R. A. (1970): Androgen and development of progesterone responsiveness in male and female rats. *Physiol. Behav.* **5**, 673—678.

DAVIDSON, J. M. (1969): Effects of estrogen on the sexual behavior of male rats. *Endocrinology* **84**, 1365—1372.

DÖRNER, G. and STAUDT, J. (1969): Perinatal structural sex differentiation of the hypothalamus in rats. *Neuroendocrinology* **5**, 103—106.

EVERETT, J. W. (1969): Neuroendocrine aspects of mammalian reproduction. *Ann. Rev. Physiol.* **31**, 383—416.

FIELD, P. M. and RAISMAN, G. (1971): Differences between amygdaloid projections to the hypothalamus and preoptic area. *Anat. Rec.* **169**, 315.

FLERKÓ, B. (1966): Control of gonadotropin secretion in the female. In: *Neuroendocrinology*. Vol. I. Ed. by L. Martini and W. P. Ganong. Academic Press, New York. pp. 613—668.

FLERKÓ, B. and MESS, B. (1968): Reduced oestradiol-binding capacity of androgen sterilized rats. *Acta physiol. Acad. Sci. hung.* **33**, 111—113.

GOLDMAN, B. D. and MAHESH, V. B. (1970): Induction of infertility in male rats by treatment with gonadotropin antiserum during neonatal life. *Biol. Reprod.* **2**, 444—451.

GORSKI, R. A. (1968): Influence of age on the response to paranatal administration of a low dose of androgen. *Endocrinology* **82**, 1001—1004.

GORSKI, R. A. (1970): Localization of hypothalamic regulation of pituitary function. *Amer. J. Anat.* **129**, 219—222.

Gorski, R. A. (1971a): Sexual differentiation of the hypothalamus. In: *The Neuroendocrinology of Human Reproduction.* Ed. by H. C. Mack and A. I. Sherman. C. Thomas, Springfield. (In press.)

Gorski, R. A. (1971b): Gonadal hormones and the perinatal development of neuroendocrine function. In: *Frontiers in Neuroendocrinology, 1971.* Ed. by L. Martini and W. F. Ganong. Oxford University Press, London. (In press.)

Gorski, R. A. (1971c): Steroid hormones and brain function: Progress, principles and problems. In: *Steroid Hormones and Brain Function.* Ed. by C. H. Sawyer and R. A. Gorski. UCLA Forum in Medical Sciences, No. 15, University of California Press, Los Angeles. (In press.)

Gorski, R. A. and Shryne, J. (1971): Intracerebral antibiotics and androgenization of the neonatal female rat. *Anat. Rec.* **169,** 327.

Grady, K. L., Phoenix, C. H. and Young, W. C. (1965): Role of the developing rat testis in differentiation of the neural tissues mediating mating behavior. *J. comp. physiol. Psychol.* **59,** 176—182.

Green, R., Luttge, W. G. and Whalen, R. E. (1969): Uptake and retention of tritiated estradiol in brain and peripheral tissues of male, female and neonatally androgenized female rats. *Endocrinology* **85,** 373—378.

Hagino, N., Wagner, J. W. and Gorski, R. A.: (1964): Ovulation induced by hypothalamic lesioning in the rat. *Anat. Rec.* **148,** 288.

Halász, B. (1969): The endocrine effects of isolation of the hypothalamus from the rest of the brain. In: *Frontiers in Neuroendocrinology, 1969.* Ed. by L. Martini and W. F. Ganong. Oxford University Press, New York. pp. 307—342.

Halász, B. and Gorski, R. A. (1967): Gonadotrophic hormone secretion in female rats after partial or total interruption of neural afferents to the medial basal hypothalamus. *Endocrinology* **80,** 608—622.

Illei-Donhoffer, A., Tima, L. and Flerkó, B. (1970): Ovulation induced by hypothalamic lesions in persistent oestrous rats. *Acta biol. Acad. Sci. hung.* **21,** 197—206.

Kikuyama, S. and Kawashima, S. (1966): Formation of corpora lutea in ovarian grafts in ovariectomized adult rats subjected to early postnatal treatment with androgen. *Sci. Papers Coll. Gen. Educ. (Tokyo)* **16,** 69—74.

Kobayashi, F. and Gorski, R. A. (1970): Effects of antibiotics on androgenization of the neonatal female rat. *Endocrinology* **86,** 285—289.

Kordon, C. (1967): Contrôle nerveux du cycle ovarien. *Arch. Anat. micr. Morph. exp.* **56,** 458—474.

Köves, K. and Halász, B. (1970): Location of the neural structures triggering ovulation in the rat. *Neuroendocrinology* **6,** 180—193.

Ladosky, W. and Gaziri, L. C. J. (1970): Brain serotonin and sexual differentiation of the nervous system. *Neuroendocrinology* **6,** 168—174.

Ladosky, W., Kesikowski, W. M. and Gaziri, I. F. (1970): Effect of a single injection of chlorpromazine into infant male rats on subsequent gonadotrophin secretion. *J. Endocr.* **48,** 151—156.

Lobl, R. T. and Gorski, R. A. (1969): Influence of age on the response to neonatal intrahypothalamic androgen administration. *Anat. Rec.* **163,** 219.

McGuire, J. L. and Lisk, R. D. (1969): Oestrogen receptors in androgen or oestrogen sterilized female rats. *Nature (London)* **221,** 1068—1069.

Nadler, R. D. (1968): Masculinization of female rats by intracranial implantation of androgen in infancy. *J. comp. physiol. Psychol.* **66,** 157—167.

Pfaff, D. W. (1968): Uptake of ^{3}H-estradiol by the female rat brain. An autoradiographic study. *Endocrinology* **82,** 1149—1155.

Ross, J., Claybaugh, C., Clemens, L. G. and Gorski, R. A. (1971): Short latency induction of estrous behavior with intracerebral progesterone in ovariectomized rats. *Endocrinology.* (In press.)

Shimada, H. and Gorbman, A. (1970): Long lasting changes in RNA synthesis in the forebrains of female rats treated with testosterone soon after birth. *Biochem. biophys. Res. Comm.* **38,** 423—430.

Stumpf, W. E. (1970): Estrogen-neurons and estrogen-neuron systems in the periventricular brain. *Amer. J. Anat.* **129,** 207—218.

Sutherland, S. D. and Gorski, R. A. (1970): Intrahypothalamic interaction of steroids and pentobarbital in the neonatal rat. *Anat. Rec.* **166,** 386.

Taleisnik, S. (1966): Influence of the cerebral cortex on the release of gonadotropin. In: *Brain and Behavior*. Vol. 3. *The Brain and Gonadal Function*. Ed. by R. A. Gorski and R. E. Whalen. UCLA Forum in Medical Sciences, University of California Press, Los Angeles. pp. 170–179.

Wagner, J. W., Erwin, W. and Critchlow, V. (1966): Androgen sterilization produced by intracerebral implants of testosterone in neonatal female rats. *Endocrinology* **79**, 1135–1142.

Whalen, R. E. (1968): Differentiation of the neural mechanisms which control gonadotropin secretion and sexual behavior. In: *Perspectives in Reproduction and Sexual Behavior*. Ed. by M. Diamond. Indiana University Press, Bloomington. pp. 303–340.

Whalen, R. E., Luttge, W. G. and Gorzalka, B. B. (1971): Neonatal androgenization and the development of estrogen responsivity in male and female rats. *Horm. Behav.* **2**, 83–90.

Zigmond, R. E. and McEwen, B. S. (1970): Selective retention of estradiol by cell nuclei in specific brain regions of the ovariectomized rat. *J Neurochem.* **17**, 889–899.

SEX HORMONE-DEPENDENT DIFFERENTIATION OF THE HYPOTHALAMUS AND SEXUALITY

G. DÖRNER

Institute of Experimental Endocrinology
Humboldt University (Charité)
Berlin, G.D.R.

In 1938 Vera Dantchakoff reported that when prenatally androgen-treated adult female guinea-pigs were given more androgen, they exhibited surprisingly strong male sexual behaviour. In 1959 this important observation was confirmed in quantitative studies by Phoenix et al., who distinguished between a sex hormone-dependent organization and activation period of the brain.

Grady and Phoenix (1963), Harris (1964) and Feder and Whalen (1965) reported that when adult male rats, which had been castrated shortly after birth, were given oestrogens, they showed surprisingly strong female sexual behaviour. The same was found by Neumann and Elger (1966) in male rats which had been treated with anti-androgens neonatally. These findings indicated that during a critical hypothalamic organization phase the direction in which the sexual instinct develops may be influenced by the sex hormone level.

In extensive animal experiments the following results were obtained in our laboratories during the last five years (Dörner 1967, 1969, 1970, 1971):

1. Male rats castrated on the first day of life showed predominantly heterotypical, i.e. homosexual behaviour, following androgen substitution in adulthood. Androgen deficiency during a critical hypothalamic differentiation phase results in predominantly female organization of the brain. The female-differentiated hypothalamus of a male is then activated postpuberally not only by oestrogens but also by androgens to female-like sexual behaviour. Thus, genotypic and phenotypic males with a female-differentiated brain are sexually far more excited by males than by females. Thus, a neuroendocrine-conditioned and androgen-activated male homosexuality was produced.

2. This male homosexuality could be completely and permanently prevented by a single androgen injection administered during the hypothalamic differentiation phase. Thus, an androgen prophylaxis of neuroendocrine-conditioned male homosexuality is possible.

3. The higher the androgen level during the hypothalamic organization period, the stronger, regardless of genetic sex, was the male and the weaker the female sexual behaviour during the hypothalamic functional period. On the basis of these findings, primary hypo-, bi- and homosexuality are based on different degrees of androgen deficiency in males and androgen (or even oestrogen) over-

dosage in females (principle of the sex hormone-dependent bipolar differentiation).

4. Neuroendocrine-conditioned male homosexuality could be repressed in adult animals by stereotaxic lesions of a female mating centre located in the central hypothalamus, i.e. in the ventromedial nucleus region. Roeder and Müller (1969) achieved similar effects in homosexual men by stereotaxic operations in the same hypothalamic region.

5. In male rats castrated on the first day of life corpus luteum formation could be induced by oestrogen injection in grafts of infantile ovaries as well as in ovaries of normal females, but not in ovaries of neonatally androgenized or oestrogenized females. Thus, an ovulation-inducing positive oestrogen feedback effect ("Hohlweg effect") could only be achieved in both sexes if low androgen and oestrogen levels were present during the differentiation of the gonadotrophin-regulating hypothalamic sex centres.

In 1961 Barraclough and Gorski had distinguished between a cyclic sex centre, located in the preoptic suprachiasmatic area, responsible for the cyclic ovulation-inducing gonadotrophin oversecretion in females, and a tonic centre, located in the arcuate-ventromedial region, responsible for the tonic gonadotrophin secretion in both sexes.

6. Hypogonadism with secondary hyposexuality was observed in adult male rats following high-dose androgen or oestrogen treatment during the critical hypothalamic organization period. This effect may be based on a defective differentiation of the tonic hypothalamic sex centre. In contrast to the testes of highly androgenized rats the testes of highly oestrogenized animals could not be stimulated by exogenous gonadotrophins in adulthood. This finding suggests that during this critical developmental stage an excessive oestrogen level may also result in direct permanent lesions of the testes.

7. A hypergonadotrophic hypergonadism in male rats caused by gonadotrophin treatment during the hypothalamic differentiation phase gave rise to a hypogonadotrophic hypogonadism during the hypothalamic functional phase.

8. High doses of progesterone compounds with antiandrogenic activity administered during the sex-specific brain differentiation produced psychic intersexuality in adult males with reduced male and increased female sexuality.

9. Significant correlations were found between the degree of androgenicity during the hypothalamic differentiation period, the nuclear volumes of the medial preoptic area and the ventromedial nucleus as well as the sexual behaviour during the hypothalamic functional period.

10. In female rats, unphysiologically high androgen and/or oestrogen levels during the hypothalamic organization phase caused a neuroendocrine predisposition for hypo-, bi-, or homosexuality. Thus, neonatally androgenized or oestrogenized females showed predominantly heterotypical, i.e. homosexual behaviour, under postpubertal androgen activation, whereas neonatally untreated females displayed hetero-, or bisexual behaviour after postpubertal androgen treatment.

11. An absolute independence of the "sex-specific" brain differentiation from the genetic sex was demonstrated. Thus, a complete inversion of sexual behaviour after postpubertal androgen activation was observed between male and female rats following androgen deficiency in the males and androgen overdosage in the females during the hypothalamic differentiation period.

12. Female rats, highly oestrogenized perinatally, showed hypogonadotrophic hypogonadism, sterility, non-evocability of a positive oestrogen feedback effect, predominantly persistent vaginal oestrus and female asexuality associated with increased attractiveness for male sexual partners in adulthood. Thus, paradoxical, i.e. androgen-like effects on brain differentiation, were produced by oestrogens (Dörner et al. 1971a).

13. Androgen or oestrogen treatment of female rats on the 10th day of life resulted in a normal or approximately normal cyclic ovarian function postpubertally. Nevertheless, these females displayed predominantly heterotypical, i.e. homosexual behaviour, under postpuberal androgen activation. This finding suggests a partial chronological dissociation in the differentiation of hypothalamic sex and mating centres.

14. In rats, the appearance of hypothalamic nuclei occurs between the 16th and 18th day of foetal life, while complete reduction of the hypothalamic matrix in the preoptic and anterior hypothalamic region is observed about two weeks after birth. Changes of sex hormone levels during this perinatal hypothalamic organization phase lead to persistent disturbances of gonadal function and/or sexual behaviour. In the human, corresponding structural alterations of the hypothalamus were found between the 4th and 7th month of foetal life (Dörner and Staudt 1971).

Our experimental results supplemented by clinical findings contribute to the explanation of neuroendocrine pathogenesis as well as to the therapy and prophylaxis of inborn sexual disturbances. The following conclusions can be drawn:

1. Changes in the androgen and/or oestrogen level during the hypothalamic organization phase may result in permanent disorders of gonadal function and/or sexual behaviour during the postpubertal hypothalamic functional phase. In gonosomal and gonadal males, androgen deficiency during the hypothalamic differentiation period leads to postpubertal hypo-, bi- or even homosexuality. In gonosomal and gonadal females, on the other hand, an unphysiological increase in the androgen and/or oestrogen level during the hypothalamic organization phase results in acyclic pituitary gonadotrophin secretion and/or hypo-, bi- or homosexuality in postpubertal life. Finally, excessively high androgen and/or oestrogen levels during the sex-specific brain differentiation give rise to postpubertal hypogonadism in both sexes.

2. The following neuroendocrine pathogenesis for inborn bi- or homosexuality in men is suggested: an absolute or relative androgen deficiency in the first, i.e. intrauterine Leydig cell-generation (during the hypothalamic organization phase) results in a predominantly female differentiation of the brain. A normal or at least approximately normal androgen level during the second, i.e. postpuberal Leydig cell-generation, then exerts a sex-nonspecific activating effect on the predominantly female-differentiated hypothalamus. Thus, a genetic and somatophenotypic male with a predominantly female-differentiated brain is sexually excited mainly by another male.

3. In females, on the other hand, unphysiologically high androgen and/or oestrogen levels during the organization of the hypothalamic mating centres lead to a predominantly male differentiation of these centres. In this case, the female

organization of the gonadotrophin-regulating hypothalamic sex centres may already have been completed or not. For this reason, a neuroendocrine conditioned predisposition for female bisexuality or even homosexuality may occur associated with normal cyclic as well as acyclic ovarian function. Postpubertally, adrenal and ovarian androgens then activate the predominantly male-differentiated hypothalamic mating centres. Thus, a genetic and somatophenotypic female with a predominantly male-differentiated brain is sexually excited mainly by another female.

4. The following neuroendocrine factors are to be considered for the aetiopathogenesis of disturbances in hypothalamic differentiation:

a) Pathological secretion of human chorionic gonadotrophin or placental sex hormones.
b) Primary disorders (e.g., enzyme deficiencies) of the foetal gonad, adrenal cortex or foetoplacental steroid metabolism.
c) Endogenous or exogenous alterations of the responsiveness of the foetal hypothalamus to sex hormones.
d) Endogenous or exogenous changes of the maternal sex hormone level.

5. During the ontogenesis of human sexuality four periods can be distinguished:

a) Determination of the gonosomal sex.
b) Organization of the gonads.
c) Differentiation, maturation and function of the somatic and psychic (hypothalamic) sex.
d) Development of sexual self-identity.

According to these periods, a pathogenetic system of sexual disturbances was established and possible aetiological factors are discussed in a monograph to be published by Gustav Fischer, Jena and Springer, Vienna and New York.

6. Most of the sexual disorders in humans are apparently based on discrepancies between the gonosomal sex and the sex-specific sex hormone status of the foetus during the differentiation of (*i*) the gonads (2nd month of foetal life), (*ii*) the internal and/or external genital organs (2nd–4th month) and/or, most frequently, (*iii*) the hypothalamus (4th–7th month of foetal life). For this reason, postnatally a mere symptomatic treatment is possible in these cases. A causal therapy or prophylaxis of somatic and/or psychic sexual differentiation disturbances, however, must be accomplished already during the corresponding organization periods. In this case, a unambiguous diagnosis of the foetal gonosomal sex is a *conditio sine qua non*.

7. The diagnosis of the gonosomal foetal sex could be established by identification of Y-chromosomes in amniotic fluid cells by means of fluorescence microscopy (Dörner et al. 1971b). Moreover, during early pregnancy significantly higher urinary values of testosterone and especially of testosterone/androstene dione ratios were found in mothers with male foetuses than in those with female foetuses (Dörner et al. 1971c). Therefore, it can be assumed that a preventive therapy of inborn sexual disorders may become possible in the future by improving these analytical methods.

REFERENCES

BARRACLOUGH, C. A. and GORSKI, R. A. (1961): Evidence that the hypothalamus is responsible for androgen-induced sterility in the female rat. *Endocrinology* **68**, 68—79.

DANTCHAKOFF, V. (1938): Rôle des hormones dans la manifestation des instincts sexuels. *C. R. Acad. Sci. (Paris)* **206**, 945—947.

DÖRNER, G. (1967): Tierexperimentelle Untersuchungen zur Frage einer hormonellen Pathogenese der Homosexualität. *Acta biol. med. germ.* **19**, 569—584.

DÖRNER, G. (1969): Zur Frage einer neuroendokrinen Pathogenese, Prophylaxe und Therapie angeborener Sexualdeviationen. *Dtsch. med. Wschr.* **94**, 390—396.

DÖRNER, G. (1970): The influence of sex hormones during the hypothalamic differentiation and maturation phases on gonadal function and sexual behaviour during the hypothalamic functional phase. *Endokrinologie* **56**, 280—291.

DÖRNER, G. (1971): *Sexualhormonabhängige Gehirndifferenzierung und Sexualität.* Fischer, Jena and Springer, Wien/New York. (In press.)

DÖRNER, G. and STAUDT, J. (1971): Vergleichende morphologische Untersuchungen der Hypothalamusdifferenzierung bei Ratte und Mensch. *Endokrinologie* (In press.)

DÖRNER, G., DÖCKE, F. and HINZ, G. (1971a): Paradoxical effects of estrogen on brain differentiation. *Neuroendocrinology* **7**, 146—155.

DÖRNER, G., ROHDE, W. and BAUMGARTEN, G. (1971b): Bestimmung des genetischen Geschlechts der Foeten durch fluoreszenzmikroskopischen Nachweis des Y-Chromosoms in Fruchtwasserzellen. *Acta biol. med. germ.* (In press.)

DÖRNER, G., STAHL, F., GÖTZ, F., RÖSSNER, P. and HALLE, H. (1971c): Der Einfluß des fötalen Geschlechts auf den Androgengehalt im Frühschwangerenharn. *Endokrinologie.* (In press.)

FEDER, H. H. and WHALEN, R. E. (1965): Feminine behavior in neonatally castrated and estrogen-treated male rats. *Science* **147**, 306—307.

GRADY, K. L. and PHOENIX, C. H. (1963): Hormonal determinants of mating behavior; the display of feminine behavior by adult male rats castrated neonatally. *Amer. Zool.* **3**, 482.

HARRIS, G. W. (1964): Sex hormones, brain development and brain function. *Endocrinology* **75**, 627—648.

NEUMANN, F. and ELGER, W. (1966): Permanent changes in gonadal function and sexual behavior as a result of early feminization of male rats by treatment with an antiandrogenic steroid. *Endokrinologie* **50**, 209—224.

PHOENIX, C. H., GOY, R. W., GERALL, A. A. and YOUNG, W. C. (1959): Organizing action of prenatally administered testosterone propionate on the tissues mediating mating behaviour in the female guinea-pig. *Endocrinology* **65**, 369—382.

ROEDER, F. and MÜLLER, D. (1969): Zur stereotaktischen Heilung der pädophilen Homosexualität. *Dtsch. med. Wschr.* **94**, 409—415.

THE ROLE OF THYROID AND ADRENOCORTICAL HORMONES IN THE BIOCHEMICAL MATURATION OF THE RAT BRAIN

S. KOVÁCS

Institute of Physiology
University Medical School
Pécs, Hungary

INTRODUCTION

In the last two decades ample evidence has accumulated to show that hypothyroidism and hyperthyroidism in infancy have serious effects on mammalian neurogenesis (Hamburgh 1969).

Irreversible morphologic changes associated with impaired behaviour (Eayrs 1954, 1955, Eayrs and Lishman 1955, Eayrs 1961, Eayrs and Levine 1963) and marked biochemical alterations in the developing brain have been observed as a result of thyroidectomy at an early age (De Guglielmone and Gómez 1966, Pasquini et al. 1967, Garcia Argiz et al. 1967, Geel and Timiras 1967, Geel et al. 1967, Balázs et al. 1968, Balázs et al. 1971a).

On the other hand, accelerated development of innately organized responses followed by impairment of adaptive behaviour in adult age, advanced maturation of electrocortical activity and accelerated formation of the dendritic spines of cortical neurons have been reported after neonatal thyroid hormone treatment (Eayrs 1964, 1968, Schapiro 1968).

It has also been reported in the past years that the administration of adrenocortical hormones after birth has a permanent effect on bodily growth and brain maturation (Howard 1965, 1968, Schapiro 1968). To a certain extent the effects of these hormones are similar to those of thyroid hormone.

In the present paper some of our results concerning the effects of neonatal triiodothyronine (T_3) and corticosteroid administration on biochemical maturation of the brain are summarized. Some of the experiments, mainly concerned with the effect of thyroid hormone, were carried out in the Neuropsychiatric Research Unit of the Medical Research Council Laboratories, Carshalton, England.

EFFECTS ON POSTNATAL CELL FORMATION

Previous publications have shown that the development of the brain in the rat takes place, to a great extent, after birth (Balázs et al. 1968, 1971a, b).

The weight of the brain increases about 8-fold and that of the cerebellum about 25-fold from birth till the 50th day of life.

Treatment with T_3 or corticosteroids in infancy markedly retarded growth of the brain. The weight of the brain was significantly reduced by T_3 treatment

(25 µg at birth and 0.5–1 µg on alternate days) in comparison to controls during the whole experimental period except at days 1–4 after birth (Fig. 1a).

Treatment with corticosteroids (1 mg cortisone or hydrocortisone subcutaneously) also decreased the weight of the brain (Fig. 1b). In these cases the reduction in weight of the brain in the treated animals appeared as early as 3 days after birth. Hydrocortisone was found to be more effective than cortisone in retarding growth of the brain.

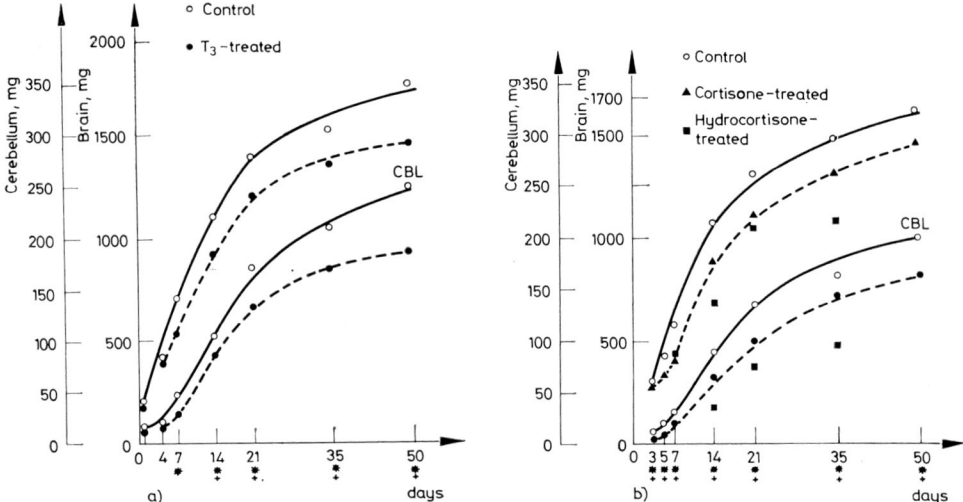

Fig. 1. Effect of treatment with T_3 (a), or corticosteroid (b) on growth of the brain. Differences between the experimental and control groups were statistically significant. * in brain weight, + in cerebellum weight

The weight of the cerebellum also decreased after T_3 or corticosteroid treatment (Fig. 1a, b). In this case the retardation in growth also appeared earlier, on day 3, in the corticosteroid treated animals.

It has been found previously that a large number of cells in the cerebrum and particularly in the cerebellum are formed after birth (Balázs et al. 1968). Assuming that the cells in the cerebrum and cerebellum are mainly diploid, the DNA content of these organs can be regarded as an index of the number of cells at different ages (Enesco and Leblond 1962).

The administration of T_3 markedly affected postnatal cell formation in the cerebrum and cerebellum. The DNA contents of the cerebrum and cerebellum were markedly less in the T_3 treated animals than in the controls. It is worth noting that the effect of T_3 on the DNA content of the cerebrum makes its appearance only after the 5th postnatal day (Fig. 2).

In the cerebellum this latent period is longer, T_3 effect manifests itself only after the second week of life. Treatment with corticosteroids having an effect similar to that of T_3 also reduced postnatal cell formation in the cerebrum and cerebellum. The total amount of DNA in the cerebrum and cerebellum was significantly decreased in the treated animals. In contrast to the above-mentioned effect of T_3, the reduction in the amount of DNA in the cerebrum as well as in the cerebellum after corticosteroid treatment appears as early as on day 5 of life. Putting off the corticosteroid injection from the day of birth until 7 days of age does not influence the effect of the hormone on DNA content either in the cerebrum or cerebellum.

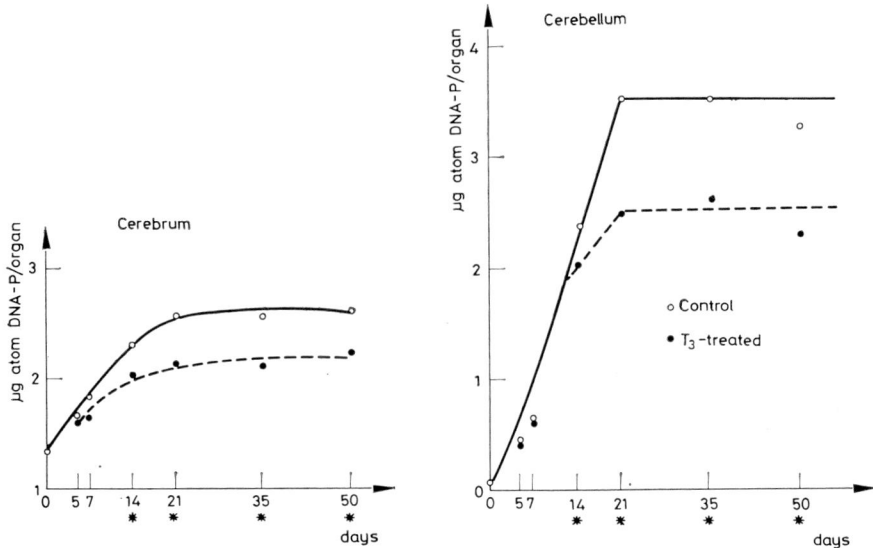

Fig. 2. Effect of T_3-treatment on the total DNA contents of cerebrum and cerebellum. * indicates when the differences between the experimental and control groups were statistically significant

Hydrocortisone given at birth seems to be more effective than cortisone on postnatal cell formation in the cerebellum but not in the cerebrum (Fig. 3).

Besides determination of the amount of DNA at different ages the rate of DNA synthesis in the brain was also studied. Our previous results had shown that the rate of incorporation of labelled thymidine into cerebral and cerebellar DNA was also affected by neonatal T_3 treatment. At 21 days of age the labelling of DNA was considerably decreased in the cerebrum and especially in the cerebellum in the T_3 treated animals, while no difference from control value was found on day 14 of life (Kovács et al. 1969a).

In the present experiments the effect of treatment with corticosteroids on DNA synthesis was investigated.

As a precursor, 6-^{3}H-thymidine was used and the animals were killed 1 hour after its subcutaneous injection. The rate of incorporation of labelled thymidine into DNA was expressed as relative specific activity (RSA), which was calculated by relating the value of the specific activity of DNA to the concentration of ^{3}H in the acid-soluble fraction.

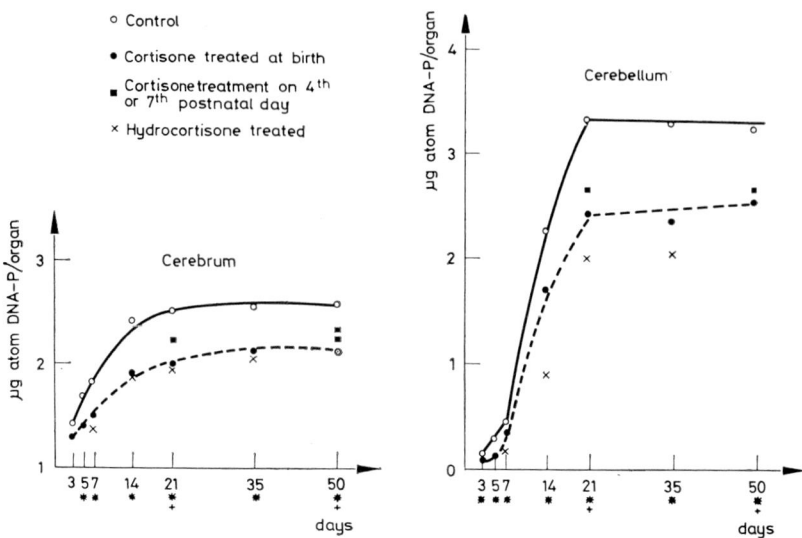

Fig. 3. Effect of corticosteroid treatment on total amount of DNA in cerebrum and cerebellum. * indicates when the difference between the animals treated with cortisone at birth and the controls was statistically significant. + statistically significant difference between the control and experimental animals treated with cortisone on the 4th or 7th postnatal day

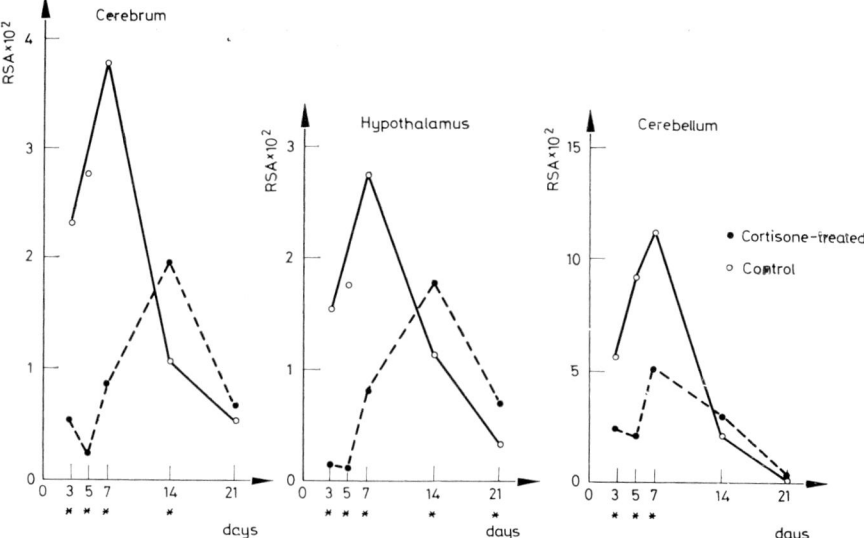

Fig. 4. Effect of corticosteroid treatment on rate of incorporation of 6-^{3}H-thymidine into DNA in cerebrum, hypothalamus and cerebellum. The results are expressed as relative specific activity:

$$\text{RSA} = \frac{\text{specific activity of DNA (d.p.m.}/\mu\text{g atom DNA-P)}}{^3\text{H content in acid-soluble fraction (d.p.m.}/\text{g wet weight)}}$$

* deviations from control values were statistically significant

In good agreement with our previous results (Kovács et al. 1969a) the rate of incorporation of thymidine into cerebral and cerebellar DNA in normal animals was considerable and varied with age. The highest rate of incorporation was found at about the 7th day of life in all three brain areas studied. After 7 days of age the rate of incorporation decreased rapidly and the very low value on day 21 showed that DNA synthesis in the brain had almost ceased. The highest rate of incorporation was found in the cerebellum, much lower values in the cerebrum and hypothalamus (Fig. 4).

Corticosteroid administration had a very pronounced effect on the rate of incorporation of labelled thymidine. In the first week, particularly in the cerebrum and hypothalamus, the rate of incorporation was very low in the treated animals, in fact it was only a fraction of the control value. The highest rate of incorporation in the cerebrum and hypothalamus was seen in the corticosteroid-treated animals on day 14. At this time the relative specific activity was higher than the control value, and a higher value for RSA was observed also on day 21 of life. Similarly to the controls the peak incorporation in the CBL of the treated animals occurred on day 7, but the subsequent decrease was much slower than in the controls and, as a result of this slower decrease, the rate of incorporation on days 14 and 21 was higher than the control value.

EFFECTS ON AVERAGE CELL SIZE AND ON AMOUNTS OF PROTEIN AND RNA IN THE BRAIN

The DNA content per unit weight of tissue may be regarded as an index of cell size. The concentration of DNA in the cerebrum and hypothalamus decreased with age, showing that the average cell size had increased. In the cerebellum an initial increase in DNA concentration was observed and the decrease appeared only after 14 days of life.

As judged by the DNA concentrations, the treatment with T_3 or corticosteroids had no significant effect on average cell size either in the cerebrum, hypothalamus or cerebellum (Figs 5 and 6).

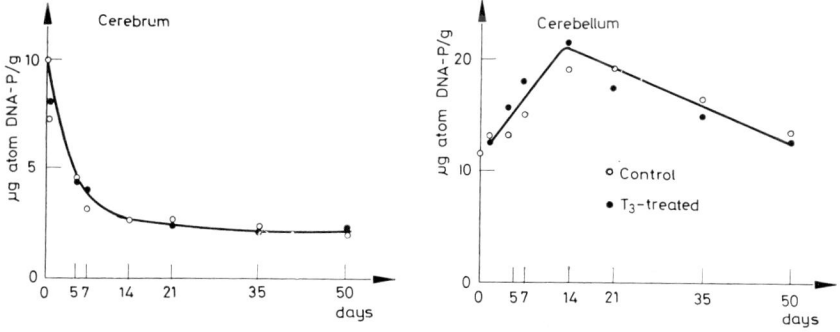

Fig. 5. Effect of T_3 treatment on DNA concentration (μg atom DNA-P/unit weight of tissue) in cerebrum and cerebellum

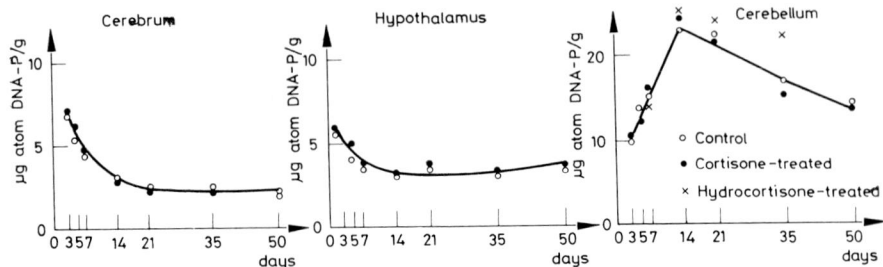

Fig. 6. Effect of treatment with corticosteroid on DNA concentration in cerebrum, hypothalamus and cerebellum

The protein concentration (protein content per unit weight of tissue) in the cerebrum, hypothalamus and cerebellum markedly increased with age after birth, reaching the level characteristic of adults at about 28–35 days of life. On the other hand, the concentration of RNA in the cerebrum and hypothalamus showed a progressive reduction with age. In the cerebellum the RNA concentration increased during the first 14 days of life and a decrease was noted only after this period.

T_3 or corticosteroid treatment had little effect on protein and RNA concentration either in the cerebrum, hypothalamus or cerebellum (Figs 7a, 8a, 9a and 10a).

As shown by the protein/DNA and RNA/DNA ratios, the average protein and RNA contents of the cells in the cerebrum, hypothalamus and cerebellum also changed during development (Figs 7b, 8b and 9b, 10b). The marked developmental

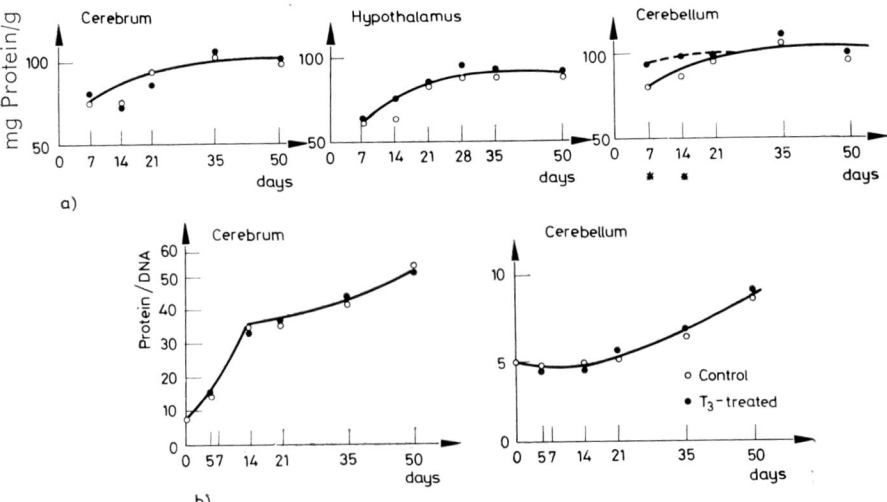

Fig. 7. Effect of T_3 treatment on protein concentration in cerebrum, hypothalamus and cerebellum (a), and on cellular content of protein (b) in cerebrum and cerebellum. Significant deviations from the control values were found only in protein concentration in the cerebellum on 7th and 14th days of age

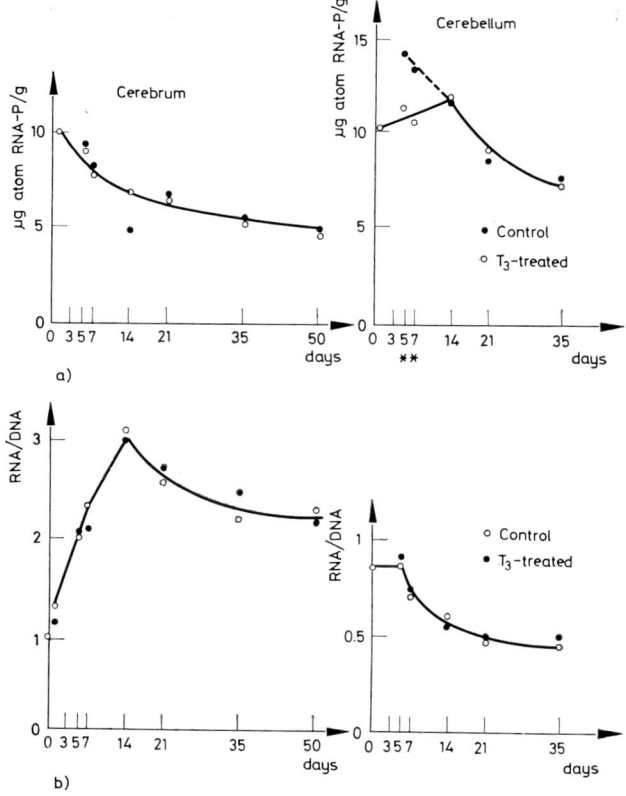

Fig. 8. Effect of T_3 treatment on RNA concentration (a), and on cellular content of RNA (b) in the cerebrum and cerebellum

changes in the mean cellular content of protein and RNA were not significantly affected by the treatment with T_3 (Figs 7b and 8b).

The treatment with corticosteroids apparently had no effect on the protein/DNA ratio either in the cerebrum, hypothalamus or cerebellum (Fig. 9b).

The RNA/DNA ratio in the cerebrum of corticosteroid-treated animals was lower during the first two weeks of life, while on days 35 and 50 the ratio was higher than the control value. No deviations from the control values were found in the RNA/DNA ratios in the hypothalamus and cerebellum (Fig. 10b).

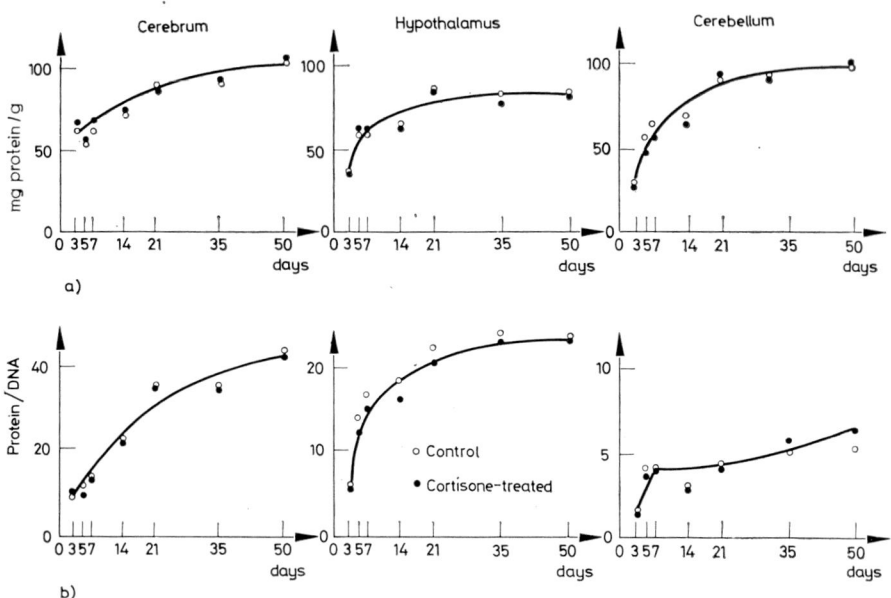

Fig. 9. Effect of corticosteroid treatment on protein concentration (a), and on protein/DNA ratios (b) in cerebrum, hypothalamus and cerebellum

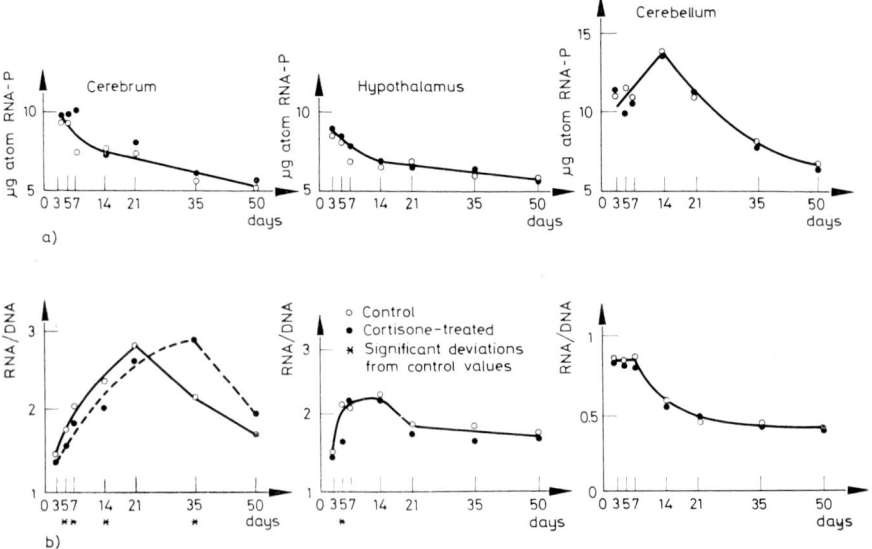

Fig. 10. Effect of corticosteroid treatment on RNA concentration (a), and on RNA/DNA ratios (b) in cerebrum, hypothalamus and cerebellum

PROTEIN AND RNA SYNTHESIS

It was reported previously that the rate of incorporation of labelled amino acid into cerebral protein is decreased in thyroid deficiency during infancy (Geel et al. 1967, Balázs et al. 1967). In the following experiments carried out likewise on male rats the effect of T_3 (also 25 µg given at birth) was investigated on the rate of incorporation of 1-^{14}C-leucine into cerebral and cerebellar protein. In view of its specific role in endocrine regulation, the hypothalamus was also studied. The animals were killed 30 minutes after the labelled leucine injection (20 $\mu C/100$ g body weight subcutaneously).

In the cerebrum and CBL of the normal as well as T_3 treated animals the rate of incorporation of labelled leucine varied with age. Between 7 and 14 days a sharp increase occurred in both groups reaching the highest rate of incorporation on the 14th day of life, and then decreasing rapidly between 14 and 21 days and much more slowly later. No significant difference in the rate of incorporation of leucine in the cerebrum and cerebellum was observed between the T_3 treated and control animals, except on day 21 of life when the rate of incorporation was lower in the T_3 treated animals.

The age curve of the rate of incorporation of labelled leucine into protein in the hypothalamus was different from the curves obtained for the cerebrum and cerebellum. In the cerebrum and cerebellum of the normal animals the highest rate of incorporation of labelled leucine into protein was observed earlier than in the hypothalamus, where it was found on the 21st day of life. Besides the age difference shown by the maximum rates of incorporation, quantitative differences were also observed: in the hypothalamus the relative specific activity of protein was much lower and the decrease after the peak incorporation was much slower than in the rest of the cerebrum or cerebellum. In the T_3 treated animals both peak incorporation and subsequent fall occurred earlier than in the controls. As a consequence, between days 21 and 35 the rate of incorporation of labelled leucine in the hypothalamus of the T_3 treated rats, as compared with the controls, was reduced by about 30 per cent (Fig. 11).

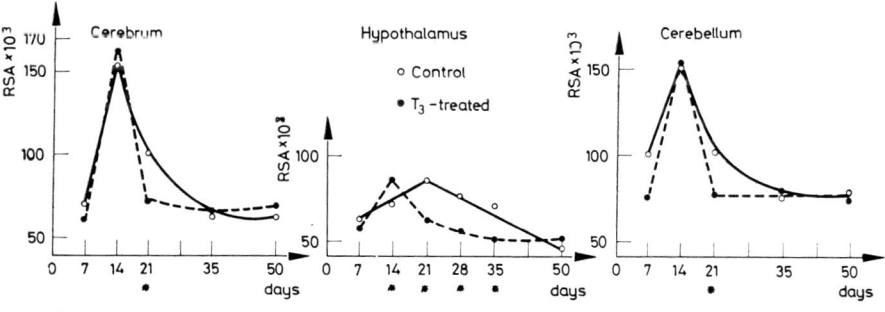

* Significant deviations from control values

Fig. 11. Effect of T_3 treatment on rate of incorporation of 1-^{14}C-leucine into protein in cerebrum, hypothalamus and cerebellum. The rate of incorporation is expressed as relative specific activity:

$$\text{RSA} = \frac{\text{specific activity of protein (dpm/mg protein)}}{^{14}\text{C content in acid soluble pool (dpm/g wet weight)}}$$

Experiments have also been commenced to investigate the effect of corticosteroid treatment on protein synthesis. Some preliminary results are shown in Fig. 12. In both age groups the rate of incorporation decreased in the three brain areas studied in the treated animals. The difference between the experimental and control groups in the CBL on day 21, however, was not significant.

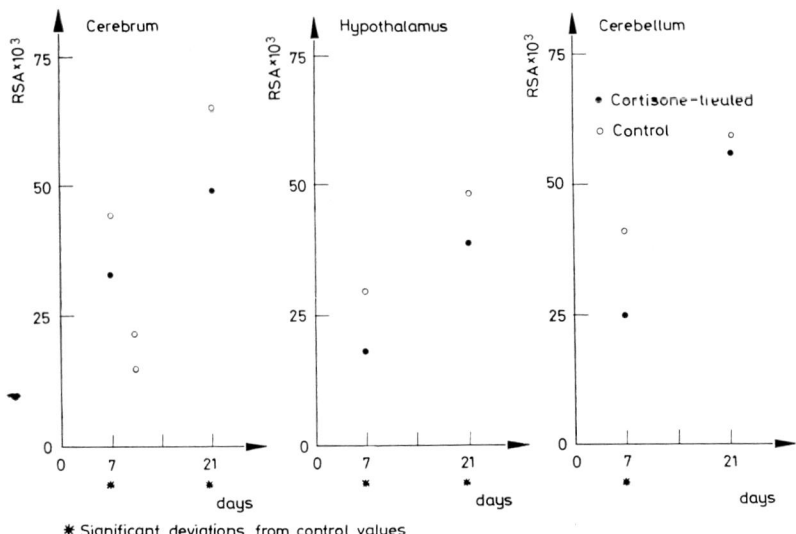

Fig. 12. Effect of corticosteroid treatment on rate of incorporation of 1-^{14}C-leucine into protein in cerebrum, hypothalamus and cerebellum. RSA as in Fig. 11

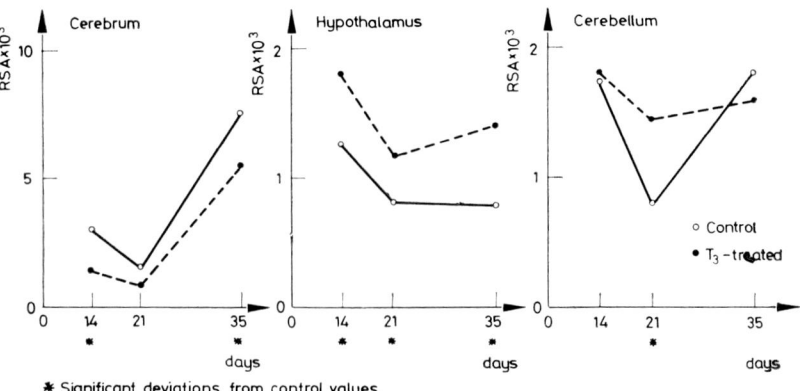

Fig. 13. Effect of T_3 treatment on rate of incorporation of 5-^{3}H-uridine into RNA in cerebrum, hypothalamus and cerebellum.

$$\text{RSA} = \frac{\text{specific activity of RNA (dpm/}\mu\text{g atom RNA-P)}}{^3\text{H content in acid soluble fraction (dpm/g wet weight)}}$$

RNA metabolism has been studied with 5-³H-uridine as a precursor. The animals were killed 1 hour after a subcutaneous injection of 5 μC/g body weight of ³H-uridine. The results are expressed as relative specific activity.

In the cerebrum the rate of incorporation of ³H-uridine was lower in the T_3 treated animals than in the controls. In contrast to this, in the hypothalamus the

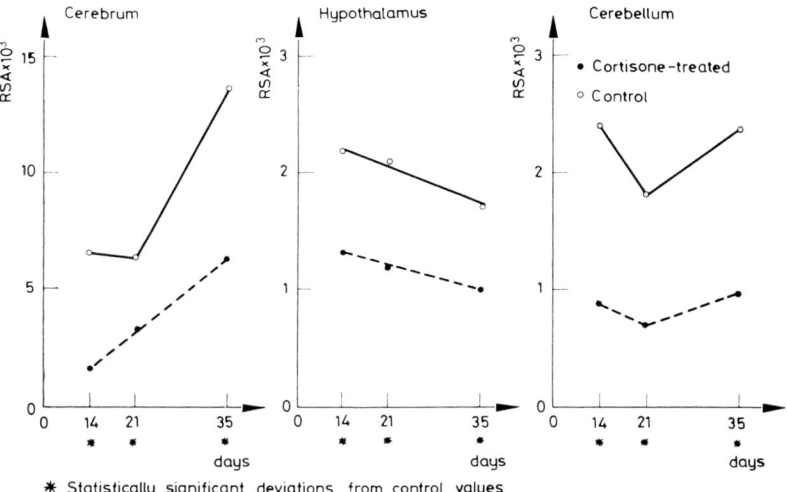

Fig. 14. Effect of corticosteroid treatment on rate of incorporation of 5-³H-uridine into RNA in cerebrum, hypothalamus and cerebellum. RSA as in Fig. 13

rate of incorporation of ³H-uridine increased in the T_3 treated rats. In the CBL not much difference can be observed between the treated and control groups, except on day 21 when the RSA was considerably higher in the T_3 treated animals than in the controls (Fig. 13).

After corticosteroid treatment in all age groups the rate of incorporation of labelled uridine into RNA was much lower in each of the three brain areas studied (Fig. 14).

DISCUSSION

The first problem I should like to deal with in particular is the effect of hormones on postnatal cell formation in the rat brain.

As it has been shown, thyroid hormone as well as corticosteroids given in infancy markedly influence postnatal cell formation in the cerebrum and cerebellum. As a result of their effect the number of cells was considerably lower in the brains of the adult experimental animals than in the controls. Although the final results of their action found in adults seem to be the same, considerable differences can be observed in timing and presumably also in the mechanism of the effects of the two hormones.

63

The effect of thyroid hormone on postnatal cell formation in the brain appears after a relatively long latent period, and a difference can be observed between the cerebrum and cerebellum in the time of manifestation of the effect of T_3. These findings and the probable mechanism of action have been discussed in detail in one of our previous publications (Balázs et al. 1971b).

In contrast to thyroid hormone, the effect of corticosteroids on postnatal cell formation in the brain is manifested very early, almost immediately after their administration, and no difference can be observed between the brain areas studied. When discussing these results one can speculate that perhaps the timing of the effect of corticosteroid treatment is restricted to the first few days after birth. The results obtained in the present experiments investigating the rate of DNA synthesis and the fact that corticosteroid given on days 4 and 7 after birth had the same effects as when injected on the day of birth contradict this assumption.

The results of our experiments with labelled thymidine show that the effect of corticosteroid on DNA synthesis is also different from that of thyroid hormone. From the present results no conclusion can be drawn as to the cell type affected or the mechanism of action of the adrenocortical hormones.

It is very interesting to note that postnatal cell formation in the brain can be influenced by different stimuli if they are applied within a certain period of time after birth. Treatment with thyroid hormone (Kovács et al. 1969a, Balázs et al. 1971b), corticosteroids (Howard 1965) and, as it has just been found in our laboratory, with gonadal hormones (Vértes et al. 1971), or undernutrition during early life (Winick and Noble 1966), have a very similar effect, viz., damage to postnatal cell formation in the brain. The question arises whether these stimuli have a specific and selective effect on the different stages of postnatal cell formation, perhaps on the formation of different cell types. Or is it rather that the brain reacts in the same way to a variety of strong stimuli only during a certain period of development.

The second problem that I should like to discuss is concerned with the effect of these hormones on cell development in the brain after birth. Besides the marked effect on postnatal cell formation, T_3 or corticosteroid administration had little, if any, effect on the average cell size in the brain. Except for the change in RNA/DNA ratio in the cerebrum after corticosteroid treatment no deviations were found from the control values for either the RNA/DNA and protein/DNA ratios or the DNA concentration in the brain after treatment with T_3 or corticosteroids. However, considerable differences were observed when the protein or RNA synthesis of the brain was studied.

The rate of protein synthesis in the brain of the control animals varied with age. In the cerebrum and cerebellum the highest rate was followed by a decrease, and the level characteristic of adults was reached at about 28–35 days of life. The protein concentration also reached the adult level at about this age. T_3 treatment had no effect on the rate of protein synthesis in the cerebrum and cerebellum during the first two weeks of life. However, the decrease after the highest rate of incorporation at 14 days was much faster in the T_3 treated animals, and as a result of this more rapid fall, the rate of labelled leucine incorporation reached the level characteristic of adults earlier than in the controls.

T_3 treatment had a much stronger effect on the development of protein synthesis in the hypothalamus. The peak incorporation occurred earlier and the value characteristic of adults was also reached earlier than in the controls. These observations suggest that T_3 treatment advances the maturation of protein synthesis first of all in the hypothalamus. The question as to the significance of this change in the rate of protein synthesis in the hypothalamus after T_3 treatment cannot be answered on the basis of the present experiments. Bearing in mind that the hypothalamus plays a very important role in the regulation of the endocrine system, one can assume that the early changes in the hypothalamus after thyroid hormone treatment might be the first step in the action of this hormone on development. This early change may effect pituitary function during development, and thus some effect observed after T_3 treatment may be related to the disturbances of development and function of the hypothalamo–pituitary system. The results of our experiments concerned with hormonal effects on the development of the pituitary gland seem to confirm this hypothesis, showing that pituitary development is affected very markedly and at a very early stage by neonatal T_3 treatment (Kovács et al. 1969b, Kovács 1971).

The rate of RNA synthesis also changes in response to T_3 treatment. The most pronounced alteration occurred, also in this case, in the hypothalamus, where the rate of labelled uridine incorporation increased in the T_3 treated rats of each age group. The relation of this finding to that observed in the rate of protein synthesis is not clear. Further work is required to answer this question. It is difficult to draw reliable conclusions from the preliminary results of the experiments concerned with protein synthesis after corticosteroid treatment because only two age groups were studied. However, it seems probable that the effect of corticosteroid hormones on protein synthesis in the brain differs from that of thyroid hormone. As it has been shown, the rate of labelled leucine incorporation decreased in both age groups studied. Similarly, decreases in RNA synthesis were found after corticosteroid treatment in the three brain regions studied in each age group. These results show that besides the reduction in postnatal cell formation, decreased rates of protein and RNA synthesis occur in the brain after corticosteroid treatment in infancy. As with DNA synthesis, the reduction in the rates of protein and RNA synthesis also seems to appear early after corticosteroid administration.

The last question I shall deal with is the specificity of the effect of thyroid and adrenocortical hormones on brain development. This question arises because it is known that treatment either with thyroid or adrenocortical hormones in infancy affects other endocrine functions which influence brain development.

Treatment with T_3, e.g., markedly reduces the production of growth hormone by the pituitary gland and, as the markedly reduced weights of the adrenal glands and testicles observed in our experiments show, probably also the production of ACTH and gonadotropic hormones (Kovács et al. 1969b). On the other hand, it has been reported that after corticosteroid treatment practically no growth hormone-releasing activity is observed in the hypothalamus and very little growth hormone and TSH activity in the pituitary (Sawano et al. 1969). Our investigations into the effect of corticosteroids on biochemical maturation of the pituitary gland also show that this gland is very markedly affected.

The present studies have demonstrated pronounced biochemical changes in the brain occurring during postnatal development in response to thyroid or adrenocortical hormones. The relationship between the biochemical changes and the morphological and behavioural alterations found by other workers after thyroid or corticosteroid treatment in early life is not yet known. Further work is also necessary to clarify the mechanism of action of these hormones on the brain, particularly at a cellular or subcellular level.

REFERENCES

BALÁZS, R., KOVÁCS, S., COCKS, W. A. and EAYRS, J. T. (1967): Effects of neonatal thyroid deficiency on the developing brain. In: *1st International Meeting of the International Society of Neurochemistry*, Strasbourg. Abstracts of Communications. p. 12.

BALÁZS, R., KOVÁCS, S., TEICHGRÄBER, P., COCKS, W. A. and EAYRS, J. T. (1968): Biochemical effects of thyroid deficiency on the developing brain. *J. Neurochem.* **15**, 1335–1349.

BALÁZS, R., COCKS, W. A., EAYRS, J. T. and KOVÁCS, S. (1971a): Biochemical effects of thyroid hormones on the developing brain. In: *Hormones in Development*. Ed. by M. Hamburg and E. J. W. Barrington. Appleton-Century-Crofts, New York. pp. 357–379.

BALÁZS, R., KOVÁCS, S., COCKS, W. A., JOHNSON, A. L. and EAYRS, J. T. (1971b): Effect of thyroid hormone on the biochemical maturation of rat brain: postnatal cell formation. *Brain Res.* **25**, 555–570.

DE GUGLIELMONE, A. E. R. and GÓMEZ, C. J. (1966): Influence of neonatal hypothyroidism on amino acids. *J. Neurochem.* **13**, 1017–1025.

EAYRS, J. T. (1954): The vascularity of the cerebral cortex in normal and cretinous rats. *J. Anat. (Lond.)* **88**, 164–173.

EAYRS, J. T. (1955): The cerebral cortex of normal and hypothyroid rats. *Acta anat. (Basel)* **25**, 160–183.

EAYRS, J. T. (1961): Age as a factor determining the severity and reversibility of the effects of thyroid deprivation in the rat. *J. Endocr.* **22**, 409–419.

EAYRS, J. T. (1964): Effect of neonatal hyperthyroidism on maturation and learning in the rat. *Anim. Behav.* **12**, 195–199.

EAYRS, J. T. (1968): Developmental relationship between brain and thyroid. In: *Endocrinology and Human Behaviour*. Ed. by R. P. Michael. Oxford Univ. Press, London. pp. 239–255.

EAYRS, J. T. and LISHMAN, W. A. (1955): The maturation of behaviour in hypothyroidism and starvation. *Brit. J. Anim. Behav.* **3**, 17–24.

EAYRS, J. T. and LEVINE, S. (1963): Influence of thyroidectomy and subsequent replacement therapy upon conditioned avoidance learning in the rat. *J. Endocr.* **25**, 505–513.

ENESCO, M. and LEBLOND, C. P. (1962): Increase in cell number as a factor on the growth of the organs of the young male rat. *J. Embryol. exp. Morph.* **10**, 530–562.

GARCIA ARGIZ, C. A., PASQUINI, J. M., KAPLUN, B. and GÓMEZ, C. J. (1967): Hormonal regulation of brain development. II. Effect of neonatal thyroidectomy on succinate dehydrogenase and other enzymes in developing cerebral cortex and cerebellum of the rat. *Brain Res.* **6**, 635–646.

GEEL, S. E. and TIMIRAS, P. S. (1967): The influence of neonatal hypothyroidism and of thyroxine on the RNA and DNA concentrations of rat cerebral cortex. *Brain Res.* **4**, 135–142.

GEEL, S. E., VALCANA, TH. and TIMIRAS, P. S. (1967): Effect of neonatal hypothyroidism and of thyroxine on L-(^{14}C)leucine incorporation in protein in vivo and the relationship to ionic levels in the developing brain. *Brain Res.* **4**, 143–150.

HAMBURGH, M. (1969): The role of thyroid and growth hormones in neurogenesis. In: *Current Topics in Developmental Biology*. Vol. 4. Ed. by A. A. Moscona and A. Monroy. Academic Press, New York and London. pp. 109–148.

HOWARD, E. (1965): Effects of corticosterone and food restriction on growth, and on DNA, RNA and cholesterol of the brain and liver in infant mice. *J. Neurochem.* **12**, 181–191.

HOWARD, E. (1968): Reductions in size and total DNA of cerebrum and cerebellum in adult mice after corticosterone treatment in infancy. *Exp. Neurol.* **22,** 191—208.

KOVÁCS, S. (1971): Pajzsmirigy hormon szerepe a hypophysis elülsőlebeny postnatalis fejlődésében (The role of thyroid hormone in the postnatal development of the anterior pituitary). In: *Annual Meeting of the Hungarian Physiological Society,* Tihany. p. 57.

KOVÁCS, S., COCKS, W. A. and BALÁZS, R. (1969a): Incorporation of 2-^{14}C thymidine into deoxyribonucleic acid of rat brain during postnatal development: Effect of thyroid hormone. *Biochem. J.* **114,** 60.

KOVÁCS, S., COCKS, W. A. and BALÁZS, R. (1969b): Effect of thyroid hormone administration on the incorporation of 1-^{14}C leucine into protein of rat pituitary and hypothalamus during development. *J. Endocr.* **45,** IX—X.

PASQUINI, J. M., KAPLUN, B., GARCIA ARGIZ, C. A. and GÓMEZ, C. J. (1967): Hormonal regulation of brain development. I. The effect of neonatal thyroidectomy upon nucleic acids, protein and two enzymes in developing cerebral cortex and cerebellum of the rat. *Brain Res.* **6,** 621—634.

SAWANO, S., ARIMURA, A., SCHALLY, A. V., REDDING, T. W. and SCHAPIRO, S. (1969): Neonatal corticoid administration: effects upon adult pituitary growth hormone and hypothalamic growth hormone-releasing hormone activity. *Acta endocr. (Kbh.)* **61,** 57—67.

SCHAPIRO, S. (1968): Some physiological, biochemical and behavioural consequences of neonatal hormone administration: cortisol and thyroxine. *Gen. comp. Endocr.* **10,** 214—228.

VÉRTES, ZS., LISSÁK, K. and KOVÁCS, S. (1971): Újszülöttkori oestradiol kezelés hatása a hypophysis elülsőlebeny és az agy fejlődésére (Effect of neonatal oestradiol treatment on the development of anterior pituitary and brain). In: *Annual Meeting of the Hungarian Physiological Society,* Tihany. p. 58.

WINICK, M. and NOBLE, A. (1966): Cellular response in rats during malnutrition at various ages. *J. Nutr.* **89,** 300—306.

DISTURBANCES OF MYELINATION IN NEONATALLY THYROIDECTOMIZED RAT BRAINS

R. TSUJIMURA, N. KARIYAMA and N. HATOTANI

Department of Psychiatry
Mie Prefectural University School of Medicine
Tsu, Japan

It is well known that thyroid deficiency in the neonatal period results in impaired development of the central nervous system. The effects in the rats of neonatal hypothyroidism have been the subject of extensive histological (Hamburgh 1969), behavioural (Eayrs and Levine 1963), electroencephalographic (Hatotani and Timiras 1967) and biochemical (Gell et al. 1967, Gómez and Ramirez de Guglielmone 1967, Balázs et al. 1968) studies. To date, however, little attention has been focussed on the cerebral lipids in the states of thyroid dysfunction. The recent works suggested that the lipid content and its fatty acid patterns in the myelin sheath were different from those in the whole brain, the gray matter and the white matter (O'Brien and Sampson 1965a, b). Despite a few studies (Cuarón et al. 1963, Walravens and Chase 1969), the data on the lipid analyses of isolated brain myelin from the hypothyroid animals are completely lacking. The present work was designed to examine in the rats the influences of neonatally induced hypothyroidism on the myelination in terms of changes in myelin lipid content and in normal fatty acid composition of the individual sphingolipid.

MATERIALS AND METHODS

The laboratory rats of Wistar strain were used in all experiments. Hypothyroidism was induced by a single intraperitoneal injection of 150 μCi of ^{131}Iodine at birth. Myelin fractions were prepared by Uyemura's procedure (1965) from both the control and the hypothyroid rat brains at the ages of 10, 15, 22, 30 and 60 days. Lipid extraction from the myelin was performed by the method of Folch and Lees (1951), and then total lipids, total phospholipids, total cholesterol and total glycolipids were determined. The total lipids were subjected to mild alkaline hydrolysis according to the method of Måtenson (1966). After hydrolysis and Folch's partition (Folch et al. 1957), the crude sphingolipid fraction was eluted from silicic acid column. This crude sphingolipid fraction was applied to silicic acid-Hyflo Super Cel (2 : 1, w/w) column and separated into cerebroside, sulphatide and sphingomyelin with chloroform containing stepwise increasing methanol concentration. Furthermore, both the cerebroside and the sulphatide fraction were subjected to Florisil column to remove the contaminated phospholipids. After identification of the individual sphingolipid by thin layer chromatography and infrared spectroscopy, cerebroside, sulphatide and sphingomyelin were estimated. These materials were methanolyzed according to the ordinary procedures. The normal fatty acid esters were separated from hydroxy fatty acid esters by thin layer chromatography and applied to gas chromatography using 10 per cent DEGS on Diasolid L packed glass column.

RESULTS

BODY AND BRAIN GROWTH IN CONTROL AND HYPOTHYROID RATS

In terms of body and brain weights, as is shown in Table 1, these increases in the experimental groups were depressed and the influence on body weight was especially striking. By 15 days of age the animals were manifestly cretinoid, as judged by the following criteria: the reduction in the size of body, skull and tail, peculiar hair and uncertainty of gait.

TABLE 1

Body and brain growth in control and hypothyroid rats

		Age (days)				
		10	15	22	30	60
Mean body weight in g	Control	21.67	34.72	53.67	98.63	161.6
	Hypothyroid	20.51	28.05	34.08	52.16	96.5
Mean brain weight in g	Control	1.17	1.27	1.44	1.55	1.75
	Hypothyroid	1.10	1.16	1.26	1.36	1.54
No. of animals	Control	82	36	32	31	12
	Hypothyroid	223	67	67	58	26

LIPID CONTENT IN BRAIN MYELIN OF CONTROL AND HYPOTHYROID RATS

As is shown in Table 2, each content of total lipids, total phospholipids, total cholesterol and total glycolipids in the brain myelin of both control and hypothyroid rats increased gradually with the developmental progress, but the aspect of the distribution within total lipids showed that both total cholesterol and total glycolipids increased relatively, while the relative decrease in total phospholipids occurred. The influences of hypothyroidism were found in all myelin lipid fractions and the reduction in both total glycolipids and total cholesterol, so essential to myelin formation, was especially prominent; in comparison with the control group at the age of 22 days, the experimental group showed a 69 per cent reduction for total glycolipids and a 43 per cent reduction for total cholesterol. Even total phospholipids revealed the disturbances due to hypothyroidism.

TABLE 2

Lipid content in myelin fraction of control and hypothyroid rat brains

		Lipid content (mg/g fresh wet weight of brain)							
		Total lipids		Total phospholipids		Total cholesterol		Total glycolipids	
		N	H	N	H	N	H	N	H
Age (days)	10	19.96	15.34	14.51	10.46	4.17	3.04	0.50	0.32
	15	33.21	23.46	22.38	16.42	7.00	4.41	1.11	0.56
	22	46.03	29.28	31.05	19.40	10.96	6.34	3.83	1.20
	30	53.33	45.25	34.34	29.73	12.49	9.50	4.64	2.35
	60	63.46	45.69	39.52	31.81	15.79	9.92	5.76	4.29
		Distribution within total lipids (%)							
Age (days)	10			72.7	68.2	20.9	19.8	2.5	2.1
	15			67.4	70.0	21.1	18.8	3.3	2.4
	22			67.5	66.2	23.8	21.6	8.3	4.1
	30			64.4	65.7	23.4	21.0	8.7	5.2
	60			62.3	69.6	24.9	21.7	9.1	9.3

N= control, H= hypothyroid.

SPHINGOLIPID CONTENT IN BRAIN MYELIN OF CONTROL AND HYPOTHYROID RATS

Regarding cerebroside, sulphatide and sphingomyelin, as given in Table 3, the gradual increase in the amount of individual sphingolipid took place in two groups with the development, but the affections caused by hypothyroidism were found in these lipids and the reduction in both cerebroside and sulphatide was especially prominent as compared with the controls in all age groups. The reduction rate in the hypothyroid rat at the age of 22 days was as follows: a 69 per cent for cerebroside, a 71 per cent for sulphatide and a 23 per cent for sphingomyelin.

TABLE 3

Sphingolipid content in myelin fraction of control and hypothyroid rat brains

		Sphingolipid content (mg/g fresh wet weight of brain)					
		Cerebrosides		Sulphatides		Sphingomyelins	
		N	H	N	H	N	H
Age (days)	10	0.32	0.25	0.20	0.06	0.24	0.19
	15	0.70	0.40	0.41	0.16	0.69	0.52
	22	3.12	0.99	0.71	0.21	1.10	0.85
	30	3.97	2.03	0.67	0.32	1.09	0.84
	60	4.99	3.52	0.77	0.76	1.12	0.87

N= control, H= hypothyroid.

UNSUBSTITUTED FATTY ACID COMPOSITION OF SPHINGOMYELIN IN BRAIN MYELIN OF CONTROL AND HYPOTHYROID RATS

As is shown in Table 4, the major fatty acids of sphingomyelin in both the control and the hypothyroid rats were stearic and palmitic acids during the early life. The relative decrease of palmitic acid and the relative increase of lignoceric and nervonic acids were found in two groups with the developmental advances, while the stearic acid remained relatively constant. As a whole, the age-dependent changes in the fatty acid composition of sphingomyelin were very slight and the changes of pattern were similar in both groups, but the chain elongation process during the course of development was slightly depressed in the experimental rats as compared with the controls.

TABLE 4

Composition of unsubstituted fatty acids in sphingomyelin of brain myelin

Fatty acids	10 days		15 days		22 days		30 days		60 days	
	N	H	N	H	N	H	N	H	N	H
14 : 0	2.6	0.6	0.7	0.9	—	0.5	0.3	0.3	0.7	tr.
15 : 1	0.6	—	—	0.8	—	—	tr.	—	0.4	0.3
16 : 0	16.9	4.1	5.4	16.2	3.0	3.2	3.3	4.0	3.1	3.3
16 : 1	1.6	tr.	4.8	1.2	tr.	0.5	1.0	tr.	tr.	0.4
17 : 0	0.4	—	0.2	tr.	0.6	—	0.5	—	—	—
17 : 1	0.9	—	tr.	1.0	—	—	—	—	0.3	0.2
18 : 0	56.4	86.7	67.9	65.2	75.5	75.8	67.2	78.5	66.7	71.3
18 : 1	8.9	tr.	5.5	6.1	tr.	3.2	5.4	2.2	tr.	3.8
19 : 0	0.9	2.3	4.0	1.4	2.5	2.8	4.6	2.0	0.5	2.0
19 : 1	0.8	—	—	—	—	—	tr.	0.6	tr.	—
20 : 0	1.8	tr.	2.1	1.0	2.9	2.3	3.1	2.4	4.2	3.3
20 : 1	0.8	—	—	—	1.4	1.1	0.8	—	tr.	—
21 : 0	1.1	—	—	—	tr.	—	tr.	—	tr.	tr.
22 : 0	2.2	1.7	2.4	4.1	3.4	2.3	3.7	1.9	5.0	2.8
22 : 1	0.1	—	1.9	0.3	0.9	tr.	1.2	1.3	2.6	2.3
23 : 0	—	—	—	tr.	tr.	—	tr.	—	tr.	—
24 : 0	1.4	0.8	1.2	0.4	2.6	1.1	1.9	2.3	3.8	1.8
24 : 1	2.5	1.1	2.9	0.4	7.1	7.2	7.0	4.4	12.7	8.5
25 : 0	—	—	—	tr.	tr.	—	tr.	—	tr.	—
25 : 1	—	—	1.1	0.7	—	—	tr.	—	tr.	—
Sum of 21 : 0—25 : 1	7.3	3.6	9.4	5.9	14.0	10.6	13.8	9.9	24.2	15.4
Sum of 24 : 0—25 : 1	3.9	1.9	5.2	1.5	9.7	8.3	8.9	6.7	16.5	10.3
Monoenes	16.2	1.1	15.1	10.5	9.4	12.1	15.4	8.5	16.0	15.5

N= normal control rats, H= hypothyroid rats.
Expressed as percentage of the total unsubstituted fatty acids.

UNSUBSTITUTED FATTY ACID COMPOSITION OF CEREBROSIDE AND SULPHATIDE IN BRAIN MYELIN OF CONTROL AND HYPOTHYROID RATS

In terms of the major fatty acids, as are given in Tables 5 and 6, both cerebroside and sulphatide in two groups had stearic, lignoceric and nervonic acids, and there were marked changes of fatty acid pattern in these lipids of both groups as the development advanced; and a wide variety of fatty acids was present, ranging in the chain length from 14 to 26 carbon atoms, and including odd-number fatty acids and both saturated and mono-unsaturated derivatives. The relative decrease of palmitic, stearic and oleic acids and the relative increase of lignoceric and nervonic acids were found in two groups with the development, therefore, these changes were responsible for a remarkable increase in the proportion of long-chain fatty acids with the developmental progress. In the earlier life, the lignoceric acid in both cerebroside and sulphatide of two groups was dominant in comparison with the nervonic acid but afterwards this ratio became reversed with the development. Regarding the chain elongation of fatty acids in both cerebroside and sulphatide, no significant differences were found between the two groups, the only difference being that the proportion of monoenes and odd-number fatty acids was considerably decreased in the experimental rats during the early life.

TABLE 5

Composition of unsubstituted fatty acids in cerebroside of brain myelin

Fatty acids	10 days		15 days		22 days		30 days		60 days	
	N	H	N	H	N	H	N	H	N	H
14 : 0	0.3	0.5	1.9	0.4	0.6	0.3	—	0.2	0.2	0.2
15 : 0	—	—	0.2	—	0.2	—	—	—	—	—
15 : 1	0.2	—	0.5	—	0.5	0.2	0.4	—	0.1	—
16 : 0	13.7	16.3	10.3	15.1	3.8	3.0	2.8	1.9	2.2	0.8
16 : 1	0.6	0.4	3.2	0.6	1.0	0.4	0.3	0.2	0.4	—
17 : 0	0.2	0.2	0.7	0.2	0.2	—	0.2	0.1	0.2	—
17 : 1	0.3	—	0.4	—	0.8	0.2	—	—	0.1	0.1
18 : 0	34.9	36.2	26.5	27.5	22.1	24.9	16.2	14.7	10.5	10.8
18 : 1	12.4	11.7	10.5	10.0	1.3	3.1	2.3	2.6	1.9	0.7
19 : 0	2.4	1.3	2.6	2.3	3.7	2.8	1.7	2.9	2.9	0.7
20 : 0	2.5	3.4	1.6	4.2	3.0	4.8	2.9	4.4	3.5	4.0
20 : 1	0.2	0.3	2.1	0.9	0.3	0.7	1.9	0.9	0.8	—
21 : 0	0.4	0.2	0.5	0.3	0.2	0.3	0.5	0.3	0.2	0.2
21 : 1	0.4	—	0.3	0.2	0.3	—	0.6	0.3	0.2	—
22 : 0	6.0	5.1	3.5	4.0	13.6	14.3	11.9	11.2	7.9	8.9
22 : 1	1.2	1.8	2.3	2.7	1.2	2.0	2.2	3.6	3.0	2.8
23 : 0	0.6	0.2	0.7	0.9	1.1	1.2	1.8	2.6	1.5	2.5
23 : 1	—	—	—	—	0.3	—	0.5	0.6	0.3	0.4
24 : 0	13.4	15.2	14.5	16.7	19.0	20.9	20.5	21.1	20.5	19.0
24 : 1	7.6	6.4	10.0	9.5	20.6	17.0	24.9	23.5	36.2	37.8
25 : 0	1.8	0.2	6.5	0.3	1.4	0.8	1.2	1.6	1.1	1.8
25 : 1	0.2	—	—	1.3	2.5	0.8	2.3	1.5	1.7	2.1
26 : 0	0.7	0.5	1.2	1.0	1.2	0.4	2.0	1.5	1.6	1.1
26 : 1	—	—	—	1.9	—	1.7	2.9	2.2	3.2	2.1
Sum of 21 : 0—26 : 1	32.3	29.6	39.5	38.8	61.4	59.4	71.3	70.1	77.4	78.7
Sum of 24 : 0—26 : 1	23.7	22.3	32.2	30.7	44.7	41.6	53.8	51.5	64.3	63.9
Monoenes	23.1	20.6	29.3	27.1	28.8	24.3	38.3	35.4	48.0	46.0
Odd number fatty acids	6.5	1.9	12.4	5.5	11.0	6.3	9.2	10.0	8.3	7.7

N = normal control rats, H = hypothyroid rats.
Expressed as percentage of the total unsubstituted fatty acids.

TABLE 6

Composition of unsubstituted fatty acids in sulphatide of brain myelin

Fatty acids	10 days		15 days		22 days		30 days		60 days	
	N	H	N	H	N	H	N	H	N	H
14 : 0	1.1	0.7	0.4	1.7	0.2	1.1	0.3	1.6	1.3	0.2
14 : 1	0.4	—	—	—	—	—	—	0.3	—	—
15 : 0	0.4	—	—	0.8	—	—	—	0.4	—	0.3
15 : 1	0.5	0.3	0.8	0.6	—	—	—	0.5	—	—
16 : 0	15.5	16.1	13.7	15.0	4.9	6.6	2.5	2.2	2.4	3.6
16 : 1	3.6	3.1	—	1.9	0.2	0.2	0.4	0.5	0.9	1.2
17 : 0	0.2	0.3	—	0.6	—	0.3	—	0.3	—	0.2
17 : 1	0.9	0.2	1.1	0.3	0.2	1.5	—	0.3	1.3	—
18 : 0	35.9	38.4	26.2	24.6	16.2	12.3	15.2	18.0	15.6	15.4
18 : 1	9.1	10.7	6.5	5.9	2.2	3.4	1.7	3.7	7.6	8.1
19 : 0	2.1	0.5	2.0	0.4	0.5	0.4	1.9	0.3	0.8	2.3
19 : 1	1.0	—	2.9	1.7	0.2	0.3	3.6	—	2.3	0.7
20 : 0	0.8	2.4	1.1	1.1	3.4	3.3	0.6	0.8	0.9	0.5
20 : 1	—	0.3	0.2	2.4	0.9	0.7	0.4	1.4	0.2	0.4
21 : 0	—	—	—	—	0.1	0.3	—	—	—	0.1
21 : 1	—	—	—	—	0.2	0.9	—	0.3	—	—
22 : 0	7.9	4.6	8.6	1.5	9.9	8.0	10.4	11.4	7.1	10.3
22 : 1	1.3	1.9	3.5	1.2	2.1	3.7	4.2	0.7	3.2	4.3
23 : 0	0.7	—	0.8	0.5	1.0	1.7	1.4	1.9	1.3	0.7
23 : 1	—	—	—	—	0.2	—	0.3	—	0.1	0.5
24 : 0	10.5	13.4	14.7	13.2	24.9	29.7	26.5	28.2	20.8	21.0
24 : 1	4.5	5.2	10.1	11.9	22.1	21.1	24.4	21.8	26.6	23.7
25 : 0	3.1	1.6	0.9	2.7	4.6	1.0	2.6	3.8	2.5	1.4
25 : 1	—	—	1.3	—	3.2	—	0.3	—	0.9	0.8
26 : 0	0.5	—	2.5	2.0	2.2	2.1	0.9	1.6	1.7	2.6
26 : 1	—	—	3.0	—	0.6	1.4	2.2	—	2.3	1.7
Sum of 21 : 0—26 : 1	28.5	26.7	45.4	43.0	71.1	69.9	73.2	69.7	66.0	67.1
Sum of 24 : 0—26 : 1	18.6	20.2	32.5	29.8	57.6	55.3	56.9	55.4	54.9	51.2
Monoenes	21.3	21.7	29.4	25.9	32.1	33.2	37.1	29.5	45.2	41.4
Odd number fatty acids	8.9	2.6	9.8	7.6	10.2	6.4	10.1	7.8	9.2	7.0

N = normal control rats, H = hypothyroid rats.
Expressed as percentage of the total unsubstituted fatty acids.

DISCUSSION

As the electron microscopic studies revealed the gradual morphological development which occurs during the myelination (De Robertis et al. 1958), the myelinogenesis is not a sudden event but rather the gradual assembly of various chemical components which appear at the same or different times to form a mature myelin structure. In the recently reported works on various species, it was indicated that the brain myelin contains 70–80 per cent lipid and 19–30 per cent protein (Norton and Autilo 1965, O'Brien and Sampson 1965a), and so the lipids are the major constituents of the myelin structure. It was demonstrated by O'Brien and Sampson (1965a, b) that the lipid component and its fatty acid composition in the myelin sheath are different from those in the whole brain, the gray matter and the white matter. Regarding the sphingolipid it was suggested (O'Brien 1965) that cerebroside and sulphatide are so essential to myelin formation and the increase in long-chain fatty acids of these lipids play a very important role in the stability of molecular arrangement in myelin structure. On the other hand, it has been revealed by histological studies (Hamburgh 1969) that the neonatally induced hypothyroid animals are in the state of myelin deficiency. Despite a few works on dysmyelination done in the whole brains of hypothyroid animals (Cuarón et al. 1963, Walravens and Chase 1969), there has been no report concerning the lipid analyses of the brain myelin isolated from the hypothyroid animals. Hence, the present work was designed to examine in the rats, using the isolated myelin fractions, the influences of neonatally induced hypothyroidism on the myelination in terms of changes in myelin lipid content and in normal fatty acid composition of individual sphingolipid.

Although the clear effects of hypothyroidism on the weight of body and brain were found, the growth of brain appeared to be less affected than that of the body and the influences of hypothyroidism became increasingly strong with age; these findings are in agreement with the observations of Cuarón et al. (1963) on rabbits and of Walravens and Chase (1969) on rats. With respect to the lipid content, the effects and influences caused by hypothyroidism were seen in all myelin lipid fractions but the diminution of glycolipid and cholesterol was especially prominent as compared with the controls in all age groups. It seems to be most important in the present experiment that the biosynthesis of both cerebroside and sulphatide was most strikingly suppressed in the hypothyroid rats. Since in the normal rats both cerebroside and sulphatide increase most strongly during the course of myelination and become to be localized mostly in the myelin sheath, it seems likely that the above-mentioned results represent the disturbances of myelin formation in the hypothyroid rats, thus confirming earlier histological (Hamburgh 1969) and electroencephalographic findings (Hatotani and Timiras 1967). These findings are generally in agreement with the results examined in the whole brain of cretinoid rats by Walravens and Chase (1969) and in the whole brain of myelin deficient mutants, the "Quaking" mouse by Baumann et al. (1968), and the "Jimpy" mouse by Galli and Re Cecconi Galli (1968) and by Nussbaum et al. (1969). Furthermore, interesting results were obtained from the calculation of maximum increase peak in myelin lipids: as is shown in Fig. 1, this increase peak in cerebroside, sulphatide and cholesterol was found in the control rats between 15 and 22 days of age, while that in the hypothyroid rats appeared between 22 and 30 days of age. This finding may make it possible to state that the onset of active myelination begins in the normal rats around 15 days of age, while in the cretinoid rats it was apparently retarded for about one week in comparison with the controls.

Regarding the phospholipid, on the basis of the observations made by Cuarón et al. (1963) on the whole brain of rabbits and by Walravens and Chase (1969) on the whole brain of rats, it has been reported that the phospholipid was less affected by hypothyroidism. In contrast to these results, however, it was suggested in the present work on the isolated myelin fractions that, although the reduction rate in phospholipid was slight as compared with glycolipid and cholesterol, the phospholipid was considerably affected due to hypothyroidism; this finding agrees with the results examined by Nomura et al. (1969) in the whole brain of cretinoid rats. As is shown in recent work (Tsujimura 1971), individual phospholipid in brain myelin has the different change patterns during the period of active myelination, and sphingomyelin, ethanolamine and serine glycerophosphatide appear in relatively high concentration within the myelin sheath in the course of development. In the present work the analyses of individual phospholipids were not performed, but it is conceivable that these myelin phospholipids were greatly affected by hypothyroidism, and consequently total phospholipids decreased considerably in the hypothyroid rats.

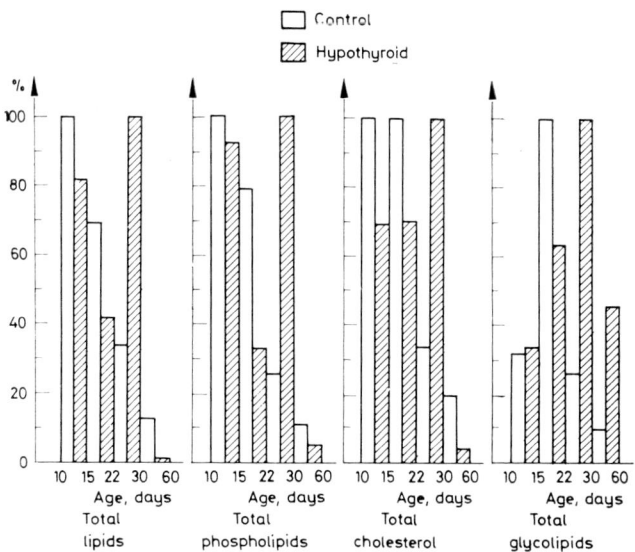

Fig. 1. Increase rate per one day

As to the fatty acid composition, the reports relevant to the present work are not available. It was demonstrated, however, by Ställberg-Stenhagen and Svennerholm (1965) on human brain with myelin disorders and by Baumann et al. (1968) on the whole brain of the "Quaking" mouse that the proportion of long-chain fatty acids in sphingomyelin, cerebroside and sulphatide decreased remarkably. In contrast to these results, the present work indicates that the chain elongation process was not disturbed by hypothyroidism: each sphingolipid with long-chain fatty acids appeared already in the early myelin of hypothyroid rats and then the proportion of long-chain fatty acids increased markedly during the course of development. It may follow that the pathology of myelin deficiency due to hypothyroidism is essentially different from that of the human disease associated with demyelination and of myelin deficiency in the "Quaking" and the "Jimpy" mice. Though little is known about the aetiology of myelin deficiency in the hypothyroid animals, the present work points to the possibility that individual sphingolipid is involved in the metabolic disorder bringing forth a remarkable decrease in cerebroside, sulphatide and sphingomyelin, hence the myelin deficiency in the hypothyroid rats. Since individual sphingolipid contains the long-chain fatty acids, which are supposed to play an important role in forming a stable membrane structure of mature myelin sheath (O'Brien 1965), the striking decrease of each sphingolipid could have caused the relative diminution of long-chain fatty acids. Consequently the membrane structure of myelin sheath became unstable.

REFERENCES

BALÁZS, R., KOVÁCS, S., TEICHGRÄBER, P., COCKS, W. A. and EAYRS, J. T. (1968): Biochemical effects of thyroid deficiency on the developing brain. *J. Neurochem.* **15**, 1335–1349.

BAUMANN, N. R., GACQUE, C. M., POLLET, S. A. and HARPIN, M. L. (1968): Fatty acid and lipid composition of the brain of a myelin deficient mutant, the "Quaking" mouse. *European J. Biochem.* **4**, 340–344.

CUARÓN, A., GAMBLE, J., MYANT, N. B. and OSORIO, C. (1963): The effect of thyroid deficiency on the growth of the brain and on the deposition of brain phospholipids in foetal and new-born rabbits. *J. Physiol.* **168**, 613–630.

DE ROBERTIS, E., GERSCHENFELD, H. M. and WALD, F. J. (1958): Cellular mechanism of myelination in the central nervous system. *J. biophys. biochem. Cytol.* **4**, 651–658.

EAYRS, J. T. and LEVINE, S. (1963): Influence of thyroidectomy and subsequent replacement therapy upon conditioned avoidance learning in the rat. *J. Endocr.* **25**, 505–513.

FOLCH, J. and LEES, M. (1951): Proteolipids, a new type of tissue lipoproteins. *J. biol. Chem.* **191**, 807–817.

FOLCH, J., LEES, M. and SLOANE-STANLEY, G. H. (1957): A simple method for the isolation and purification of total lipids from animal tissues. *J. biol. Chem.* **226**, 497–509.

GALLI, C. and RE CECCONI GALLI, D. (1968): Cerebroside and sulphatide deficiency in the brain of "Jimpy Mice", a mutant strain of mice exhibiting neurological symptoms. *Nature (Lond.)* **220**, 165–166.

GELL, S. E., VALCANA, T. and TIMIRAS, P. S. (1967): Effect of neonatal hypothyroidism and of thyroxine on L-[^{14}C] leucine incorporation in protein in vivo and the relationship to ionic levels in the developing brain of the rat. *Brain Res.* **4**, 143–150.

GÓMEZ, C. J. and RAMIREZ DE GUGLIELMONE, A. E. (1967): Influence of neonatal thyroidectomy on glucose-amino acids interrelations in developing rat cerebral cortex. *J. Neurochem.* **14**, 1119–1128.

HAMBURGH, M (1969): In: *Current Topics in Developmental Biology.* Vol. 4. Ed. by A. A. Moscona and A. Monroy. Academic Press, New York and London. pp. 109–148.

HATOTANI, N. and TIMIRAS, P. S. (1967): Influence of thyroid function on the postnatal development of the transcallosal response in the rat. *Neuroendocrinology* **2**, 147–156.

MÅTENSON, E. (1966): Neutral glycolipids of human kidney: isolation, identification, and fatty acid composition. *Biochim. biophys. Acta (Amst.)* **166**, 296–308.

NOMURA, M., NAGAI, K., MORI, K. and TSUKADA, Y. (1969): Neurochemical studies on the experimental hypothyroidism. *Bull. Jap. Neurochem. Soc.* **8**, 56–59. (In Japanese.)

NORTON, W. T. and AUTILO, L. A. (1965): The chemical composition of bovine CNS myelin. *Ann. N. Y. Acad. Sci.* **122**, 77–85.

NUSSBAUM, J. L., NESKOVIC, N. and MANDEL, P. (1969): A study of lipid components in brain of the "Jimpy" mouse, a mutant with myelin deficiency. *J. Neurochem.* **16**, 927–934.

O'BRIEN, J. S. (1965): Stability of the myelin membrane. *Science* **147**, 1099–1107.

O'BRIEN, J. S. and SAMPSON, E. L. (1965a): Lipid composition of the normal human brain: gray matter, white matter and myelin. *J. Lipid Res.* **6**, 537–544.

O'BRIEN, J. S. and SAMPSON, E. L. (1965b): Fatty acid and fatty aldehyde composition of the major brain lipids in normal human gray matter, white matter and myelin. *J. Lipid Res.* **6,** 545—551.

STÄLLBERG-STENHAGEN, S. and SVENNERHOLM, L. (1965): Fatty acid composition of human brain sphingomyelins: normal variation with age and changes during myelin disorders. *J. Lipid Res.* **6,** 146—155.

TSUJIMURA, R. (1971): Immunological and biochemical studies on myelination in the brain of chick embryo. *J. Embryol. exp. Morph.* (In press.)

UYEMURA, K. (1965): Biochemical studies on subcellular units of guinea-pig brain cortex. *Ad. Neurol. Sci.* **9,** 121—124. (In Japanese.)

WALRAVENS, P. and CHASE, H. P. (1969): Influence of thyroid on formation of myelin lipids. *J. Neurochem.* **16,** 1477—1484.

RNA SYNTHESIS IN EMBRYONIC CEREBELLAR EXPLANTS CULTURED WITH ESTRADIOL*

A. VERNADAKIS

Department of Psychiatry
University of Colorado Medical Center
Denver, Col., U.S.A.

INTRODUCTION

Studies from this laboratory and associate laboratories have shown that steroid hormones play a regulatory role in CNS maturation (Timiras et al. 1968, Vernadakis and Woodbury 1971a, b; Vernadakis 1971a, b).

In an attempt to elucidate some of the mechanisms by which steroid hormones influence brain growth we have used tissue culture techniques. The potential value of tissue culture as a tool to investigate growth patterns as well as cellular interrelationships in several tissues including the brain has become apparent during the last few years.

In our laboratory we are using two types of tissue culture: organotypic and cell cultures which are described in detail elsewhere (Vernadakis 1971b). In previous studies using the organotypic culture technique we have found that in cerebellar explants removed from 16-day-old chick embryos and maintained in culture for 24 hours total RNA content was higher when steroid hormones such as cortisol or estradiol were added to the culture medium (Vernadakis 1971a). To investigate whether this increase in RNA content was a result of increased RNA synthesis, incorporation of ^{3}H-uridine into RNA was studied.

METHODS

ORGANOTYPIC CULTURE PROCEDURE

Cerebellar explants were removed from 16-day-old chick embryos washed in Earle's balanced salt solution (Earle 1943) and oriented on a triangular stainless steel organ culture grid. The molecular surface of the cerebellum rested against the grid. Platforms with explant (1 explant per grid) were placed in organ culture dishes with a center well and an absorbent ring. The medium, 0.5 ml, was added to the center well of the organ culture dish and did not reach the top of the plat-

---

* Supported by a USPHS Research grant MH-15931 and a Research Scientist Development Award MH-42479, from the National Institute of Mental Health.

form. Humidity was maintained by saturating the absorbent ring with distilled water. The culture medium was Eagle's basal medium with Earle's balanced salt solution (Eagle 1955).

Explants were cultured for 30, 60, 90, 150 and 240 min in the presence of ^{3}H-uridine (1 μC; specific activity, 28 C/mM, Schwarz BioResearch) and estradiol dipropionate, 2.65×10^{-5} M, in the medium.

After each incubation period explants were weighed and extracted for nucleic acids according to the method of Schneider (1945) as modified by Geel and Timiras (1967). Determination of RNA from portions of the nucleic acid extract was made according to the orcinol procedure of Ceriotti (1955) as modified by Geel and Timiras (1967). Another portion of the nucleic acid extract was transferred to a vial containing 10 ml of Bray's solution (Bray 1970) and radioactivity was counted by liquid scintillation spectrometry. Results were expressed as cpm/μg of RNA.

RESULTS AND DISCUSSION

Incorporation of ^{3}H-uridine into RNA progressively increased with time in both control and estradiol-treated explants. However, after 90 min in culture incorporation of ^{3}H-uridine was significantly higher in the hormone-treated explants as compared to those cultured in basal medium (Table 1).

TABLE 1

Incorporation of ^{3}H-uridine into RNA of cerebellar explants removed from 16-day-old chick embryos and cultured in estradiol dipropionate

Culture medium	^{3}H-Uridine (cpm/μg RNA)				
	Time (min) of incubation				
	30	60	90	150	240
Eagle's Basal	36 ± 2*	63 ± 5	103 ± 4	157 ± 4	320 ± 41
Estradiol	37 ± 4	76 ± 7	135 ± 10	194 ± 11	426 ± 23
(2.65×10^{-5} M)			($p < 0.01$)**	($p < 0.01$)	($p < 0.05$)

* Mean ± S.E.
** Numbers in parentheses are p values for comparison to basal control.

This increase in RNA synthesis by estradiol may represent both increased cellular activity and increase in cell number, specifically of glial cells. That this increase may represent proliferation of glial cells is indirectly supported by other studies in our laboratory. For example, we have found, using the Maximow double coverslip assembly culture, that some steroid hormones accelerate the migration rate of cells into the neuroglial zone (Vernadakis 1971 b). This is interpreted to reflect proliferation of glial cells since neurons do not proliferate in culture (Murray 1965).

Steroid hormones, e.g., have been shown to increase RNA in the liver (Kenney et al. 1965). Thus, the present data, although still in a preliminary phase, suggest that steroid hormones may also increase RNA synthesis in embryonic neural tissue. In view of the role of RNA in the functional activity of cells, the possibility that steroid hormones may influence RNA synthesis is of importance. Estrogens have been proposed as "organizers" of behavioral activity during critical periods of brain development (Timiras 1971). The present data offer further evidence of this hypothesis.

ACKNOWLEDGEMENT

The able technical assistance of Mrs. Judith Shearer is gratefully acknowledged.

REFERENCES

Bray, G. A. (1970): Determination of radioactivity in aqueous samples. In: *The Current Status of Liquid Scintillation Counting*. Ed. by E. D. Bransome. Grune and Stratton, New York. pp. 171–180.

Eagle, H. (1955): Nutrition needs of mammalian cells in tissue culture. *Science* **122**, 501–504.

Earle, W. R. (1943): Production of malignancy in vitro. IV. The mouse fibroblast cultures and changes seen in living cells. *J. nat. Cancer Inst.* **4**, 165–212.

Geel, S. and Timiras, P. S. (1967): The influences of neonatal hypothyroidism and of thyroxine on the ribonucleic acid and deoxyribonucleic acid concentrations of rat cerebral cortex. *Brain Res.* **4**, 135–142.

Kenney, F. T., Greenman, D. L., Wicks, W. D. and Albritton, W. L. (1965): RNA synthesis and enzyme induction by hydrocortisone. *Adv. Enzyme Reg.* **3**, 1–10.

Murray, M. R. (1965): Nervous tissues *in vitro*. In: *Cells and Tissues in Culture*. Vol. 2. *Methods, Biology and Physiology*. Ed. by E. N. Willmer. Academic Press, New York. pp. 373–455.

Schneider, W. C. (1945): Phosphorus compounds in animal tissues. I. Extractions and estimation of deoxypentose nucleic acid and of pentose nucleic acid. *J. biol. Chem.* **161**, 293–303.

Timiras, P. S. (1971): The role of hormones in the development of seizure activity. In: *Influence of Hormones on the Nervous System*. Proceedings of the first meeting of the International Society of Psychoneuroendocrinology. June 22–25, 1970, Brooklyn, N. Y. Ed. by D. H. Ford. Karger, Basel. (In press.)

Timiras, P. S., Vernadakis, A. and Sherwood, N. (1968): Development and plasticity of the nervous system. In: *Biology of Gestation*. Vol. 2. *The Fetus and Neonate*. Ed. by N. S. Assali. Academic Press, New York. pp. 261–319.

Vernadakis, A. (1971a): Hormonal dependence of embryonic neural tissue in culture. In: *Hormones in Development*. Ed. by M. Hamburgh and E. J. Barrington. Appleton-Century-Crofts, New York. pp. 67–74.

Vernadakis, A. (1971b): Hormonal factors in the proliferation of glial cells in culture. In: *Influence of Hormones on the Nervous System*. Proceedings of the first meeting of the International Society of Psychoneuroendocrinology, June 22–25, 1970, Brooklyn, N. Y. Ed. by D. H. Ford. Karger, Basel. (In press.)

Vernadakis, A. and Woodbury, D. M. (1971a): Influence of cortisol on brain and spinal cord excitability in developing rats. In: *Steroid Hormones and Brain Function*. UCLA Forum in Medical Sciences. (In press.)

Vernadakis, A. and Woodbury, D. M. (1971b): Effects of cortisol on maturation of the central nervous system. In: *Influence of Hormones on the Nervous System*. Proceedings of the first meeting of the International Society of Psychoneuroendocrinology, June 22–25, 1970, Brooklyn, N. Y. Ed. by D. H. Ford. Karger, Basel. (In press.)

INFLUENCE OF CORTICOSTERONE AND ACTH ON THE POSTNATAL DEVELOPMENT OF LEARNING AND MEMORY FUNCTIONS

CS. NYAKAS

Central Research Division
Postgraduate Medical School
Budapest, Hungary

In recent years, on the analogy of the hormonal background of sexual differentiation, attempts have been made to analyse the postnatal influence of adrenocortical hormones on the maturation of the psychoneuroendocrine processes. The influence of adrenocortical hormones as well as ACTH on the central nervous system have widely been studied in adult animals (Cleghorn 1957, Lissák and Endrőczi 1960, de Wied 1966, 1969).

It is well known from the early works in connection with the response of the hypothalamic–pituitary–adrenal axis that there is a relatively stress-nonresponsive period up to the end of the first postnatal week (Jailer 1950, Endrőczi and Tóth 1955, Milkovic and Milkovic 1959, Schapiro et al. 1962, Eguchi and Wells 1965, etc.). In contrast to these findings a stress-responsive period was postulated in the first postnatal five days by other authors (Haltmeyer et al. 1966, Denenberg et al. 1967, Levine 1968). It was assumed by Levine (1970) that endocrine changes occurring in the first postnatal days play a significant role in the early hormonal control of developing neuroendocrine mechanisms. Nevertheless, a handling of infant rats for 20 days proved as a modulating factor for the open field activity and plasma corticosterone response in adulthood (Levine et al. 1967). Taking into consideration that a decreased response of the plasma corticosterone to environmental stimuli in adulthood can be obtained when the animals are handled either before or after the weaning period (Ader 1970), the effect of handling on the later behaviour cannot be entirely regarded as a corticosteroid-mediated action on the maturation of the central nervous system.

From another respect early cortisol treatment was used to investigate the effect of adrenal hormones on the development of the central nervous system (Schapiro 1968). In this experiment 1 mg cortisol was given on the first postnatal day which led to a marked body weight retardation, a decreased activity in the open field box and a delayed development of the cortical neurones, but which did not cause changes in the ether-induced plasma corticosterone response levels.

The aim of the present investigations was to study the effect of corticosterone and ACTH administration given in the early postnatal period on the development of brain and behaviour relationships.

EFFECT OF EARLY POSTNATAL ADMINISTRATION OF CORTICOSTERONE ON PASSIVE AVOIDANCE LEARNING, EXPLORATION AND PITUITARY–ADRENOCORTICAL RESPONSE IN THE PREWEANING PERIOD

Influence of the early postnatal corticosterone administration on the central nervous system was investigated by a single subcutaneous injection of 100, respectively, 300 µg corticosterone dissolved in 15 per cent ethanol in saline on the fourth postnatal day. In the second series of the experiment the rats received 100, respectively, 300 µg corticosterone daily from the third to the fifth postnatal days. The rate of passive avoidance learning was investigated on the 12th and 22nd postnatal days. In the 12-day-old, the conflict situation was produced between the approaching response of the young rats to the mother and the presentation of an electric shock before reaching the mother's compartment. At this age only the filial drive was enough strong to create a conflict situation for studying passive avoidance learning. At the age of 22 days, a 16- to 18-hour food deprivation was necessary to maintain a high intensity of the approaching behaviour and this was conflicted with an electric shock. In both cases passive avoidance learning was studied during a 1,000 sec observation period. Other details of the procedures have been described elsewhere (Nyakas and Endrőczi 1970, 1972). The learning capability of the animals was characterized by the slope of the curves obtained by plotting the consecutive intertrial intervals on the sequence of trials (Dupont et al. 1970, Endrőczi and Nyakas 1972).

The exploratory activity was tested on the 14th and 23rd postnatal days in a 12-cell box of 40×30 cm footing area with 17 gates on the separating walls during a 10-minute period. Scoring was based on the number of gates being crossed, and on the standing-up activity of the animals.

The plasma corticosterone determination was carried out by a slightly modified technique of Givner and Rochefort (1965) on the 15th and 24th postnatal days.

It was found that the administration of 100 µg corticosterone did not change the rate of passive avoidance learning, the exploration and plasma corticosterone level which were tested on the 22nd, 23rd and 24th postnatal days. In contrast to this observation a similar injection of 300 µg corticosterone on the 4th postnatal day resulted in an increase in the exploratory activity and a significant decrease in the plasma corticosterone response level to the exposure of the animals to a new environmental situation for 30 minutes (Fig. 1). It is necessary to remark that neither the lower nor the higher dose of corticosterone failed to produce changes in these parameters between the 12th and 15th postnatal days.

In the other experimental series the infant rats received 100, respectively, 300 µg corticosterone on the 3rd to 5th postnatal days. Testing passive avoidance learning rate, the exploration and plasma corticosterone response level on the 12th to 15th days it was found that administration of 100 µg corticosterone produced a moderate and a 300 µg corticosterone pretreatment a marked decrease in the rate of passive avoidance learning, although it did not change the exploratory activity and the pituitary–adrenocortical function (Fig. 2). At the age of 22 to 24 days the 3-day corticosterone treatment after birth led to a marked suppression of the learning rate and the plasma corticosterone level and to a significant

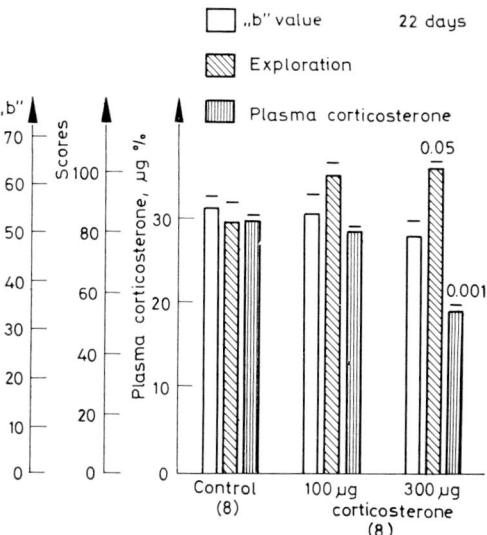

Fig. 1. Effect of a single injection of 100 or 300 µg corticosterone on the passive avoidance learning rate, exploration and plasma corticosterone response level in 22–24-day-old animals

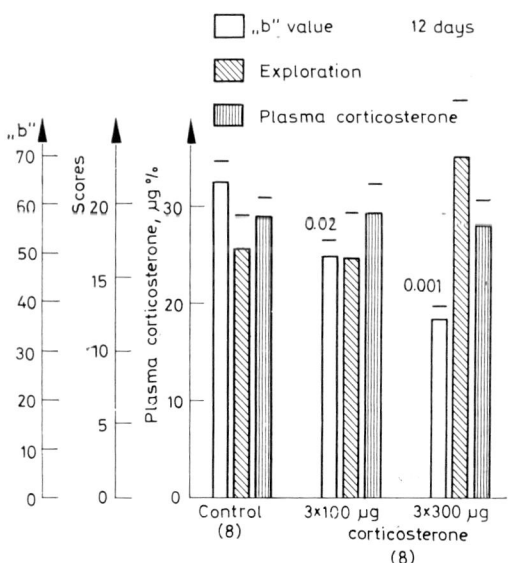

Fig. 2. Effect of administration of 100 or 300 µg corticosterone from the 3rd to 5th postnatal days on the three parameters investigated at 12–15 days of age

increase in the exploratory activity (Fig. 3). It is worth to mention that body weight and the adrenal weight per 100 g body weight did not change in any of the groups pretreated with corticosterone.

With regard to a suppressed pituitary–adrenal response level of the rats receiving corticosterone in the early postnatal period the sensitivity of the adrenal corticosterone production was tested by 0.05 IU ACTH per 100 g administration. Figure 4 shows a decreased responsiveness in the rats with 3×300 μg corti-

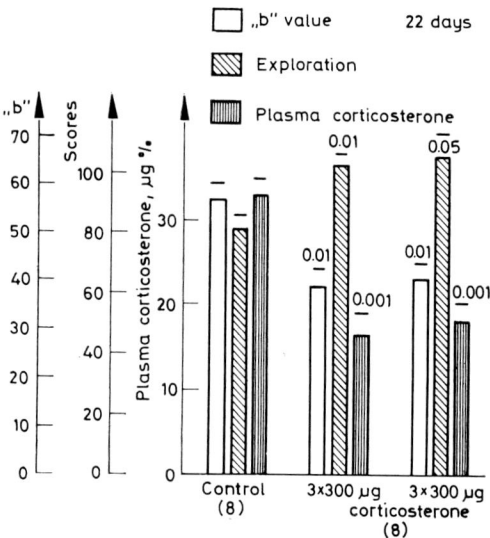

Fig. 3. Effect of administration of 100 or 300 μg corticosterone from the 3rd to 5th postnatal days on the three parameters investigated at the age of 22 to 24 days

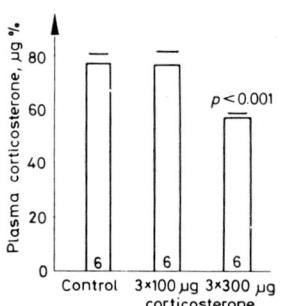

Fig. 4. Effect of administration of 0.05 IU ACTH per 100 g body weight on plasma corticosterone response level in the control and pretreated groups

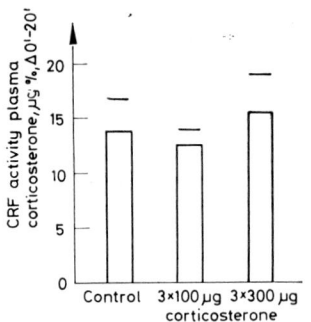

Fig. 5. CRF activity of the control and 3×100 or 3×300 μg corticosterone-pretreated animals

costerone pretreatment in comparison to lower corticosterone treatment or vehicle injection. When studying the mechanism of the altered pituitary–adrenocortical function of corticosterone-pretreated rats the CRF activity of the median eminence extracts, which were obtained at the end of the investigation on the 24th postnatal day, did not show a remarkable difference from the control value (Fig. 5).

EFFECT OF ACTH ON THE POSTNATAL DEVELOPMENT OF THE CENTRAL NERVOUS SYSTEM

In this experiment 2 IU ACTH was injected daily in physiological saline from the 3rd to 5th postnatal days. No effect of ACTH treatment could be observed on the investigated three parameters in the 12- to 15-day-old rats. On the 22nd to 24th postnatal days the rate of passive avoidance learning increased significantly but without a concomitant change in the exploration and the adrenocortical response level after an environmental stress (Fig. 6). It would be too early to draw final conclusions on the effect of ACTH administration on the development of the central nervous system and the infant adrenal cortex, but the results suggest the importance of the ACTH peptide in the maturation of the infant neuroendocrine system.

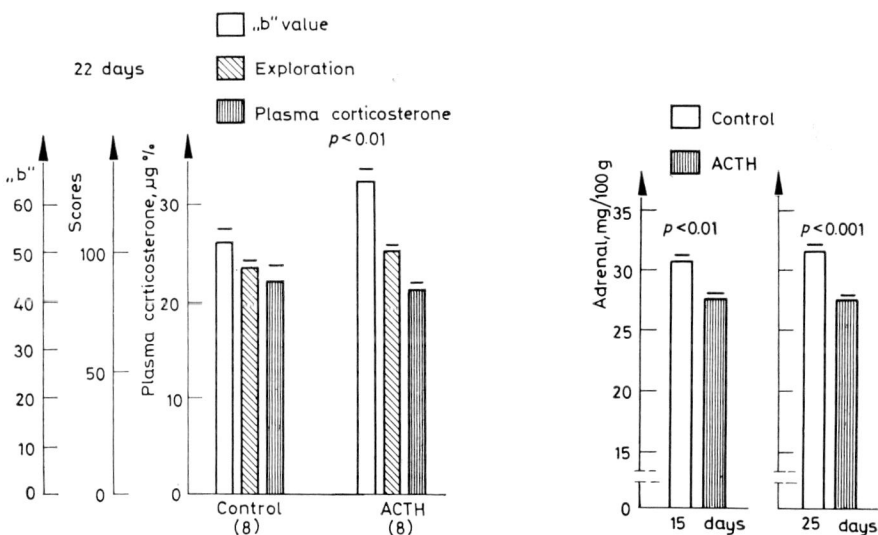

Fig. 6. Effect of 2 IU ACTH administered daily from the 3rd to 5th postnatal days on the rate of passive avoidance learning, exploration and plasma corticosterone response level

CONCLUSION

The present findings indicate that an excess supply of infant rats with adreno cortical hormone during the early postnatal days results in a change of the maturation of brain and behaviour relations. Our behavioural observations have led us to assume that the early administration of corticosterone produces a permanent change in the corticosteroid-adjusted behavioural reactions. The specific binding property of the central nervous system in adult rats is well known and interference of the high corticosterone level with the maturation of this binding site merits some considerations (McEwen et al. 1969, McEwen and Weiss 1970).

An inverse correlation between the plasma corticosterone level and the exploratory activity, on the one hand, and a linear relationship of the plasma corticosterone response level and passive avoidance learning rates, on the other, have been demonstrated in adult rats (Endrőczi 1970, Dupont et al. 1971, Endrőczi and Nyakas 1972). It seems that early corticosterone administration produces a functional damage of the neuroanatomical substrate necessary for the integration of corticosterone-sensitive behavioural reactions. This assumption seems to be confirmed by an increased exploration and a decreased rate of passive avoidance learning. However, a decreased plasma corticosterone response level to environmental stimuli may also explain the deficit in passive avoidance learning and the higher exploratory activity of the corticosterone-pretreated animals.

REFERENCES

ADER, R. (1970): The effect of early experience on the adrenocortical response to different magnitudes of stimulation. *Physiol. Behav.* **5**, 837–839.

CLEGHORN, R. A. (1957): Steroid hormones in relation to neuropsychiatric disorders. In: *Hormones. Brain Function, and Behavior*. Ed. by H. Hoagland. Academic Press, New York. pp. 3–19.

DENENBERG, V. H., BRUMAGHIM, J. T., HALTMEYER, G. C. and ZARROW, M. X. (1967): Increased adrenocortical activity in the neonatal rat following handling. *Endocrinology* **81**, 1047–1052.

DUPONT, A., ENDRŐCZI, E. and FORTIER, C. (1970): Relationships of pituitary–thyroid and pituitary–adrenocortical activities to conditioned behaviour in the rat. In: *Influence of Hormones on the Nervous System*. Ed. by D. H. Ford. Karger, Basel and New York.

EGUCHI, Y. and WELLS, L. (1965): Response of the hypothalamic–hypophyseal adrenal axis to stress: observation in fetal and caesarean newborn rats. *Proc. Soc. exp. Biol. (N. Y.)* **120**, 675–678.

ENDRŐCZI, E. (1970): Pituitary–adrenocortical activity, exploration and avoidance behaviour in the rat. UCLA Workshop Conference, Los Angeles. Ed. by C. H. Sawyer and R. Gorski. Univ. Calif. Press. (In press.)

ENDRŐCZI, E. and TÓTH, K. (1955): Analytical studies on the ontogenetical development of humoral adaptation. *Acta physiol. Acad. Sci. hung.* **8**, 33–42.

ENDRŐCZI, E. and NYAKAS, C. (1972): Correlation of pituitary–adrenal function to exploratory activity and passive avoidance learning in the rat. *Acta physiol. Acad. Sci. hung.* (In press.)

GIVNER, M. and ROCHEFORT, J. (1965): An improved assay of corticosterone in rat serum and adrenal tissue. *Steroids* **6**, 486–489.

HALTMEYER, G. C., DENENBERG, V. H., THATCHER, J. and ZARROW, M. X. (1966): Response of the adrenal cortex of the neonatal rat after subjection to stress. *Nature (Lond.)* **212**, 1371–1373.

JAILER, J. W. (1950): The maturation of the pituitary–adrenal axis in the newborn rat. *Endocrinology* **46**, 420–425.

Levine, S. (1968): Influence of infantile stimulation on the response to stress during preweaning development. *Developmental Psychobiology* **1**, 67–70.

Levine, S. (1970): The pituitary–adrenal system and the developing brain. In: *Progress in Brain Research*. Vol. 32. Ed. by D. de Wied and J. A. W. M. Weijnen. Elsevier, Amsterdam. pp. 79–85.

Levine, S., Haltmeyer, G. C., Karas, G. G. and Denenberg, V. H. (1967): Physiological and behavioral effects of infantile stimulation. *Physiol. Behav.* **2**, 55–59.

Lissák, K. and Endrőczi, E. (1960): *Die neuroendokrine Steuerung der Adaptationstätigkeit*. Akadémiai Kiadó, Budapest.

McEwen, B. S. and Weiss, J. M. (1970): The uptake and action of corticosterone: regional and subcellular studies on rat brain. In: *Progress in Brain Research*. Vol. 32. Ed. by D. de Wied and J. A. W. M. Weijnen. Elsevier, Amsterdam. pp. 200–212.

McEwen, B. S., Weiss, J. M. and Schwartz, L. (1969): Uptake of corticosterone by rat brain and its concentration by certain limbic structures. *Brain Res.* **16**, 227–241.

Milkovic, K. and Milkovic, S. (1959): Reactiveness of the pituitary–adrenal system of the first postnatal period in some laboratory mammals. *Endokrinologie* **37**, 301–310.

Nyakas, C. and Endrőczi, E. (1970): Olfaction guided approaching behaviour of infantile rats to the mother in maze box. *Acta physiol. Acad. Sci. hung.* **38**, 59–65.

Nyakas, C. and Endrőczi, E. (1972): Passive avoidance learning and memory as a function of age and food deprivation in young rats. *Acta physiol. Acad. Sci. hung.* (In press.)

Schapiro, S. (1968): Some physiological, biochemical, and behavioral consequences of neonatal hormone administration: cortisol and thyroxine. *Gen. comp. Endocr.* **10**, 214–228.

Schapiro, S., Geller, E. and Eiduson, S. (1962): Neonatal adrenal cortical response to stress and vasopressin. *Proc. Soc. exp. Biol. (N. Y.)* **109**, 937–941.

Wied, D. de (1966): Inhibitory effect of ACTH and related peptides on extinction of conditioned behavior in rats. *Proc. Soc. exp. Biol. (N.Y.)* **122**, 28–32.

Wied, D. de (1969): Effect of peptide hormones on behavior. In: *Frontiers in Neuroendocrinology*. Ed. by W. F. Ganong and L. Martini. Oxford University Press, New York. pp. 97–140.

SECTION II

CONTROL, BIOSYNTHESIS AND RELEASE OF PITUITARY HORMONES

Chairman: C. FORTIER

INTERRELATIONSHIPS IN THE CONTROL OF ACTH AND TSH SECRETION*

C. FORTIER

Department of Physiology
Medical Faculty of Laval University
Quebec, Canada

The possibility of an inverse relationship between ACTH and TSH secretion was suggested by the inhibition of TSH secretion observed concurrently with enhanced release of ACTH as a result of non-specific stress.

This stress-induced inhibition of TSH secretion, first postulated on the basis of depressed thyroid activity by Bogoroch and Timiras in 1951 and by Brown-Grant et al. in 1954, was later confirmed in our laboratory by Kraicer et al. (1965) who showed that, 15 minutes after exposure to stress (surgical trauma), a sharp fall in plasma TSH coincided with maximal ACTH stimulation, in both intact and adrenalectomized rats.

The shift from TSH to ACTH secretion elicited by stress could conceivably be ordered by a center exerting opposite influences on the hypothalamic areas independently involved in the control of TRF and of CRF release. It could result, alternatively, from a competition between CRF and TRF, at the hypothalamic level, so that enhanced release of one principle would necessarily depress the release of the other. A third possibility could involve a competition of a similar type, at the pituitary level, between ACTH and TSH secretion; the two processes being inversely related, so that stimulation or inhibition of one would have the opposite effect on the other.

The third alternative, implying a competition between ACTH and TSH for a common precursor or cofactor, at the pituitary level, though difficult to reconcile with prevalent views on the specificity of the cellular sites of ACTH and of TSH secretion, was supported by reports on the allegedly opposite effects of non-specific stress and of pharmacological blockade of ACTH release on the plasma TSH responses to cold exposure (Ducommun et al. 1966) and to TRF (Sakiz and Guillemin 1965). The findings to be presently outlined are inconsistent with this viewpoint and indicate, furthermore, that the dorsal hippocampus exerts opposite influences on TSH and ACTH secretion and may be involved, in association with other components of the limbic system, in the stress-induced shift of these secretory activities.

I am deeply indebted to the many investigators who have pursued, in my laboratory, the studies which I shall review.

* Supported by grants (MT-1205 and 1555) from the Medical Research Council of Canada.

EVIDENCE AGAINST A COMPETITION BETWEEN CRF AND TRF OR BETWEEN ACTH AND TSH

1. *Prolonged enhancement or depression of ACTH secretion fails to alter the TSH secretion rate* (Delgado, in prep., Delgado et al. 1970, Fortier et al. 1970). Rats were either adrenalectomized or subjected to twice-daily injections of corticosterone; procedures were found to result respectively in enhancement or depression of

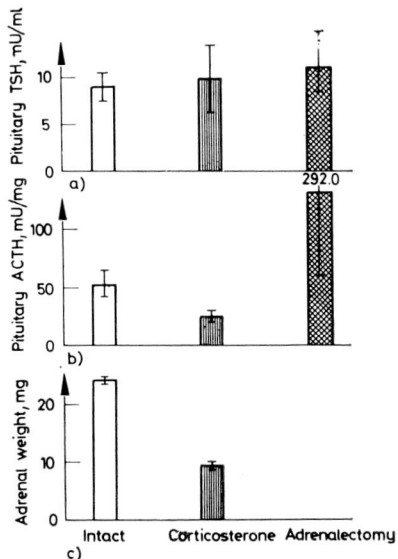

Fig. 1. Comparative effects of corticosterone administration (1.35 mg/100 g b.w. in two daily s.c. injections for 14 days) and of bilateral adrenalectomy (30 days prior to killing) on pituitary TSH (a), pituitary ACTH (b) and adrenal weight (c) in the adult male rat. The columns and T-shaped bars correspond to the weighed means and 95% confidence limits from four assays for TSH and three assays for ACTH, and to the means and standard errors of eight determinations of adrenal weight

ACTH secretion, reflected by a 250 per cent increase of the pituitary ACTH concentration four weeks after bilateral adrenalectomy, and by a 50 per cent decrease of this parameter after two weeks of corticosterone administration (Fig. 1).

A comparative study of the disappearance characteristics of exogenous TSH in intact, adrenalectomized and corticosterone-treated animals revealed that, in spite of significant alterations of the metabolic clearance rate which was depressed by adrenalectomy and increased by corticosterone administration, the TSH secretion rates were nearly identical in the three groups (Fig. 2). This clearly suggests that ACTH and TSH are secreted independently.

2. *Exposure to cold concurrently enhances ACTH and TSH secretion* (Delgado, in press, Fortier et al. 1970, Jobin 1971). Figure 3 illustrates the inversely related plasma TSH response patterns elicited by cold (exposure to $-5°C$ for 20 minutes) and by a faradic stimulus (applied for 2 minutes), in spite of nearly superimpos-

able plasma corticosterone responses to the two stimuli. The simultaneous stimulation of ACTH and of TSH secretion by cold is difficult to reconcile with a competition between the two hormones or between CRF and TRF.

3. *Prolonged enhancement of ACTH secretion fails to alter the plasma TSH response to thyroidectomy and to acute exposure to cold* (Fortier et al. 1970, Jobin 1971).

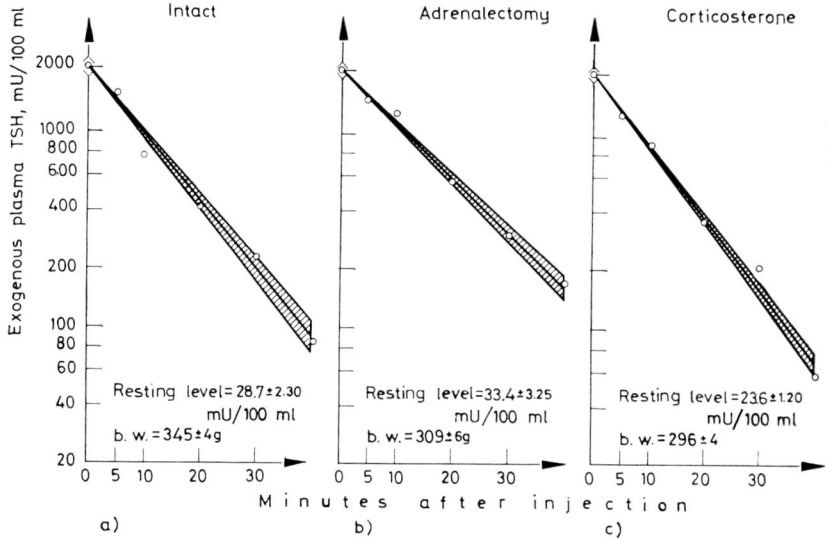

Fig. 2. Comparison of the plasma disappearance characteristics. $T^1/_2$ = half-life; V = virtual volume of distribution; MCR = metabolic clearance rate; SR = secretion rate of "exogenous" TSH in intact, bilaterally adrenalectomized (30 days prior to killing) and corticosterone-treated (1.25 mg/100 g b.w. in two daily s.c. injections for 14 days) adult male rats. The plasma TSH concentrations (weighed means of six independent potency estimates of the pooled samples of ten rats, for each time interval) recorded after the intravenous injection of 157 mU of TSH and of its vehicle and respectively corresponding to total and to endogenous levels provide the basis for evaluation of the disappearance characteristics of the "exogenous" hormone by "regression" and the "trapezoid" rule, as outlined by Normand and Fortier (1970). Whereas the metabolic clearance rate (MCR) is yielded by the two techniques, determination of the half-life ($T^1/_2$) and volume of distribution (V) is restricted to regression. The secretion rate (SR) corresponds to the product of the MCR and the TSH concentration recorded at "zero" time. The shaded areas and double-pointed arrows respectively correspond to the standard errors for the slopes and for their origins on the "y" axis

Adrenalectomy, by resulting, after four weeks, in markedly increased ACTH secretion, did not depress the plasma TSH rise induced by concurrent thyroidectomy or by a short (40 minutes) exposure to cold (Fig. 4).

4. *Pharmacological blockade of ACTH secretion fails to enhance the plasma TSH response to cold and does not prevent the plasma TSH fall induced by non-specific stress* (Delgado, in prep., Delgado et al. 1970, Fortier et al. 1970).

As shown in Fig. 5, complete blockade of ACTH secretion through pretreatment with dexamethasone (0.5 mg subcutaneously, five hours before killing) depressed

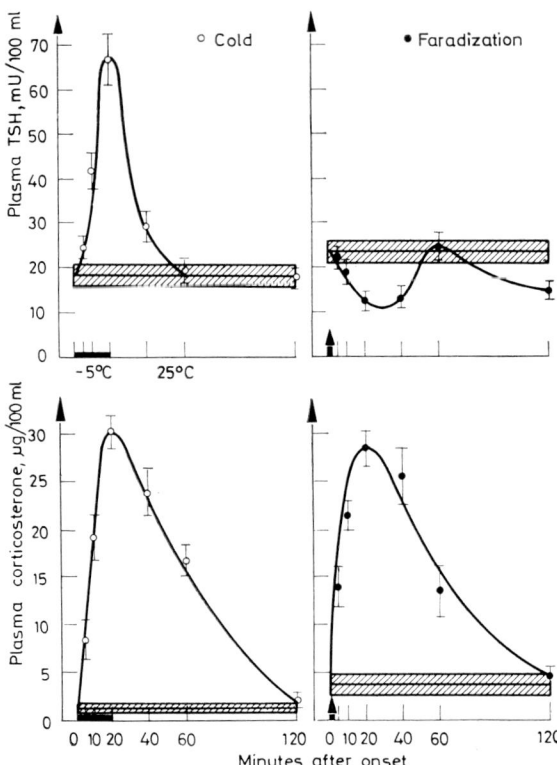

Fig. 3. Comparative time-response patterns of plasma TSH and corticosterone to cold exposure (20 min at —5°C) and to faradization (exposure for 150 seconds to alternating 30-second periods of faradic stimulation, through a grid floor). The dots and T-shaped bars, as well as the baselines and their parallel stippled areas, correspond to the weighed means and standard errors from four to five assays for TSH, and to the means and standard errors of eight individual determinations for corticosterone. The baselines represent the mean values of samples collected immediately before the onset of stimulation

the resting plasma TSH level and failed to alter the inversely related plasma TSH responses to cold (30 minutes at 5°C) and to faradic stimulation (2 minutes). It appears likely that the enhancement of the TSH response to cold, ascribed by Ducommun et al. (1966) to blockade of endogenous ACTH secretion, was in fact related to the utilization by these authors of pentobarbital in association with dexamethasone. Barbiturate anesthesia could enhance the TSH response to cold through suppression of a TSH-inhibitory "anxiety component" of this stimulus.

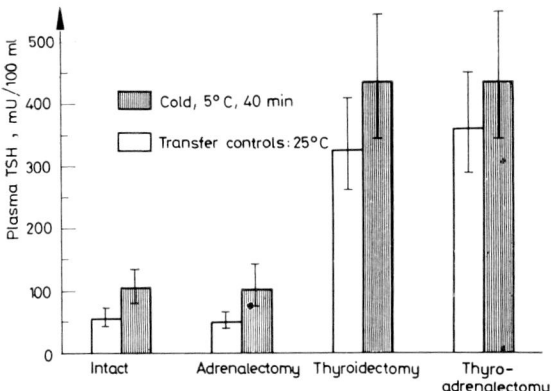

Fig. 4. Effects of adrenalectomy, thyroidectomy, and thyroadrenalectomy (performed one month previously) on the plasma TSH response to cold. Columns and T-shaped bars correspond to the weighed means and 95% confidence limits from six to seven assays

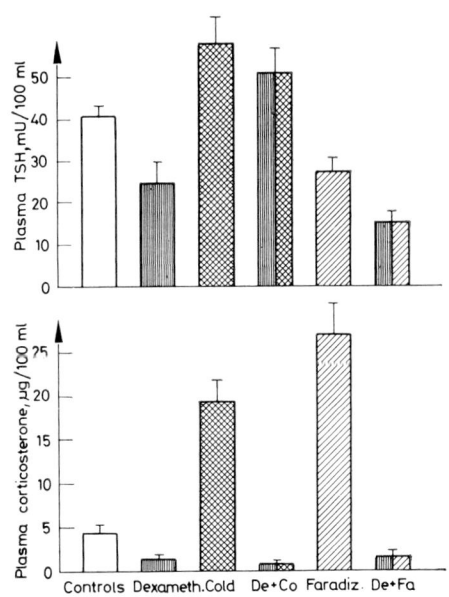

Fig. 5. Effect of dexamethasone pretreatment (0.5 mg, s.c., five hours prior to killing) on the plasma TSH and corticosterone responses to cold (30 min at 5°C) and to faradization (150 sec; sacrifice 15 minutes after onset), in the adult male rat. In this graph, as in Figs 6, 7 and 10, the columns and T-shaped bars correspond to the means and standard errors of four to five assays for TSH and of eight individual determinations for corticosterone

SPECIFIC EVIDENCE AGAINST A COMPETITION BETWEEN ACTH AND TSH AT THE PITUITARY LEVEL

1. *Pharmacological blockade of ACTH secretion fails to enhance the plasma TSH response to synthetic TRF* (Koch, Jobin, Dulac and Fortier, unpublished observations). In contradistinction with the alleged enhancement of the plasma TSH response to TRF through blockade of endogenous ACTH secretion (Sakiz and Guillemin 1965), pretreatment of rats with dexamethasone (0.5 mg, subcutaneously, five

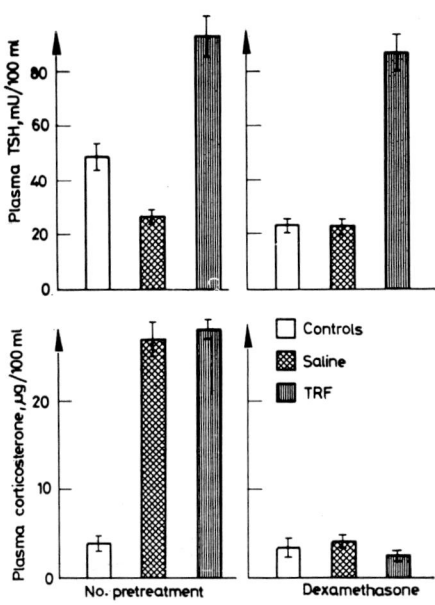

Fig. 6. Effect of dexamethasone pretreatment (0.5 mg, s.c., five hours prior to killing) on the plasma TSH and corticosterone responses of adult male rats to saline and to synthetic TRF (200 mµg) injected intravenously under ether anesthesia. The animals were killed 10 minutes after the injection

hours before killing), though completely suppressing the rise in plasma corticosterone associated with the intravenous injection of either saline or synthetic TRF (Abbott laboratories; 200 mµg) under ether anesthesia, failed to alter the plasma TSH response to TRF recorded 10 minutes after the injection (Fig. 6).

In connection with the claim of Sakiz and Guillemin (1965) that "When the pituitary is induced to secrete TSH by TRF, it concomitantly secretes less ACTH in response to stress", it is interesting to note that the plasma corticosterone response to the combined stress of ether anesthesia and intravenous injection was of the same order in the animals injected with TRF as in the saline-injected controls.

The hypothesis of a competition between ACTH and TSH, at the pituitary level, did not fare better in an analogous experiment in which ACTH secretion was strongly stimulated by the combined stress of intravenous injection and ether, slightly enhanced by an intravenous injection under nembutal anesthesia or completely blocked by pretreatment with chlorpromazine, morphine and pentobarbital, as prescribed by Arimura et al. (1967). In spite of these different levels of ACTH secretion, no significant difference was observed in the plasma TSH responses to TRF (Fig. 7). No difference was observed either in the plasma corticosterone response to stress of the animals in which TSH secretion was depressed by stress or enhanced by TRF.

2. *The TRF-induced enhancement of TSH release from the incubated anterior pituitary is not accompanied by depressed release of ACTH* (Koch, Jobin, Dulac and

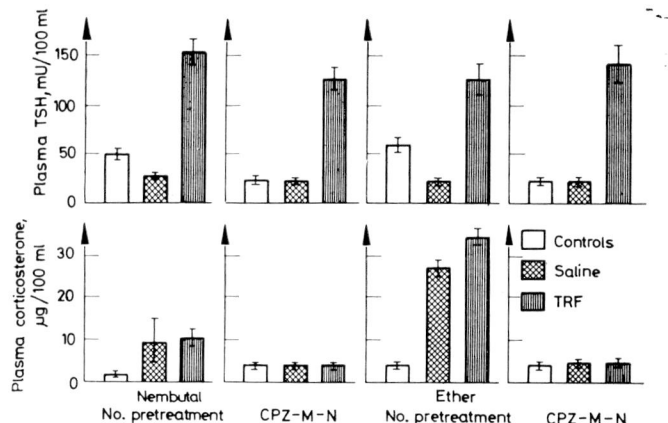

Fig. 7. Effect of pretreatment with chlorpromazine, morphine and nembutal (CPZ-M-N), according to the procedure of Arimura et al. (1967), on the plasma TSH and corticosterone responses of adult male rats to the intravenous injection of saline and of synthetic TRF (200 mμg). The effects of nembutal and of ether anesthesia are compared in the non-pretreated groups of two independent experiments

Fortier, unpublished observations). Sets of rat hemi-pituitaries, preincubated in KRBG for 30 minutes, were incubated with or without graded amounts of synthetic TRF (Abbott laboratories) for a further period of one hour at the end of which the TSH and ACTH concentrations of the media were determined. The hormonal secretion of the stimulated sets was expressed in percentage of the secretion of their non-stimulated controls. Though TRF enhanced the release of TSH from the incubated glands, no concomitant depression of ACTH release was observed (Fig. 8). This finding further supports our conclusion that the secretion of ACTH and of TSH are independent processes.

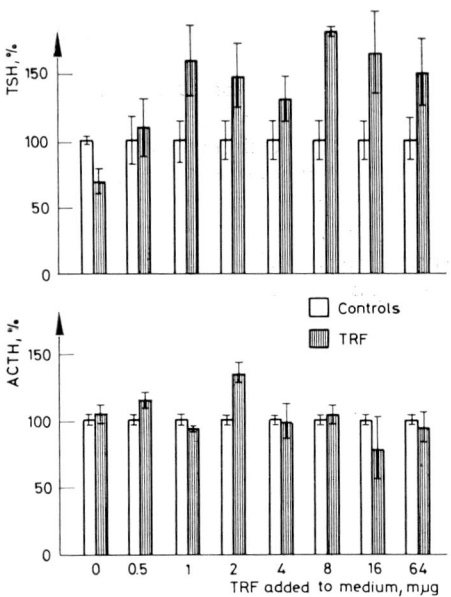

Fig. 8. Effect of graded amounts of synthetic TRF on the in vitro release of TSH and of ACTH by incubated rat hemi-pituitaries. Matching sets of three hemi-pituitaries were used in the control and experimental beakers. The columns and T-shaped bars correspond to the weighed means and standard errors of the assays

OPPOSITE INFLUENCE OF THE HIPPOCAMPUS ON ACTH AND TSH SECRETION

Electrical stimulation of the dorsal hippocampus prevents the inhibition of the plasma TSH response to cold and the rise of plasma corticosterone induced by non-specific stress (Dupont et al. 1971). It may be inferred from the foregoing that neither an inverse relationship between CRF and TRF release from the hypothalamus nor a competition between ACTH and TSH at the pituitary level can account for the stress-induced shift from TSH to ACTH secretion. Hence the interest of a recent study by our group which suggests the possible involvement therein of the hippocampus, a structure whose inhibitory influence upon the pituitary–adrenocortical system is well documented (Endrőczi and Lissák 1962, Kawakami et al. 1968, Moberg et al. 1971).

Seven days after the stereotaxic implantation of bipolar electrodes in the dorsal hippocampus, according to coordinates borrowed from de Groot's atlas (Fig. 9), adult male rats were respectively subjected, with the exception of a group of absolute controls, to minor forms of non-specific stress (presence of an observer or nicking of the tail), exposure to cold ($-5°C$ for 20 minutes) associated or not with a minor stress (presence of an observer) and stimulation of the hippocampus (with a current of 1.3–1.5 V, 10 cps and 0.1 msec pulse duration) either paired with a minor stress (nicking of the tail) or with the association of cold exposure and a minor stress.

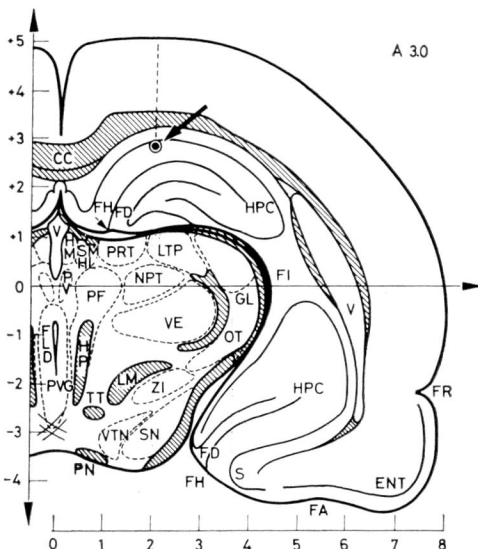

Fig. 9. The effective site of stimulation in the gyrus dentatus of the hippocampal formation is indicated by a concentric circle; the electrode tract, by interrupted line.
After de Groot (1959)

As shown in Fig. 10, the sheer presence of an observer in the experimental room induced a slight rise of the plasma corticosterone level without affecting the plasma TSH concentration. Nicking of the tail elicited a greater rise of plasma corticosterone without affecting plasma TSH. Exposure to cold, in the absence of additional disturbance, resulted in concomitant rises of the plasma TSH and corticosterone concentrations. When cold was associated, however, with such a minor disturbance as the presence of an observer in the experimental room, no plasma TSH rise was recorded, whereas the rise in plasma corticosterone was higher than in the animals exposed to cold alone. Stimulation of the hippocampus resulted in nearly complete suppression of the plasma corticosterone response to minor stress, but had no effect on the plasma TSH level. When the hippocampus was stimulated, on the other hand, concomitantly with exposure to cold and minor stress, the plasma TSH response to cold, otherwise suppressed by the associated disturbance, was fully restored, whereas the plasma corticosterone response to the combined stimuli (cold + minor stress) was almost completely prevented.

These findings confirm in the rat the observation by other groups (Endrőczi and Lissák 1962, Kawakami et al. 1968) that stimulation of the hippocampus inhibits the pituitary–adrenocortical response to stress in cats and rabbits. They suggest, furthermore, that the concurrent enhancement of ACTH release and inhibition of TSH secretion induced by non-specific stress are possibly related to depressed hippocampal activity and underline the interest of a systemic reassessment of the role of the hippocampus and of other components of the limbic system in the control of ACTH and TSH secretion.

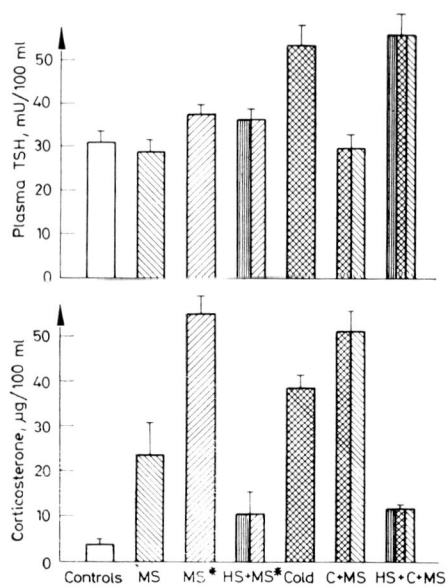

Fig. 10. Plasma TSH and corticosterone responses to the presence of an observer in the experimental rooms (MS), nicking of the tail (MS*) in association or not with electrical stimulation of the dorsal hippocampus (HS) and exposure to cold (20 min at —5°C) associated or not with the presence of an observer and with or without concomitant stimulation of the hippocampus. The animals (adult male rats) were killed 20 min after the onset of these procedures. Note that hippocampal stimulation resulted in nearly complete suppression of the plasma corticosterone rise elicited by nicking of the tail or by exposure to cold in the presence of an observer and fully restored the plasma TSH response to cold, otherwise prevented by the associated disturbance

ACKNOWLEDGEMENT

The synthetic TRF utilized in this investigation was generously supplied by Abbott Laboratories (Scientific Divisions), through the courtesy of Drs Wilfrid F. White and Michael S. Anderson.

REFERENCES

Arimura, A., Saito, T. and Schally, A. V. (1967): Assays for corticotropin-releasing factor (CRF) using rats treated with morphine, chlorpromazine, dexamethasone and nembutal. *Endocrinology* **81**, 235—245.

Bogoroch, R. and Timiras, P. (1951): The response of the thyroid gland of the rat to severe stress. *Endocrinology* **49**, 548—556.

Brown-Grant, K., Harris G. W. and Reichlin, S. (1954): The effect of emotional and physical stress on thyroid activity in the rabbit. *J. Physiol.* **126**, 29—40.

De Groot, J. (1959): The rat forebrain in stereotaxic coordinates. *Trans. Roy. Neth. Acad. Sci.* **52**, 1—40.

Delgado, A.: Relations entre la sécrétion d'ACTH et de TSH par l'adénohypophyse. Thèse de doctorat ès sciences, Université Laval, Québec. (In preparation).

Delgado, A., Marceau, H. and Fortier, C. (1970): Absence of interrelationship between ACTH and TSH secretion. *Fed. Proc.* **29,** 509.

Ducommun, P., Sakiz, E. and Guillemin, R. (1966): Dissociation of the acute secretions of thyrotropin and adrenocorticotropin. *Amer. J. Physiol.* **210,** 1257—1259.

Dupont, A., Bastarache, E., Endrőczi, E. and Fortier, C. (1971): Effect of hippocampal stimulation on the plasma TSH and corticosterone responses to acute exposure to cold in the rat. In: *Proc. XXVth International Congress of Physiological Sciences*, Munich.

Endrőczi, E. and Lissák, K. (1962): Interrelations between paleocortical activity and pituitary–adrenocortical function. *Acta physiol. Acad. Sci. hung.* **21,** 257—263.

Fortier, C., Delgado, A., Ducommun, P., Ducommun, S., Dupont, A., Jobin, M., Kraicer, J., MacIntosh-Hardt, B., Marceau, H., Mialhe, P., Mialhe-Voloss, C., Rerup, C. and Van Rees, G. P. (1970): Functional interrelationships between the adenohypophysis, thyroid, adrenal cortex and gonads. *Canad. med. Ass. J.* **103,** 864—874.

Jobin, M. (1971): Interrelations hypophyso-thyroido-surrénaliennes au cours de l'exposition au froid. Thèse de doctorat ès sciences, Université Laval, Québec.

Jobin, M. and Fortier, C. (1965): Pituitary-thyroid-adrenocortical interactions during cold exposure in the rat. *Fed. Proc.* **24,** 149.

Kawakami, M., Seto, K., Terasawa, E., Yoshida, K., Miyamoto, T., Sekiguchi, M. and Hattori, Y. (1968): Influence of electrical stimulation and lesion in limbic structure upon biosynthesis of adrenocorticoid in the rabbit. *Neuroendocrinology* **3,** 337—348.

Kraicer, J., Ducommun, P., Jobin, M., Rerup, C., Van Rees, G. P. and Fortier, C. (1965): Pituitary and plasma TSH response to stress in the intact and adrenalectomized rat. *Fed. Proc.* **22,** 507.

Moberg, G. P., Scapagnini, U., De Groot, J. and Ganong, W. F. (1971): Effect of sectioning the fornix on diurnal fluctuation in plasma corticosterone levels in the rat. *Neuroendocrinology* **7,** 11—15.

Normand, M. and Fortier, C. (1970): Numerical versus analytical integration of hormonal disappearance data. *Can. J. Physiol. Pharmacol.* **48,** 274—281.

Sakiz, E. and Guillemin, R. (1965): Inverse effects of purified hypothalamic TRF on the acute secretion of TSH and ACTH. *Endocrinology* **77,** 797—801.

RELATIONSHIP OF ACTIVE AVOIDANCE LEARNING TO THE PITUITARY–THYROID AND PITUITARY–ADRENOCORTICAL RESPONSES TO COLD EXPOSURE IN THE RAT*

A. DUPONT, E. BASTARACHE, I. BERNATCHEZ-LEMAIRE, E. ENDRŐCZI**
and C. FORTIER

Laboratories of Endocrinology
Department of Physiology
Medical Faculty of Laval University
Quebec, Canada

As shown by previous findings, enhanced ACTH release and depressed TSH secretion are useful parameters of emotional disturbances, such as fear or anxiety. A positive correlation was observed between passive avoidance learning and the plasma corticosterone concentration, used as an index of ACTH release (Dupont et al. 1971b). Contrariwise, active avoidance learning proved inversely related to the plasma corticosterone level and positively related to the plasma TSH concentration (Dupont et al. 1971 a, b). From the opposite correlations recorded between these endocrine parameters and the two forms of avoidance learning, it was inferred that "fear tension", which is reflected by the endocrine responses, plays opposite roles in the two situations. Passive avoidance learning would represent the inhibition by shock-induced fear of the goal-directed motor activity. Active avoidance learning, by contrast, requires the initiation of a goal-directed motor response which would be inhibited by the fear tension.

As opposed to other environmental stimuli which simultaneously enhance ACTH release and depress TSH secretion, exposure to cold concurrently stimulates the secretion of the two tropic hormones (Fortier et al. 1970, Jobin 1971). On the other hand, fear or anxiety was shown by our group to depress the plasma TSH response to cold, while enhancing the plasma corticosterone response to this stimulus (Fortier 1972, Fortier et al. 1970). It therefore appeared of interest, in order to test our hypothesis of an inverse relationship between anxiety and active avoidance learning ability, to relate the latter to the endocrine response to cold exposure.

MATERIALS AND METHODS

Active avoidance learning was developed in male adult rats by repeated associations of a conditional signal with an unconditional stimulus, in a two-way shuttle box. Beeps of 10 cps and 5 sec duration, used as conditional signals, were immediately followed by short (1 sec) electric shocks (unconditional stimuli) repeated

---

* Supported by grants (MT-1205 and 1555) from the Medical Research Council of Canada.
** Present adress: Central Research Division, Postgraduate Medical School, Budapest, Hungary.

at 1–2 sec intervals until the animal escaped from the electrified to the "safe" compartment. The daily sessions, repeated over a 10-day period, involved 10 successive associations at 1 min intervals. On the 11th day, the animals were presented with the conditional signal alone repeated 10 times at 1 min intervals and their CR (for conditioned response) performance was assessed in terms of the number of conditioned responses (escapes into the "safe" compartment elicited by the conditional signal) recorded during this test session.

Five days later, the animals were exposed to a temperature of −5°C for 20 min, at the end of which they were killed for determination of plasma TSH by McKenzie's (1958) technique and of plasma corticosterone by the competitive protein binding method of Murphy (1967). Non-tested controls were also killed, for comparison, before and after exposure to cold.

RESULTS AND CONCLUSION

To facilitate the interpretation of the results obtained in this experiment, it may be useful to recall the previously observed relationship between the CR performance and the plasma TSH and corticosterone concentrations determined 10 min after the test session.

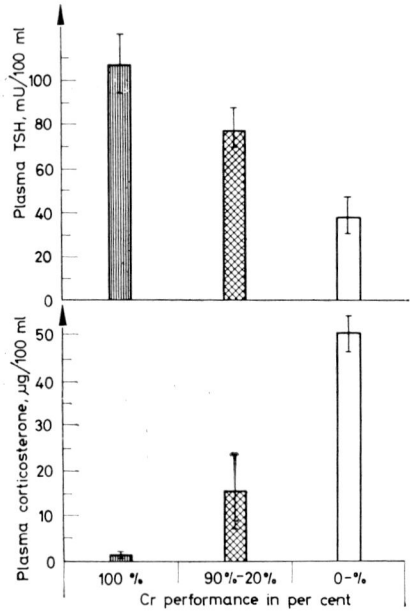

Fig. 1. Relationship between the plasma TSH and corticosterone concentrations (determined 10 min after the test session for active avoidance learning) and the CR (conditioned response) performance (as defined in the text) in adult male rats. Corticosterone was determined in individual samples; TSH, in pooled samples of the individuals grouped according to learning performance. Columns and T-shaped bars correspond to means and standard errors (weighed means ± S.E. of three independent assays for TSH). From Dupont et al. 1971b

As shown in Fig. 1, the plasma TSH and corticosterone concentrations evidenced opposite relationships to the CR performance, high TSH and low corticosterone levels being associated with optimal performance, while low TSH and elevated corticosterone, with poor performance.

Figure 2 illustrates the relationship between the CR performance and the endocrine response to cold exposure, ascertained 5 days after the test session for active avoidance learning.

The plasma TSH and corticosterone responses to cold of the non-tested control population are represented in this graph by the distance between two horizontal bars, respectively, corresponding to the baseline and to the postexposure level. The latter was the only value obtained in the pretested animals, which have been grouped according to their learning performance.

Only one animal out of twenty had a score of 100 per cent, three had scores ranging from 20 to 40 per cent and the remainder failed to perform a single conditioned response (0 per cent).

In agreement with our hypothesis, the best student evidenced the highest TSH and the lowest corticosterone response to cold, inversely related responses

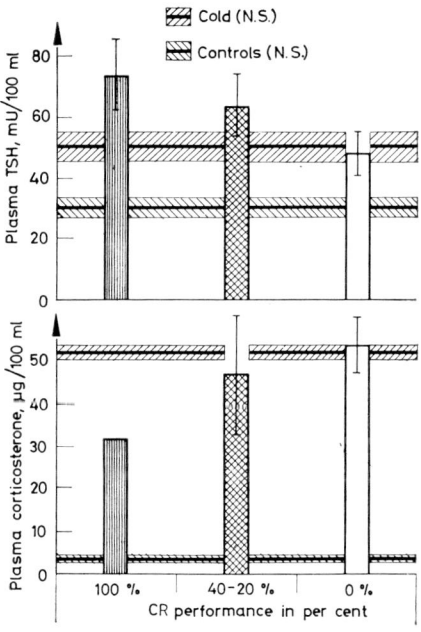

Fig. 2. Relationship between the plasma TSH and corticosterone responses to cold exposure (20 min at —5 °C) and the CR performance in adult male rats. The columns and T-shaped bars correspond to the means and standard errors of the values recorded after exposure to cold in the tested animals; the horizontal lines and parallel hatched areas, to the means and standard errors of the values recorded before and after exposure to cold in the non-tested (N.S.) population. Corticosterone was determined in individual samples; TSH, in pooled samples of the individuals grouped according to learning performance, with the exception of the sample corresponding to the single subject with a 100% score

were recorded for the drop-outs and an intermediate pattern, for the remainder of the class.

Though, in view of the limited population and skewed performance distribution, no definitive conclusion can be drawn from this experiment, our findings tend to support the postulated inverse relationship between anxiety and active avoidance learning ability and illustrate, moreover, the possible contribution of endocrinology to the interpretation of behavioural reactions.

REFERENCES

Dupont, A., Bastarache, E., Bernatchez, I., Endrőczi, E. and Fortier, C. (1971a): Endocrine correlates of conditioned behaviour in the rat. *Proc. Can. Fed. Biol. Soc.* **14**, 112.

Dupont, A., Endrőczi, E. and Fortier, C. (1971b): Relationship of pituitary–thyroid and pituitary–adrenocortical activities to conditioned behaviour in the rat. In: *The Influence of Hormones on the Nervous System*. Proceedings of the first meeting of the International Society of Psychoneuroendocrinology. Ed. by D. H. Ford. Karger, Basel. (In press.)

Fortier, C. (1972): Interrelationships in the control of ACTH and TSH secretion. In: *Hormones and Brain Function*. Proceedings of the Second Congress of the International Society of Psychoneuroendocrinology. Budapest, 1971. Ed. by K. Lissák. Akadémiai Kiadó, Budapest. pp. 93—103.

Fortier, C., Delgado, A., Ducommun, P., Ducommun, S., Dupont, A., Jobin, M., Kraicer, J., MacIntosh-Hardt, B., Marceau, H., Mialhe, P., Mialhe-Voloss, C., Rerup, C. and Van Rees, G. P. (1970): Functional interrelationships between the adenohypophysis, thyroid, adrenal cortex and gonads. *Canad. med. Ass. J.* **103**, 864—874.

Jobin, M. (1971): Interrelations hypophyso-thyroido-surrénaliennes au cours de l'adaptation au froid. Thèse de doctorat ès sciences, Université Laval, Québec.

McKenzie, J. M. (1958): The bioassay of thyrotropin in serum. *Endocrinology* **58**, 372—382.

Murphy, B. E. P. (1967): Some studies of the protein-binding of steroids and their application to the routine micro and ultramicro measurement of various steroids in body fluids by competitive protein-binding radioassay. *J. clin. Endocr.* **27**, 973—990.

FOETAL STEROIDOGENESIS

GY. TELEGDY

Department of Physiology
University Medical School
Pécs, Hungary

During human pregnancy the foetus develops in a specific hormonal environment. Foetal distress or intrauterine death of the foetus are usually associated with remarkable hormonal changes. From the results of the past years it has become evident that the foetus as part of the integrated foeto-placental unit, introduced by Diczfalusy (1962, 1964), plays an important role in the hormonal balance of pregnancy. Since 1964 the foeto-placental unit concept has gained a general acceptance (e.g., Pecile and Finzi 1969). According to this concept the midgestation foetus and placenta form a steroid synthesizing functional unit capable of elaborating all steroid hormones that the placenta or the foetus alone is unable to produce.

The present paper deals mainly with steroidogenesis occurring in the foetal part of the human foeto-placental unit. The results are based mainly on in vivo experiments carried out in Diczfalusy's laboratory, in the Reproductive Endocrinology Research Unit at Karolinska Sjukhuset in Stockholm. The material was obtained from the interruption of pregnancy authorized by the Royal Medical Board of Sweden under the statute of 1938 amended in 1946 and 1963. The period of gestation was between the 17th and 20th weeks.

In order to study the de novo steroid synthesis from a small molecule such as acetate, or from cholesterol, we perfused midterm foeto-placental units with 5 mCi of sodium acetate and tritium-labelled cholesterol and isolated foetuses with 2.5 mCi of each compound (Telegdy et al. 1970a, c). The labelled material was introduced into the umbilical artery in the foeto-placental unit and in the umbilical vein of the isolated foetuses. The perfusion was carried out at 36–37°C for 90–120 minutes, the blood was oxygenated with 95.0 per cent oxygen and 5 per cent CO_2 or with air and CO_2 mixture, 23.1 per cent oxygen and 3.7 per cent CO_2 (Lerner and Diczfalusy 1968). The pH was maintained constant during the perfusion. During the experiments the perfusate was collected and after completion of the study the different foetal organs and perfusate were analysed and radiochemically homogeneous sterols and steroids were isolated.

The results of isolated placenta perfusion, carried out with ^{14}C-labelled acetate in other experiments, indicated that the midterm placenta cannot utilize acetate for sterol and steroid synthesis (Telegdy et al. 1970b, Van Leusden et al. 1971). In this case in the perfusion of the complete foeto-placental unit with ^{14}C-labelled acetate, only the foetus was able to utilize acetate for sterol and steroid synthesis. From acetate a considerable amount of squalene, lanosterol and cholesterol was formed (Telegdy et al. 1970a, Mathur et al. 1970, Van Leusden et al. 1971) and isolated from different foetal organs. Foetal liver and adrenals are the most active sterol-synthesizing organs. In addition some ^{14}C-labelled cholesterol from foetal brain and residual foetal tissue and some lanosterol from the latter could be isolated.

TABLE 1

Sterols isolated from different foetal organs following perfusion with ^{14}C-labelled acetate

	Squalene	Lanosterol	Cholesterol
Adrenal	+	+	+
Liver	+	+	+
Brain	−	−	+
Testis	−	+	+
Residual foetal tissue	−	+	+
Perfusate	−	−	+

According to Telegdy et al. 1970a, Mathur et al. 1970, Van Leusden et al. 1971.

In the foetus acetate was further metabolized to pregnenolone and dehydroepiandrosterone. The incorporation of ^{14}C-labelled acetate in these steroids was much higher in the conjugated fraction than in the free fraction. This indicated that the acetate in the foetus is metabolized mainly via a conjugated pathway (Telegdy et al. 1970c).

In the same experiment cholesterol-7α-^{3}H introduced into the foetal circulation is metabolized differently from that of cholesterol formed de novo from acetate. More free than conjugated pregnenolone could be found. It seems that circulating cholesterol is metabolized mainly via an unconjugated pathway (Telegdy et al. 1970c).

From acetate and cholesterol a major amount of pregnenolone and dehydroepiandrosterone, a small amount of progesterone, 17α-hydroxy-progesterone and androstenedione could be isolated from different tissues. In the adrenal small amount of progesterone and androstenedione, derived from acetate, could be demonstrated. From cholesterol only progesterone was formed. From the perfusate, in addition to progesterone and androstenedione, 17α-hydroxy-progesterone, derived from both precursors, could be isolated. In the liver only pregnenolone and dehydroepiandrosterone were found. The presence of other steroids formed either from acetate or from cholesterol, such as 20α- and 20β-dihydroprogesterone, cortisol and corticosterone in the adrenal, progesterone, 20α- and 20β-dihydroprogesterone and androstenedione in the liver, 20α- and 20β-dihydroprogesterone, 16α-hydroxy-dehydroepiandrosterone, oestrone in the perfusate could be excluded (Telegdy et al. 1970c).

The exact quantity of different steroids and cholesterol formed from acetate was measured in other experiments carried out by Archer et al. (1971) and Mathur et al. (1970) in the same laboratory. ^{14}C-labelled acetate was used as precursor and

TABLE 2

Steroids isolated from foetal adrenal, liver and perfusate following perfusion with ^{14}C-labelled acetate and tritiated cholesterol

	Adrenal	Liver	Perfusate
Pregnenolone	+	+	+
Dehydroepiandrosterone	+	+	+
Progesterone	+	—	+
17α-hydroxy-progesterone			+
Androstenedione	+*	—	+

According to Telegdy et al. 1970c.
* Only from acetate.

tritiated steroids and cholesterol were used as internal standards to monitor the losses occurring in the course of isolation procedure (Table 3).

Table 3 indicates that from acetate cholesterol is formed in a major quantity, while cholesterol sulphate is found to a much lesser extent. Among the $\varDelta^5$-steroids isolated, dehydroepiandrosterone, dehydroepiandrosterone sulphate, pregnenolone and pregnenolone sulphate were the major yield. As much as 0.07 per cent of the total precursor perfused is converted to these compounds. $\varDelta^4$-compounds such as androstenedione progesterone and 17α-hydroxyprogesterone in a total of 0.0003 per cent were formed. In addition to all the above compounds, a small amount of testosterone and cholesterol esters have also been found (Archer et al. 1971, Cekan and Diczfalusy 1970).

It seems the foetal $\varDelta^4$—$\varDelta^5$-isomerase 3β-hydroxysteroid dehydrogenase system is lacking or it has an insufficient capacity in the foetus during midgestation period. Therefore, the foetus is unable to convert pregnenolone to progesterone or dehydroepiandrosterone to androstenedione to a significant degree (Solomon et al. 1967, Bolte et al. 1966).

Progesterone in a significant amount is derived from the placenta. This is the most important precursor in corticoid synthesis in foetal adrenal. The adrenal

TABLE 3

Average amounts (μCi) of sterols and steroids formed by four human foetuses perfused with 3–6 μCi of [^{14}C] sodium acetate

Progesterone	0.001
17α-hydroxy-progesterone	0.005
Androstenedione	0.006
Pregnenolone	0.044
Pregnenolone sulphate	0.664
Dehydroepiandrosterone	0.270
Dehydroepiandrosterone sulphate	2.161
Cholesterol	29.650
Cholesterol sulphate	0.410

According to Mathur et al. 1970, and Archer et al. 1971.

converts progesterone to desoxycorticosterone, corticosterone and cortisol (Bird et al. 1965, 1966) and corticosterone to aldosterone (Pasqualini et al. 1966).

In the foetal liver from progesterone a large quantity of pregnanediol, 3α-hydroxy-5β-pregnan-20-one and 20α-dihydroxyprogesterone (Bird et al. 1966) and 3-sulphates of the last two compounds were metabolized (Bird et al. 1965). Progesterone in foetal tissues can be hydroxylated in 6β, 11β, 16α and 17α positions (Bird et al. 1966). 11β and 21-hydroxylation can take place only in the presence of the adrenals (Wilson et al. 1966).

Pregnenolone formed by the foetus or reaching the foetus from the placenta will be sulphurylated to a large extent and converted to dehydroepiandrosterone and dehydroepiandrosterone sulphate. In the foetal adrenal hydroxylation takes place in the 17α position and in the liver in the 16α position (Solomon et al. 1967).

It has been shown that 17α and/or 21-hydroxy-pregnenolone can also be converted to corticoids (Pasqualini and Lowy 1968, Pasqualini et al. 1968, Jackanicz et al. 1969). The quantitative importance of this corticoid synthetic pathway has to be assessed.

In the foeto-placental unit dehydroepiandrosterone and dehydroepiandrosterone sulphate are the most important precursors of oestrogens. In the placenta extensive conversion of dehydroepiandrosterone and dehydroepiandrosterone sulphate to androstenedione and testosterone occurs after hydrolysis of the sulphate ester, followed by aromatization to oestrone and oestradiol-17β (Bolte et al. 1964, Lamb et al. 1967, Dell'Acqua et al. 1967, Reynolds et al. 1968, Schwers et al. 1971). From dehydroepiandrosterone very little if any androstenedione and testosterone are formed in the foetus, because of insufficient activity of the Δ^4–Δ^5-isomerase-3β-hydroxysteroid dehydrogenase enzyme system (Mancuso et al. 1965, 1968). In our experiments androstenedione and testosterone may be derived from the minute amount of progesterone produced by the adrenal or by the testis (Telegdy et al. 1970c, Archer et al. 1971). Therefore, the oestrogen formation in the foetus from dehydroepiandrosterone via foetal androstenedione and testosterone has a very limited significance if any. However, androgens reaching the foetus from the placenta will be aromatized by the foetal liver to oestrone and oestradiol-17β (Mancuso et al. 1965, 1968).

Some of the androstenedione will be converted to testosterone by the liver and gastrointestinal tract. In all other tissues more testosterone is converted to androstenedione than vice versa (Benagiano et al. 1967). In the foetal adrenal androstenedione and testosterone are converted to 11β-hydroxylated forms and testosterone to testosterone sulphate (Mancuso et al. 1968).

Reductive pathways of androstenedione and testosterone seem to have a very high organ specificity. In the liver 5β-oriented reduction is predominant, whereas 5α prevails in all other tissues (Benagiano et al. 1967).

Dehydroepiandrosterone and dehydroepiandrosterone sulphate are extensively hydroxylated in the 16α position in the foetal liver (Bolte et al. 1966). This reaction does not take place in the placenta (Dell'Acqua et al. 1967, Reynolds et al. 1968). For oestriol synthesis this is the most important biosynthetic neutral pathway. Since the foetus has a very limited aromatizing capability of Δ^5-compounds (Mancuso et al. 1965, 1968) via Δ^4-intermediates, this reaction takes place mainly in the placenta using foetal precursor. Any major disturbance of the foetal liver may lead to decreased activity of the 16α-hydroxylase enzyme system, which would effect overall oestriol production.

Oestrone and oestradiol-17β reaching the foetus from the placenta or small amounts synthesized by the foetal liver from androgens of mainly placental origin, can be hydroxylated in 16α position. In this way the oestriol will be formed from oestradiol-17β and with subsequent reduction of 17-oxo group from oestrone (Benagiano et al. 1967, Schwers et al. 1965a). This phenolic pathway of oestriol synthesis in the foetus is of much less importance.

The oestrogens in the foetus are rapidly sulphurylated in almost all tissues (Diczfalusy 1953, Diczfalusy et al. 1961a, b, c) and the foetal liver seems to have a well-developed oestrogen glucosiduronating system also (Engel et al. 1962). From oestriol the synthesis leads to oestriol-3-sulphate, oestriol-16-glucosiduronate and sulpho-glucosiduronate double conjugate (Mikhail et al. 1963).

In the liver, besides extensive 16-hydroxylation, other hydroxylating reactions can take place such as the formation of 2-methoxy-oestradiol 6α-hydroxy-oestrone, 6α-hydroxy-oestradiol-17β, 17-epioestriol, 15α-hydroxy-oestradiol, 15α-hydroxy-oestriol (Schwers et al. 1965b, Knuppen et al. 1966, Zucconi et al. 1967).

In summary foetal steroidogenesis, in contrast to the placental steroidogenesis, can be characterized as follows:

1. Sterol and steroid formation from acetate.
2. Predominance of the conjugated pathways (sulphate and glucosiduronate formation).
3. Insufficient activity of the Δ^4–Δ^5-isomerase and 3β-hydroxysteroid dehydrogenase system.
4. 16α-hydroxylation.

CONCLUSION

Although much information concerning foetal steroidogenesis has been accumulated, very little is known about the regulation of different steroidogenetic and metabolic pathways. The physiological role of the different conjugation processes and the role of the conjugates upon foetal development and maturation, and the biological role of different hydroxylated and reduced compounds remain to be explored. In spite of the delicate nature of the human foeto-placental unit and the difficulty in extrapolating animal data to human foetal endocrine function, appropriate solution to these problems hopefully will be found in the near future.

REFERENCES

Archer, D. F., Mathur, R. S., Wiqvist, N. and Diczfalusy, E. (1971): Quantitative assessment of the de novo sterol and steroid synthesis in the human foeto-placental unit. 2. Synthesis and secretion of steroids and steroid sulphates by the midgestation foetus. *Acta endocr. (Kbh.)* **66**, 666.

Benagiano, G., Kincl, F. A., Zielska, F., Wiqvist, N. and Diczfalusy, E. (1967): Studies on the metabolism of C-19 steroids in the human foeto-placental unit. Metabolism of androstenedione and testosterone in the intact foeto-placental unit. *Acta endocr. (Kbh.)* **56**, 203.

BIRD, C. E., SOLOMON, S., WIQVIST, N. and DICZFALUSY, E. (1965): Formation of C-21 steroid sulphates and glucosiduronates by previable human foetuses perfused with [4-^{14}C] progesterone. *Biochim. biophys. Acta (Amst.)* **104**, 623.

BIRD, C. E., WIQVIST, N., DICZFALUSY, E. and SOLOMON, S. (1966): Metabolism of progesterone by the perfused previable human foetus. *J. clin. Endocr.* **26**, 1144.

BOLTE, E., MANCUSO, S., ERIKSSON, G., WIQVIST, N. and DICZFALUSY, E. (1964): Studies on the aromatization of neutral steroids in pregnant women. 1. Aromatization of C-19 steroids by the placentas perfused in situ. *Acta endocr. (Kbh.)* **45**, 535.

BOLTE, E., WIQVIST, N. and DICZFALUSY, E. (1966): Metabolism of dehydroepiandrosterone sulphate by the human foetus at midpregnancy. *Acta endocr. (Kbh.)* **52**, 583.

CEKAN, Z. and DICZFALUSY, E. (1970): De novo synthesis of cholesterol esters by human foetuses. In: *Abstracts of the IIIrd International Congress on Hormonal Steroids.* Hamburg. Ed. by V. H. T. James. Excerpta Medica, International Congress Series, **110**. p. 185.

DELL'ACQUA, S., MANCUSO, S., ERIKSSON, G., RUSE, J. L., SOLOMON, S. and DICZFALUSY, E. (1967): Studies on the aromatization of neutral steroids in pregnant women. Aromatization of 16α-hydroxylated C-19 steroids by midterm placentas perfused in situ. *Acta endocr. (Kbh.)* **55**, 401.

DICZFALUSY, E. (1953): Chorionic gonadotrophin and oestrogens in the human placenta. *Acta endocr. (Kbh.) Suppl.* **12**, 1.

DICZFALUSY, E. (1962): Endocrinology of the foetus. *Acta obstet. gynec. scand.* **41**, Suppl. **1**, 45.

DICZFALUSY, E. (1964): Endocrine function of the human foeto-placental unit. *Fed. Proc.* **23**, 791.

DICZFALUSY, E., CASSMER, O., ALONSO, C. and DE MIQUEL, M. (1961a): Estrogen metabolism in the human foetus and newborn. *Recent Progr. Hormone Res.* **17**, 147.

DICZFALUSY, E., CASSMER, O., ALONSO, C. and DE MIQUEL, M. (1961b): Oestrogen metabolism in the human foetus. I. Tissue levels following the administration of 17β-oestradiol and oestriol. *Acta endocr. (Kbh.)* **37**, 353.

DICZFALUSY, E., CASSMER, O., ALONSO, C., DE MIQUEL, M. and WESTIN, B. (1961c): Oestrogen metabolism in the human foetus. II. Oestrogen conjugation by foetal organs in vitro and in vivo. *Acta endocr. (Kbh.)* **37**, 516.

ENGEL, L. L., BAGGETT, B. and HALLA, M. (1962): In vitro metabolism of estradiol-17β by human foetal liver: formation of estriol, 16-epiestriol, estrone and estriol glucosiduronic acid. *Endocrinology* **70**, 907.

JACKANICZ, T. M., WIQVIST, N. and DICZFALUSY, E. (1969): Conversion of 17α-hydroxypregnenolone to αβ-unsaturated 3-ketosteroids by the previable human foetus. *Biochim. biophys. Acta (Amst.)* **175**, 883.

KIRSCHNER, M. A., WIQVIST, N. and DICZFALUSY, E. (1966): Studies on oestriol synthesis from dehydroepiandrosterone sulphate in human pregnancy. *Acta endocr. (Kbh.)* **53**, 584.

KNUPPEN, R., BREUER, H. and DICZFALUSY, E. (1966): Comparative studies on the metabolism of oestrogens by the human foetus during perfusion and in vitro. In: *Abstracts of the IInd International Congress on Hormonal Steroids*, Milan, 1966. Ed. by E. B. Romanoff and L. Martini. Excerpta Medica, International Congress Series **111**. p. 171.

LAMB, E., MANCUSO, S., DELL'ACQUA, S., WIQVIST, N. and DICZFALUSY, E. (1967): Studies on the metabolism of C-19 steroids in the human foeto-placental unit. 1. Neutral metabolites formed from dehydroepiandrosterone and dehydroepiandrosterone sulphate by the placenta at midpregnancy. *Acta endocr. (Kbh.)* **55**, 263.

LERNER, U. and DICZFALUSY, E. (1968): A new method for the in vitro perfusion of the human foeto-placental unit. In: *Abstracts of the International Symposium on Foeto-placental Unit*. Milan, 1968. Ed. by A. Pecile and G. B. Carruthers. Excerpta Medica, International Congress Series *170*. p. 19.

MANCUSO, S., DELL'ACQUA, S., ERIKSSON, G., WIQVIST, N. and DICZFALUSY, E. (1965): Aromatisation of androsteronedione and testosterone by the human foetus. *Steroids* **5**, 183.

MANCUSO, S., BENAGIANO, G., DELL'ACQUA, S., SHAPIRO, M., WIQVIST, N. and DICZFALUSY, E. (1968): Studies on the metabolism of C-19 steroids in the human foeto-placental unit. 4. Aromatization and hydroxylation products formed by previable foetuses perfused with androstenedione and testosterone. *Acta endocr. (Kbh.)* **57**, 208.

MATHUR, R. S., ARCHER, D. F., WIQVIST, N. and DICZFALUSY, E. (1970): Quantitative assessment of the de novo sterol and steroid synthesis in the human foetoplacental unit. 1. Synthesis and secretion of cholesterol and cholesterol sulphate. *Acta endocr. (Kbh.)* **65**, 663.

MIKHAIL, G., WIQVIST, N. and DICZFALUSY, E. (1963): Oestriol metabolism in the previable human foetus. *Acta endocr. (Kbh.)* **42**, 519.

PASQUALINI, J. R. and LOWY, J. (1968): New pathway of corticosteroid synthesis in the human foetus. In: *Abstracts of the IIIrd International Congress of Endocrinology*, Mexico, Ed. by C. Gual. Excerpta Medica, International Congress Series, *157*, p. 29.

PASQUALINI, J. R., WIQVIST N. and DICZFALUSY, E. (1966): Biosynthesis of aldosterone by human foetuses perfused with corticosterone at mid-term. *Biochim. biophys. Acta (Amst.)* **121**, 430.

PASQUALINI, J. R., LOWY, J., WIQVIST, N. and DICZFALUSY, E. (1968): Biosynthesis of cortisol from 3β, 17α, 21-trihydroxypregn-5-en-20-one by the intact human foetus at midpregnancy. *Biochim. biophys. Acta (Amst.)* **152**, 648.

PECILE, A. and FINZI, C. (1969): The foeto-placental unit. Excerpta Medica, International Congress Series, *183*.

PION, R. J., JAFFE, R. B., WIQVIST, N. and DICZFALUSY, E. (1967): Formation of dehydroepiandrosterone sulphate by the previable human foetuses. *Biochem. biophys. Acta (Amst.)* **137**, 584.

REYNOLDS, J. W., MANCUSO, S., WIQVIST, N. and DICZFALUSY, E. (1968): Studies on aromatization of neutral steroids in pregnant women. 7. Aromatization of 3β, 17β-dihydroxy-androst-5-en-16-one by placenta perfused in situ at midpregnancy. *Acta endocr. (Kbh.)* **58**, 377.

SCHWERS, J., ERIKSSON, G. and DICZFALUSY, E. (1965a): Metabolism of oestrone and oestradiol in the human foeto-placental unit at midpregnancy. *Acta endocr. (Kbh.)* **49**, 75.

SCHWERS, J., ERIKSSON, G., WIQVIST, N. and DICZFALUSY, E. (1965b): 15α-Hydroxylation: a new pathway of estrogen metabolism in the human foetus and newborn. *Biochim. biophys. Acta (Amst.)* **100**, 313.

SCHWERS, J., VANCROMBREUCQ, T., GOVAERTS, M., ERIKSSON, G. and DICZFALUSY, E. (1971): Metabolism of dehydroepiandrosterone sulphate following in situ placental perfusion at midpregnancy. *Acta endocr. (Kbh.)* **66**, 637.

SOLOMON, S., BIRD, C. E., LING, W., IWAMIYA, M. and YOUNG, P. C. (1967): Formation and metabolism of steroids in the foetus and placenta. *Recent Progr. Hormone Res.* **23**, 297.

TELEGDY, G., WEEKS, J. W., LERNER, U., STAKEMAN, G. and DICZFALUSY, E. (1970a): Acetate and cholesterol metabolism in the human foeto-placental unit at midgestation. 1. Synthesis of cholesterol. *Acta endocr. (Kbh.)* **63**, 91.

TELEGDY, G., WEEKS, J. W., WIQVIST, N. and DICZFALUSY, E. (1970b): Acetate and cholesterol metabolism in the human foeto-placental unit at midgestation. 2. Steroids synthesized and secreted by the placenta. *Acta endocr. (Kbh.)* **63**, 105.

TELEGDY, G., WEEKS, J. W., ARCHER, D. F., WIQVIST, N. and DICZFALUSY, E. (1970c): Acetate and cholesterol metabolism in the human foeto-placental unit at midgestation. 3. Steroids synthesized and secreted by the foetus. *Acta endocr. (Kbh.)* **63**, 119.

VAN LEUSDEN, H. A., SIEMERINK, M., TELEGDY, G. and DICZFALUSY, E. (1971): Squalene and lanosterol synthesis in the foeto-placental unit at midgestation. *Acta endocr. (Kbh.)* **66**, 711.

WILSON, R., BIRD, C. E., WIQVIST, N., SOLOMON, S. and DICZFALUSY, E. (1966): Metabolism of progesterone by the perfused adrenalectomized human foetus. *J. clin. Endocr.* **26**, 1155.

ZUCCONI, G., LISBOA, B. P., SIMONITSCH, E., ROTH, L., HAGEN, A. A. and DICZFALUSY, E. (1967): Isolation of 15α-hydroxy-oestriol from pregnancy urine and from the urine of newborn infants. *Acta endocr. (Kbh.)* **56**, 413.

ON THE LOCATION OF THE NEURAL STRUCTURES INVOLVED IN THE RESERPINE-INDUCED HYPERSECRETION OF ACTH

B. HALÁSZ* and I. LENGVÁRI

Department of Anatomy
University Medical School
Pécs, Hungary

It is well known that reserpine causes an increase in pituitary ACTH secretion. A single injection of the drug results in a marked decrease of hypothalamic CRF (corticotrophic releasing factor, Bhattacharya and Marks 1969) and pituitary ACTH content (Kitay et al. 1959, Saffran and Vogt 1960, Maickel et al. 1961, Bhattacharya and Marks 1969) and a simultaneous elevation in plasma corticosterone levels (Maickel et al. 1961, Bhattacharya and Marks 1969). Administration of reserpine for several days leads to adrenal hypertrophy (Gaunt et al. 1954, Hertting and Hornykiewicz 1957, Montanari and Stockham 1962).

There is practically no information about the site of reserpine action, more specifically we do not know at present which neural structures are primarily responsible for the pituitary ACTH response to the drug.

The present investigations were concerned with this question. Various hypothalamic deafferentations, fornix transection or mesencephalic lesion were made and the mentioned reserpine effect studied.

The experiments were performed on adult male rats of our inbred strain (originally Wistar), kept on standard diet, under constant environment and controlled light and dark periods. The rats were subjected to the following operative interferences:

1. *Complete deafferentation of the medial basal hypothalamus* (Fig. 1a, b, c; Group 1). All neural connections of the region were interrupted, but the area was left in contact with the pituitary by the unbroken pituitary stalk. The reason for deafferenting this part of the hypothalamus was that this region (called hypophysiotrophic area) appears to produce the hypothalamic releasing and inhibiting factors, among others CRF essential for pituitary ACTH function (Halász et al. 1962, 1965, Flament-Durand 1965).

2. *Frontal cut behind the optic chiasma* (Fig. 1d, e; Group 2). A half-dome-shaped cut was made directly behind the optic chiasma, extending laterally 1.3 mm from the midline on both sides, and dorsally to the paraventricular nuclei (Table 1, subgroup 2a). Thus, only the anterior connections to the medial basal hypo-

---

* Present address: 1st Department of Anatomy, Semmelweis Medical University, Hungary.

thalamus were severed. In some animals the whole cut was placed unilaterally interrupting the afferents to the mentioned region only on one side (Table 1, subgroup 2b).

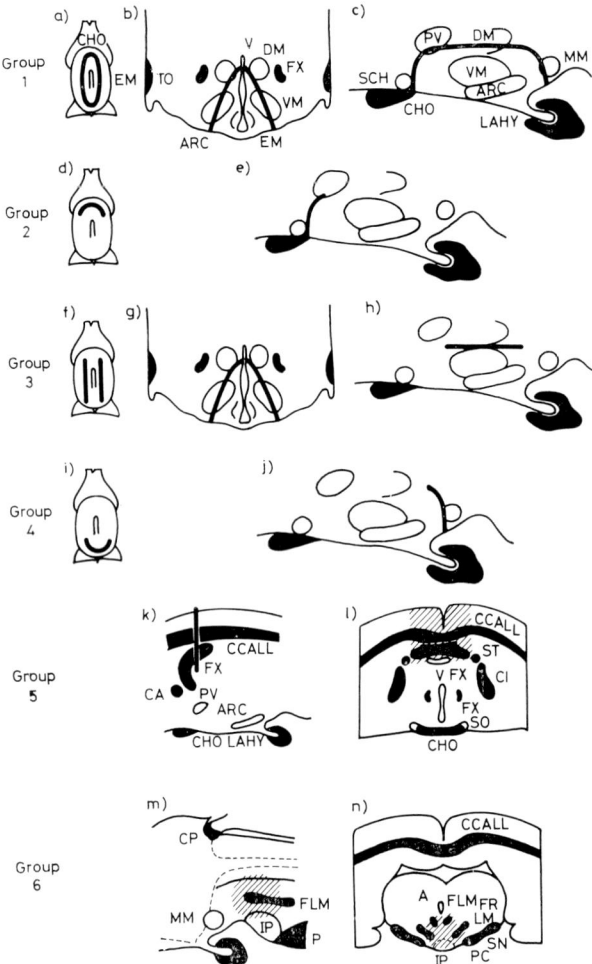

Fig. 1. Schematic drawings of the location and extent of the various operations. a, d, f, i: the knife cut as seen from the base of the brain; b, g, l, n: the cut or lesion as seen in frontal section and c, e, h, j, k, m: as projected upon a midsagittal section of the brain. Heavy line indicates the cut, hatched area the lesioned region. A: aqueduct; ARC: arcuate nucleus; CA: anterior commissure; CCALL: corpus callosum; CHO: optic chiasm; CI: internal capsule; CP: posterior commissure; DM: dorsomedial nucleus; EM: median eminence; FLM: fasciculus longitudinalis medialis; FR: reticular formation; FX: fornix; IP: interpeduncular nucleus; LAHY: anterior lobe of the hypohysis; LM: medial lemniscus; MM: medial mamillary nucleus; P: pons; PC: cerebral peduncle; PV: paraventricular nucleus; SCH: suprachiasmatic nucleus; SN: substantia nigra; SO: supraoptic nucleus; ST: stria terminalis; TO: optic tract; V: third ventricle; VM: ventromedial nucleus

3. *Parasagittal cuts passing through the medial part of the ventromedial nuclei* (Fig. 1f, g, h; Group 3). These cuts disrupted the bilateral and superior connections to the medial basal hypothalamus.

4. *Posterior arched cut* (Fig. 1i, j; Group 4). A half-dome-shaped cut was made at the level of the mamillary nuclei, extending 1.3 mm from the midline on both sides. This intervention deafferented the medial basal hypothalamus from posterior.

5. *Fornix transection at the level of the optic chiasma* (Fig. 1k, l; Group 5).

6. *Destruction of the medial ventral tegmentum of the mesencephalon* (Fig. 1m, n; Group 6).

Hypothalamic deafferentations were made by means of a small, bayonet-shaped knife fixed in the holder of a stereotaxic instrument (for technical details *see* Halász and Pupp 1965, Halász and Gorski 1967). A small piece of a razor blade (3.0 mm wide) fixed in the stereotaxic instrument was used for fornix transection. Through a transverse fissure drilled on the top of the skull the blade was lowered in the brain 5.5 mm at the midline, and then moved laterally 3.0 mm.

In the morning, 10–14 days after operation 2.0 ml blood was taken under ether anaesthesia by heart puncture (within less than a minute) into a syringe rinsed with heparin (except Group 1, in which this happened thirty days following surgery). Two days later, again in the morning, reserpine (Rausedyl, G. Richter, Budapest) was given (3.0–3.5 mg/kg) intraperitoneally. Four hours after drug administration a second blood sample was withdrawn from the abdominal aorta under ether anaesthesia. Afterwards the animals were sacrificed by decapitation, their brains were removed, fixed and prepared for histology. Both blood samples were centrifuged, the plasma removed and its corticosterone content determined by the spectrofluorimetric method of Silber et al. (1958) as modified by Guillemin et al. (1958).

In the rats with complete deafferentation of the medial basal hypothalamus the chronic effect of reserpine on the pituitary–adrenal system was also studied. These animals were treated for 9 days with reserpine (0.7 mg/kg was injected i.p. daily) and sacrificed on the next day. Treatment started one week after surgery. At autopsy the weight of the pituitary and of the adrenal glands was measured and the brain was removed for histological control of the isolation.

RESULTS

In the control animals the well-known rise in plasma corticosterone levels following reserpine treatment occurred; two to three times more corticosterone was detected in the plasma after reserpine than before (Table 1).

Complete deafferentation of the medial basal hypothalamus blocked this response completely. When comparing the corticoid content of the two blood samples of this group, it appears that the drug did not cause any change in blood corticosterone levels (Table 1).

The chronic effect of reserpine on pituitary ACTH secretion was also inhibited in the animals with a medial basal hypothalamic island. The findings are shown

TABLE 1

Effect of reserpine on plasma corticosterone levels
of control animals and of rats with partial or total deafferentation of the medial basal
hypothalamus (MBH), with fornix transection or mesencephalic lesion

Group	No. of animals	Plasma corticosterone μg/100 ml			p values*
		Before reserpine	After reserpine	Increase %	
Intact	14	16.6 ± 0.82**	65.3 ± 2.81	293	< 0.001
1 Complete deaff. of MBH	10	27.0 ± 1.44	26.5 ± 1.40	0	—
2a Bilateral frontal cut behind the optic chiasma	8	25.3 ± 2.32	28.7 ± 0.94	13	N.S.
2b Unilateral frontal cut behind the optic chiasma	11	25.7 ± 2.14	46.2 ± 1.31	79	< 0.001
3 Parasagittal cuts through the hypothalamus	14	13.6 ± 0.68	57.7 ± 5.02	324	< 0.001
4 Posterior arched cut in the mamillary region	13	23.2 ± 1.40	55.0 ± 4.15	137	< 0.001
5 Fornix transection	14	22.3 ± 1.04	77.7 ± 1.47	248	< 0.001
6 Mesencephalic lesion	16	20.3 ± 1.45	71.7 ± 3.00	251	< 0.001

* Comparing the two corticosterone values of the group.
** Mean ± standard error of the mean.

in Table 2. In the control rats reserpine induced a significant increase in adrenal weight, while this effect failed to take place in the operated rats.

These observations indicate that after neural isolation of the medial basal hypothalamus reserpine presumably did not induce any ACTH release.

TABLE 2

Adrenal weight of untreated
and of reserpine-treated (for 9 days) intact rats
and of animals with complete deafferentation of the medial basal
hypothalamus (MBH)

Group	No. of animals	Body weight g	Adrenal weight mg
Intact	10	154 ± 4*	39.0 ± 1.6
Intact + reserpine	10	152 ± 4	53.5 ± 1.5[a]
Deafferentation of MBH	13	160 ± 5	40.3 ± 2.0
Deafferentation of MBH + reserpine	13	152 ± 7	45.0 ± 1.4[b]

* Mean ± standard error of the mean.
a: $p < 0.01$ compared to untreated controls.
b: $p < 0.05$ compared to untreated group with deafferentation.

Interruption of the anterior connections to the medial basal hypothalamus on both sides (Table 1, subgroup 2a) and leaving intact all the other pathways had a fairly similar effect as complete deafferentation of the area; in these rats there was almost no rise in plasma corticosterone levels following drug administration.

In those animals in which the frontal cut was unilateral (Table 1, subgroup 2b) the blockade of the reserpine response was only partial.

Parasagittal cuts through the ventromedial nuclei, disconnecting the medial basal hypothalamus from the rest of the brain on both sides and from above (Group 3), did not interfere with the action of the drug; elevation in blood corticosterone content occurred, and the degree of rise was close to that found in the controls (Table 1).

The reserpine effect was also evident in the rats with a posterior arched cut (Group 4) interrupting the posterior connections of the medial basal hypothalamus (Table 1).

Fornix transection (Group 5) as well as electrolytic lesions placed in the mesencephalon (Group 6) did not alter the pituitary response to reserpine (Table 1). In both these groups the plasma corticosterone content rose to the same level as in the controls.

In the light of the data presented it is not clear whether the results obtained in Group 4 can be considered a normal ACTH response to reserpine or a slightly reduced one. When comparing the second corticoid value of this group with the intact, fornix-transected or mesencephalon-lesioned groups, it appears that the rise in corticosterone levels was in the animals with a posterior arched cut less than in the other mentioned groups. However, if one compares Group 4 with Group 3, the second values of these two groups are practically the same. The only difference is that in Group 3 the "resting" levels were low, while in Group 4 they were elevated, consequently the per cent increase in plasma corticosterone content following reserpine is in the former group very high (more than 320 per cent), whereas in the latter it is relatively low (only 137 per cent).

In all experimental groups, except Group 3, the initial blood corticoid levels were higher than in the controls. The complete blockade of the reserpine response in the animals with an isolated medial basal hypothalamus, or a bilateral frontal cut behind the optic chiasma cannot be due to this fact, because plasma corticosterone levels were elevated also following unilateral frontal cut, fornix transection or mesencephalic lesion, and in spite of this, these latter groups showed a normal response.

Our observations suggest, first of all, that reserpine when inducing pituitary ACTH hypersecretion does not act directly on the medial basal hypothalamus but might exert its influence on neural structures outside this region. This assumption is consistent with Smelik's (1967) finding according to which reserpine, if implanted into the mentioned hypothalamic area, does not affect pituitary ACTH secretion.

Our data indicate further that the critical afferents causing the reserpine-induced release of CRF from the hypophysiotrophic area reach this region from the anterior direction. One half of these fibres is not enough to elicit a normal reaction of the CRF-producing neurons.

The origin of the fibres in question is not known yet. All we can say is that those neurons in the mesencephalon and in the hippocampus which are directly connected with the medial basal hypothalamus are probably not responsible for the reserpine effect, because neither the interruption of the nervous connections between the mesencephalon and the medial basal hypothalamus (Groups 3 and 4) (see for detailed discussion of mesencephalic afferents to the hypothalamus Szentágothai 1968), nor transection of the fornix, including also the transection of the medial corticohypothalamic tract — which pathways represent the most important connections between the hippocampus and the medial basal hypothalamus (Nauta 1956, Raisman 1970) — blocked the drug-induced ACTH hypersecretion.

REFERENCES

BHATTACHARYA, A. N. and MARKS, B. H. (1969): Reserpine- and chlorpromazine-induced changes in hypothalamo–hypophyseal–adrenal system in rats in the presence and absence of hypothermia. *J. Pharmacol. exp. Ther.* **165**, 108—116.

FLAMENT-DURAND, J. (1965): Observations on pituitary transplants into the hypothalamus of the rat. *Endocrinology* **77**, 446—454.

GAUNT, R., RENZI, A. A., ANTONCHAK, N., MILLER, G. J. and GILMAN, M. (1954): Endocrine aspects of the pharmacology of reserpine. *Ann. N.Y. Acad. Sci.* **59**, 22—35.

GUILLEMIN, R., CLAYTON, G. W., SMITH, J. D. and LIPSCOMB, H. S. (1958): Measurement of free corticosteroids in rat plasma. Physiological validation of a method. *Endocrinology* **63**, 349—358.

HALÁSZ, B. and GORSKI, R. A. (1967): Gonadotrophic hormone secretion in female rats after partial or total interruption of neural afferents to the medial basal hypothalamus. *Endocrinology* **80**, 608—622.

HALÁSZ, B. and PUPP, L. (1965): Hormone secretion of the anterior pituitary gland after physical interruption of all nervous pathways to the hypophysiotrophic area. *Endocrinology* **77**, 553—562.

HALÁSZ, B., PUPP, L. and UHLARIK, S. (1962): Hypophysiotrophic area in the hypothalamus. *J. Endocr.* **25**, 147—154.

HALÁSZ, B., PUPP, L., UHLARIK, S. and TIMA, L. (1965): Further studies on the hormone secretion of the anterior pituitary transplanted into the hypophysiotrophic area of the rat hypothalamus. *Endocrinology* **77**, 343—355.

HERTTING, G. and HORNYKIEWICZ, O. (1957): Beeinflussung der durch Reserpin hervorgerufenen Nebennierenrinde Hypertrophie durch Cortison. *Acta endocr. (Kbh.)* **26**, 204—208.

KITAY, J. I., HOLUB, D. A. and JAILER, J. W. (1959): "Inhibition" of pituitary ACTH release after administration of reserpine and epinephrine. *Endocrinology* **65**, 548—554.

MAICKEL, R. F., WESTERMANN, E. O. and BRODIE, B. B. (1961): Effects of reserpine and cold-exposure on pituitary–adrenocortical function in rats. *J. Pharmacol. exp. Ther.* **134**, 167—175.

MONTANARI, R. and STOCKHAM, M. A. (1962): Effects of single and repeated doses of reserpine on the secretion of adrenocorticotrophic hormone. *Brit. J. Pharmacol.* **18**, 337—345.

NAUTA, W. (1956): An experimental study of the fornix system in the rat. *J. comp. Neurol.* **104**, 247—270.

RAISMAN, G. (1970): An evaluation of the basic pattern of connections between the limbic system and the hypothalamus. *Amer. J. Anat.* **129**, 197—202.

SAFFRAN, M. and VOGT, M. (1960): Depletion of pituitary corticotrophin by reserpine and by nitrogen mustard. *Brit. J. Pharmacol.* **15**, 165—169.

SILBER, R. H., BUSCH, R. D. and OSLAPAS, R. (1958): Practical procedure for estimation of corticosterone or hydrocortisone. *Clin. Chem.* **4**, 278—285.

SMELIK, P. G. (1967): ACTH secretion after depletion of hypothalamic monoamines by reserpine implants. *Neuroendocrinology* **2**, 247—254.

SZENTÁGOTHAI, J. (1968): Anatomical considerations. In: *Hypothalamic Control of the Anterior Pituitary. An Experimental-Morphological Study.* Ed. by J. Szentágothai, B. Flerkó, B. Mess and B. Halász. Akadémiai Kiadó, Budapest, pp. 22—109.

HYPOTHALAMIC MECHANISMS CONTROLLING ANTERIOR PITUITARY FUNCTIONS

L. MARTINI

Department of Pharmacology
University of Milan
Milan, Italy

INTRODUCTION

It is now generally accepted that the central nervous system (CNS) plays an essential role in the regulation of many endocrine functions and that the hypothalamus is the crucial element of such regulation (Mangili et al. 1966, Martini et al. 1968a, Mess and Martini 1968, Motta et al. 1969a). The key position of the hypothalamus is due to its strategic location in close contact with the anterior pituitary gland, and to the fact that this region of the brain contains particular neurons which synthesize the chemical messengers necessary for stimulating or for inhibiting the anterior pituitary (the so-called hypothalamic releasing and inhibitory factors), as well as feedback receptors whose activity is modified by hormonal influences (Mangili et al. 1966, Martini et al. 1968a, Mess and Martini 1968; Motta et al. 1969a).

This paper will summarize the data obtained in the author's laboratory aimed at clarifying:

1. the site of production of the hypothalamic gonadotropin-releasing factors;
2. the possible existence of hypothalamic gonadotropin-synthesizing factors, separated from the classical releasing factors;
3. the type of mediators which are involved in the control of the secretion of the gonadotropin-releasing factors;
4. the mode of operation of the feedback mechanisms which control gonadotropin secretion.

LOCALIZATION OF THE NUCLEI WHICH SYNTHESIZE GONADOTROPIN-RELEASING FACTOR

Three groups of experiments have been performed in order to clarify which region of the hypothalamus synthesizes the releasing factors (RFs) which control the secretion of pituitary gonadotropins in the rat.

The first technique used was that of placing separate electrolytic lesions in each of the hypothalamic areas which are believed to play some role in the control of gonadotropin secretion (Szentágothai et al. 1968), in order to study whether such lesions modify the concentrations of the FSH-releasing factor (FSH-RF) and of the LH-releasing factor (LH-RF) at the level of the median eminence (ME), i.e. of the region of the hypothalamus which is specifically responsible for the storage of hypophysiotropic principles, and for their delivery to the anterior pituitary through the portal circulation. It was assumed that a lesion placed exactly in an area in which RF is produced would prevent its synthesis, and consequently reduce its accumulation in the ME.

Three independent areas of the brain were bilaterally lesioned; they will be referred to as (*i*) paraventricular area, (*ii*) suprachiasmatic area, and (*iii*) arcuate–ventromedial area. Five days following placement of the lesions the animals were killed and their ME were collected in order to evaluate their content in FSH-RF and in LH-RF. For the assays of these principles the "pituitary depletion methods" described by Fraschini et al. (1966) and by Motta et al. (1970a) were used. Using this approach it has been possible to localize, within the hypothalamus of the rat, a circumscribed region in which FSH-RF is synthesized; it has actually been shown that lesions in or around the paraventricular nuclei are the only ones which reduce the concentration of this RF at ME level (Fig. 1). The synthesis of LH-RF takes place apparently in two different regions, since the content of this RF in the ME is reduced when lesions are placed either in the suprachiasmatic area or in the arcuate–ventromedial nuclei (Fig. 1; Mess et al. 1967, Martini et al. 1968a).

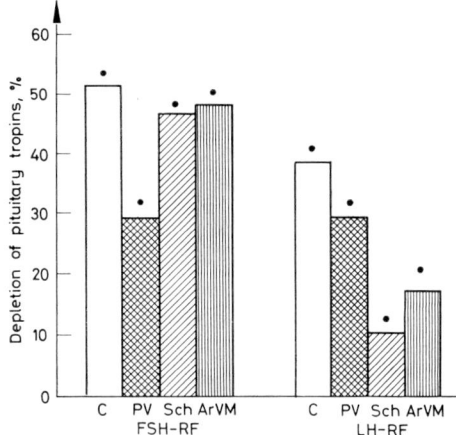

Fig. 1. Effect of lesions localized in the paraventricular (PV), suprachiasmatic (Sch) and arcuate–ventromedial (ArVM) areas on FSH-RF and LH-RF activity of the median eminence of male rats. Columns represent the depletion of pituitary tropins induced in normal male rats by the intracarotid injection of hypothalamic extracts prepared from non-lesioned controls (C) or from animals with different hypothalamic lesions

HYPOTHALAMIC DEAFFERENTATION

The second approach devised to study the localization of the nuclei which synthesize the RFs controlling the secretion of gonadotropins was that of evaluating the concentrations of FSH-RF and of LH-RF in the hypothalamic islands of rats submitted to a complete hypothalamic deafferentation (Halász 1969). This operation permits a total separation of the paraventricular region from the rest of the hypothalamus (Fig. 2); consequently, if it is true that FSH-RF originates in the paraventricular area, the complete disappearance of FSH-RF from the island a few days after the operation would be expected. On the other hand, the suprachiasmatic and the arcuate ventromedial regions are still included within the hypothalamic island; consequently, if LH-RF is really produced by these two zones, its concentrations in the island should not be reduced following the operation.

The content of FSH-RF and of LH-RF in the deafferented island of adult rats was measured eight and fifteen days following the operation, using the techniques

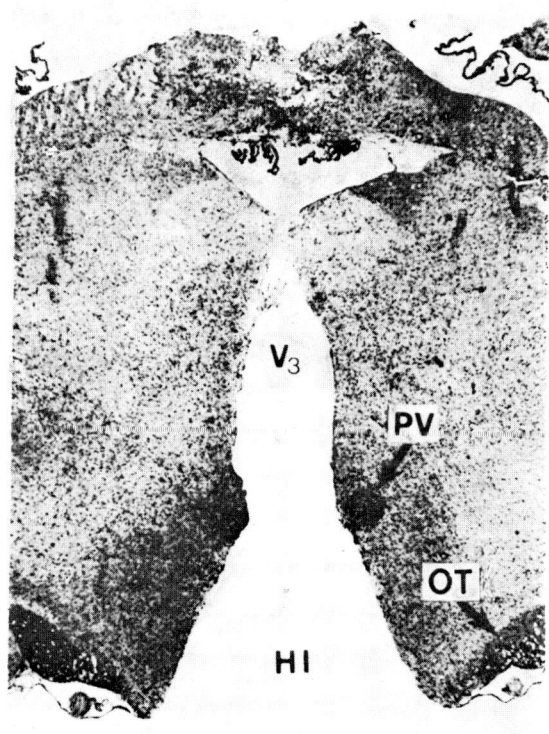

Fig. 2. Frontal section of the rat brain following total hypothalamic deafferentation and removal of the hypothalamic island. OT = optic tracts; PV = paraventricular nuclei; V_3 = 3rd ventricle; HI = removed hypothalamic island

described by Fraschini et al. (1966) and by Motta et al. (1970a). The results shown in Fig. 3 indicate that FSH-RF stores are significantly reduced in the hypothalamic island eight days after a complete deafferentation; FSH-RF disappears completely from the isolated hypothalamus fifteen days after the operation. Eight and fifteen days after deafferentation LH-RF is still present in the isolated island (Fig. 4); surprisingly, the concentration of this RF in deafferented animals is even higher than usual (Tima et al. 1969, Motta et al. 1970b).

These data confirm with a new technique that FSH-RF is synthesized in the paraventricular region and that LH-RF is probably manufactured in the suprachiasmatic and in the arcuate ventromedial regions. The fact that the stores of LH-RF are increased following deafferentation suggests that, after the operation,

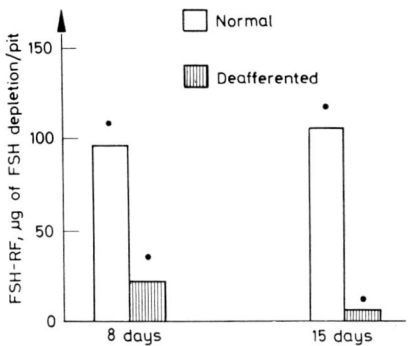

Fig. 3. Effect of hypothalamic deafferentation on the FSH-RF content of the hypothalamic island of adult male rats (8 and 15 days after the operation). Columns represent the depletion of pituitary FSH induced in normal male rats by the intracarotid injection of hypothalamic extracts prepared from normal or from deafferented animals

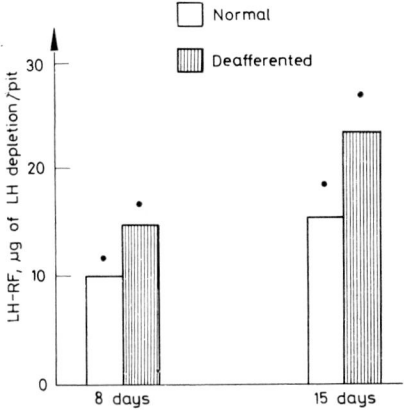

Fig. 4. Effect of hypothalamic deafferentation on the LH-RF content of the hypothalamic island of adult male rats (8 and 15 days after the operation). Columns represent the depletion of pituitary LH induced in normal male rats by the intracarotid injection of hypothalamic extracts prepared from normal or from deafferented animals

all the LH-RF synthesized is accumulated in the island, because the extrahypothalamic neural stimuli necessary for its release are no longer transmitted to the hypothalamus (see below; Tima et al. 1969, Motta et al. 1970b).

HYPOTHALAMIC IMPLANTS OF INHIBITORS OF PROTEIN SYNTHESIS

In the third group of experiments, the hypothesis that FSH-RF might be synthesized in the paraventricular nuclei was tested by implanting cycloheximide (Actidione), an inhibitor of protein synthesis, into the paraventricular region of adult, castrated, male rats, and by evaluating the effects of such implants on FSH-RF stores in the ME. Cycloheximide was implanted either unilaterally or bilaterally. When unilateral implants were performed, at time of autopsy ME tissue was collected in a way which permitted to separate the half ME corresponding to the implanted side, from the half corresponding to the non-implanted one; the two halves of the ME were then tested separately for their content in FSH-RF and in LH-RF (Fraschini et al. 1966, Motta et al. 1970a).

Data shown in Fig. 5 indicate that, five days after unilateral implantation of cycloheximide, FSH-RF disappears only from the ipsilateral half of the ME; complete disappearance of FSH-RF from the ME is induced by bilateral implants. It may be concluded from these results that inhibition of protein synthesis in the cells of the paraventricular nuclei interfere with some biochemical process which is essential for the synthesis of FSH-RF in this region; these data, however, are not taken as indicating that FSH-RF itself is a protein or a polypeptide (McCann and Dhariwal 1966). It is also clear from the results that fibres originating in one paraventricular nucleus do not cross and carry FSH-RF only to the ipsilateral half of the ME.

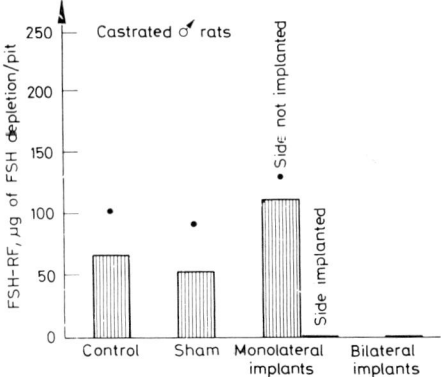

Fig. 5. Effect of implants of cycloheximide (Actidione) in the paraventricular region on the FSH-RF content of the median eminence of adult, castrated, male rats. See text for more details. Columns represent the depletion of pituitary FSH induced in normal male rats by the intracarotid injection of hypothalamic extracts prepared from controls or from implanted animals. Control: unimplanted animals. Sham: animals implanted with empty cannulae. Monolateral implants: animals implanted with cycloheximide in one paraventricular nucleus. Bilateral implants: animals implanted with cycloheximide in both paraventricular nuclei

Figure 6 shows once more that the paraventricular region is not strictly involved in the synthesis of LH-RF. Animals bearing cycloheximide either unilaterally or bilaterally in this region of the brain have normal amounts of LH-RF in the ME. These results, when considered in conjunction with the evidence previously described indicating that LH-RF is synthesized in the suprachiasmatic region, suggest that the effect of cycloheximide is very localized and that no significant diffusion of the drug toward the basal hypothalamus takes place.

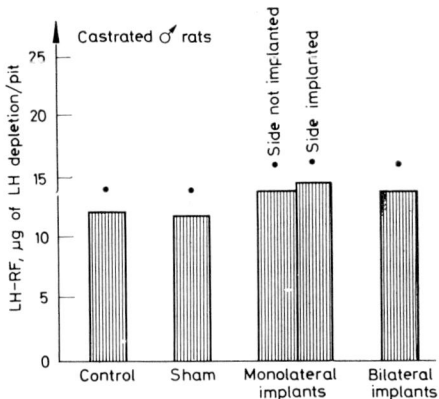

Fig. 6. Effect of implants of cycloheximide (Actidione) in the paraventricular region on the LH-RF content of the median eminence of adult, castrated male rats. See text for more details. Columns represent the depletion of pituitary LH induced in normal male rats by the intracarotid injection of hypothalamic extracts prepared from controls or from implanted animals. Control: unimplanted animals. Sham: animals implanted with empty cannulae. Monolateral implants: animals implanted with cycloheximide in one paraventricular nucleus. Bilateral implants: animals implanted with cycloheximide in both paraventricular nuclei.

DATA SUGGESTING THE EXISTENCE OF A FOLLICLE-STIMULATING HORMONE-SYNTHESIZING FACTOR

The three sets of results presented in the preceding sections of this paper agree in indicating that, in the rat, FSH-RF is synthesized in the area of the paraventricular nuclei. It is interesting that, both following paraventricular lesions and after hypothalamic deafferentation, the concentration of FSH in the anterior pituitary of the operated animals was perfectly normal, though the synthesis of FSH-RF had been considerably reduced. This result is surprising, since it is generally believed that RFs control not only the release of anterior pituitary hormones, but also their synthesis (Geschwind 1969); in accordance with this view, one should expect the synthesis of a pituitary hormone to be interrupted, when the corresponding RF is no longer available.

The presence of normal amounts of FSH in the anterior pituitary of animals in which the synthesis of FSH-RF had been experimentally suppressed, might be tentatively explained by suggesting that the hypothalamus controls FSH secretion through the production of two independent humoral factors: one devoted to the control of FSH release (FSH-RF), the other to the control of FSH synthesis (FSH-synthesizing factor or FSH-SF). It was believed that such a hypothesis might be tested by evaluating whether hypothalamic extracts prepared from animals submitted to a complete hypothalamic deafferentation (and consequently devoid of any FSH-RF activity) might induce the synthesis of FSH in animals in which this had been interrupted by appropriate experimental manipulations. Corbin and Daniels (personal communication) have recently shown that ME lesions, performed in adult male rats, result in 1–2 weeks in a significant decrease of the amounts of FSH stored in the anterior pituitary. The decrease of FSH in the pituitary of lesioned animals has been interpreted as being due to the impossibility, for hypophysiotropic principles endowed with synthesizing capacities, to be transported to the anterior pituitary. Daniels and Corbin (personal communication) have also shown that the intravenous injection of crude hypothalamic extracts prepared from the brain of normal rats induces a rapid and significant increase of FSH stores in ME-lesioned recipient animals. They have concluded that, under the conditions of their experiments, crude hypothalamic extracts are able to facilitate the resynthesis of FSH.

A similar approach has been recently used by Daniels, Motta and Martini (unpublished observations). First of all, they have confirmed that electrolytic lesions placed in the ME region of adult male rats are followed in 10 days by a significant decrease in pituitary FSH concentration (Table 1). Like in the experiments of Daniels and Corbin, the intravenous injection of a hypothalamic extract prepared from the brain of normal animals induced, in 45 minutes, a significant increase in the amounts of FSH stores in the pituitary of ME-lesioned rats. Daniels, Motta and Martini have shown in addition that the concentration of FSH in the pituitary of lesioned animals is brought back to normal also by the intravenous injection of a hypothalamic extract prepared from the brain of deafferented animals (Table 1); this is in spite of the fact that this hypothalamic extract does not contain any FSH-RF.

The results indicate that both normal hypothalamic extracts and hypothalamic extracts prepared from animals submitted to complete hypothalamic deafferenta-

TABLE 1

Effect of median eminence (ME) lesions and of intravenous injections of median eminence extracts (MEE) on pituitary concentrations of FSH in adult male rat

Groups	No. of animals	Intravenous treatment	Pituitary FSH[a] $\mu g/mg$	Significance
Normal	20	Saline	42.54 ± 3.82[b]	
ME-lesioned	25	Saline	32.27 ± 3.38	$p < 0.05$ vs normal
ME-lesioned	18	2 MEE from normal rat	43.19 ± 3.10	$p < 0.05$ vs ME-lesioned saline treated
ME-lesioned	18	2 MEE from deafferented rat	45.68 ± 5.21	$p < 0.05$ vs ME-lesioned saline treated

[a] Microgram equivalents of NIH-FSH-S-5 per mg wet weight of pituitary tissue.
[b] Values are means $\pm$ SE.

tion contain a factor which is able to increase the concentration of FSH in the pituitary of ME-lesioned animals. There are two mechanisms through which this factor may operate: one that facilitates the synthesis of new FSH; or the other which inhibits the release of stored FSH. The first possibility is the one favoured by the authors, since it is not believed that in ME-lesioned animals release of FSH occurs so rapidly as to permit a significant reaccumulation of the hormone 45 minutes after blockade of the release process. In addition, no factors able to suppress FSH release have been described so far; inhibiting factors have been recognized to exist for the control of the secretion of prolactin (Meites 1966), melanocyte-stimulating hormone (Kastin and Schally 1967) and growth hormone (Krulich et al. 1968).

The results obtained using the hypothalamic extract prepared from the deafferented animals suggest that the hypothetical FSH-RF is different and independent from FSH-RF; moreover, its site of origin is within the deafferented island and not in the paraventricular region.

MEDIATORS INFLUENCING THE NUCLEI WHICH SYNTHESIZE THE LUTEINIZING HORMONE-RELEASING FACTOR

It is a generally accepted concept that extrahypothalamic nervous structures (e.g., amygdala, cortex, hippocampus, midbrain) may influence the neurons which secrete the gonadotropin-releasing factors (Szentágothai et al. 1968, Halász 1969, Mess and Martini 1968). The validity of this concept is proved once more by the observation, reported in a previous section of this paper, that LH-RF is accumulated in the deafferented hypothalamic island when all inputs from extrahypothalamic structures are eliminated. The chemical nature of the humoral mediator(s) involved in transferring the information from extrahypothalamic centres to the hypothalamic nuclei has not been fully clarified so far. Considerable data seem to suggest that traditional central nervous system mediators (e.g., epinephrine, norepinephrine, serotonin, dopamine, acetylcholine, etc.) may be involved in such a process (Kobayashi and Matsui 1969, Fuxe and Hökfelt 1969, Ganong and Lorenzen 1967, Piva et al. 1969).

The possibility that acetylcholine (ACh) might be the mediator involved in transmitting extrahypothalamic influences to the nuclei synthesizing LH-RF, has been tested recently using an "in vitro" procedure by Fiorindo and Martini (unpublished observations). They have shown that the anterior pituitary of normal adult male rats, when incubated alone, secretes very low amounts of LH. The release of LH from the incubated pituitaries is increased, though not significantly, by the addition of fragments of rat hypothalamus; such fragments have been prepared in a way to include the ME and the arcuate–ventromedial region, i.e., one of the areas in which LH-RF is synthesized. ACh, added to incubation flasks containing only anterior pituitary tissue, does not increase LH output. The cholinergic mediator does increase LH secretion in flasks containing simultaneously hypothalamic fragments and anterior pituitary tissue; under these circumstances, the increase in LH release is proportional to the dose of ACh added to the medium. The data have been interpreted as indicating that ACh stimulates the release of

LH-RF from the hypothalamic fragments; the LH-RF released under the influence of the drug enhances the secretion of LH from the incubated pituitary.

This interpretation is supported by the results of additional experiments performed by Fiorindo and Martini (unpublished observations) using drugs which either counteract or prolong ACh action. Atropine, a drug inhibiting the peripheral effects of ACh, has been shown to counteract in vitro the LH-releasing effect of ACh added to the medium containing anterior pituitary tissue and hypothalamic fragments. It is interesting that atropine also inhibits the small release of LH which is observed when hypothalamic tissue is added to anterior pituitaries in the absence of ACh; this result may suggest that atropine is able to block the effects on LH-RF release of endogenous ACh present in the incubated hypothalamic tissue. Prostigmine, a drug which inhibits cholinesterases, enhances the LH-releasing effect of ACh, when this mediator is added to media in which hypothalamic fragments are incubated together with anterior pituitary tissue. Prostigmine also increases the release of LH from anterior pituitaries incubated with hypothalamic fragments, but without exogenous ACh. This result may be explained by admitting that prostigmine enhances the activity of the endogenous ACh present in the hypothalamic tissue incubated.

In a similar set of experiments, Schneider and McCann (1969) have found that the adrenergic mediator dopamine is able to release LH in vitro when added to incubation media containing hypothalamic fragments and anterior pituitary tissue. They have suggested that dopamine might be the mediator liberating LH-RF. The possibility then exists that both cholinergic and adrenergic mechanisms participate in the control of the release of LH-RF from the neurons in which this factor is synthesized. The relative role of the two types of mediators remains to be ascertained.

FEEDBACK MECHANISMS AND THE CONTROL OF GONADOTROPIN SECRETION

A summary of the different types of endocrine feedback mechanisms that have been studied in this laboratory is provided in Table 2. It appears that there are at least three levels of feedback control of pituitary gonadotropins.

TABLE 2
Different types of endocrine feedback mechanisms

"*Long*" *Feedback Mechanisms*
  "Negative" feedback effect of corticosteroids (Corbin et al. 1965)
  "Negative" feedback effect of oestrogen (Martini et al. 1968)
  "Negative" feedback effect of progesterone (Martini et al. 1968)
  "Negative" feedback effect of testosterone (Martini et al. 1968)
  "Positive" feedback effect of oestrogen (Motta et al. 1968)
  "Positive" feedback effect of progesterone (Motta et al. 1970c)

"*Short*" *Feedback Mechanisms*
  "Negative" feedback effect of ACTH (Motta et al. 1965)
  "Negative" feedback effect of LH (David et al. 1966)
  "Negative" feedback effect of FSH (Fraschini et al. 1968)
  "Positive" [feedback effect of TSH (Motta et al. 1969b)

"*Ultrashort*" *Feedback Mechanisms*
  "Negative" feedback effect of FSH-RF (Hyyppä and Motta 1969, Motta 1969)

1. "Long" feedback systems: the controlling (inhibiting or activating) messages are provided by the hormone produced in the peripheral target glands.
2. "Short" feedback systems: the controlling signals are the hormones synthesized in the anterior pituitary gland.
3. "Ultrashort" feedback systems: the releasing factors directly influence their rate of production.

Because of the limitation of space, this paper will present only one single example for each category of feedback mechanisms.

"LONG" FEEDBACK SYSTEMS

A description of the classic findings about the "long" feedback control of the hypothalamo–pituitary complex may be found in the original papers quoted in Table 2, and in the review articles by Mess and Martini (1968), Reichlin (1966), Davidson (1969), Beyer and Sawyer (1969) and Sawyer (1967). Only one particular problem will be dealt with in detail here.

Several recent data indicate that some of the hormones produced in and secreted by the peripheral endocrine glands are not directly active on their target organs. Apparently, some hormones, in order to be able to initiate the response of their target tissues, must be transformed into an "active" metabolite. This possibility has been extensively investigated in the last few years with regard to the mode of action of testosterone on androgen-dependent peripheral target structures. It has been suggested that the potent androgenic steroid 17-beta-hydroxy-5-alpha-androstan-3-one (androstanolone, dihydrotestosterone, DHT Fig. 7), may be the "active" form of testosterone at tissue level (Bruchovsky and Wilson 1968, Gloyna and Wilson 1969, Tveter and Aakvag 1969). Conversion of testosterone into DHT has been reported to occur in the prostate, the seminal vesicles, the preputial glands and the other accessory organs of male reproduction (Bruchovsky and Wilson 1968, Gloyna and Wilson 1969, Tveter and Aakvag 1969). The enzyme 5-alpha-reductase involved in this transformation has been shown to exist both in the chromatin (Bruchovsky and Wilson 1968) and in the micro-

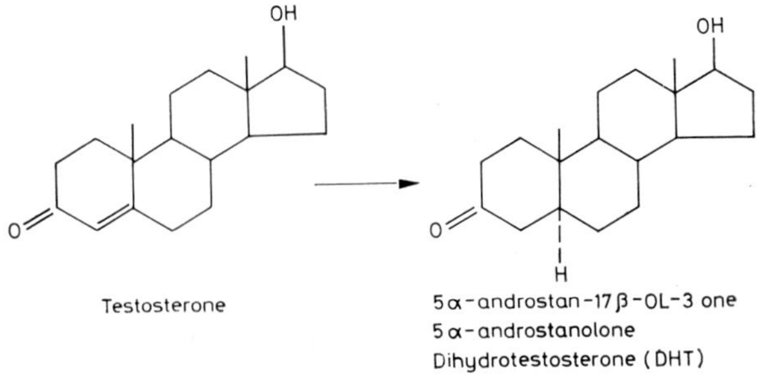

Fig. 7. Conversion of testosterone into its "active metabolites"

somal fractions (Shimazaki et al. 1965) for peripheral androgen-sensitive structures. In addition, the cytoplasm (Mainwaring 1969) and the nuclei (Fang and Liao 1969) of these structures contain receptor proteins with a particular binding specificity towards DHT.

If the formation of DHT is a general feature of testosterone action, one might expect this derivative to be formed also at the sites where androgen exerts its feedback effect on gonadotropin secretion. This hypothesis has been recently tested by Kniewald et al. (1971).

^{14}C-labelled testosterone was incubated in vitro with slices of hypothalamus (basal part, including the median eminence region), pituitary gland, amygdala, cerebral cortex, prostate and seminal vesicles, taken from adult, male rats. After three hours of incubation the metabolites formed were extracted, purified and identified using the procedures briefly summarized in Table 3.

TABLE 3

Outline of procedure

1. Incubation of tissue in Krebs—Ringer solution for 3 hours with testosterone 4-^{14}C
2. Extraction of the incubation media with diethyl ether
3. Evaporation of solvent
4. Dry residue transferred to thin layer chromatography (TLC) plates
5. TLC in heptane
6. TLC in cyclohexane : ethyl acetate : N heptane (5 : 5 : 1)
7. Autoradiographic localization of labelled compounds
8. Collection of spots and elution with diethyl ether
9. Identification of metabolites by means of:
   a) TLC
   b) gas chromatography with electron capture detector
   c) recrystallization to constant specific activity

The results obtained indicate that testosterone is converted into DHT by all tissues examined; however, the rate of conversion appears to vary considerably from tissue to tissue (Table 4). The formation of DHT occurs at a very large extent in the two peripheral androgen-dependent structures (prostate and seminal vesicles); this is confirmatory of previous findings (Bruchovsky and Wilson 1968, Gloyna and Wilson 1969, Tveter and Aakvag 1969). Very little DHT is formed by the cerebral cortex and by the amygdala; these cerebral zones have been included in this study as "control" tissues, since they are not supposed to be androgen-sensitive. Testosterone is converted into its "active" metabolite by the anterior pituitary; the amounts of DHT formed by the gland are significantly higher than those formed by the two "control" tissues; however, they do not reach the very elevated levels found in the media in which the peripheral androgen-sensitive organs have been incubated. The hypothalamus is also able to reduce testosteron' in the 5-alpha-position in a fashion significantly higher than that of the "control' tissues; however, the reducing capacity of the hypothalamus appears significantly lower than that of the anterior pituitary.

DHT is not the only metabolite formed by the different tissues examined so far: delta-4-androstene-3,17-dione, 5-alpha-androstan-3,17-dione and 5-alpha-androstan-3,17-diol have been identified practically in all incubation media. The for-

TABLE 4

Conversion of testosterone to 5α-androstan-17-β-ol-3-one (DHT) by the basal hypothalamus, anterior pituitary, cerebral cortex, amygdala, prostate and seminal vesicles of normal adult male rats[a]

Tissue	No. of animals	DHT pg/mg[b]
Basal hypothalamus	14	265.0 ± 22.2[c]
Anterior pituitary	7	744.1 ± 137.6[c,d]
Cerebral cortex	5	138.2 ± 7.9
Amygdala	5	128.0 ± 19.8
Prostate	5	$1,703.8 \pm 143.0$
Seminal vesicles	4	$1,536.0 \pm 199.0$

[a] Values are means $\pm$ SE.
[b] Picrograms of steroid formed per mg of wet tissue following a 3-hour incubation with 160 ng of testosterone 4-^{14}C (specific activity: 56.6 mCi/mM).
[c] $p < 0.001$ vs cerebral cortex, amygdala, prostate and seminal vesicles.
[d] $p < 0.005$ vs basal hypothalamus.

mation of some of these metabolites has been previously demonstrated to occur in the peripheral androgen-sensitive structures (Baulieu et al. 1969, Harding and Samuels 1962).

Results similar to the ones here described have been reported by Jaffe (1969), who incubated ^{3}H-labelled testosterone with rat anterior pituitary and hypothalamic slices. Moreover, Sholiton and Werk (1969) have recently found that the conversion of testosterone into DHT is effected in vitro also by the bovine brain; it is noteworthy that these authors did not detect any quantitative difference between the amounts of DHT formed by the hypothalamus and those formed by other cerebral structures (cerebral cortex and cerebral peduncles).

The data presented here suggest then that the transformation of testosterone into DHT is probably necessary also for initiating androgen-induced feedback responses; they also suggest that androgen exerts its feedback effect both on the hypothalamus and on the anterior pituitary. From the data, one would probably be inclined to assign a prominent role in this process to the anterior pituitary. This is contrary to previous physiological evidence emphasizing a hypothalamic site of action of androgen (Davidson 1969, Davidson and Smith 1967). A major role of the pituitary in androgen feedback responses is suggested also by some recent data which indicate that the gland has a much higher capacity than the hypothalamus for binding androgenic molecules (Samperez et al. 1969); preliminary evidence indicating that intrapituitary implants of testosterone may modify FSH secretion has recently appeared (Kamberi and McCann 1969).

After having shown that the anterior pituitary and the hypothalamus are able to convert testosterone into DHT, it was promising to investigate whether the conversion process might be modified by experimental manipulations which activate the hypothalamo–pituitary axis. Consequently, the conversion capacity of the anterior pituitary and of the hypothalamus of gonadectomized, adult, male rats has been studied in vitro. Animals were killed 2, 14 and 21 days following castration.

Castration considerably activates the transformation of testosterone into DHT at the pituitary level; the rate of conversion has been found to be three times higher than normal in pituitaries taken two days after the operation; it was still significantly increased in the pituitaries of animals which had been castrated two weeks before (Table 5). The conversion process is activated by castration also at the hypothalamic level; however, increase in the activity of the 5-alpha-reductase in this tissue appears to be slower (two weeks following the operation) and is not as marked as that found at the pituitary level (Table 6).

TABLE 5

Conversion of testosterone to 5α-androstan-17-β-ol-3-one (DHT) by the anterior pituitary (AP) of normal and castrated adult male rats[a]

Tissue	No. of animals	DHT pg/mg[b]
AP-normal	7	744.1 ± 137.6
AP-castrated		
2 days	3	2,169.1 ± 397.0
14 days	3	1,788.2 ± 178.3[c]

[a] Values are means ± SE.
[b] Picrograms of steroid formed per mg of wet tissue following a 3-hour incubation with 160 ng of testosterone 4-^{14}C (specific activity: 56.6 mCi/mM).
[c] $p < 0.05$ vs AP-normal.

TABLE 6

Conversion of testosterone to 5α-androstan-17-β-ol-3-one (DHT) by the basal hypothalamus (BH) of normal and castrated adult male rats[a]

Tissue	No. of animals	DHT pg/mg[b]
BH-normal	14	265.0 ± 22.2
BH-castrated		
2 days	3	331.7 ± 14.7
14 days	4	404.5 ± 28.6[c]
21 days	3	284.0 ± 8.0

[a] Values are means ± SE.
[b] Picrograms of steroid formed per mg of wet tissue following a 3-hour incubation with 160 ng of testosterone 4-^{14}C (specific activity: 56.6 mCi/mM).
[c] $p < 0.05$ vs BH-normal.

The data obtained following castration may be taken as additional evidence in support of the hypothesis that testosterone must be converted into "active" metabolite before initiating feedback responses; they also reinforce the conclusion that both the anterior pituitary and the hypothalamus are the sites on which androgen exerts its feedback effect on gonadotropin secretion. It appears again from the data that the pituitary probably plays a more important role than the hypothalamus in this process. It is interesting that following castration a higher uptake of radioactive testosterone has been reported to occur both in the anterior pituitary and in the hypothalamus (Roy and Laumas 1969).

"SHORT" FEEDBACK SYSTEMS

Background information on the physiological significance of "short" feedback mechanisms and on their interplay with the other types of feedback systems is provided in the papers quoted in Table 2 as well as in the articles by Motta (1969), Motta et al. (1969a), Kobayashi and Kato (1968), Desjardins (1969), Katz et al. (1969), Ojeda and Ramirez (1970), Corbin et al. (1970). Recent data on possible electrophysiological and biochemical correlates of the "short" feedback effects of anterior pituitary hormones have been reported by Steiner et al. (1967), Kawakami and Sawyer (1969), Terasawa et al. (1969), Libertun et al. (1969), Anton-Tay et al. (1969) and Hyyppä and Valavaara (1970).

The most recent efforts of our laboratory in the "short" feedback area have been devoted to clarifying the mode of operation of the "short" feedback mechanism controlling the secretion of the follicle-stimulating hormone (FSH). Two sets of experiments have been performed; in the first one, the effects of increased levels of exogenous FSH on the hypothalamo–pituitary complex have been evaluated; in the second the consequences of the elimination of endogenous FSH have been studied.

Fraschini et al. (1968) have studied the effects of the administration of exogenous FSH on the pituitary stores of FSH and on the hypothalamic content of the FSH-releasing factor (FSH-RF) in adult, castrated, male rats. Orchidectomized animals have been used in order to avoid the possibility that the injected FSH might activate the gonads, and operate through a "long" feedback effect. FSH was measured with the bioassay of Steelman and Pohley (1953) and FSH-RF with the "pituitary depletion method" described by David et al. (1965a). The data summarized in Fig. 8 indicate that treatment with exogenous FSH results in a significant drop in the pituitary stores of FSH and of the hypothalamic content of FSH-RF. These data have been interpreted as indicating that exogenous FSH may depress the synthesis of both FSH-RF and FSH. The data shown in Fig. 8 also suggest that the inhibitory signal provided by FSH is specific; it has been impossible to duplicate its effects by injecting Corticotropin (ACTH) and luteinizing hormone (LH) into the castrated animals.

The effects of endogenous FSH elimination on hypothalamic stores of FSH-RF have been reported by Motta and co-workers (Motta 1969, Motta et al. 1969a). Different groups of adult male rats have been subjected to castration, hypophysectomy, or castration followed by hypophysectomy; their hypothalamic stores of FSH-RF have been then evaluated utilizing the "pituitary depletion method" of David et al. (1965a). Three weeks following castration a significant increase in the amounts of FSH-RF stores in the hypothalamus was observed (Fig. 9). One week following hypophysectomy a slight, but not significant, increase of FSH-RF was detected. It is uncertain whether this small increase was due to the elimination of the "short" FSH signal, or to the reduction of testosterone secretion brought about by hypophysectomy. The latter appears a likely explantaion, since all testosterone-dependent structures

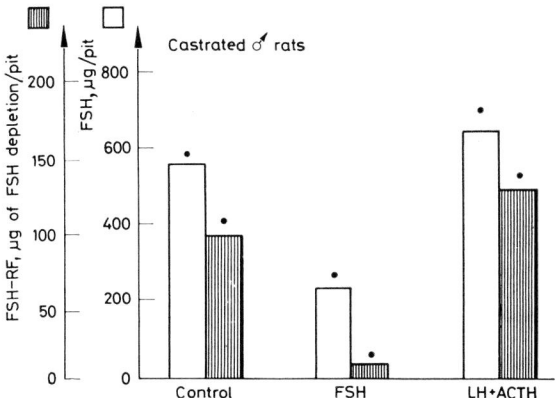

Fig. 8. Effect of systemic administration of FSH on pituitary FSH content and on hypothalamic FSH-RF stores of castrated male rats

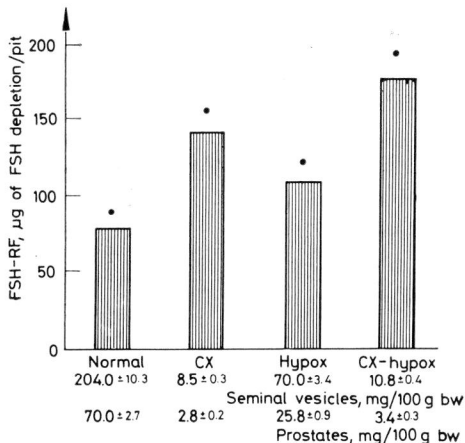

Fig. 9. Effect of castration (CX), hypophysectomy (Hypox) and castration plus hypophysectomy (CX+Hypox) on hypothalamic FSH-RF stores and on seminal vesicles and prostate weight of male rats

(prostate and seminal vesicles) were atrophied in this group of rats. In the animals subjected to the removal of the pituitary and of the testes, hypothalamic FSH-RF stores reached a level well above that observed following the elimination of either gland alone. These data indicate then that the elimination of the inhibiting signal, normally provided by FSH, probably stimulates FSH-RF synthesis; release is probably also enhanced as shown by the fact that after hypophysectomy, FSH-RF appears in the peripheral plasma (Negro-Vilar et al. 1969, Saito et al. 1967). The data indicate in addition that the effects of castration and of hypophysectomy are additive; it is also clear that in castrated animals, FSH-RF stores do not reach the high levels found following castration plus hypophysectomy because of the "short" negative feedback signal provided by FSH.

"ULTRASHORT" FEEDBACK CONTROL

It has recently been decided to explore the possibility that the synthesis, storage and release of the releasing factors might be influenced also by changes in the levels of the releasing factors themselves in the general circulation. The first experiments in this area performed by Hyyppä and Motta (Hyyppä and Motta 1969, Hyyppä et al. 1971) were planned in order to study whether the increase in the circulating levels of FSH-RF (obtained by chronically administering a crude hypothalamic extract containing FSH-RF) might influence the storage of FSH-RF at the hypothalamic level. In order to avoid the possibility that the administration of exogenous FSH-RF might activate the secretion of FSH, and consequently of sex steroids, and operate via the traditional "short" and "long" feedback mechanisms, the experiments were performed in hypophysectomized–castrated animals. Three separate experiments were run, in each of them two groups of male rats, castrated for three weeks and hypophysectomized for one week, were used; one of these groups was injected subcutaneously with an extract of rat hypothalamus (1 hypothalamus per rat per day for 5 days); the other was treated in a similar way with saline solution. Normal controls were also studied. The content of FSH-RF in the hypothalami of the different groups of animals was measured as previously described (David et al. 1965a). Figure 10, which provides a summary of the three experiments performed so far, indicates that the treatment with the hypothalamic extract results in a considerable reduction of hypothalamic stores of FSH-RF. As expected, these were particularly elevated in castrated–hypophysectomized controls (Motta 1969, Motta et al. 1969a). Since the hypothalamic extract used was not contaminated with sex steroids or with FSH, the effect observed cannot be due to the "long" and "short" feedback effects of these hormones. The data, then, suggest that some unknown factor present in the hypothalamic extract is able to reduce hypothalamic stores of FSH-RF. Since the hypothalamic extract injected contained high amounts of FSH-RF, it has been tentatively suggested that the administration of exogenous FSH-RF is responsible

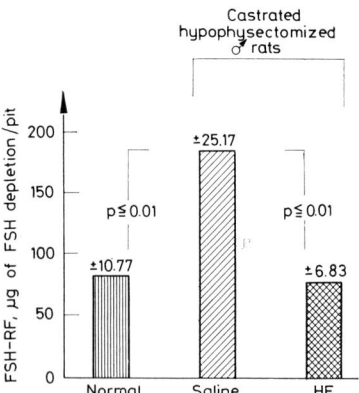

Fig. 10. Effect of hypothalamic extracts (HE) on hypothalamic FSH-RF stores of castrated–hypophysectomized male rats; columns represent means ± SE of the results obtained in 3 individual experiments

for the effect observed. It is important to recall in this connection that, in another set of experiments, it has been shown that cerebrocortical or liver extracts do not modify FSH-RF stores in castrated–hypophysectomized rats. Even if it is difficult, on the basis of this preliminary evidence, to establish whether the reduction of FSH-RF stores observed following treatment with hypothalamic extracts is due to inhibition of synthesis of FSH-RF or to stimulation of its release, it seems reasonable to suggest that the brain contains elements that are sensitive to changing levels of releasing factors. Work now in progress in the author's laboratory (Piva, Motta and Martini, unpublished observations) indicates that also the thyrotropin-releasing factor (TSH-RF) exerts an "ultrashort" feedback effect on hypothalamic stores of TSH-RF when administered to hypophysectomized–thyroidectomized animals. These data, if confirmed, will be particularly conclusive, since a synthetic preparation of TSH-RF has been used; this obviously rules out the possibility of non-specific effects due to the presence of contaminants in the crude hypothalamic extracts.

ACKNOWLEDGEMENTS

The experimental work performed in the author's laboratory and here described has been supported by the following grants: 67–530 of the Ford Foundation, New York; AM 11783–01–02–03 and AM 10119–01–02–03 of the National Institutes of Health, Bethesda, Maryland. Gifts of FSH and LH were made by the National Institutes of Health, Bethesda, Maryland.

All such support is gratefully acknowledged.

REFERENCES

ANTON-TAY, F., PELHAM, R. W. and WURTMAN, R. J. (1969): Increased turnover of ^{3}H-norepinephrine in rat brain following castration or treatment with ovine follicle-stimulating hormone. *Endocrinology* **84,** 489–492.

BAULIEU, E. E., LASNITZKI, J. and ROBEL, P. (1969): Testosterone metabolism in rat prostate grown in organ culture and hormone action. In: *Advances in the Biosciences*. Vol. III. Ed. by G. Raspé. Pergamon, Oxford–Vieweg, Braunschweig. pp. 169–174.

BEYER, C. and SAWYER, C. H. (1969): Hypothalamic unit activity related to control of the pituitary gland. In: *Frontiers in Neuroendocrinology*. Ed. by W. F. Ganong and L. Martini. Oxford University Press, New York. pp. 255–287.

BRUCHOVSKY, N. and WILSON, J. D. (1968): The conversion of testosterone to 5-androstan-17β-ol-3-one by rat prostate "in vivo" and "in vitro". *J. biol. Chem.* **243,** 2012–2021.

CORBIN, A., MANGILI, G., MOTTA, M. and MARTINI, L. (1965): Effect of hypothalamic and mesencephalic steroid implantations on ACTH feedback mechanisms. *Endocrinology* **76,** 811–818.

CORBIN, A., DANIELS, E. L. and MILMORE, J. E. (1970): An "internal" feedback mechanism controlling follicle stimulating hormone releasing factor. *Endocrinology* **86,** 735–743.

DAVID, M. A., FRASCHINI, F. and MARTINI, L. (1965a): An in vivo method for evaluating the hypothalamic follicle stimulating hormone releasing factor. *Experientia (Basel)* **21,** 483.

DAVID, M. A., FRASCHINI, F. and MARTINI, L. (1965b): Control of LH secretion: role of a "short" feedback mechanism. *Endocrinology* **78,** 55–60.

DAVIDSON, J. M. (1969): Feedback control of gonadotropin secretion. In: *Frontiers in Neuroendocrinology*, 1969. Ed. by W. F. Ganong and L. Martini. Oxford University Press, New York. pp. 343—388.

DAVIDSON, J. M. and SMITH, E. R. (1967): Testosterone feedback in the control of somatic and behavioral aspects of male reproduction. In: *Hormonal Steroids*. Ed. by L. Martini, F. Fraschini and M. Motta. Excerpta Medica, Amsterdam. pp. 805—813.

DESJARDINS, C. (1969): Alteration of hypophyseal LH and FSH release by exogenous LH and FSH in orchidectomized mice. *Proc. Soc. exp. Biol. (N.Y.)* **130**, 535—538.

FANG, S. and LIAO, S. (1969): Dihydrotestosterone binding by androphilic proteins of rat ventral prostate. *Fed. Proc.* **28**, 846.

FRASCHINI, F., MOTTA, M. and MARTINI, L. (1966): Methods for the evaluation of hypothalamic hypophysiotropic principles. In: *Methods in Drug Evaluation*. Ed. by P. Mantegazza and F. Piccinini. North-Holland Publishing Company, Amsterdam. pp. 424—457.

FRASCHINI, F., MOTTA, M. and MARTINI, L. (1968): A "short" feedback mechanism controlling FSH secretion. *Experientia (Basel)* **24**, 270—271.

FUXE, K. and HÖKFELT, T. (1969): Catecholamines in the hypothalamus and the pituitary gland. In: *Frontiers in Neuroendocrinology*, 1969. Ed. by W. F. Ganong and L. Martini. Oxford University Press, New York. pp. 47—96.

GANONG, W. F. and LORENZEN, L. (1967): Brain neurohumors and endocrine function. In: *Neuroendocrinology*. Vol. 2. Ed. by L. Martini and W. F. Ganong. Academic Press, New York. pp. 583—640.

GESCHWIND, I. I. (1969): Mechanism of action of releasing factors. In: *Frontiers in Neuroendocrinology*, 1969. Ed. by W. F. Ganong and L. Martini. Oxford University Press, New York. pp. 389—431.

GLOYNA, R. E. and WILSON, J. D. (1969): A comparative study of the conversion of testosterone to 17β-hydroxy-5α-androstan-3-one (dihydroxy-testosterone) by prostate and epididymis. *J. clin. Endocr.* **29**, 970—977.

HALÁSZ, B. (1969): The endocrine effects of isolation of the hypothalamus from the rest of the brain. In: *Frontiers in Neuroendocrinology*, 1969. Ed. by W. F. Ganong and L. Martini. Oxford University Press, New York. pp. 307—342.

HARDING, B. W. and SAMUELS, L. T. (1962): The uptake and subcellular distribution of C^{14} labelled steroid in rat ventral prostate following "in vivo" administration of testosterone-4-C^{14}. *Endocrinology* **70**, 109—118.

HYYPPÄ, M. and MOTTA, M. (1969): "Ultra-short" feedback control of the secretion of hypothalamic releasing factors. *Scand. J. clin. Lab. Invest.* **23**, Suppl. **108**, 39.

HYYPPÄ, M. and VALAVAARA, M. (1970): The effect of castration and hypophysectomy on the content of noradrenaline and serotonin in the hypothalamus of the rat. *Experientia (Basel)* **26**, 193—194.

HYYPPÄ, M., MOTTA, M. and MARTINI, L. (1971): Ultrashort feedback control of follicle stimulating hormone releasing factor secretion. *Neuroendocrinology* **7**, 227—235.

JAFFE, R. B. (1969): Testosterone metabolism in target tissues: hypothalamic and pituitary tissues of the adult rat and human fetus, and the immature rat epiphysis. *Steroids* **14**, 483—499.

KAMBERI, I. A. and McCANN, S. M. (1969): Effect of testosterone implants in the anterior pituitary (AP) of FSH secretion. *Fed. Proc.* **28**, 382.

KASTIN, A. J. and SCHALLY, A. V. (1967): MSH activity in pituitaries of rats treated with hypothalamic extracts from various animals. *Gen. comp. Endocr.* **8**, 344—347.

KATZ, S. H., MOLITCH, M. and McCANN, S. M. (1969): Effect of hypothalamic implants of GH on anterior pituitary weight and GH concentration. *Endocrinology* **85**, 725—734.

KAWAKAMI, M. and SAWYER, C. H. (1969): Effects of FSH on multiple unit activity in the rat hypothalamus. *Anat. Rec.* **163**, 308—315.

KNIEWALD, Z., MASSA, R. and MARTINI, L. (1971): Conversion of testosterone into 5α-androstan-17β-ol-3-one at the anterior pituitary and hypothalamic level. In: *Hormonal Steroids*. Ed. by V. H. T. James and L. Martini. Excerpta Medica, Amsterdam. pp. 946—953.

KOBAYASHY, H. and MATSUI, T. (1969): Fine structure of the median eminence and its functional significance. In: *Frontiers in Neuroendocrinology*, 1969. Ed. by W. F. Ganong and L. Martini. Oxford University Press, New York. pp. 3—46.

KOBAYASHY, T. and KATO, J. (1968): Short feedback mechanisms in the control of pituitary hormone secretion. *Saishin Jgaku* **23**, 1037–1047.

KRULICH, L., DHARIWAL, A. P. S. and McCANN, S. M. (1968): Stimulatory and inhibitory effects of purified hypothalamic extracts on growth hormone release from rat pituitary "in vitro". *Endocrinology* **83**, 783–790.

LIBERTUN, C., MOGUILEVSKY, J. A., SCHIAFFINI, O. and FOGLIA, V. (1969): Effect of hypophysectomy on the oxidative and glycolytic metabolism of hypothalamus. *Experientia (Basel)* **25**, 196–197.

MAINWARING, W. I. P. (1969): A soluble androgen receptor in the cytoplasm of rat prostate. *J. Endocr.* **45**, 531–541.

MANGILI, G., MOTTA, M. and MARTINI, L. (1966): Control of adrenocorticotropic hormone secretion. In: *Neuroendocrinology*. Vol. 1. Ed. by L. Martini and W. F. Ganong. Academic Press, New York. pp. 297–370.

MARTINI, L., FRASCHINI, F. and MOTTA, M. (1968a): Neural control of anterior pituitary functions. *Recent. Progr. Hormone Res.* **24**, 439–496.

MARTINI, L., FRASCHINI, F. and MOTTA, M. (1968b): Comments on "long" and "short" feedback loops. In: *Endocrinology and Human Behaviour*. Ed. by R. P. Michael. Oxford University Press, London. pp. 175–187.

McCANN, S. M. and DHARIWAL, A. P. S. (1966): Hypothalamic releasing factors and the neurovascular link between the brain and the anterior pituitary. In: *Neuroendocrinology*. Vol. 1. Ed. by L. Martini and W. F. Ganong. Academic Press, New York. pp. 261–296.

MEITES, J. (1966): Control of mammary growth and lactation. In: *Neuroendocrinology*. Vol. 1. Ed. by L. Martini and W. F. Ganong. Academic Press, New York. pp. 669–707.

MESS, B. and MARTINI, L. (1968): The central nervous system and the secretion of anterior pituitary trophic hormones. In: *Recent Advances in Endocrinology*. Ed. by V. M. T. James. Churchill, London. pp. 1–49.

MESS, B., FRASCHINI, F., MOTTA, M. and MARTINI, L. (1967): The topography of the neurons synthesizing the hypothalamic releasing factors. In: *Hormonal Steroids*. Ed. by L. Martini, F. Fraschini and M. Motta. Excerpta Medica, Amsterdam. pp. 1004–1013.

MOTTA, M. (1969): The brain and the physiological interplay of long and short feedback systems. In: *Progress in Endocrinology*. Ed. by C. Gual. Excerpta Medica, Amsterdam. pp. 523–531.

MOTTA, M., MANGILI, G. and MARTINI, L. (1965): A "short" feedback loop in the control of ACTH secretion. *Endocrinology* **77**, 392–395.

MOTTA, M., FRASCHINI, F., GIULIANI, G. and MARTINI, L. (1968): The central nervous system, estrogen and puberty. *Endocrinology* **83**, 1101–1107.

MOTTA, M., FRASCHINI, F. and MARTINI, L. (1969a): "Short" feedback mechanisms in the control of anterior pituitary function. In: *Frontiers in Neuroendocrinology, 1969*. Ed. by W. F. Ganong and L. Martini. Oxford University Press, New York. pp. 211–253.

MOTTA, M., STERESCU, N., PIVA, F. and MARTINI, L. (1969b): The participation of "short" feedback mechanisms in the control of ACTH and TSH secretion. *Acta neurol. belg.* **69**, 501–507.

MOTTA, M., PIVA, F., FRASCHINI, F. and MARTINI, L. (1970a): "Pituitary depletion methods" for the bioassay of hypothalamic releasing factors. In: *Hypophysiotropic Hormones of the Hypothalamus: Assay and Chemistry*. Ed. by J. Meites. Williams and Wilkins, Baltimore. pp. 44–59.

MOTTA, M., PIVA, F., TIMA, L., ZANISI, M. and MARTINI, L. (1970b): Feedback mechanisms and the control of the secretion of the hypothalamic releasing factors. *Mem. Soc. Endocr.* **18**, 407–422.

MOTTA, M., PIVA, F. and MARTINI, L. (1970c): The hypothalamus as the center of endocrine feedback mechanisms. In: *The Hypothalamus*. Ed. by L. Martini, M. Motta and F. Fraschini. Academic Press, New York. pp. 463–489.

NEGRO-VILAR, A., DICKERMAN, E. and MEITES, J. (1968): FSH releasing factor activity in plasma of rats after hypophysectomy and continuous light. *Endocrinology* **82**, 939–944.

NEGRO-VILAR, A., DICKERMAN, E. and MEITES, J. (1969): Removal of plasma FSH-

RF activity in hypophysectomized rats by testosterone propionate or reserpine. *Endocrinology* **83,** 1349—1352.
OJEDA, S. R. and RAMIREZ, V. D. (1970): Failure of estrogen to block compensatory ovarian hypertrophy in prepuberal rats bearing medial basal hypothalamic FSH implants. *Endocrinology* **86,** 50—56.
PIVA, F., STERESCU, N., ZANISI, M. and MARTINI, L. (1969): Non-steroidal antifertility agents affecting brain mechanisms. *Bull. Wld. Hlth. Org.* **41,** 275—288.
REICHLIN, S. (1966): Control of thyrotropic hormone secretion. In: *Neuroendocrinology.* Vol. 1. Ed. by L. Martini and W. F. Ganong. Academic Press, New York. pp. 445—536.
ROY, S. F., JR. and LAUMAS, K. R. (1969): 1,2-^{3}H-Testosterone: distribution and uptake in neural and genital tissues of intact male, castrated male and female rats. *Acta Endocr. (Kbh.)* **61,** 629—640.
SAITO, T., SAWANO, S., ARIMURA, A. and SCHALLY, A. V. (1967): Follicle stimulating hormone-releasing activity in peripheral blood. *Endocrinology* **81,** 1226—1230.
SAMPEREZ, S., THIEULANT, M. L. and JOUAN, P. (1969): Mise en évidence d'une association macromoléculaire de la testostérone 1-2-^{3}H- dans l'hypophyse antérieure et l'hypothalamus du rat normal et castré. *C.R. Acad. Sci. (Paris)* **268,** 2967.
SAWYER, C. H. (1967): Effects of hormonal steroids on certain mechanisms in the adult brain. In: *Hormonal Steroids.* Ed. by L. Martini, F. Fraschini and M. Motta. Excerpta Medica, Amsterdam. pp. 123—135.
SCHNEIDER, H. P. G. and McCANN, S. M. (1969): Possible role of dopamine as transmitter to promote discharge of LH-releasing factor. *Endocrinology* **85,** 121—132.
SHIMAZAKI, J., KURIHARA, H., ITO, Y. and SHIDA, K. (1965): Testosterone metabolism in prostate; formation of androstan-17β-ol-3-one and androst-4-ene-3,17-dione and the inhibitory effect of natural and synthetic oestrogens. *Gunma J. med. Sci.* **14,** 313—323.
SHOLITON, L. J. and WERK, E. E. (1969): The less-polar metabolites produced by incubation of testosterone-4-^{14}C with rat on bovine brain. *Acta Endocr. (Kbh.)* **61,** 641—648.
STEELMAN, S. L. and POHLEY, F. M. (1953): Assay of the follicle stimulating hormone based on the augmentation with human chorionic gonadotropin. *Endocrinology* **53,** 604—616.
STEINER, F. A., RUF, K. and AKERT, K. (1967): Steroid sensitive neurones in rat brain: anatomical localization and response to neurohumours and ACTH. *Brain Res.* **12,** 74—85.
SZENTÁGOTHAI, J., FLERKÓ, B., MESS, B. and HALÁSZ, B. (1968): *Hypothalamic Control of the Anterior Pituitary.* Akadémiai Kiadó, Budapest.
TERASAWA, E., WHITMOYER, D. I. and SAWYER, C. H. (1969): Effects of luteinizing hormone on multiple unit activity in the rat hypothalamus. *Amer. J. Physiol.* **217,** 1119—1126.
TIMA, L., MOTTA, M. and MARTINI, L. (1969): Effect of "hypothalamic deafferentation" on hypothalamic follicle stimulating hormone releasing factor (FSH-RF) and on pituitary FSH. In: *Program of the 51st Meeting of Endocrine Society.* p. 194.
TVETER, K. J. and AAKVAG, A. (1969): Uptake and metabolism "in vivo" of testosterone-1,2-^{3}H by accessory sex organs of male rats: influence of some hormonal compounds. *Endocrinology* **85,** 683—689.

THYROXINE BINDING TO ANTERIOR PITUITARY PROTEINS IN VITRO: CORRELATION WITH ANTERIOR PITUITARY GROWTH

V. SCHREIBER

Laboratory for Endocrinology and Metabolism
IIIrd Medical Clinic
Faculty of General Medicine
Charles University
Prague, Czechoslovakia

The main role in the regulation of anterior pituitary function is played by the hypothalamic hypophysiotrophic factors or hormones (Guillemin 1964, 1967, Schally et al. 1968, McCann et al. 1968, McCann and Porter 1969, Harris and George 1969, Schreiber 1969, Campbell 1970, Meites 1970). Most of the available evidence shows that the primary effect of these factors is the release of anterior pituitary hormones into the blood, i.e., their secretion, and not their increased synthesis. The whole question is still awaiting a final answer and it will probably not be long before it is demonstrated that the hypothalamic hypophysiotrophic hormones directly influence biosynthesis of the anterior pituitary hormones, as preliminary evidence already exists (Geschwind 1970).

At present we know nothing of the factors regulating the growth and histological and histochemical properties of the anterior pituitary and the differentiation of its individual types of cells. In studies investigating the hypothalamic hypophysiotrophic hormones, structural changes in anterior pituitary grafts directly exposed to the action of hypothalamic extracts were described (Nikitovitch-Winer and Evans 1964, Ducommun and Guillemin 1966, Evans and Nikitovitch-Winer 1969). The structural differentiation of anterior pituitary grafts in the "adenohypophysiotrophic" area of the hypothalamus is also evidence of the trophic and differentiative effects of hypothalamic factors on the anterior pituitary (Halász et al. 1962, Halász et al. 1965, Flament-Durand 1965). Studies with purified individual hypothalamic hypophysiotrophic hormones, however, testify mainly to a primary effect on secretion.

The anterior pituitary, in association with its function, undergoes marked morphological, histological and histochemical changes, which presumably require regulatory mechanisms. We can hardly follow these changes in peripheral blood, as in the presence of a diminished peripheral hormone level, trophic and biochemical changes in the anterior pituitary are not infrequently the reverse of changes in other tissues. Examples can be found in the studies of Tonoue and Yamamoto (1967) and Matsuzaki (1968) showing differences in the reaction of pituitary and liver enzymes to thyroidectomy or substitutive thyroxine administration. We must therefore conclude that there is another regulatory factor, or that this additional factor acts in combination with a change in the blood level of the hormones of the peripheral endocrine glands.

Some authors are of the opinion that the factors regulating secretion of the anterior pituitary hormones are different from those responsible for growth of the anterior pituitary. Purves (1963), e.g., concluded: "Certainly, there would appear to be trophic influences which come down the stalk by way of the blood vessels and which are important for the preservation of cytological appearance and function of the cells. I do not think that the trophic effect is the regulatory mechanism, however". Florsheim (1969), in a review of hypothalamic regulation of TSH secretion, analysed findings on the role of the specific thyrotrophin-releasing hormone (TRH or TRF) and went on: ". . . we have to postulate a second hypothalamic factor involved in pituitary thyrotrophic function. This second factor, probably identical with Halász's hypophysiotrophic substance, maintains normal pituitary architecture . . ." Despite this, the existence of hypothalamic hypophysiotrophic (growth) factors is still purely hypothetical.

The strongest anterior pituitary growth reaction is the hypertrophy following chronic oestrogen treatment. This type of hypertrophy was chosen as an experimental model for this study because it was found previously that this type of anterior pituitary hypertrophy can be blocked by simultaneous treatment with excess thyroid hormones (Zbuzková-Kmentová and Schreiber 1966, 1967). The finding of increased thyroxine binding to the proteins of oestrogenized anterior pituitary in vitro forms a connecting link between the present study and the studies on the key role of thyroxine in anterior pituitary growth reactions reviewed previously (Schreiber 1967).

There is no time here to discuss the history of the study of oestrogenized anterior pituitary. The first report on this type of hypertrophy is probably that of Selye et al. (1935) and several dozens of papers on this subject have appeared since that time. The effect of oestrogens in the anterior pituitary seems to be a direct one (e.g., Palka et al. 1966, Lisk 1969). Morphologically the basic characteristic of oestrogen-induced anterior pituitary hypertrophy is proliferation of the acidophilic prolactin (LTH) cells. The tumours formed by the action of oestrogens in the anterior pituitary are also composed of this type of cells and are sometimes known as mammo-somatotrophic tumours (e.g., Farquhar and Furth 1959).

The most significant evidence of the direct action of oestrogens in the anterior pituitary is furnished by studies investigating their distribution, which show that the anterior pituitary behaves like a target tissue for oestrogens (e.g., Jensen and Jacobsohn 1962, Eisenfeld and Axelrod 1966 and many others). The uptake of labelled oestradiol in the anterior pituitary can be inhibited by pre-administration of unlabelled oestradiol (e.g., Kato and Villee 1967) but not with testosterone (Eisenfeld 1970, Eisenfeld and Axelrod 1966). The negative results with testosterone present an interesting problem. It has long been known that testosterone inhibits anterior pituitary hypertrophy after oestrogens (Haour and Selye 1948, Oberling et al. 1950). As will be shown later, in our experiments testosterone not only inhibited anterior pituitary hypertrophy after oestrogens, but also inhibited the increase in thyroxine binding to anterior pituitary proteins in vitro. Testosterone (Emmens and Miller 1969) belongs to the anti-oestrogens which do not inhibit or reduce the oestrogen concentration in the target tissues, but exert their influence by some unknown way.

Another point which should be discussed here is the binding of thyroxine by proteins. This is known for more than 30 years (Trevorrov 1939) and it is impossible to review it here in detail. Suffice it here to say that thyroxine is bound not only by serum proteins but also by proteins of the tissues. Tata (1958) demonstrated binding of the thyroid hormones to several tissue proteins extracted from the skeletal muscles of the rat. Cellular binding protein was also found in rabbit skeletal muscle and brain. It strongly inhibited thyroxine deiodase activity, evidently as a result of competition for thyroxine (Robbins and Rall 1960). There are also several reports on thyroxine binding by the proteins of the anterior pituitary and of anterior pituitary tumours (Grinberg 1964, 1965) and relatively much was reported on the binding of thyroid hormones by the anterior pituitary in vivo (Ford and Gross 1958, Ford et al. 1959, Ford et al. 1962).

MATERIAL AND METHODS

Adult male and female albino rats (descendants of the Wistar strain, Velaz, Prague) were used throughout the experiments. The animals were fed on a standard laboratory diet (Larsen diet, Velaz, Prague) and tap water ad libitum, the environmental temperature was $22 \pm 2°C$ and the illumination as by indirect daylight. All experiments lasted 3–4 weeks and the following substances and dosages were used:

Oestradiol dipropionate (Agofolin, SPOFA), 50 or 100 μg daily in 0.1 or 0.2 ml olive oil, intramuscularly.
Oestradiol benzoate (Agofolin depot, SPOFA), microcrystalline water suspension, 1 mg twice weekly subcutaneously or intramuscularly.
Testosterone isobutyrate (Agovirin depot, SPOFA), microcrystalline water suspension, 2.5 mg weekly subcutaneously.
Cyproterone (6-chloro-Δ^6-1,2α-methylene-17α-hydroxyprogesterone, Schering SH 80881), 0.166‰ in the food, i.e. about 5 mg/rat/day.
Cyproterone acetate (Schering 80714), the same dosage.
Progesterone (Aggolutin depot, SPOFA), microcrystalline water suspension, 5 mg twice weekly intramuscularly.
16-methylene-6-dehydro-17α-acetoxyprogesterone (Superlutin, SPOFA), 0.083 ‰ in the food, i.e. about 2.5 mg/rat/day.
Hydrocortisone acetate ((Hydrocortison, SPOFA suspension per injection), 5 mg weekly subcutaneously.
Clomiphene citrate (2-[p-(2-chloro-1,2-diphenyl-vinyl)phenoxy] triethylamine dihydrogen citrate (Clomid Merrell) 0.042 ‰ in the food, i.e. about 1.25 mg/rat/day (Clomiphene citrate, SPOFA), the same dosage.
Dried thyroid powder (Thyreoidin, SPOFA), 0.2% in the food.
Methylthiouracil (Alkiron, SPOFA), 0.2% in the food.

On the day of termination of the experiment (3–4 weeks after the beginning) the animals were killed by exsanguination, the anterior pituitaries weighed and homogenized in 0.1 N NaCl solution (0.5 ml for 1 mg tissue). The homogenate was filtered through filter paper (Filtrak No. 388) and frozen at $-18°C$; 0.6 ml filtrate was used for the determination of proteins (Lowry et al. 1951) and 1 ml for the determination of the binding of thyroxine by anterior pituitary proteins in vitro (Schreiber et al. 1970a). The solution of ^{125}I-thyroxine (The Radiochemical

Centre, Amersham, England) mixed with stable thyroxine (Thyroxine, Roche) was used for 1 hour incubation. After precipitation with 20 per cent trichloracetic acid, centrifugation, washing the sediment with trichloracetic acid and the second centrifugation, the radioactivity of the sediment was measured in a well detector connected with NK 108 amplitude analyser (Gamma, Budapest). The percentage of radioactivity taken up by the protein in 1 ml homogenate was determined and binding was calculated as the number of μg thyroxine per mg fresh anterior pituitary and per mg protein in the solution. Means $\pm$ 95 per cent confidence limits were calculated and the results were evaluated statistically by variance analysis and the significance of differences of means was determined by Duncan's (Duncan 1955) test.

RESULTS

All experiments reported here were repeated at least twice and most of them three or four times. Only representative examples of the results are given here and full information can be found in the original publications, cited in the relevant paragraphs. These original papers also contain the additional information on radioiodine uptake in the thyroid gland, weights of the other endocrine glands and other organs, etc. The biochemical characteristics of thyroxine binding by anterior pituitary protein in vitro are dealt with in separate communications (Přibyl et al. 1971, 1972): thyroxine binds to the proteins and not to the nucleic acids; the binding can be demonstrated also by gel filtration on Sephadex columns; the bound substance is probably thyroxine and not iodide split from thyroxine by deiodination; some substances known as inhibitors of the binding of thyroxine to plasma proteins are effective also in our in vitro system (oleate, dinitrophenol). It should be mentioned that of course thyroxine is bound by proteins of all tissues of the body. On the other hand, the increase observed after oestrogen treatment occurs in the adrenals and salivary glands, and also in the anterior pituitary, plasma and spleen.

FUNDAMENTAL OBSERVATION: THE EFFECT OF OESTRADIOL

Two to four weeks' treatment of male and female rats with oestradiol dipropionate was found to increase anterior pituitary weight and the binding of thyroxine by anterior pituitary proteins in vitro simultaneously (Schreiber et al. 1970a, 1970b). An example of this reaction is shown in Fig. 1. The increase of thyroxine binding is both quantitative (per mg wet weight) and qualitative (per mg protein): this shows possible qualitative alterations of the proteins of the oestrogenized anterior pituitary.

INHIBITORY EFFECT OF EXCESS THYROID HORMONES

Simultaneous treatment of the oestrogenized rats with excess thyroid hormones produced a decrease in anterior pituitary hypertrophy as well as in thyroxine binding (Schreiber et al. 1970a, 1970b) as shown in Fig. 2. It is obvious that simultaneous as well as previous+simultaneous treatment with thyroid hormones inhibited both reactions of the anterior pituitary to oestrogens. There was no

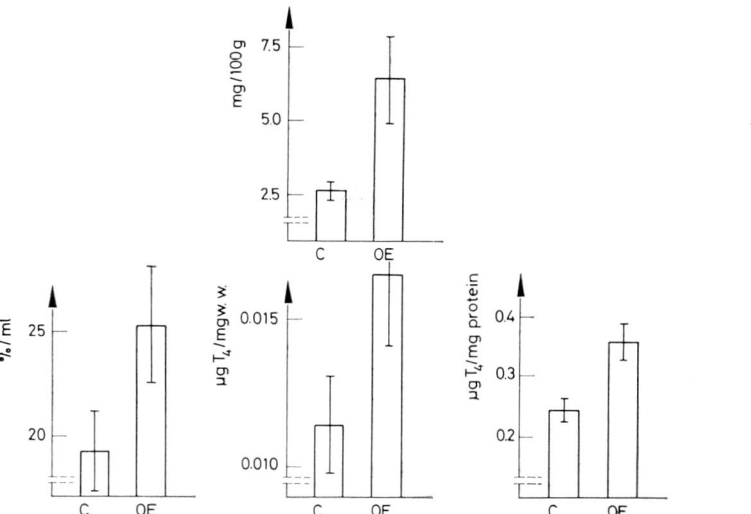

Fig. 1. Anterior pituitary weights (above) and thyroxine binding by anterior pituitary proteins in vitro (% dose/ml homogenate, µg T_4/mg wet weight, µg T_4/mg protein) in control (C) and oestradiol dipropionate-treated (100 µg daily for 3 weeks) male rats (OE). Means ± 95% confidence limits

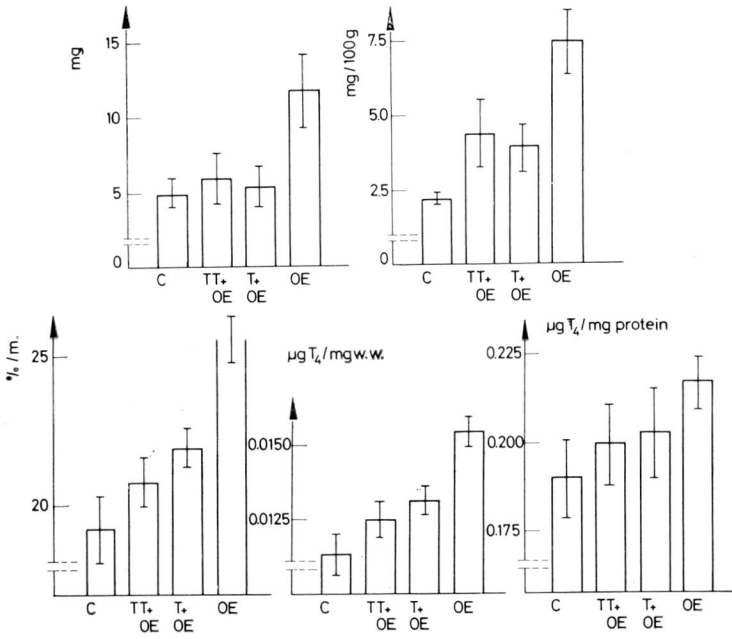

Fig. 2. Anterior pituitary weights (above) and thyroxine binding by anterior pituitary proteins in vitro in control (C) and oestradiol dipropionate-treated rats (OE), in rats treated simultaneously with dried thyroid and oestradiol (T+OE) and in rats treated previously+simultaneously with dried thyroid (TT+OE). Means±95% confidence limits

difference in either treatment as far as anterior pituitary weight is concerned, but the previous+simultaneous treatment was slightly more effective in influencing the binding of thyroxine: the difference between these two groups was not statistically significant, however. Another finding, not mentioned here, was that treatment of control (not oestrogenized) rats with thyroxine slightly decreased and treatment with methylthiouracil slightly increased thyroxine binding.

INHIBITORY EFFECT OF TESTOSTERONE

Simultaneous treatment of oestrogenized rats with testosterone inhibited simultaneously anterior pituitary growth and the increase in thyroxine binding (Schreiber et al. 1970c, 1971a) as shown in Fig. 3. Castration itself produced an increase in anterior pituitary weight but not in thyroxine binding. Castration potentiated the effect of oestrogen on anterior pituitary weight but not on thyroxine binding.

EFFECT OF THE ANTIANDROGEN CYPROTERONE AND CYPROTERONE ACETATE

As testosterone had an inhibitory effect on the reaction of the anterior pituitary, as to oestrogen treatment, a potentiating effect of the antiandrogen could be anticipated. This was not found to be true (Schreiber et al. 1971b, c) as shown in Fig. 4. Cyproterone acetate slightly increased anterior pituitary weight and both antiandrogens slightly increased thyroxine binding, but they partially blocked the stimulating effect of oestradiol treatment. This shows that possibly oestrogens, androgens and antiandrogens compete for identical protein binding sites in the anterior pituitary.

EFFECT OF PROGESTERONE AND HYDROCORTISONE: COMPARISON WITH TESTOSTERONE

Since the gestagenic or corticoid effects of the antiandrogens could be the cause of their action in our testing system, we also tested progesterone and hydrocortisone, and for control, again testosterone (Schreiber et al. 1971a). Oestrogen again produced an increase in anterior pituitary weight and thyroxine binding as shown in Fig. 5. Its effect was again blocked by testosterone. Progesterone had in males a similar effect as oestradiol, i.e. it increased anterior pituitary weight and thyroxine binding. Progesterone did not, however, inhibit the reaction to oestrogen. Hydrocortisone was without effect. This shows that the anterior pituitary effect of the antiandrogens was not caused by their gestagenic or corticoid properties. The similarity between the effect of progesterone and effect of oestradiol was possibly caused by the conversion of progesterone to oestrogens in vivo.

A similar experiment on females gave identical results (Fig. 6) except that progesterone did not increase anterior pituitary weight although it still increased thyroxine binding. Again, neither progesterone nor hydrocortisone blocked the effect of oestradiol.

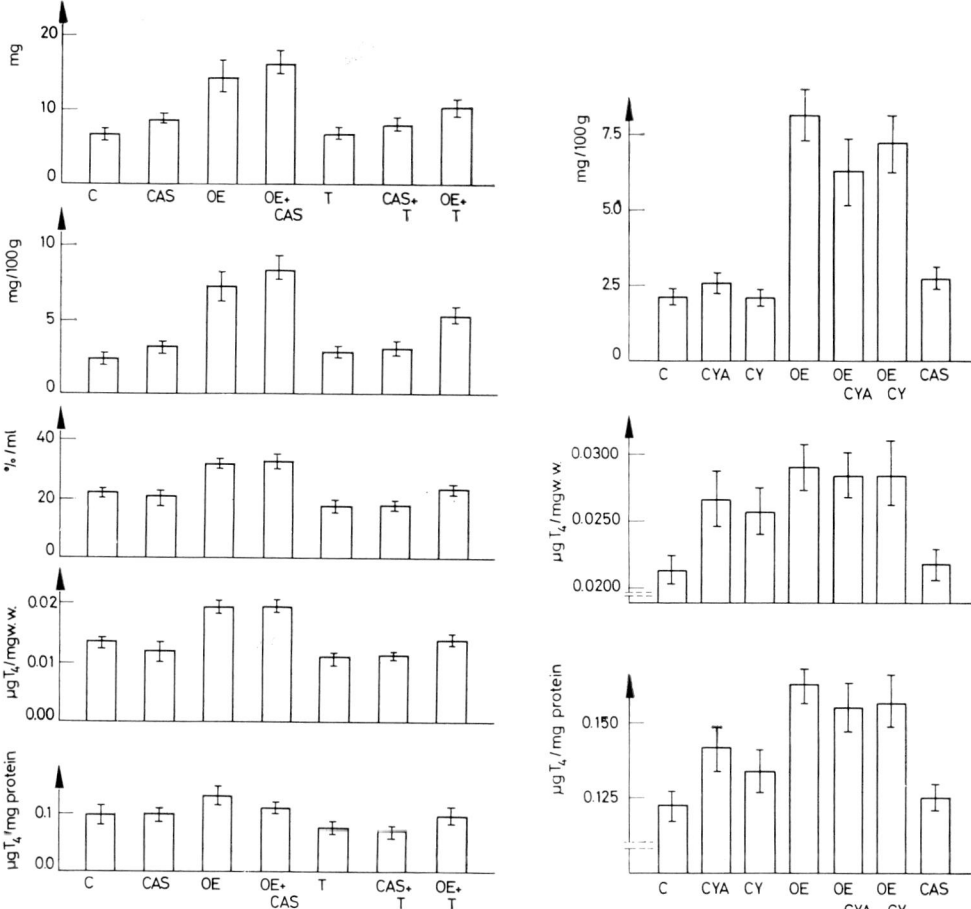

Fig. 3. Absolute (mg) and relative (mg/100 g) anterior pituitary weights and thyroxine binding by anterior pituitary proteins in vitro in control male rats (C), castrated (CAS), oestradiol dipropionate-treated (OE) and testosterone-treated rats (T), as well as after combined treatments. Means ± 95% confidence limits

Fig. 4. Relative anterior pituitary weights (mg/100 g) and thyroxine binding by anterior pituitary proteins in vitro (μg T_4/mg wet weight, μg T_4/mg protein) in control male rats (C), rats treated with cyproterone (CY), cyproterone acetate (CYA), oestradiol benzoate (OE) and after castration (CAS). Means ± 95% confidence limits

149

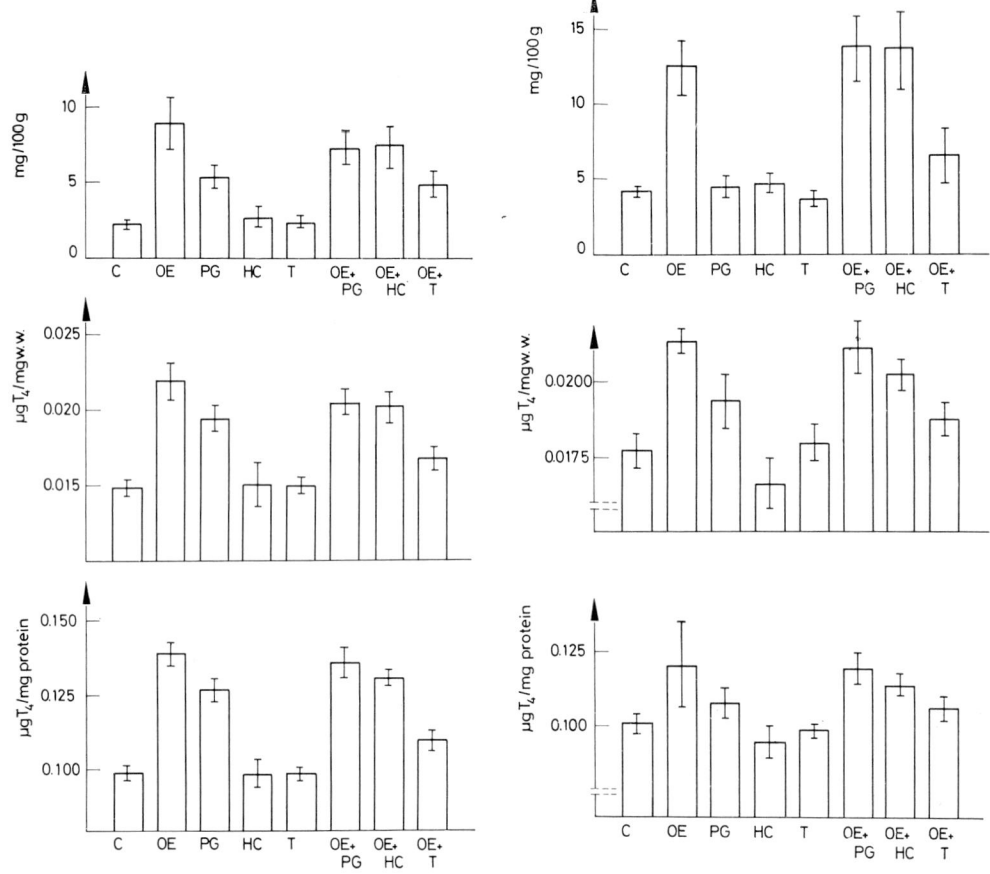

Fig. 5. Relative anterior pituitary weights and thyroxine binding in male control rats (C), rats treated with oestradiol benzoate (OE), progesterone (PG), hydrocortisone (HC), testosterone (T) and their combinations. Means ± 95% confidence limits

Fig. 6. Relative anterior pituitary weights and thyroxine binding in female control rats (C), rats treated with oestradiol benzoate (OE), progesterone (PG), hydrocortisone (HC), testosterone (T) and their combinations. Means ± 95% confidence limits

EFFECT OF 16-METHYLENE-6-DEHYDRO-17α-ACETOXYPROGESTERONE

This synthetic gestagen, which is not a precursor of oestrogens in vivo, was used in the same series of experiments (Schreiber et al. 1971d). An example of its action is given in Fig. 7. This hormone had no effect on anterior pituitary weight and thyroxine binding, but it blocked partially the effect of oestradiol. Since the antiandrogens had an effect on thyroxine binding it seems that their anterior pituitary effects cannot be ascribed to their gestagenic activity.

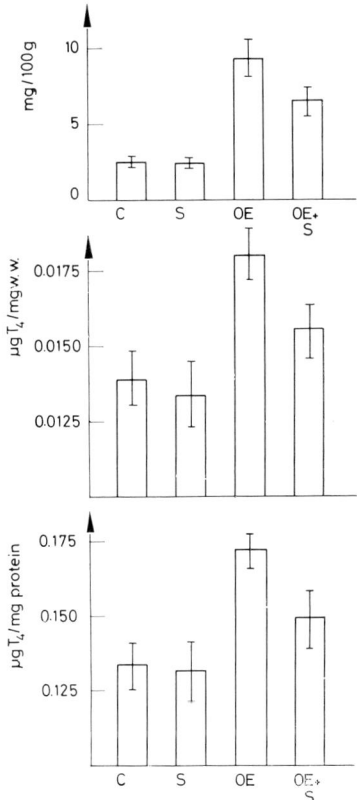

Fig. 7. Relative anterior pituitary weights and thyroxine binding in control male rats (C), rats treated with 16-methylene-6-dehydro-17α-acetoxyprogesterone (S), rats treated with oestradiol benzoate (OE) and after combined treatment (OE+S). Means ± 95% confidence limits

EFFECT OF THE ANTIOESTROGEN CLOMIPHENE

The last substance which was used in our in vitro system up to now is antioestrogen clomiphene (Schreiber et al. 1972). The results in male rats are shown in Fig. 8. Neither preparation of clomiphene changed anterior pituitary weight and thyroxine binding but significantly inhibited the effect of oestradiol benzoate.

They behaved as true antioestrogens in this respect and did not show any oestrogenic activity, although they increased adrenal weight (like oestrogens) and did not block the effect of the given (high) dose of oestradiol on uterine weight.

The results of a similar experiment on female rats are shown in Fig. 9. The results are practically the same with the exception that the antioestrogens produced a complete block of the oestrogenic effect both on anterior pituitary weight and thyroxine binding and one of the clomiphene preparations decreased also normal (not oestrogenized) anterior pituitary weight and thyroxine binding.

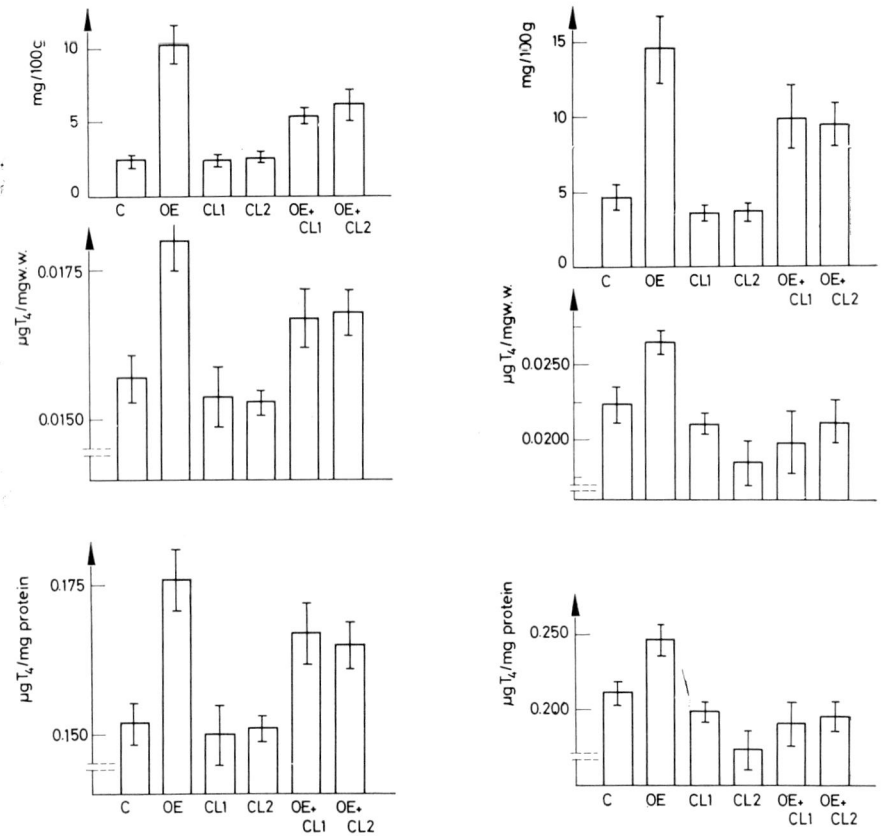

Fig. 8. Relative anterior pituitary weights and thyroxine binding in control male rats (C), rats treated with oestradiol benzoate (OE), rats treated with two preparations of clomiphene citrate (CL1, CL2) and after combined treatments. Means ± 95% confidence limits

Fig. 9. Relative anterior pituitary weights and thyroxine binding in control female rats (C), rats treated with oestradiol benzoate (OE), rats treated with two different preparations of clomiphene citrate (CL1, CL2) and after combined treatments. Means ± 95% confidence limits

DISCUSSION

The results of effects of the various hormones and antihormones used in this study can be summarized in Table 1.

TABLE 1

Isolated effects		
Treatment	Anterior pituitary weight	Thyroxine binding
Oestrogen (oestradiol dipropionate or benzoate)	++++	++++
Androgen (testosterone isobutyrate)	0	—
Gestagen (progesterone) (16-methylene-6-dehydro-17α-acetoxyprogesterone)	++ (males) 0	++ 0
Corticoid (hydrocortisone)	0	0
Antiandrogen (cyproterone acetate)	++	++
Antioestrogen (clomiphene citrate)	0 (females)	0

Modification of effect of oestradiol		
Treatment (in addition to oestradiol)	Anterior pituitary weight	Thyroxine binding
Androgen (testosterone isobutyrate)	—	—
Gestagen (progesterone) (16-methylene-6-dehydro-17α-acetoxyprogesterone)	0 —	0 —
Corticoid (hydrocortisone)	0	0
Antiandrogen (cyproterone acetate)	—	—
Antioestrogen (clomiphene citrate)	—	—

Since the growth effect of oestrogens in the anterior pituitary is probably a direct one, the most probable explanation of our findings is the competition of the steroids and antihormones for protein binding sites in the anterior pituitary. There is a striking parallelity between anterior pituitary growth reaction and changes in thyroxine binding by anterior pituitary proteins in vitro. There are, however, several exceptions to this parallelity: castration produced anterior pituitary growth but not an increase in thyroxine binding; cyproterone increased thyroxine binding but not anterior pituitary weight; progesterone increased thyroxine binding in females but not anterior pituitary weight. The biochemical basis of the observed association of thyroxine with anterior pituitary protein in vitro still remains unclear but it seems that this phenomenon could be of considerable physiological importance In addition, our results suggest that thyroxine behaves in the anterior pituitary model used as an antigrowth (and possibly antitumorous) agent.

SUMMARY

Chronic oestrogen treatment produced increase in anterior pituitary weight and simultaneously an increase in thyroxine binding by anterior pituitary proteins in vitro. This effect could be inhibited by simultaneous treatment with excess thyroxine hormones and with testosterone. The antiandrogen cyproterone acetate slightly increased anterior pituitary weight and thyroxine binding but it partly inhibited both reactions to oestradiol. Progesterone increased anterior pituitary weight in males and thyroxine binding in both sexes. The anterior pituitary reaction to oestradiol was not changed by simultaneous progesterone treatment. Hydrocortisone was without any effect. 16-Methylene-6-dehydro-17α-acetoxyprogesterone itself had no effect but it inhibited both reactions of the anterior pituitary to oestradiol. The antioestrogen clomiphene itself had no effect but it blocked the anterior pituitary response (growth and increase in thyroxine binding in vitro) to oestradiol.

REFERENCES

CAMPBELL, H. J. (1970): Control of anterior pituitary gland by hypothalamic releasing factors. *Sci. Basis Med. Ann. Rev.* **152**.

DUCOMMUN, S. and GUILLEMIN, R. (1966): Maintenance of normal morphology in adenohypophysial transplants by topical administration of hypothalamic extract with a simple method for transplantation in a pneumoderma pouch. *Proc. Soc. exp. Biol.* (N.Y.) **122**, 1251.

DUNCAN, D. B. (1955): Multiple range and multiple F tests. *Biometrics* **11**, 1.

EISENFELD, A. J. (1970): ^{3}H-oestradiol: in vitro binding to macromolecules from the rat hypothalamus, anterior pituitary and uterus. *Endocrinology* **86**, 1313.

EISENFELD, A. J. and AXELROD, J. (1966): Selectivity of estrogen distribution in tissues. *J. Pharmacol. exp. Ther.* **150**, 469.

EMMENS, C. W. and MILLER, B. G. (1969): Estrogens, proestrogens and antiestrogens. *Steroids* **13**, 725.

EVANS, J. S. and NIKITOVITCH-WINER, M. B. (1969): Functional reactivation and cytological restoration of pituitary grafts by continuous local intravenous infusion of median eminence extracts. *Neuroendocrinology* **4**, 83.

FARQUHAR, M. G. and FURTH, J. (1959): Electron microscopy of experimental pituitary tumors. *Amer. J. Path.* **35**, 698.

FLAMENT-DURAND, J. (1965): Observations on pituitary transplants into the hypothalamus of the rat. *Endocrinology* **77**, 446.

FLORSHEIM, W. H. (1969): Hypothalamic influences on pituitary thyrotrophic function. In: *Physiology and Pathology of Adaptation Mechanisms*. Ed. by E. Bajusz. Pergamon Press, Oxford.

FORD, D. H. and GROSS, J. (1958): The metabolism of ^{131}I-labelled thyroid hormones in the hypophysis and brain of the rabbit. *Endocrinology* **62**, 416.

FORD, D. H., KANTOUNIS, S. and LAWRENCE, R. (1959): The localization of ^{131}I-labelled triiodothyronine in the pituitary and brain of normal and thyroidectomized male rats. *Endocrinology* **64**, 977.

FORD, D. H., FISHMAN, S. K. and RHINES, R. (1962): The uptake of ^{131}I-labelled L-triiodothyronine by the brain, pituitary and muscle of diestrous and estrous female rats as compared with the uptake in male rats. *Gen. comp. Endocr.* **2**, 480.

GESCHWIND, I. I. (1970): Mechanism of action of hypothalamic adenohypophysiotropic factors. In: *Hypophysiotropic Hormones of the Hypothalamus: Assay and Chemistry*. Ed. by J. Meites. Williams and Wilkins Co., Baltimore.

GRINBERG, R. (1964): Effect of epinephrine on metabolism of thyroxine by pituitary and brain. *Proc. Soc. exp. Biol.* (N.Y.) **116**, 35.

GRINBERG, R. (1965): Binding of thyroxine and triiodothyronine by heart and pituitary proteins. *Nature* (Lond.) **205**, 701.

GUILLEMIN, R. (1964): Hypothalamic factors releasing pituitary hormones. *Recent Progr. Hormone Res.* **20,** 89.
GUILLEMIN, R. (1967): The adenohypophysis and its hypothalamic control. *Ann. Rev. Physiol.* **29,** 313.
HALÁSZ, B., PUPP, L. and UHLARIK, S. (1962): Hypophysiotrophic area in the hypothalamus. *J. Endocr.* **25,** 147.
HALÁSZ, B., PUPP, L., UHLARIK, S. and TIMA, L. (1965): Further studies on the hormone secretion of the anterior pituitary transplanted into the hypophysiotrophic area of the rat hypothalamus. *Endocrinology* **77,** 343.
HAOUR, P. and SELYE, H. (1948): Inhibition des effets morphogènes produits par les folliculoïdes sur l'hypophyse du rat. *Ann. Endocr. (Paris)* **9,** 154.
HARRIS, G. W. and GEORGE, R. (1969): Neurohormonal control of the adenohypophysis and the regulation of the secretion of TSH, ACTH and growth hormone. In: *The Hypothalamus.* Ed. by W. Haymaker, E. Anderson and W. J. H. Nauta. C. C. Thomas, Springfield, Ill.
JENSEN, E. V. and JACOBSOHN, H. I. (1962): Basic guides to the mechanism of estrogen action. *Recent Progr. Hormone Res.* **18,** 387.
KATO, J. and VILLEE, C. A. (1967): Factors affecting uptake of estradiol-6,7-^{3}H by the hypophysis and hypothalamus. *Endocrinology* **80,** 1133.
LISK, R. D. (1969): Oestrogen: direct effects on hypothalamus or pituitary in relation to pituitary weight changes. *Neuroendocrinology* **4,** 368.
LOWRY, O. H., ROSEBROUGH, N. J., FARR, A. L. and RANDALL, R. J. (1951): Protein measurement with the Folin phenol reagent. *J. biol. Chem.* **193,** 265.
MATSUZAKI, S. (1968): Difference in effects of thyroidectomy and thyroxine supplements on hepatic and anterior pituitary enzymes in the rat. *Endocr. jap.* **15,** 223.
McCANN, S. M. and PORTER, J. C. (1969): Hypothalamic-pituitary stimulating and inhibiting hormones. *Physiol. Rev.* **49,** 240.
McCANN, S. M., DHARIWAL, A. P. S. and PORTER, J. C. (1968): Regulation of the adenohypophysis. *Ann. Rev. Physiol.* **30,** 589.
MEITES, J. (Ed.) (1970): *Hypophysiotropic Hormones of the Hypothalamus: Assay and Chemistry.* Williams and Wilkins, Baltimore.
NIKITOVITCH-WINER, M. B. and EVANS, J. S. (1964): Reactivation of hypophysial grafts by continued perfusion with median eminence extracts. In: *Proceedings of 2nd International Congress of Endocrinology.* Excerpta Medica, Amsterdam. p. 1278.
OBERLING, C., GUÉRIN, M., SÈZE, L. DE and LACOUR (1950): Production de tumeurs hypophysaires et mammaires chez le rat par injection de folliculine seule où associée à d'autres hormones. *Bull. Ass. franç. Cancer* **37,** 176.
PALKA, Y. S., RAMIREZ, V. D. and SAWYER, C. H. (1966): Distribution and biological effects of tritiated estradiol implanted in the hypothalamo-hypophysial region of female rats. *Endocrinology* **78,** 487.
PŘIBYL, T., SCHREIBER, V. and ROHÁČOVÁ, J. (1971): Binding of thyroxine by rat tissue proteins. *Physiol. bohemoslov.* **20.**
PŘIBYL, T., SCHREIBER, V. and ROHÁČOVÁ, J. (1972): Further characteristic of the binding of thyroxine by adenohypophysial proteins in vitro. (In press.)
PURVES, H. D. (1963): Discussion. In: *Thyrotropin.* Ed. by S. C. Werner. Thomas, Springfield, Ill. p. 73.
ROBBINS, J. and RALL, J. E. (1960): Protein associated with thyroid hormones. *Physiol. Rev.* **40,** 415.
SCHALLY, A. V., ARIMURA, A., BOWERS, C. Y., KASTIN, A. J., SAWANO, S. and REDDING, T. W. (1968): Hypothalamic neurohormones regulating anterior pituitary function. *Recent Progr. Hormone Res.* **24,** 497.
SCHREIBER, V. (1967): Functions of the adenohypophysis: special position of thyrotrophic function. *Acta Univ. Carol. Med. (Praha)* **13,** 493.
SCHREIBER, V. (1969): Chemistry of hypothalamic releasing factors. Excerpta Medica International Congress Series **184,** 555.
SCHREIBER, V., PŘIBYL, T. and ROHÁČOVÁ, J. (1970a): Adenohypophysial growth after oestrogens in rats: binding of ^{125}I-thyroxine by adenohypophysial proteins. *Physiol. bohemoslov.* **19,** 501.
SCHREIBER, V., PŘIBYL, T. and ROHÁČOVÁ, J. (1970b): Hypertrofie adenohypofysy

po estrogenech: vazba ^{125}I-thyroxinu na adenohypofysární proteiny. *Čs. Fysiol.* **19,** 275.

SCHREIBER, V., PŘIBYL, T. and ROHÁČOVÁ, J. (1970c): Sex hormones and adenohypophysial weight: interaction of gonadectomy, oestradiol and testosterone in rats. *Physiol. bohemoslov.* **19,** 511.

SCHREIBER, V., PŘIBYL, T. and ROHÁČOVÁ, J. (1971a): Hypertrofie adenohypofysy u krys po estrogenu: interakce s testosterone. *Sborn. lék.* **73,** 49.

SCHREIBER, V., PŘIBYL, T. and ROHÁČOVÁ, J. (1971b): Effect of the anti-androgen cyproterone acetate on the action of oestrogen on the rat endocrine system. *Physiol. bohemoslov.* **20,** 255—261.

SCHREIBER, V., PŘIBYL, T. and ROHÁČOVÁ, J. (1971c): Vergleich der Wirkung der Antiandrogene Cyproteron und Cyproteron Acetat auf das endokrine System der Ratten. *Endokrinologie.* (In press.)

SCHREIBER, V., PŘIBYL, T. and ROHÁČOVÁ, J. (1971d): Adenohypophysial weight and thyroxine binding by adenohypophysial proteins in vitro: interaction of oestradiol with gestagens, hydrocortisone and testosterone. *Physiol. bohemoslov.* (In press.)

SCHREIBER, V., PŘIBYL, T. and ROHÁČOVÁ, J. (1972): Der Einfluß des Anti-Oestrogens Clomiphen auf die adenohypophysäre Reaktion auf Oestradiol. *Endokrinologie.* (In press.)

SELYE, H., COLLIP, J. B. and THOMSON, D. L. (1935): Effect of oestrin on ovaries and adrenals. *Proc. Soc. exp. Biol. (N.Y.)* **32,** 1377.

TATA, J. R. (1958): A cellular thyroxine-binding protein fraction. *Biochim. biophys. Acta (Amst.)* **28,** 91.

TONOUE, T. and YAMAMOTO, K. (1967): Effect of thyroidectomy and a thyroxine supplement on amino acid incorporation into proteins of rat anterior pituitary. *Endocrinology* **81,** 1029.

TREVORROV, V. (1939): Studies on the nature of the iodine in blood. *J. biol. Chem.* **127,** 737.

ZBUZKOVÁ-KMENTOVÁ, V. and SCHREIBER, V. (1966): Empêchement par les hormones thyroïdiennes de l'hypertrophie hypophysaire causée par l'oestrogène. *C.R. Acad. Sci. (Paris)* **262,** 1565.

ZBUZKOVÁ-KMENTOVÁ, V. and SCHREIBER, V. (1967): Gonado-thyroidal relationships: interactions of oestrogens and thyroid hormones in infantile rats. *Endocr. Exp.* **1,** 29.

HYPOPHYSIOTROPIC HORMONES, CYCLIC AMP AND ANTERIOR PITUITARY PROTEIN SYNTHESIS AND RELEASE

F. LABRIE, G. PELLETIER, A. LEMAY, S. LEMAIRE, G. POIRIER,
N. BARDEN, G. BÉRAUD, R. BOUCHER, M. GAUTHIER and A. DELÉAN

Department of Physiology
Medical Faculty of Laval University
Quebec, Canada

INTRODUCTION

Physiological and anatomical evidence has established for quite some time that the secretion of the anterior pituitary hormones is under the control of substances originating from the hypothalamus and transported, via a portal system, to the anterior pituitary (Fig. 1 — Meites and Nicoll 1966, Guillemin 1967, McCann and Porter 1969, Meites 1970). Very important knowledge on the mechanism of action of the hypothalamic hypophysiotropic hormones (also called hypothalamic releasing factors) has been gained using hypothalamic extracts at various stages of the purification, but the recent availability of a pure releasing factor of known molecular structure, TRF (Burgus et al. 1969, Boler et al. 1969), brings more confidence and opens new possibilities for this area of investigation.

POSSIBLE ROLES OF ADENOSINE 3',5'-MONOPHOSPHATE IN ANTERIOR PITUITARY FUNCTION

The action of many polypeptide hormones and of catecholamines is at least partly mediated by changes of the levels of cyclic AMP in target cells (Robison et al. 1969) and much effort is currently devoted to the elucidation of the role of the cyclic nucleotide in a wide variety of biological systems (Robison et al. 1969, Greengard and Costa 1970). Recent evidence suggested that cyclic AMP might also be involved in the mechanism of action of the hypothalamic releasing factors in the anterior pituitary gland (Zor et al. 1969, Bowers et al. 1968). A crude hypothalamic extract (Zor et al. 1969, 1970) and purified thyrotropin-releasing factor (Bowers et al. 1968) stimulated adenyl cyclase activity in rat anterior pituitary gland in vitro.

As mediator of the action of the hypothalamic hypophysiotropic hormones, cyclic AMP could act at many sites, including among others, the synthesis, intracisternal transport, packaging, storage and release of proteins, activity of the lysosomes, supply of energy and RNA synthesis or transport (Fig. 2). Our first studies were aimed at investigating the effect of cyclic AMP on protein synthesis and release in the rat anterior pituitary gland in vitro.

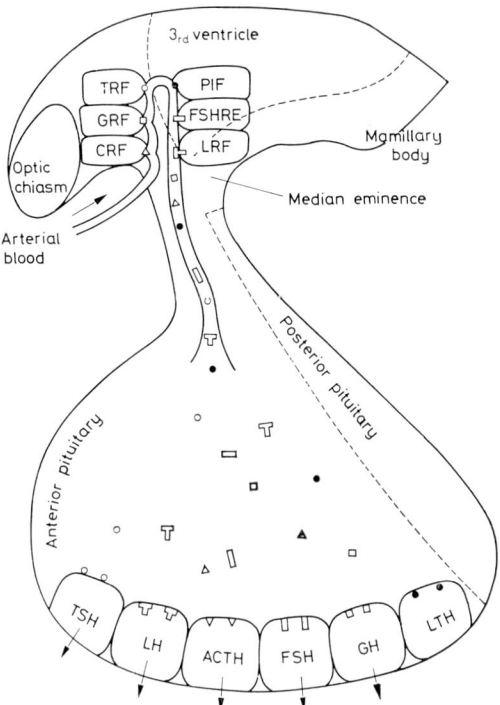

Fig. 1. Schematic representation of the hypothalamo-anterior pituitary complex. TSH, thyrotropic hormone; LH, luteinizing hormone; ACTH, adrenocorticotropic hormone; FSH, follicle-stimulating hormone; GH, growth hormone; LTH, prolactin; TRF, thyrotropin-releasing factor; GRF, growth hormone-releasing factor; CRF, corticotropin-releasing factor; PIF, prolactin-inhibiting factor; FSHRF, follicle-stimulating hormone-releasing factor; LRF, luteinizing hormone-releasing factor

CYCLIC AMP AND TOTAL PROTEIN SYNTHESIS

The rates of protein synthesis at different times after addition of dibutyryl cyclic AMP (dbcAMP) were measured by 45-min pulses with ^{14}C-leucine beginning at various times after addition of the cyclic nucleotide (Labrie et al. 1971). Figure 3 shows that the maximal rate of increase is found after 150 min of incubation with dbcAMP (5 mM), the level of stimulation ranging between 50 and 80 per cent in different experiments. Under these conditions, there was no change of the radioactive amino acid pool, suggesting that true stimulation of protein synthesis occurs with cyclic AMP. Signs of increased activity of the Golgi apparatus after incubation with dbcAMP were evidenced in both the somatotrophs (Fig. 4) and prolactin-secreting cells. DbcAMP has also been shown to stimulate the synthesis of total cellular proteins and amylase in the rat parotid gland (Wicks et al. 1971) and to induce rat liver tyrosine transaminase in the intact animal (Jolicœur and Labrie, in press, Wicks 1968) and in foetal organ maintained in culture (Wicks 1968).

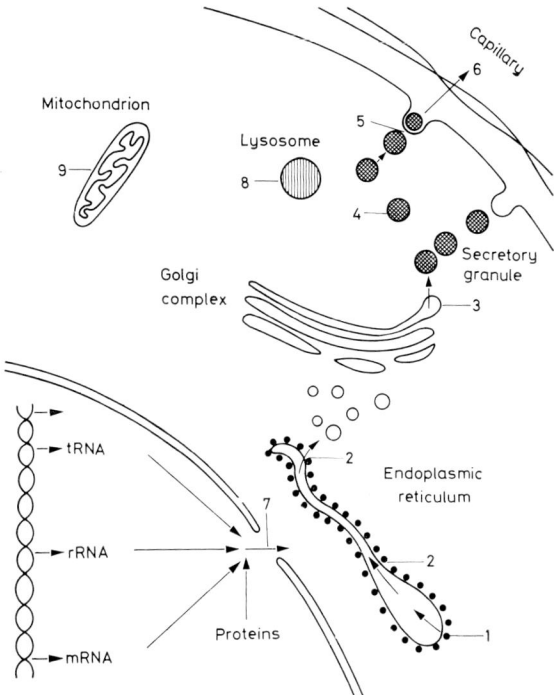

Fig. 2. Diagram of the probable sequence of intracellular processing of secretory proteins in the anterior-pituitary cell and some possible sites of control: 1, polypeptide synthesis on the rough endoplasmic reticulum (RER); 2, transport through the cisternae of the endoplasmic reticulum to the Golgi complex; 3, formation of secretory granules; 4, storage of exportable material; 5, release; 6, transport from the basement membrane to the general circulation; 7, RNA synthesis and transport to the cytoplasm; 8, lysosomal activity and, 9, supply of energy (modified from Smith and Farquhar, *J. cell. Biol.* **31**, 319, 1966)

The role of RNA synthesis in the stimulatory effect of cyclic AMP on protein synthesis was investigated with Actinomycin D, an inhibitor of DNA-dependent RNA synthesis. Actinomycin D, at a dose (25 μg/ml) that inhibits total RNA synthesis to 10 per cent of its control rate during a 5-hour incubation period, is without apparent effect on the stimulatory action of cyclic AMP on either total protein synthesis or release (Fig. 5).

Since maximal stimulation of protein synthesis by dbcAMP occurs between $1\frac{1}{2}$ and $2\frac{1}{2}$ hours after addition of dbcAMP, a possible effect of cyclic AMP on RNA synthesis was studied during a $2\frac{1}{4}$ hour period in the presence of the cyclic nucleotide. There was no detectable effect of dbcAMP on the incorporation of ^{3}H-uridine into total RNA or into the individual species of cytoplasmic RNA as separated on sucrose gradients (Fig. 6). Similar results were obtained with nuclear RNA extracted with phenol-sodium dodecyl sulphate (Labrie 1969) at room temperature (Fig. 7) or at 65°C (data not shown). These findings suggest that

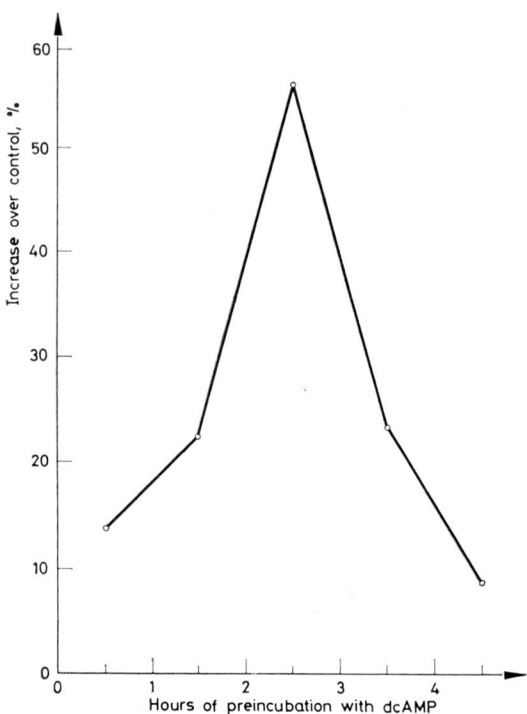

Fig. 3. Time course of the stimulatory effect of dibutyryl cyclic AMP on the rates of anterior pituitary protein synthesis. The pooled results of two similar experiments are presented. Pituitary halves (four per group) of male rats (300 to 500 g) were incubated in KRBG in the presence or absence of dibutyryl cyclic AMP (5 mM) and, at the times shown, 0.5 µCi of ^{14}C-leucine was added for 45 min. Pituitary halves from the same animal served as control. Tissue was homogenized and the trichloracetic-insoluble radioactivity was measured. (Reproduced from Labrie et al., *J. biol. Chem.* **246,** 1902, 1971)

cyclic AMP stimulates protein synthesis in the anterior pituitary gland, at the translation level, through activation of a stable messenger RNA. It remains, however, possible that a small fraction of DNA-dependent RNA synthesis is refractory to such doses of Actinomycin or cannot be detected by our separation techniques and that this small fraction is responsible for the cyclic AMP-dependent stimulation of protein synthesis.

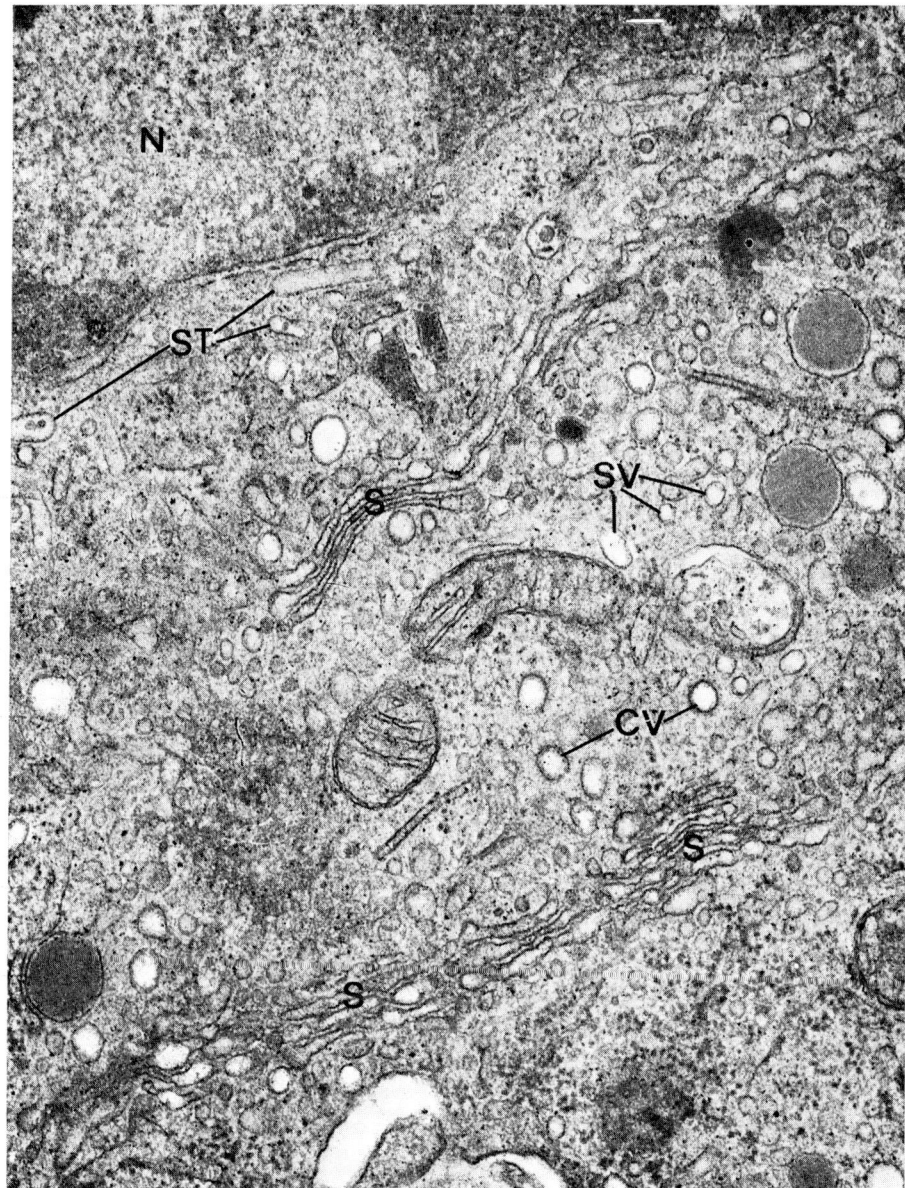

Fig. 4. Somatotrophic cell after 6 hours of incubation in the presence of dbcAMP (5 mM). The Golgi area occupies a volume larger than in the control cell. The parallel saccules (S) are longer than in normal cells. The striking feature is the appearance of a large number of smooth vesicles (SV) associated with the saccules. Coated vesicles (CV) typically associated with the Golgi apparatus are moderately increased in number. It is also important to note the appearance of smooth tubular (ST) structures in the vicinity of the Golgi complex. These tubules have a diameter close to that of the smooth vesicles. (N) nucleus ($\times$ 36,000)

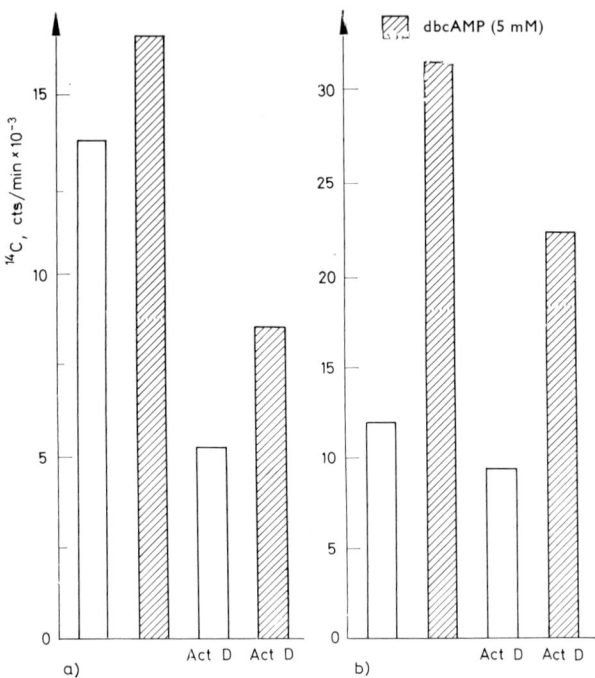

Fig. 5. Effect of Actinomycin D on in vitro dibutyryl cyclic AMP-stimulated protein synthesis and release in the anterior pituitary gland. Pituitary halves from male rats (350–375 g) were pre-incubated in groups of five with or without Actinomycin D (25 μg/ml) for 30 min. Pituitary halves were then transferred into medium either consisting of KRBG alone or with the addition of Actinomycin D (25 μg/ml), dibutyryl cyclic AMP (5 mM) or Actinomycin D + dibutyryl cyclic AMP; the incubation being continued for 2 hrs before addition of ^{14}C-leucine (0.6 μCi/ml) for an additional period of $3^{1}/_{2}$ hrs. Samples were prepared as described in Fig. 3. Panel *a* represents total protein synthesis and panel *b* illustrates release of radioactive TCA-precipitable material. The CPMs are expressed per mg wet weight of tissue. (Reproduced from Labrie et al., *J. biol. Chem.* **246**, 1902, 1971)

Fig. 7. Effect of dibutyryl cyclic AMP (5 mM) on the pattern of labelling of anterior pituitary nuclear RNA extracted at 24°C. Rat anterior pituitary halves were prepared, incubated as in Fig. 6. Detergent-treated nuclei were prepared and RNA was extracted at 24°C with phenol-SDS and separated on sucrose gradients as described in Fig. 6

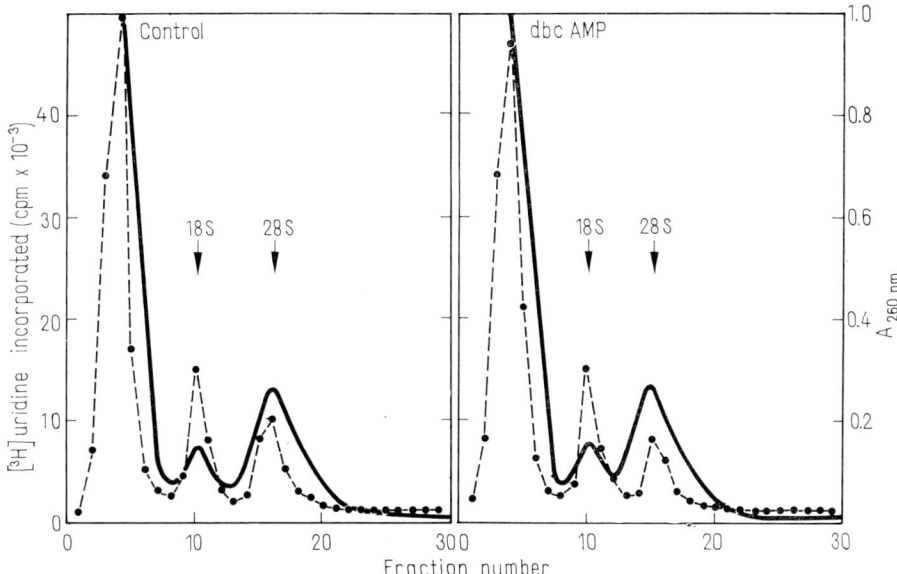

Fig. 6. Effect of dibutyryl cyclic AMP (5 mM) on the pattern of labelling of anterior pituitary cytoplasmic RNA. Rat pituitary halves (40/group) were prepared and incubated for 2 hrs and 15 min at 37°C as described under "Materials and Methods" (Labrie et al. 1971) with ^{3}H-uridine (160 μCi/ml) in the absence or presence of dibutyryl cyclic AMP (dbc AMP). The tissue was homogenized and the RNA was extracted from the 25,000 ×g supernatant with phenol-SDS at room temperature. The RNA was sedimented in a 12–34% linear sucrose gradient for 12 hours at 27,000 rpm in a SW 27 rotor. TCA-precipitable radioactivity was measured in thirty-drop fractions. Broken line means O.D.; continuous line represents ^{3}H, as described by Labrie (1969)

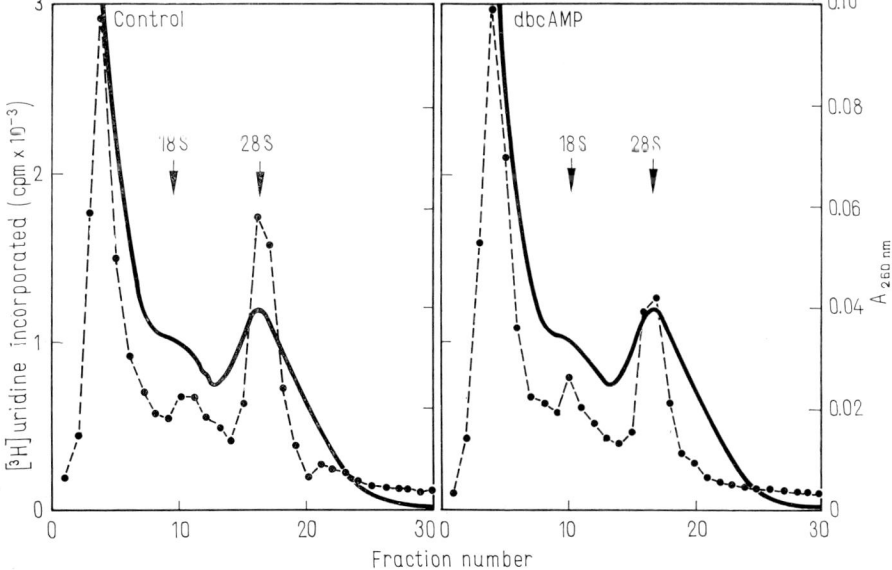

CYCLIC AMP AND PROTEIN RELEASE

In our in vitro system, the time required for the complete processing of radioactive proteins (between the addition of labelled amino acids to the incubation medium and the first appearance of radioactive proteins into the medium) is usually 1½ to 2 hours. In order to study the release of newly-synthesized proteins under various experimental conditions, secretory proteins were first labelled during a 2½-hour preliminary incubation period with radioactive leucine before addition of the agents to be tested and measurement of the trichloracetic acid-precipitable radioactivity released into the incubation medium or of the radioactivity associated with proteins separated on polyacrylamide gels (Labrie et al. 1971). As shown in Fig. 8, growth hormone and prolactin account, respectively, for 60 and 95 per cent of the radioactivity incorporated into released proteins from anterior pituitary of male and female animals. DbcAMP (5 mM) leads to a marked stimulation of the release of labelled proteins (Fig. 9), the effect being already maximal at 4 min (Labrie et al. 1971) and 95 per cent accounted for by the induced release of both growth hormone and prolactin.

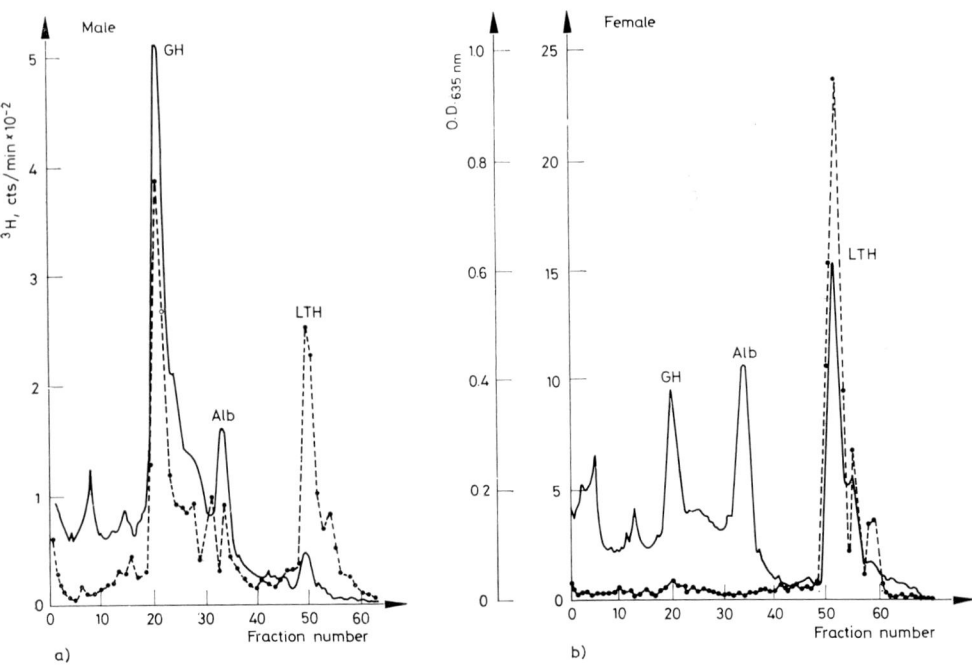

Fig. 8. Comparison of the unlabelled and newly-synthesized proteins released from anterior pituitary glands of male (a) and female (b) adult rats. Six pituitary halves were incubated in KRBG containing 5.0 µCi of ^{3}H-leucine/ml for 5 hrs as described by Labrie et al. (1971). Aliquots of 100 µl of the incubation media were run on 12% polyacrylamide gels. The gels were scanned at 635 nm (———) and then sliced for determination of radioactivity (— — —). GH, growth hormone; Alb, albumin; LTH, prolactin (luteotropic hormone). (Reproduced from Labrie et al., J. biol. Chem. **246**, 1902, 1971)

Morphologic studies indicate that release of secretory proteins from the anterior pituitary gland involves fusion of the membrane of the secretory granule with that of the cell surface and extrusion of the content by exocytosis into the adjacent basement membrane (Pelletier et al. 1971), as observed in the parotid gland (Jamieson and Palade 1967) and the exocrine pancreas (McShan and Hartley 1965). Active extrusion of the secretory granules is already evident at the shortest time studied, 5 min after addition of dbcAMP (5 mM) to the incubation medium (Fig. 10).

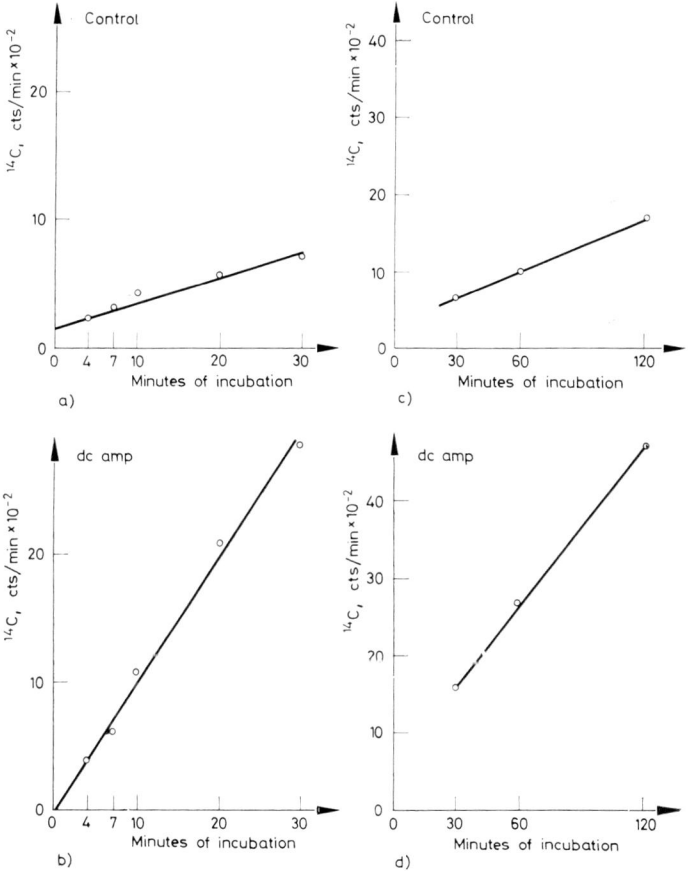

Fig. 9. Time characteristics of the stimulatory effect of dibutyryl cyclic AMP on the release of newly synthesized protein in rat anterior pituitary tissue. Pituitary halves (8/group) from male rats (225–250 g) were preincubated for 30 min in KRBG and incubated for $2^1/_2$ hrs in KRBG containing ^{14}C-leucine (0.5 µCi/ml). Pituitary halves were then washed with KRBG and transferred respectively in 2.2 ml of KRBG or 2.2 ml of KRBG containing dibutyryl cyclic AMP (5 mM). Aliquots of 50 µl of the incubation medium were removed at the specified times for measurement of TCA-precipitable radioactivity

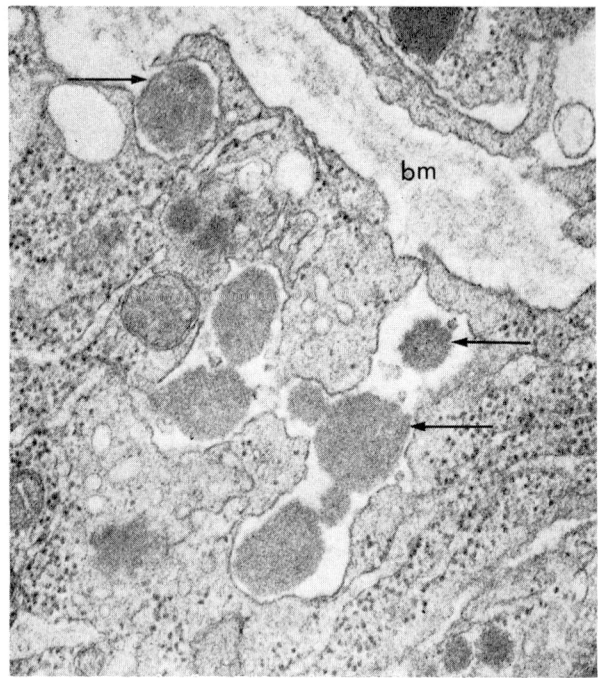

Fig. 10. A portion of somatotrophic cell fixed after 5 min in the presence of dbcAMP, shows the release of many secretory granules (→) into the basement membrane (bm). Exocytosis at multiple sites is seen in both somatotrophic and mammotropic cells (× 42,000)

The morphological appearance of a normal somatotroph after 6 hours of incubation is shown in Fig. 11. The cell contains a large number of secretory granules. The dbcAMP-induced release of GH and LTH during a 6-hour incubation period is accompanied by an almost complete depletion of the content of secretory granules in both somatotrophs (Fig. 12) and prolactin-secreting cells (Fig. 13). No marked depletion of secretory granules was observed in the corticotrophs; thyrotrophs or gonadotrophs. Coupled with other data (Beraud and Labrie, in prep., Gagliardino and Martin 1968, Schofield 1967, Wilber et al. 1968, Cehovic 1969, Fleischer et al. 1969, Parsons and Nicoll 1970), it seems clear that cyclic AMP stimulates the release of all six anterior pituitary hormones.

DISSOCIATION OF PROTEIN SYNTHESIS AND RELEASE

We have previously shown that dbcAMP stimulates both protein synthesis and release in anterior pituitary gland (Labrie et al. 1971) but there remained the problem of whether increased synthesis was a direct effect or was secondary to depletion of the stores of intrapituitary hormones. Moreover, as the maximal stimulatory effect of dbcAMP on protein release could be measured after 4 min of

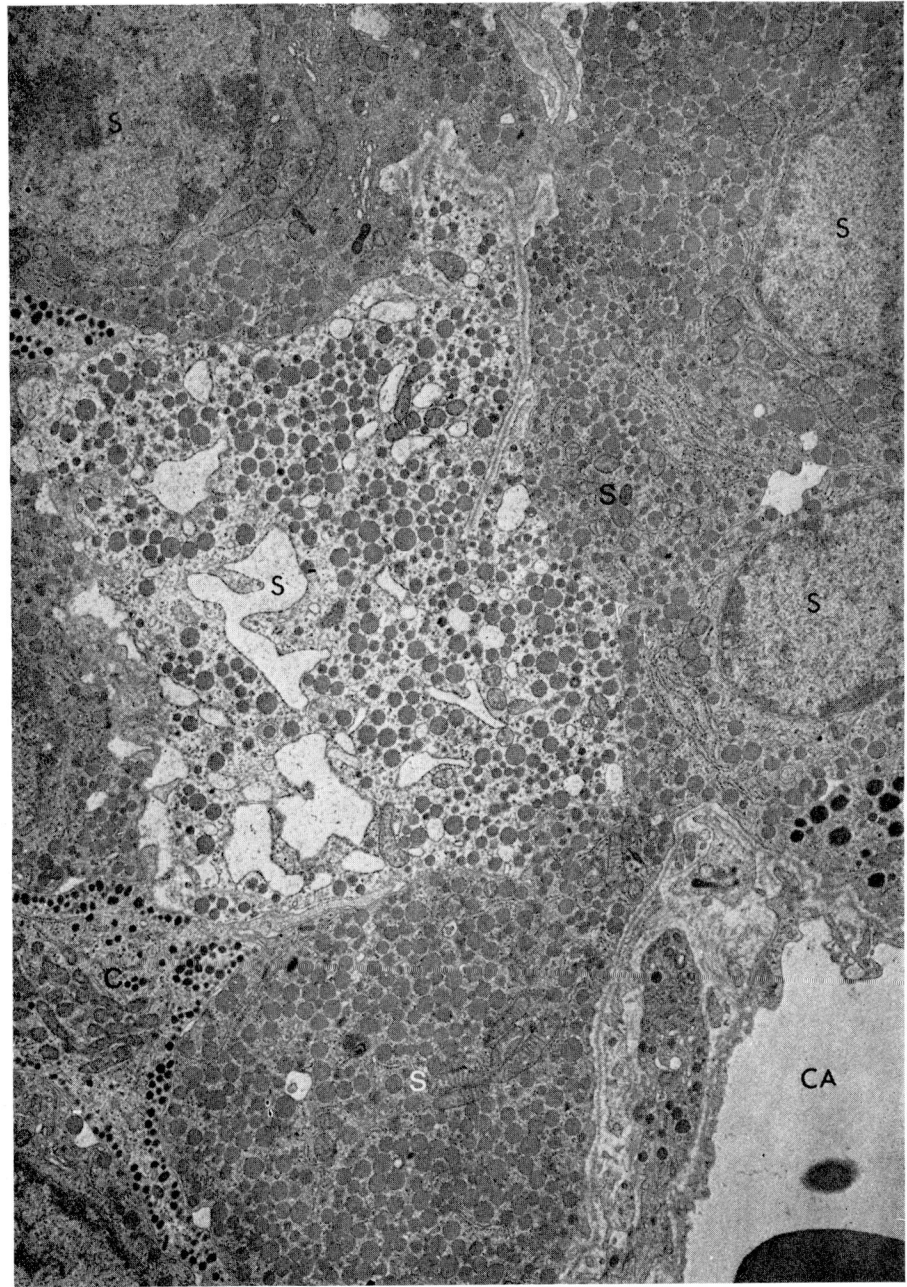

Fig. 11. Low magnification of a control pituitary after six hours of incubation in the Krebs–Ringer medium. The somatotrophs (S) are well granulated and show no evident exocytosis. Part of a corticotroph (C) is identified by the typical position of the secretory granules along the plasma membrane. (CA) capillary ($\times 7{,}200$)

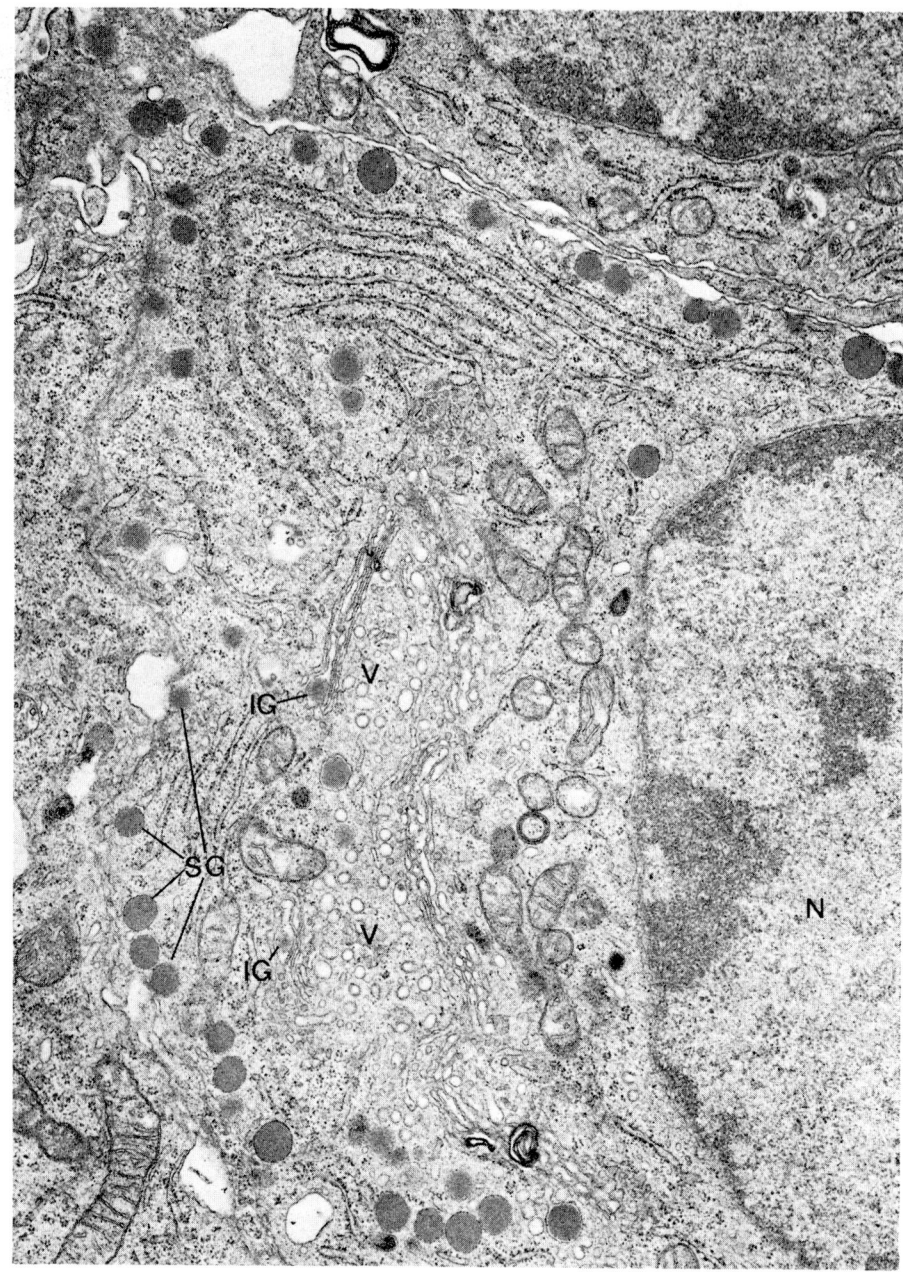

Fig. 12. Somatotroph 6 hrs after the addition of dbcAMP in the incubation medium. The cell is almost completely degranulated. The remaining secretory granules (SG) are located along the plasma membrane. The Golgi apparatus is very well developed and associated with a large number of vesicles (V). Immature granules (IG) are seen in the Golgi saccules. (N) nucleus ($\times 20,000$)

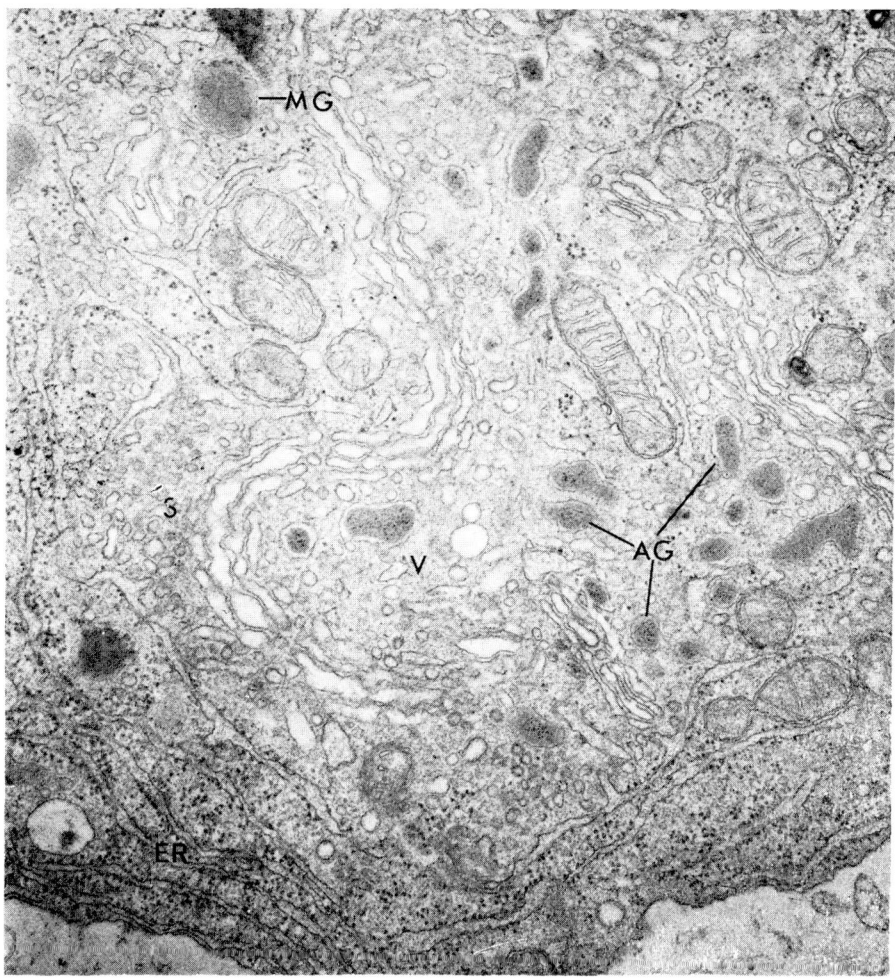

Fig. 13. Mammotrophic cell. After 6 hrs of incubation with dbcAMP, the cytoplasm is almost completely devoid of mature secretory granules (MG). The Golgi apparatus is composed of many saccules (S) and associated vesicles (V). Secretory granules (AG) at different stages of maturation are abundant, indicating active granule formation. ($\times 35{,}000$)

incubation, it was quite conceivable that the maximal stimulatory effect on protein synthesis observed 2 to 3 hours later (Labrie et al. 1971) could be secondary to release. To gain information on this problem, the effects of dbcAMP and elevated potassium ion concentration on synthesis and release were studied under normal incubation conditions or during selective inhibition of either synthesis (with cycloheximide) or release (with elevated Mg^{2+} in the absence of Ca^{2+}).

Combined omission of calcium and increased concentration of magnesium (12.5 mM) inhibits spontaneous release of newly-synthesized anterior pituitary protein to 35 per cent of the control rate (Fig. 14a and b) while the dbcAMP-induced release is inhibited by 80 per cent (Fig. 14c and d). These simple modifications of the concentrations of calcium and magnesium gave very marked inhibition of protein release and thus satisfied the requirements for a study of a possible direct effect of dbcAMP on protein synthesis.

Figure 15 shows clearly that 80 per cent inhibition of the dbcAMP-induced release does not interfere with the stimulation of protein synthesis. The stimulation

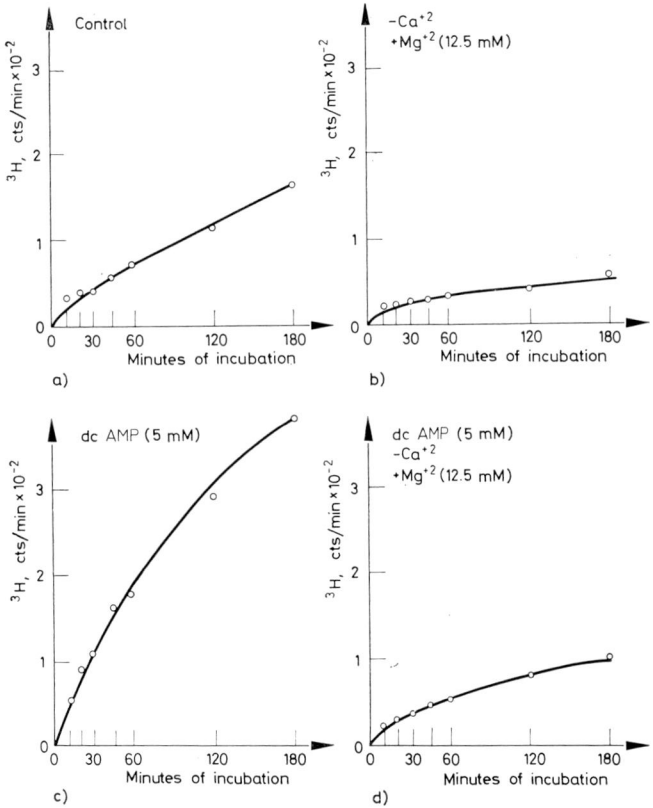

Fig. 14. Effect of calcium-free and high-magnesium (12.5 mM) incubation medium on spontaneous and dibutyryl cyclic AMP (dbcAMP)-induced protein release in rat anterior pituitary gland. Pituitary halves (8/group) of male rats (225–250 g) were initially incubated for 30 min in KRBG and incubated at 37°C for $2^{1}/_{2}$ hours in KRBG containing ^{3}H-leucine (3.0 µCi/ml) as described by Labrie et al. (1971). Pituitary halves were then washed with KRBG and transferred to KRBG containing either 2.5 mM Ca^{2+}—1.25 mM Mg^{2+} (a), no Ca^{2+}—12.5 mM Mg^{2+} (b), 2.5 mM Ca^{2+}—1.25 mM Mg^{2+}—5 mM dibutyryl cyclic AMP (c) and no Ca^{2+}—12.5 mM Mg^{2+}—5 mM dibutyryl cyclic AMP (d). Aliquots of 50 µl of the incubation medium were removed at the specified times for measurement of trichloracetic acid-precipitable radioactivity

was consistently of higher magnitude and duration in modified KRBG (no Ca^{2+} and 12.5 mM Mg^{2+}) than in normal KRBG medium (Fig. 3).

In view of the well-known stimulatory effect of elevated K^+ on the in vitro release of anterior pituitary hormones (Jutisz 1970, Kraicer et al. 1968, 1969, MacLeod and Lehmeyer 1970, MacLeod et al. 1970, Samli and Geschwind 1968, Schofield and Stead 1971, Vale et al. 1967, Wakabayashi and McCann 1970,

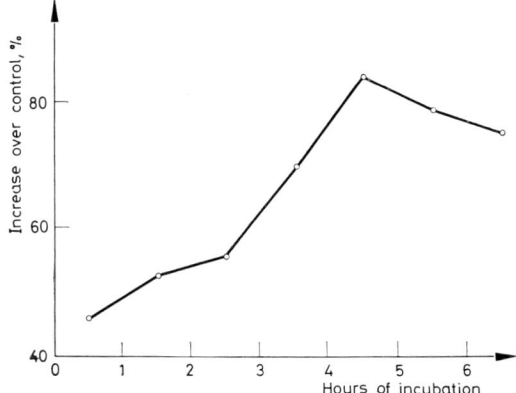

Fig. 15. Time course of the stimulatory effect of dibutyryl cyclic AMP on the rate of anterior pituitary protein synthesis in calcium-free and high-magnesium (12.5 mM) KRBG medium. The pooled results of three similar experiments are presented. Pituitary halves (4/group) of male rats (250–275 g) were initially incubated for 30 min in KRBG and transferred to medium consisting either of modified KRBG alone or containing dibutyryl cyclic AMP (5 mM). At the times shown, 2.0 µCi of ^{3}H-leucine were added for 45 min. Pituitary halves were then washed with KRBG, homogenized and aliquots taken for measurement of trichloracetic acid-precipitable radioactivity. Pituitary halves from the same animals served as control

Wakabayashi et al. 1968) it seemed of interest to investigate the possible effect of K^+-induced depletion of the intrapituitary stores of secretory proteins on the rate of protein synthesis. Figure 16b shows the K^+-induced release of newly-synthesized proteins. This effect of 23 mM K^+ is accounted for by stimulation of growth hormone release while the release of prolactin was not affected up to the longest time interval studied (2 hrs), as recently reported (Parsons 1970, Schofield and Stead 1971, Lemay et al. in press). Figure 16a shows clearly that the depletion of intracellular stores of pituitary hormones by high K^+ concentration has no stimulatory effect on the rates of protein synthesis measured up to 5 hours of incubation. We have also observed that 90 per cent inhibition of protein synthesis by cycloheximide has no appreciable effect on either the spontaneous or dbcAMP-induced release of growth hormone and prolactin (Lemay et al., in press). These data suggest strongly independent control of protein synthesis and release in the anterior pituitary gland.

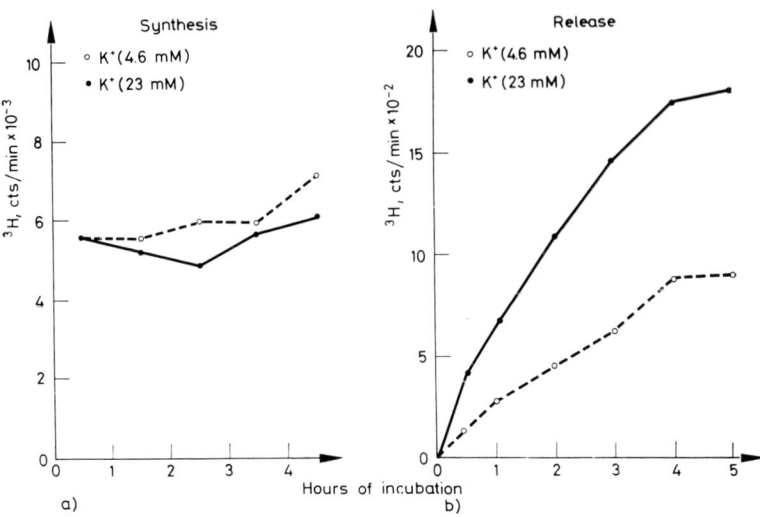

Fig. 16. Effect of 23 mM K$^+$ on the rates of protein synthesis and release in anterior pituitary gland. In the experiment on synthesis (a), pituitary halves (3/group) of male rats (225–250 g) were initially incubated for 30 min in 1.0 ml of KRBG and transferred to KRBG containing either 4.6 mM K$^+$ or 23 mM K$^+$. At the times shown, 2.0 μCi of ^{3}H-leucine were added for a further 45-min incubation period. Pituitary halves were then washed with KRBG, homogenized and aliquots taken for measurement of trichloracetic acid-precipitable radioactivity. Results are expressed as cpm/mg of tissue, wet weight. In the experiment on release (b), pituitary halves (6/group) of male rats (325–350 g) were initially incubated for 30 min in 2.0 ml of KRBG and for $2^1/_2$ hrs in KRBG containing ^{3}H-leucine (0.9 μCi/ml). Pituitary halves were then washed with KRBG and transferred to KRBG containing cycloheximide (10^{-3} M) and K$^+$ at either 4.6 or 23 mM. Aliquots of 50 μl of the incubation medium were removed at the specified times for measurement of trichloracetic acid-precipitable radioactivity

ANTERIOR PITUITARY ADENYL CYCLASE

Since cyclic AMP mimics at least some of the effects of the hypophysiotropic hormones of the hypothalamus, understanding of their mechanism of action will require detailed investigation of the properties of the enzymes involved with cyclic AMP metabolism and action in the anterior pituitary gland.

Adenyl cyclase, the enzyme which catalyses the reaction ATP → cyclic AMP + PPi is part of a membrane-bound enzyme system in mammalian tissues (Sutherland et al. 1962, Rall and Sutherland 1962, Pohl et al. 1969, 1971). Plasma membranes from bovine anterior pituitary tissue were isolated by our modification (Poirier et al., in press) of Neville's technique originally designed for the purification of plasma membranes from rat liver (Neville 1960). This technique is based essentially on differential and isopicnic centrifugation and, as now applied to homogenates of bovine anterior pituitary tissue, yields simultaneous plasma membranes (Fig. 17), microsomes and secretory granules. As shown in Fig. 18, maximal basal and NaF-stimulated adenyl cyclase activity was found in the membrane fractions sedimenting at 1.14 to 1.16 and 1.16 to 1.18 in a step-sucrose

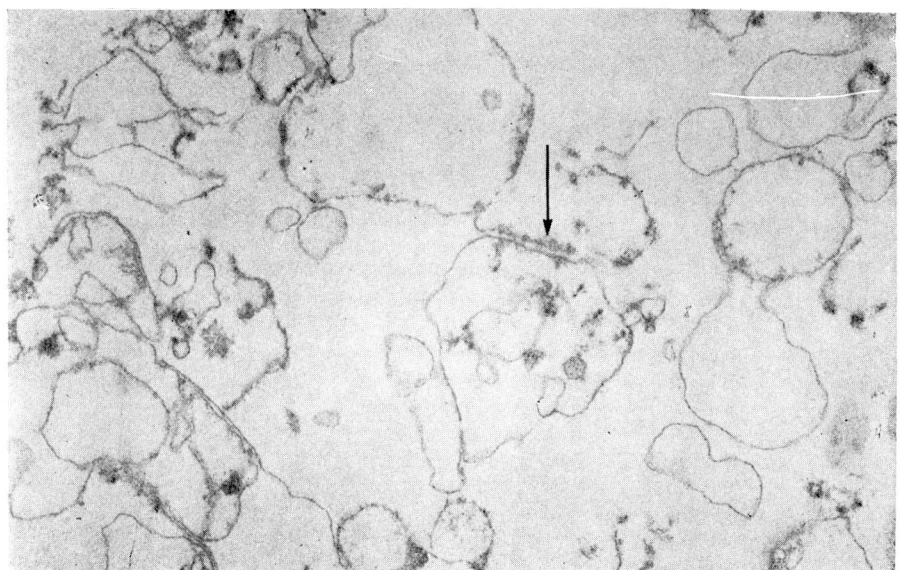

Fig. 17. Fraction sedimenting at density 1.16 to 1.81 in a discontinuous sucrose gradient. This fraction consists essentially of vacuolar membranes. A desmosome (→) is present. No contaminants were found (×30,000)

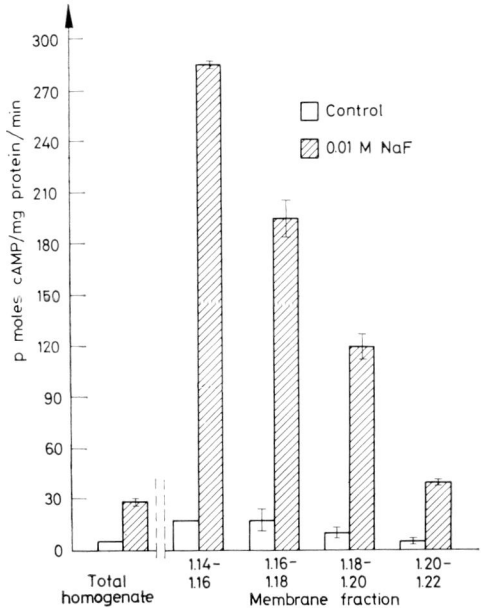

Fig. 18. Adenyl cyclase activity of total homogenate of bovine anterior pituitary gland and of various membrane fractions prepared by a modification (Poirier et al. in press) of the original technique of Neville (1960) sedimenting at the indicated densities in a discontinuous sucrose gradient. Adenyl cyclase activity was measured according to Krishna et al. (1968)

gradient. Adenyl cyclase activity was usually ten times greater in the plasma membrane fraction than in the original homogenate. NaF (10 mM) gives a 4- to 10-fold stimulation of enzymatic activity in all fractions.

ANTERIOR PITUITARY PROTEIN KINASE

The demonstration of a cyclic AMP-dependent protein kinase in many tissues in which 3',5'AMP is presumed second messenger has led to the original proposal (Koo and Greengard 1969) that protein kinases mediate the various effects of cyclic AMP. This enzyme was first discovered in muscle (Walsh et al. 1968) and its study has led to the explanation of how cyclic AMP acts on glycogen breakdown at the chemical level. A similar enzyme has been found in many mammalian tissues and in other sources, including representatives of invertebrate phyla and in bacteria.

We have purified a cyclic AMP-dependent protein kinase from bovine anterior pituitary gland (Courte et al., in press) and we have studied some of its properties. Figure 19 shows the activation of protein kinase activity by increasing concentrations of the various cyclic nucleotides. Cyclic AMP is the most potent of the

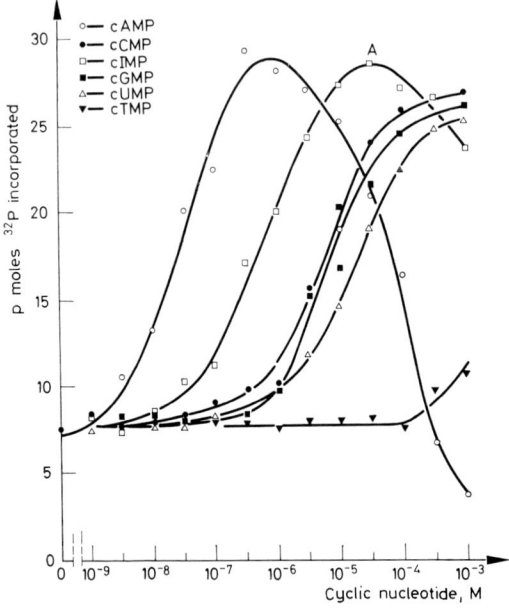

Fig. 19. Effect of increasing concentrations of cyclic AMP (cAMP), cyclic IMP, (cIMP), cyclic CMP (cCMP), cyclic GMP (cGMP), cyclic UMP (cUMP) and cyclic TMP (cTMP) on anterior pituitary protein kinase activity. The incubation mixture contained, in a final volume of 0.2 ml, 0.050 M sodium acetate, 0.010 M $MgCl_2$, 5 μg of enzyme fraction SEa_1, 100 μg of histones, 0.8×10^{-5} M ($\gamma^{32}P$) ATP and the indicated concentration of cyclic nucleotides. The reaction was carried out for 5 min at 30°C in the trichloracetic acid-precipitable radioactivity measured

cyclic nucleotides tested with an apparent Km of 2.5×10^{-8} M. The apparent Kms for the other cyclic nucleotides are: cyclic IMP, 5.0×10^{-7} M; cyclic CMP, 0.83×10^{-5} M; cyclic UMP, 2.0×10^{-5} M; and cyclic GMP, 1×10^{-5} M. The increased enzymatic activity induced by cyclic AMP is not due to increased affinity of the enzyme for ATP or for the histones but results from an increased V_{max}.

The sedimentation profile of anterior pituitary protein kinase activity in a 5 to 20 per cent sucrose gradient in the absence of cyclic AMP is shown in Fig. 20a, while the effect of the cyclic nucleotide on sedimentation characteristics is illustrated in Fig. 20b. The purified protein kinase used in these studies consistently shows two peaks of cyclic AMP-dependent activity after sedimentation on sucrose gradients while a single peak is found after dissociation with cyclic AMP. These results are similar to those recently reported for the enzyme isolated from rabbit skeletal muscle (Reimann et al. 1971) and suggest that a single enzyme may bind to more than one type of inhibitory component leading to inactive complexes of different sedimentation velocities. Other evidence suggests that cyclic AMP activates adenohypophyseal protein kinase by binding to the receptor component of the inactive receptor-catalytic complex and releasing the active catalytic subunit. Such a mechanism of activation has been proposed for the cyclic AMP-dependent protein kinases isolated from adrenal cortex (Cehovic 1969), rabbit

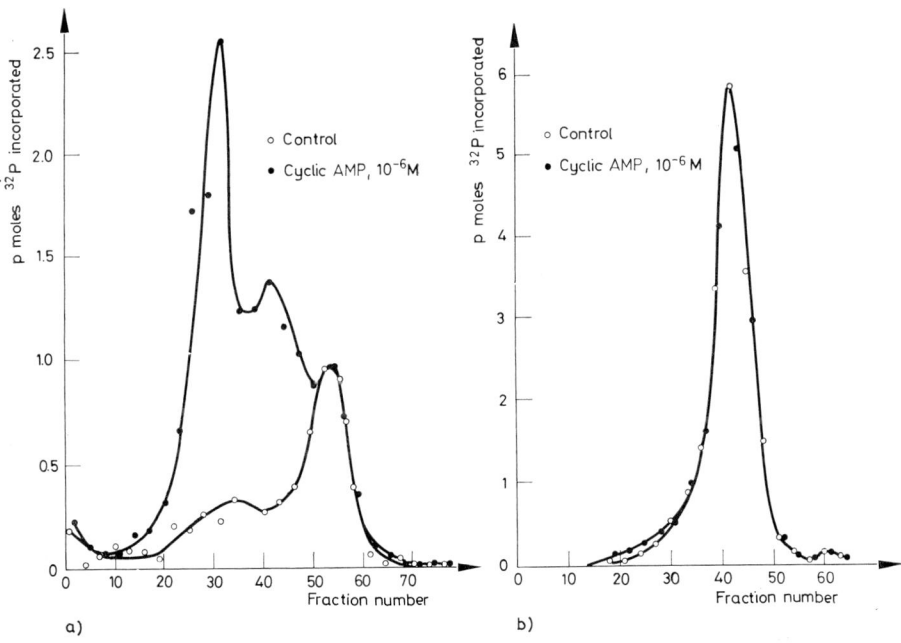

Fig. 20. Sedimentation profile of protein kinase fraction SEa_1 in a 5 to 20% sucrose gradient in buffer A (0.020 M Tris-HCl, pH 7.4, 0.1 M KCl, 0.005 M $MgCl_2$ and 0.006 M mercaptoethanol) run for 15 hrs at 2–4°C in a SW-56 rotor. Alternative drops were collected from the bottom of the tubes for measurement of protein kinase activity in the presence or absence of 10^{-6} M cyclic AMP (as described in Fig. 19) and measurement of protein concentration according to Lowry and his team using bovine serum albumin as standard

reticulocytes (Tao et al. 1970), rat liver (Kumon et al. 1970), cardiac muscle (Takeda et al. 1971), and rat skeletal muscle (Reimann et al. 1971).

Figure 21 shows the subcellular distribution of protein kinase in bovine anterior pituitary gland. Of particular significance is the wide distribution of enzymatic activity among the particulate subcellular fractions and the presence of 50 per cent of the total cyclic AMP-dependent enzymatic activity in the 200,000 g supernatant.

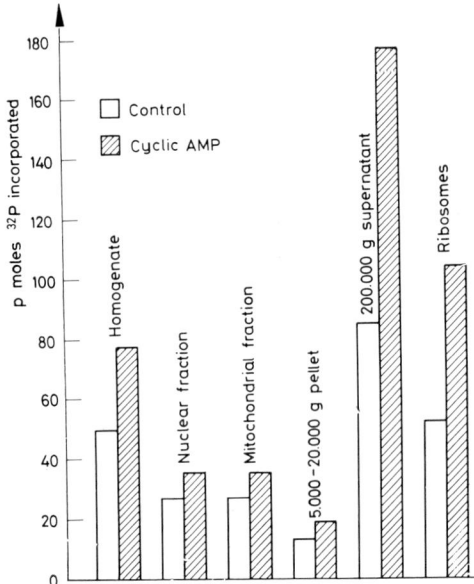

Fig. 21. Subcellular distribution of anterior pituitary protein kinase. Incubation conditions were as described in Fig. 19 and activity was measured in the presence or absence of 10^{-6} M cyclic AMP. Data are expressed as pM ^{32}P incorporated/mg protein/8 min

PHOSPHORYLATION OF ENDOGENOUS SUBSTRATES

Understanding of the action of protein kinases in anterior pituitary tissue will require identification of the endogenous substrate or substrates. Since cyclic AMP stimulates both protein synthesis and release in anterior pituitary gland, it seemed important to study the possible phosphorylation of structures immediately involved in the synthetic and release processes: microsomes, membranes of the secretory granules and plasma membranes. Figure 22 shows that plasma membranes sedimenting at densities of 1.16 to 1.18 and rough microsomes equilibrating at densities 1.18 to 1.22 are phosphorylated to an appreciable extent in the presence of endogenous protein kinase (Fig. 22a) and after addition of exogenous protein kinase (Fig. 22b). Similar results were obtained with isolated secretory granules. Electrophoresis of an acid hydrolysate of the incubation mixtures of plasma membranes, microsomes and secretory granules illustrates that ^{32}P is incorporated

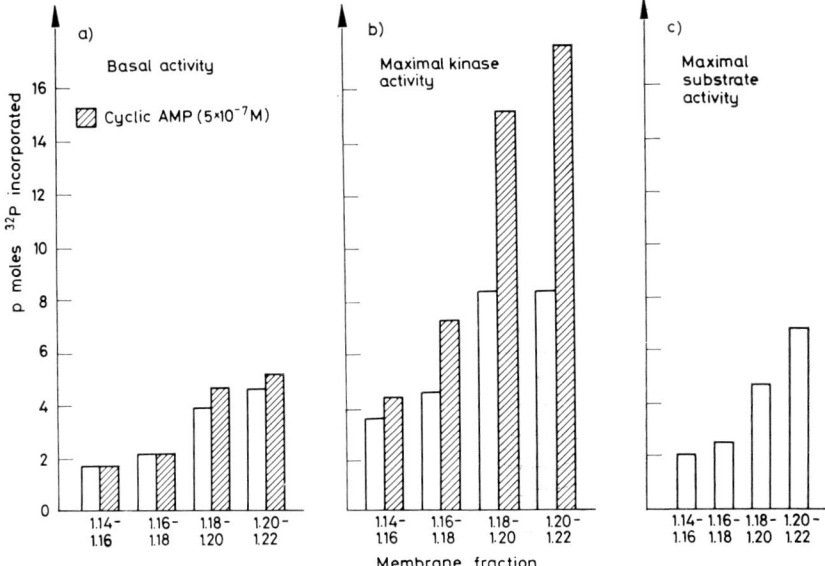

Fig. 22. Distribution of protein kinase activity and substrate in membrane fractions sedimenting at the indicated densities in discontinuous sucrose gradient. Preparation of fractions was as described in Fig. 19. Assay of protein kinase activity was as described in Fig. 19 except that no histones or protein kinase were added (a), 100 µg of histones were added (b) or 20 µg of SEa_t protein kinase were added (c). 100 µg of protein of the membrane fraction was present in all incubations

as phosphoserine while little incorporation occurs as phosphothreonine in the three subcellular fractions (Fig. 23). Figure 24 shows the activation of protein kinase activity from the secretory granules by cyclic AMP and cyclic IMP. Identical results were obtained with isolated microsomes and ribosomes. Table 1 shows the phosphorylation of unwashed and 0.5 M NH_4Cl-washed ribosomes in the presence or absence of 2.5×10^{-7} M cyclic AMP or exogenous protein kinase.

One remarkable feature of the protein kinase associated with all the particulate subcellular fractions studied is the low level of stimulation by cyclic AMP in the absence of added histones compared with the enzyme isolated from the soluble part of the cell. This might be due to the presence of different protein kinases in the various subcellular compartments, to the relative inaccessibility of cyclic AMP to the receptor subunit of the enzymic complex of the particulate fractions or the almost exclusive presence of the catalytic subunit at these sites of action. This would then suggest that cyclic AMP acts in the soluble compartments of the cell, releasing the free catalytic subunit and making it available for binding to the various subcellular substrates according to the scheme of Fig. 25.

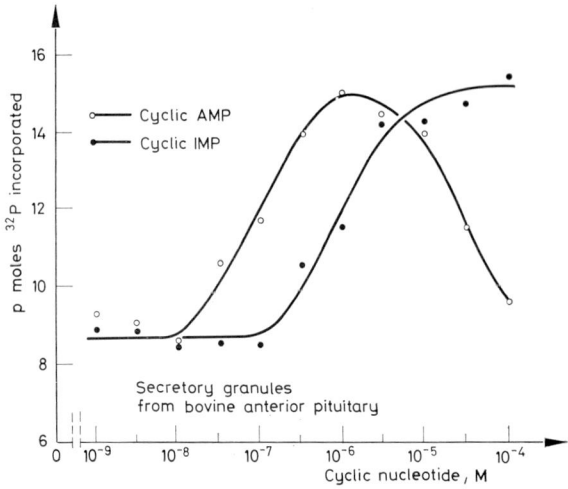

Fig. 23. Activation of protein kinase activity of secretory granules by increasing concentrations of cyclic AMP or cyclic IMP. The protein kinase assay was performed in the presence of 100 μg of histones as described in Fig. 19

TABLE 1

Phosphorylation of ribosomal proteins[a]

Incubation	pmoles ^{32}P incorporated
Unwashed ribosomes	1.24
Unwashed ribosomes + cyclic AMP	1.59
Unwashed ribosomes + protein kinase	1.32
Unwashed ribosomes + protein kinase + cyclic AMP	1.65
Protein kinase	0.13
Protein kinase + cyclic AMP	0.12
Washed ribosomes	0.24
Washed ribosomes + cyclic AMP	0.43
Washed ribosomes + protein kinase	0.42
Washed ribosomes + protein kinase + cyclic AMP	0.59
Protein kinase	0.13
Protein kinase + cyclic AMP	0.12

[a] Unwashed or 0.5 M NH_4Cl-washed ribosomes (50 μg) were incubated for 5 min at 30°C in 0.2 ml of buffer (20 mM Na acetate, 10 mM Mg acetate, pH 6.5) with (γ^{32} P)-ATP (16×10^{-5} M) and, where indicated, cyclic AMP (2.5×10^{-7} M) or a purified anterior pituitary soluble fraction of protein kinase (10 μg). ^{32}P incorporated into ribosomal constituents was measured as described in legend to Fig. 19

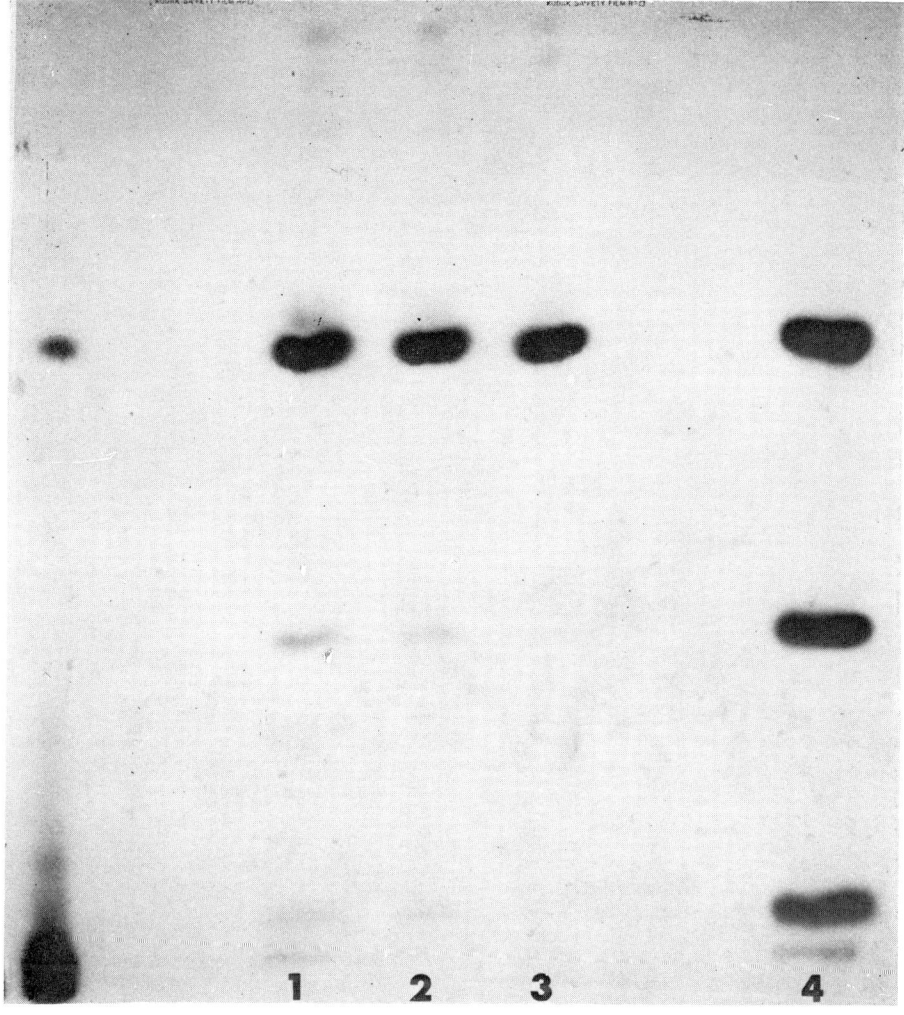

Fig. 24. Autoradiograph of an electropherogram (pH 1.85) of acid hydrolysates of protein kinase incubation mixtures of secretory granules (1), rough microsomes (2), plasma membranes (3) and histones (4)

Our data on the effect of cyclic AMP on protein synthesis and release and on enzymes involved in the metabolism and presumed action of the cyclic nucleotide suggest strongly that cyclic AMP is involved in anterior pituitary gland function and that detailed study of its mechanism of action may be basic to an understanding of the action of the hypophysiotropic hormone of the hypothalamus.

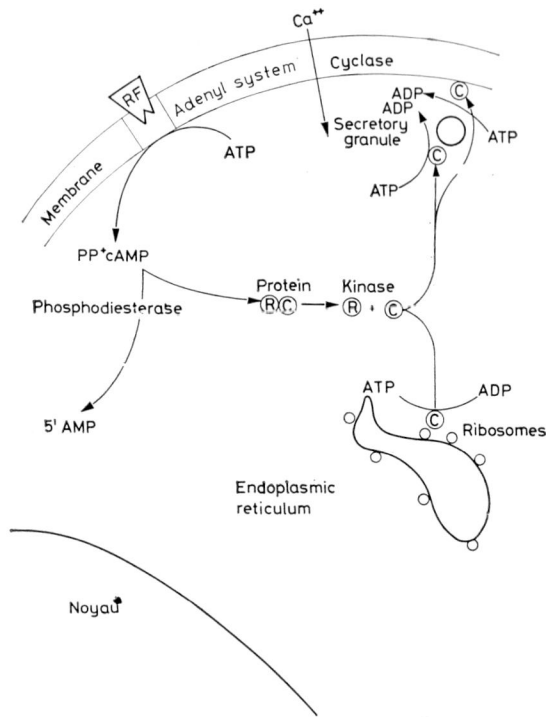

Fig. 25. Schematic representation of a possible mode of action of cyclic AMP in the anterior pituitary cell. Elevation of the cyclic AMP level would, in the cytosol, release the catalytic subunit of protein kinase which would then be free to bind to and phosphorylate its various subcellular substrates

The abbrevations used are: cyclic AMP = adenosine 3',5'-monophosphate; cyclic IMP = inosine 3',5'-monophosphate; cyclic CMP = cytidine 3',5'-monophosphate; cyclic GMP = guanosine 3',5'-monophosphate; cyclic UMP = uridine 3',5'-monophosphate; dibutyryl cyclic AMP = $N^6,O^{2'}$-dibutyryl adenosine 3',5'-monophosphate; monobutyryl cyclic AMP = N^6-butyryl adenosine 3',5'-monophosphate; buffer KRBG = Krebs-Ringer bicarbonate containing 11 mM D-glucose

REFERENCES

BERAUD, G. and LABRIE, F.: (In preparation).
BOLER, J., ENZMANN, F., FOLKERS, K., BOWERS, C. Y. and SCHALLY, A. V. (1969): Biochem. biophys. Res. Commun. **37**, 705.
BOWERS, C. Y., ROBISON, G. A., LEE, K. L., VERSTER, F. and SCHALLY, A. V. (1968): In: Program of the American Thyroid Association, Washington, D.C. p. 55.
BURGUS, R., DUNN, T. F., DESIDERIO, D. and GUILLEMIN, R. (1969): C.R. Acad. Sci. (Paris) **269**, 1870.
CEHOVIC, G. (1969): C.R. Acad. Sci. (Paris) **268**, 2929.
CORBIN, J. D. and KREBS, E. G. (1969): Biochem. biophys. Res. Commun. **36**, 328.
COURTE, C., LEMAIRE, S. and LABRIE, F.: (In press).
FLEISCHER, H., DONALD, R. A. and BUTCHER, R. W. (1969): Amer. J. Physiol. **5**, 1287.

GAGLIARDINO, J. J. and MARTIN, J. M. (1968): *Acta endocr. (Kbh.)* **59,** 390.
GILL, G. N. and GARREN, L. D. (1970): *Biochem. biophys. Res. Commun.* **39,** 335.
GREENGARD, P. and COSTA, E. (Eds) (1970): Role of Cyclic AMP in Cell Function. In: *Advances in Biochemical Psychopharmacology.* Vol. 3. Raven Press, New York.
GUILLEMIN, R. (1967): *Ann. Rev. Physiol.* **29,** 313.
JAMIESON, J. D. and PALADE, G. E. (1967): *J. cell Biol.* **34,** 577.
JARD, S. and BASTIDE, F. (1970): *Biochem. biophys. Res. Commun.* **39,** 559.
JERGIL, B. and DIXON, G. (1970): *J. biol. Chem.* **245,** 425.
JOLICŒUR, P. and LABRIE, F.: (In press).
JUTISZ, M. (1970): In: *Mécanismes d'action intracellulaires des hormones.* Ed. by R. Vokau. Masson, Paris. p. 93.
KOO, J. F. and GREENGARD, P. (1969): *Proc. nat. Acad. Sci. (Wash.)* **64,** 1349.
KRAICER, J., MILLIGAN, J. V., GOSBEE, J. L., CONRAD, R. G. and BRANSON, C. M. (1968): *Science* **164,** 426.
KRAICER, J., MILLIGAN, J. V., GOSBEE, J. L., CONRAD, R. G. and BRANSON, C. M. (1969): *Endocrinology* **85,** 1144.
KRISHNA, G., WEISS, B. and BRODIE, B. B. (1968): *J. Pharmacol. exp. Ther.* **163,** 379.
KUMON, A., YAMAMURA, H. and NISHIZUKA, Y. (1970): *Biochem. biophys. Res. Commun.* **41,** 1290.
KUO, J. F. and GREENGARD, P. (1969): *J. biol. Chem.* **244,** 3417.
LABRIE, F. (1969): *Nature (Lond.)* **221,** 1217.
LABRIE, F., BERAUD, G., GAUTHIER, M. and LEMAY, A. (1971): *J. biol. Chem.* **246,** 1902.
LANGAN, T. A. (1968): *Science* **162,** 579.
LANGAN, T. A. and SMITH, L. K. (1967): *Fed. Proc.* **26,** 603.
LEMAY, A., GAUTHIER, M. and LABRIE, F.: (In press).
LOWRY, O. H., ROSEBROUGH, N. J., FARR, A. L. and RANDALL, R. J. (1951): *J. biol. Chem.* **193,** 265.
MACLEOD, R. M. and LEHMEYER, J. E. (1970): *Proc. nat. Acad. Sci. (Wash.)* **67,** 1172.
MACLEOD, R. M., FONTHAM, E. H. and PACE, R. C. (1970): *Endocrinology* **86,** 863.
MAJUNDER, G. C. and TURKINGTON, R. W. (1971): *J. biol. Chem.* **246,** 2650.
MCCANN, S. M. and PORTER, J. C. (1969): *Physiol. Rev.* **49,** 249.
MCSHAN, W. H. and HARTLEY, H. W. (1965): *Ergebn. Physiol.* **56,** 264.
MEITES, J. (Ed.) (1970): *Hypothalamic Hypophysiotropic Hormones.* Williams and Wilkins, Baltimore.
MEITES, J. and NICOLL, C. S. (1966): *Ann. Rev. Physiol.* **28,** 57.
MIYAMOTO, E., KUO, J. F. and GREENGARD, P. (1969a): *Science* **165,** 63.
MIYAMOTO, E., KUO, J. F. and GREENGARD, P. (1969b): *J. biol. Chem.* **244,** 6395.
NEVILLE, D. M. (1960): *J. biophys. biochem. Cytol.* **8,** 413.
PARSONS, J. A. (1970): *J. Physiol.* **210,** 973.
PARSONS, J. A. and NICOLL, C. S. (1970): *Fed. Proc.* **29,** 750.
PELLETIER, G., PEILLON, F. and VILA-PORCILE, E. (1971): *Z. Zellforsch.* **115,** 501.
POHL, S. L., BIRNBAUMER, L. and RODBELL, M. (1969): *Science* **164,** 566.
POHL, S. L., BIRNBAUMER, L. and RODBELL, M. (1971): *J. biol. Chem.* **246,** 1849.
POIRIER, G., DELEAN, A. and LABRIE, F.: (In press).
RALL, T. W. and SUTHERLAND, E. W. (1962): *J. biol. Chem.* **237,** 1228.
REIMANN, E. M., BROSTROM, C. O., CORBIN, J. D., KING, C. A. and KREBS, E. G. (1971): *Biochem. biophys. Res. Commun.* **42,** 187.
ROBISON, G. A., BUTCHER, R. W. and SUTHERLAND, E. W. (1969): *Ann. Rev. Biochem.* **34,** 149.
ROBISON, G. A., SUTHERLAND, E. W. and BUTCHER, R. W. Eds. (1969): *Cyclic AMP.* Academic Press, New York.
SAMLI, M. and GESCHWIND, I. I. (1968): *Endocrinology* **82,** 225.
SCHLENDER, K. K., WEI, S. H. and VILLAR-PALASI, C. (1969): *Biochim. biophys. Acta (Amst.)* **191,** 272.
SCHOFIELD, J. G. (1967): *Nature (Lond.)* **215,** 1382.
SCHOFIELD, J. G. and STEAD, M. (1971): *FEBS Letters* **13,** 149.
SODERLING, T. R., HICKENBOTTOM, J. P., REIMANN, E. M., HUNKELER, F. L., WALSH, D. A. and KREBS, E. G. (1970): *J. biol. Chem.* **245,** 6317.
SUTHERLAND, E. W., RALL, T. W. and MENON, T. (1962): *J. biol. Chem.* **237,** 1220.

Takeda, M., Yamamura, H. and Ohga, Y. (1971): *Biochem. biophys. Res. Commun.* **42,** 103.
Tao, M., Salas, M. L. and Lipmann, F. (1970): *Proc. nat. Acad. Sci. (Wash.)* **67** 408.
Vale, W., Burgus, R. and Guillemin, R. (1967): *Experientia (Basel)* **23,** 855.
Walsh, D. A., Perkins, J. P. and Krebs, E. G. (1968): *J. biol. Chem.* **243,** 3763.
Wakabayashi, K. and McCann, S. M. (1970): *Endocrinology* **87,** 771.
Wakabayashi, K., Schneider, H. P. G., Watanabe, S., Crighton, D. B. and McCann, S. W. (1968): *Fed. Proc.* **27,** 269.
Weller, M. and Rodnight, R. (1970): *Nature (Lond.)* **225,** 187.
Wilber, J., Peake, G. T. and Utiger, R. (1968): *Endocrinology* **84,** 758.
Wicks, W. D. (1968): *Science* **160,** 997.
Wicks, W. D., Kenney, F. T. and Lee, K. L. (1971): *J. biol. Chem.* **246,** 1902.
Yamamura, H., Takeda, M., Kumon, A. and Nishzuka, Y. (1970): *Biochem. biophys. Res. Commun.* **40,** 675.
Zor, U., Kaneko, T., Schneider, H. P. G., McCann, S. M., Lowe, I. P., Bloom, G., Borland, B. and Field, J. B. (1969): *Proc. nat. Acad. Sci. (Wash.)* **63,** 918.
Zor, U., Kaneko, T., Schneider, H. P. G., McCann, S. M. and Field, J. B. (1970): *J. biol. Chem.* **245,** 2883.

PSYCHONEUROENDOCRINE INTERACTIONS IN A REFLEX OVULATOR

J. HILLIARD and Ch. H. SAWYER

Medical Research Programs
Long Beach VA Hospital
Long Beach, Cal., U.S.A.
and
Department of Anatomy
UCLA School of Medicine
Los Angeles, Cal., U.S.A.

Within the past two years, radioimmuno- and protein-binding assays have provided new information concerning steroid–gonadotrophin levels in cyclic-ovulating mammals. In all species studied so far, the normal preovulatory rise in plasma luteinizing hormone (LH) is preceded by an elevation in urinary or plasma estrogen. Scaramuzzi et al. (1970) obtained evidence to support a causal relationship between high estrogen secretion and LH discharge in the ewe by simultaneous radioimmunoassays of plasma LH and ovarian venous estrogen. In their studies, an elevation in estrogen concentration was measurable 24 hours before the proestrus rise in circulating LH. A similar estrogen–LH relationship has been demonstrated in the rat by several investigators (Exley and Dutton 1970, Brown-Grant et al. 1970, Neill et al. 1971).

Baird and Guevara (1969) and Abraham and Klaiber (1970), using radioimmunoassays, and Korenman and associates (1969), using the uterine cytosol protein-binding assay, likewise concluded that an elevation in plasma estrogen precedes the presumed ovulatory surge of LH in women. Baird and Guevara (1969) noted that changes in both estrone and estradiol could be positively correlated with increased plasma LH during the normal menstrual cycle, suggesting that a certain critical level of estrogen may be necessary to trigger the midcycle LH discharge.

The role of progestin in cyclic ovulation has been controversial, but evidence that it is required to synergize with estrogen in some species is accumulating. Although recent studies in women by Ross and associates (1970) failed to show definite elevations in plasma progesterone until after the midcycle LH surge, rises in 17-hydroprogesterone (17-OH P), which they considered to be evidence of follicular maturation, did precede the LH peak. The progressive increase in plasma 17-OH P has also been reported by Abraham and coworkers (1971) who suggest that 17-OH P acts with estradiol to stimulate the LH-FSH ovulatory surge in women. The classical studies of Everett (1948) have shown that a single injection of progesterone, administered to 5-day cycling rats on the third day of diestrus, will advance ovulation by 24 hours; and persistent-estrous rats will ovulate in response to progesterone treatment. More recently Krey and Everett (1971) have advanced ovulation in 4-day cycling rats by injecting estradiol benzoate on diestrus-1, and since progesterone release was always increased in diestrus-2 in all animals which later ovulated, they propose that both estrogen and a consequential release of progesterone are required to trigger the LH ovulatory surge. The adrenals have been implicated as a source of preovulatory progestin on the rat: Resko (1969) found that plasma progesterone persisted following ovariectomy but fell very rapidly to undetectable levels after adrenalectomy. Moreover, Lawton (1970) has reported that adrenalectomy totally prevents the LH surge in cycling rats.

Although these studies have implicated progestin as well as estrogen in the cyclic discharge of ovulating hormone, the mechanisms involved are yet to be resolved fully. Considerable evidence has shown, however, that electrochemical stimulation and steroid treatment will alter multiple unit electrical activity of the hypothalamus, and positive responses in the rat and rabbit have been correlated with subsequent ovulation in the same animals (Sawyer 1970, Kawakami et al. 1971). In addition, Arimura and Schally (1971) have found that estrogen augments the responsiveness of the pituitary to LH-releasing hormone.

So far the list of species in which radioimmunoassays and protein-binding procedures have been used to investigate steroid–gonadotrophin relationships has failed to include any of the reflex ovulators, such as the rabbit, cat, ferret, mink, vole and thirteen-lined ground squirrel. Yet this highly diversified group of mammals provide the clearest examples of psychoneuroendocrine interaction, since, under natural circumstances, the ovulatory surge of LH is triggered by sensory and emotional stimuli generated at copulation. In the rabbit, coitus is the neurogenic stimulus responsible for triggering the hypothalamic release of LH-releasing hormone which is then transported by the pituitary portal vessels directly to the anterior pituitary (Fig. 1). Because ovulation occurs about 10 hours later, and can be predicted with greater accuracy than is possible in any other species, the doe has contributed generously to our progressive understanding of hypothalamo–pituitary–ovarian interactions. More than 40 years ago, Fee and Parkes (1929) and Smith and White (1931) were able to establish a temporal relationship between coitus and discharge of ovulating hormone from the pituitary gland by hypophysectomizing female rabbits at various intervals after mating. Whereas they provided evidence that the pituitary requires an hour to discharge an ovulatory amount of gonadotrophin, subsequent bleeding and transfusing experiments of Westman and Jacobsohn (1937) indicated that the discharged gonadotrophin was ineffective when removed from the circulation within 90 minutes. It is evident, therefore, that if ovulation is to occur, a certain level of gonadotrophin must act on the ovary for an extended period of time.

The manner in which brief emotional and proprioceptive stimuli, initiated by a copulation lasting but a few seconds, can induce the prolonged period of pituitary discharge required to insure ovulation is difficult to understand without the concept of a positive steroid-feedback mechanism. The ovary of the estrous rabbit is especially adapted in this respect; in addition to containing vesicular follicles which synthesize and release the estrogen required to bring the rabbit into behavioral estrus (Eaton and Hilliard 1971), it contains an abundance of opaque, creamy interstitial tissue which stores cholesterol and cholesterol esters. In 1961, Hilliard, Endrőczi and Sawyer demonstrated that, following coitus or the injection of LH or HCG, the estrous rabbit ovary synthesizes and releases substantial amounts of a progestin, 20_α-hydroxypregn-4-en-3-one (20_α-OH), which is closely related to progesterone in structure but which possesses only a fraction of its progestational activity. After the removal of follicles by cautery, it became clear that the ovarian interstitial tissue was the source of this steroid. Immediately after copulation the ovarian venous levels of 20_α-OH mount rapidly and remain elevated for several hours (Fig. 2). Moreover, LH is the pituitary gonadotrophin responsible for stimulating 20_α-OH release, and a dose–response relationship is obtained when increasing amounts of exogenous LH are injected or infused (Hayward et al. 1964, Endrőczi and Hilliard 1965).

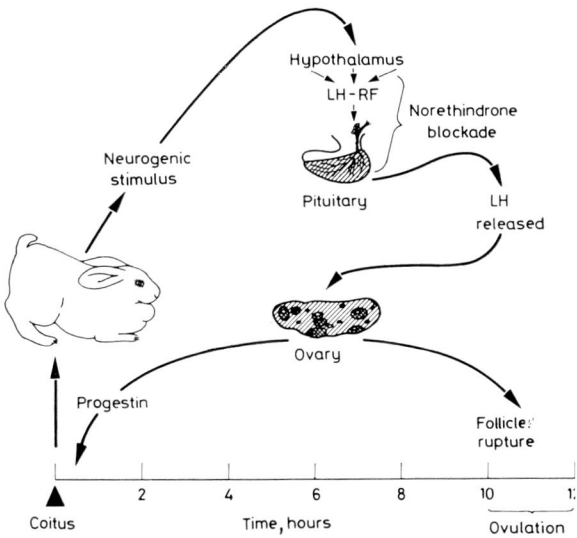

Fig. 1. In the reflectory-ovulating rabbit, coitus excites the hypothalamus to secrete LH-releasing factor (LH-RF), which is carried directly to the anterior pituitary by the pituitary-portal vessels to accelerate LH discharge. Although ovarian follicles do not rupture until 10 to 12 hrs later, plasma LH levels are sufficiently elevated within minutes after copulation to stimulate progestin (20_α-OH) secretion from the ovarian interstitial tissue (Hilliard et al. 1969. In: *The Gonads*. Ed. by K. W. McKers. p. 55. Courtesy of Appleton-Century-Crofts, Meredith Corporation, New York)

In subsequent studies we were also able to demonstrate elevated plasma LH levels in response to electrical stimulation of the medial amygdala and hypothalamus as shown in Fig. 3 (Hayward et al. 1964) or to intrapituitary infusion of median eminence extracts which resulted in ovulation (Fig. 4). Before radioimmuno- and protein-binding assays were available, this 20_α-OH response was used to assess plasma LH content by infusing peripheral blood through the ovaries of recipient rabbits. Figure 5 shows that pooled blood from mated donors contains sufficiently elevated levels of LH to stimulate 20_α-OH release from the infused ovary, whereas the gonadotrophic content of blood from estrous donors, infused simultaneously through the opposite ovary, is insufficient to do so (Hilliard et al. 1964).

The first evidence that 20_α-OH might act as a positive feedback agent to prolong and heighten LH discharge was obtained by ovariectomizing rabbits

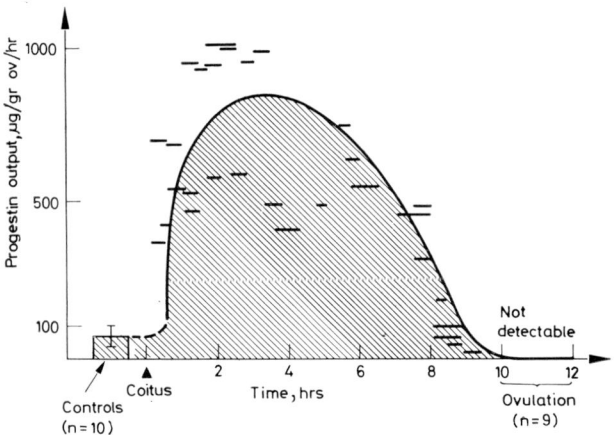

Fig. 2. Progestin (20_α-OH) levels in ovarian venous blood samples collected from 49 individual rabbits before and at varying intervals after coitus. Horizontal lines represent progestin levels obtained in different animals and the length of each line shows the duration of the collection (15 to 60 min). The bars over "Controls" represent the mean level of 10 unmated animals $\pm$ standard error of mean (adapted from Hilliard et al. 1964. *Endocrinology* **75**, 957. Courtesy of J. B. Lippincott Company)

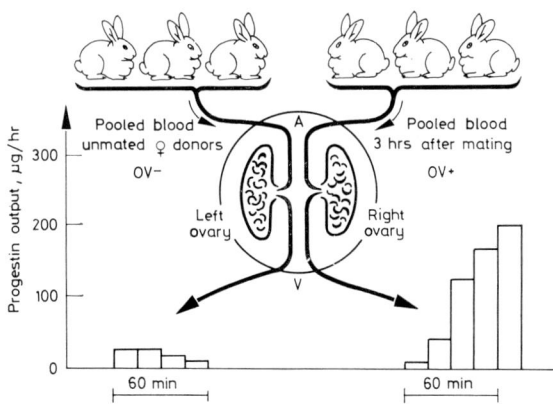

Fig. 3. Ovarian progestin output in 4 rabbits in response to 4 different ovulation-inducing procedures. The uncannulated ovary ovulated (OV^+) to the stimulus in all 4 cases. Electrical excitation was applied under chloralosane anesthesia through bipolar concentric electrodes implanted chronically (adapted from Hayward et al. 1964. *Endocrinology* **74**, 108. Courtesy of J. B. Lippincott Company)

within 30 minutes after mating. In the absence of the ovaries, peripheral blood had lost its capacity to increase 20_α-OH release by four hours after mating, although blood from sham-ovariectomized, mated rabbits, infused simultaneously through the opposite ovary, still contained sufficient LH to elicit the 20_α-OH response (Fig. 6). Similar results were obtained in chronologically ovariectomized

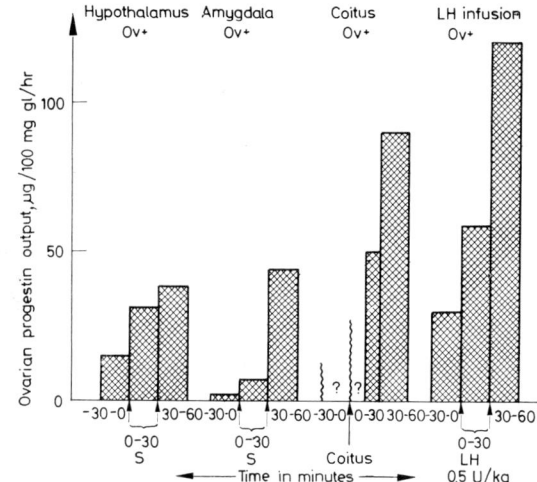

Fig. 4. Ovarian progestin output during intrapituitary infusion of extracts prepared from rabbit brain. Extracts of white matter were inactive, but median eminence extracts stimulated progestin release and induced ovulation

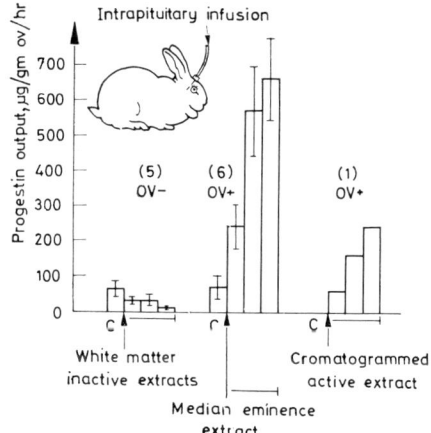

Fig. 5. Progestin outputs obtained from the 2 ovaries of a recipient rabbit following intra-arterial infusion of heart blood drawn from unmated and mated donor rabbits. The mated donors all ovulated (OV⁺) (adapted from Hilliard et al. 1964. *Endocrinology* **74**, 957. Courtesy of J. B. Lippincott Company)

rabbits which had been primed with estrogen to induce estrous behavior. In intact mated controls, plasma levels of endogenous LH remained sufficiently elevated for six hours after mating to stimulate 20_α-OH release from infused ovaries, but blood from chronically ovariectomized rabbits had lost its initial small spurt of gonadotrophic activity within the first two to three hours (Fig. 7).

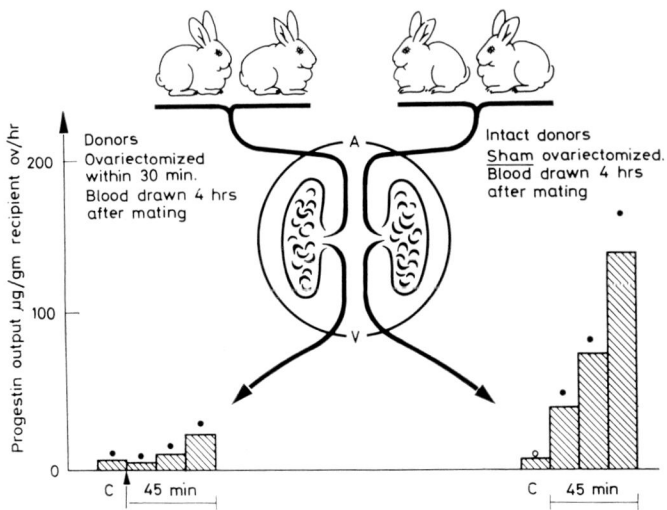

Fig. 6. Effect of *acute ovariectomy* on postcoital LH release. Ovariectomy or sham ovariectomy was performed within 30 min after mating. Samples of heart blood, withdrawn from both groups 4 hrs after mating, were tested for their ability to stimulate progestin (20_α-OH) output from the ovaries of an estrous recipient rabbit during 3 continuous 15-min infusion periods preceded by a 15-min control period (C) during which recipient ovaries received pooled blood from ovariectomized donors. Standard errors of the means are shown. (From Hilliard et al. 1967. *Endocrinology* **80**, 901. Courtesy of J. B. Lippincott Company)

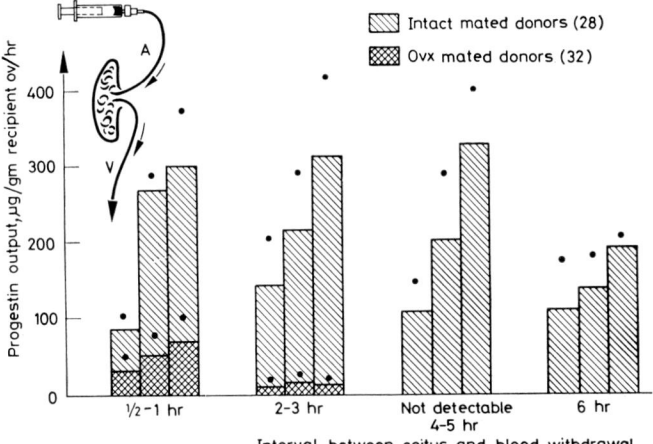

Fig. 7. Gonadotrophic activity in peripheral blood of *intact* and *chronically-ovariectomized* donors at various intervals after mating. Ovariectomized donors had been primed with estrogen to induce estrous behaviour. Gonadotrophic activity, assessed by infusing the blood through the ovaries of recipient rabbits, is expressed in terms of progestin (20_α-OH) output. Standard deviations of the means are shown (From Hilliard et al., 1967. *Endocrinology* **80**, 901. Courtesy of J. B. Lippincott Company)

In the final experiment of this series, mating alone, 20_α-OH alone, and 20_α-OH injected immediately after mating were tested for their ability to maintain LH discharge in estrogen-primed, chronically-ovariectomized rabbits (Hilliard et al. 1967). Our results indicate that copulation triggers a brief spurt of LH discharge sufficient to stimulate the release of 20_α-OH from the ovarian interstitial tissue, and that this progestin, in synergy with estrogen, exerts a positive feedback action to heighten and prolong LH release (Fig. 8). Although priming doses of estrogen failed to sustain postcoital LH levels in ovariectomized rabbits in the absence of 20_α-OH, the probable synergistic role of estrogen is unequivocal since mating does not occur in its absence. Sawyer and Markee (1959) have shown that low doses of estrogen facilitate the induction of reflex ovulation in rabbits by lowering the hypothalamic–pituitary threshold for LH release; and, as mentioned earlier, Arimura and Schally (1971) have demonstrated an increase in pituitary sensitivity to purified LH-RH in rats treated with estrogen.

During the past year, Dr. Linn W. Eaton, Jr. and Dr. Rex Scaramuzzi, working in our Long Beach VA laboratory, have used both protein binding and radio-immunoassays to quantitate and qualify estrogen secretion from the rabbit ovary during estrus and following copulation. In addition to stimulating the release of 20_α-OH from the interstitial tissue, physiological doses of LH increase the release of estradiol-17β from the ovarian follicles (Eaton and Hilliard 1971). Endogenous LH has the same effect: within minutes after coitus, concentrations of estradiol-17β and 20_α-OH in the ovarian venous plasma of intact rabbits begin to rise, and reach peak values between $1\frac{1}{2}$ and 4 hours later (Hilliard and Eaton 1971).

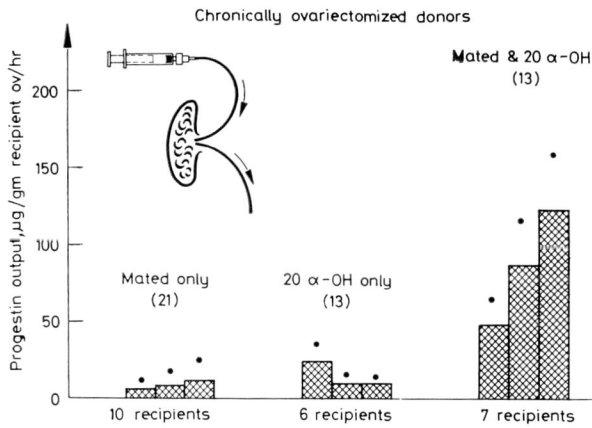

Fig. 8. Effect of exogenous 20_α-OH on postcoital LH discharge in *chronically ovariectomized rabbits*. The steroid (20_α-OH) was injected s.c. in oil immediately after mating. Blood for infusion was obtained by heart puncture 2 hrs later. Progestin outputs elicited by blood drawn from mated rabbits which had not received 20_α-OH and from unmated rabbits which had been injected with 20_α-OH 2 hrs earlier are also shown. The gonadotrophic (LH) activities present in the respective blood samples are assessed by infusion through the ovaries of estrous recipient rabbits. Bar graphs depict the progestin outputs from the recipient ovaries during 3 continuous 15-min infusion periods. Standard errors of the means are shown (adapted from Hilliard et al. 1967. *Endocrinology* **80**, 901. Courtesy of J. B. Lippincott Company)

The preovulatory release of estrogen and progestin undoubtedly serves a variety of functions. By the use of EEG recordings, Kawakami and Sawyer (1959) demonstrated a biphasic synergistic effect of estrogen and progesterone on electrical excitability and activity of the central nervous system, correlated with an initial facilitatory and a later inhibitory effect on LH discharge. In addition, LH stimulates follicular swelling and growth and renders the follicles more sensitive to gonadotrophin (Young 1961). Rondell (1970) has used exquisite microtechniques to show that a progestin, secreted in response to the preovulatory surge of LH, is responsible for the activation of a collagenase-like enzyme which increases follicular distensibility to the point of rupture.

Because the rabbit is a reflex ovulator, pregnancy is the expected result of ovulation. By four to five hours after mating, sufficient capacited sperm will have reached the ampullar ends of the oviducts to fertilize all ova, and fertilization is usually completed within 1 to $1\frac{1}{2}$ hours after ovulation (Austin and Braden 1959). Forty-five years ago, Westman (1926) observed the movements of the reproductive tract in unanesthetized rabbits by means of surgically-implanted windows. He noted that the contractile activities of the ampulla and mesotubarium became more pronounced following copulation, but that soon after the ova had entered the ampulla, ovarian and tubal movements began to subside. According to the elegant time-lapse, photomicrographic studies of Boling and Blandau (1971), extruded ova in cumulus are swept from the surface of the ovary into the Fallopian tube by highly activated infundibular fimbria and traverse the ampulla within six minutes, then remain at the isthmoampullar constriction for several hours before continuing a precisely-timed, 3-day journey down the oviduct.

It is now well established that transport of ova through the oviduct requires a period of three days in most mammals (Blandau 1969), and that the retention of ova within the oviduct for this period has definite physiological significance. Chang (1955) has shown that ova transplanted prematurely to the uterus fail to develop; and, conversely, after three days within the oviduct, eggs must be transferred to the uterus if development is to continue (McLaren 1969).

Since the action of the oviduct is hormone-dependent, a remarkable programming of steroid secretion must occur to control the rapid ascent of sperm from the uterus and the subsequent 3-day descent of the zygotes down the tube (Blandau and Boling 1970). But many data in this area have been inconclusive and often contradictory. Greenwald (1961) noted that small doses of estradiol injected at mating accelerated egg transport, but that large doses caused ova to be retained in the oviducts for as long as six days. Burdick and Pincus (1935) reported that injected estrogen prevents egg transport in pseudopregnant rabbits, whereas Harper (1966) found that estrogen treatment restores the rate of ova transport in ovariectomized rabbits. Progestin, likewise, appears to have a role in oviductal activity. Adams (1958) noted that progesterone delays egg passage in newly spayed rabbits, but Boling and Blandau (1971) have found that the mean transport time is much reduced in normal estrous rabbits 12 to 14 hours after an injection of either progesterone or 20_α-OH. Based on observations in which supravitally stained donor eggs were introduced into the oviducts of recipient rabbits, Boling and Blandau (1970) have offered the hypothesis that acute estrogen withdrawal may be responsible for the hyperactivity of the oviductal musculature at ovulation and during the initial transport of the ova through the ampulla.

In view of this interesting estrogen-withdrawal hypothesis, we have extended our studies of ovarian estrogen and progestin release after mating to include the period of tubal transport and implantation in order to establish the minimal steroid requirements during these processes (Fig. 9). Immediately after mating, there is a transient rise in the ovarian venous levels of estradiol-17β, which occurs concurrently with elevations in plasma LH as assayed by Dr. E. M. Bogdanove at Indiana University. Dr. Bogdanove is using a radioimmunoassay in which rabbit LH competes with I^{131}-labeled sheep LH for binding to an antiserum against ovine LH generated in a guinea-pig. In his hands the competition has proved effective: pituitary extract added to rabbit serum is recovered quantitatively. Moreover, repeated estimates of pituitary/blood activity ratios are indistinguishable from ratios obtained through bioassay of the same material (Bogdanove et al. 1971). Elevated levels of estradiol-17β also parallel the dramatic increase in 20_α-

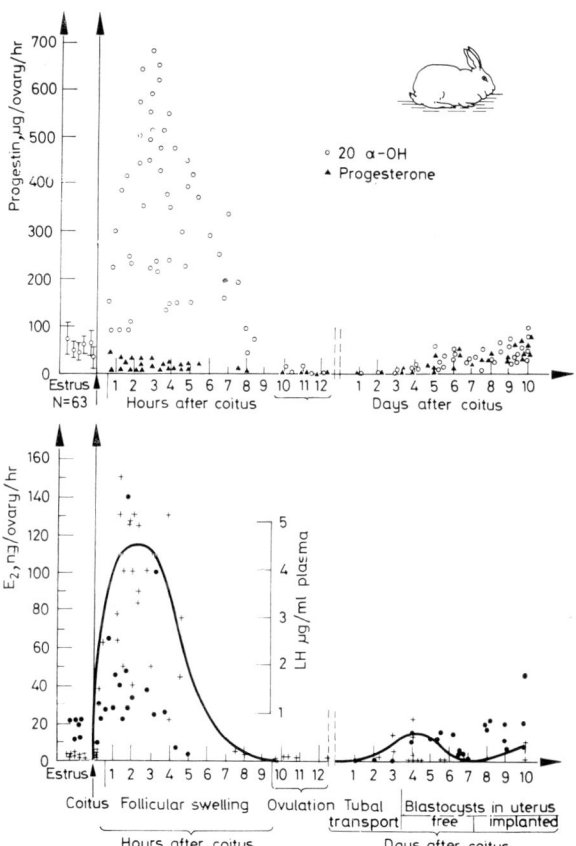

Fig. 9. Ovarian release of 20_α-OH, progesterone (top graph), estradiol-17β (o) and plasma LH levels (+) (bottom graph) in rabbits before and after mating, at ovulation, and during tubal transport and implantation. Steroid levels were obtained from ovarian venous plasma. Note low levels of steroids and LH at ovulation and during initial period of tubal transport (Hilliard et al., unpublished)

OH output obtained in the same blood samples as well as in those reported previously (Hilliard et al. 1964, 1968a, b). On the other hand, progesterone output remains essentially unchanged until about four hours after mating when the release of all three steroids begins to decline. By eight hours, estrogen is no longer detectable and progestin output has dropped sharply, and at ovulation, when the tubal musculature is most active and the fimbria are sweeping the extruded ova into the ampulla (Blandau 1969), the output of all three steroids is at nadir. Moreover, they continue to remain low during the subsequent 3-day period while ova are traversing the oviduct, data which fully support the Boling and Blandau (1971) steroid-withdrawal hypothesis.

Following a 3-day sojourn in the oviduct, fertilized blastocysts proceed into the uterus where they remain free for an additional four days before implanting on the endometrium. Our composite estrogen, LH and progestin data suggest that estrogen secretion is gradually increasing during the final 24 hours within the oviduct (Fig. 9). There is also some indication that a small rise in estrogen release may occur prior to implantation on the seventh or eighth post-mating day. Since estrogen is luteotrophic in the rabbit, it is not fortuitous that progesterone release from the developing corpora lutea also begins to increase steadily as estrogen output rises. The inhibition of ovulation by progesterone during pregnancy is itself an action involving a wide circuit of psychoneuroendocrine interactions, exerted at the level of the central nervous system as well as the pituitary gland and possibly at the ovary (Hilliard et al. 1971).

REFERENCES

ABRAHAM, G. E. and KLAIBER, E. L. (1970): Plasma immunoreactive estrogens and LH during the menstrual cycle. *Amer. J. Obstet. Gynec.* **108**, 528.

ABRAHAM, G. E., ODELL, W. D., SWERDLOFF, R. S. and HOPPER, K. (1971): Simultaneous radioimmunoassay of plasma progesterone (P), 17-hydroxyprogesterone (17-OH P), Estradiol (E-2), LH and FSH during the menstrual cycle. In: *Program of the 53rd Meeting of the Endocrine Society*, A-160, Abst. 236.

ADAMS, C. E. (1958): Egg development in the rabbit: The influence of post-coital ligation of the uterine tube and of ovariectomy. *J. Endocr.* **16**, 283.

ARIMURA, A. and SCHALLY, A. V. (1971): Augmentation of pituitary responsiveness to LH-releasing hormone (LH-RH) by estrogen. *Proc. Soc. exp. Biol. (N.Y.)* **136**, 290.

AUSTIN, C. R. and BRADEN, A. W. H. (1954): Time relations and their significance in the ovulation and penetration of eggs in rats and rabbits. *Austr. J. biol. Sci.* **7**, 179.

BAIRD, D. T. and GUEVARA, A. (1969): Plasma estrogens in non-pregnant women and in men. *J. clin. Endocr.* **29**, 149.

BLANDAU, R. J. (1969): Gamete transport—comparative aspects. In: *The Mammalian Oviduct.* Ed. by E. S. E. Hafez and R. J. Blandau. University of Chicago Press, Chicago—London, p. 164.

BLANDAU, R. J. and BOLING, J. L. (1970): An experimental approach to the study of egg transport through the oviducts of mammals. Conference on the Regulation of Mammalian Reproduction, NIH, Bethesda, Md. USA. (In press).

BOGDANOVE, E. M., HILLIARD, J. and SAWYER, C. H. (1971): Serum LH patterns in the female rabbit as determined by radioimmunoassay. In: *Program of the 53rd Meeting of the Endocrine Society.* A-76, Abst. 68.

BOLING, J. L. and BLANDAU, R. J. (1971): Egg transport through the ampullae of the oviducts of normal estrous rabbits, rabbits injected with gonadotrophins, progestins and CN-55, 945-27. *Biol. Abst.* (In press).

Brown-Grant, K., Exley, D. and Naftolin, F. (1970): Peripheral plasma oestradiol and luteinizing hormone concentrations during the oestrous cycle in the rat. *J. Endocr.* **48,** 295.

Bryans, F. E. (1951): Progesterone of the blood in the menstrual cycle of the monkey. *Endocrinology* **48,** 733.

Burdick, H. O. and Pincus, G. (1935): The effect of oestrin injection upon the developing ova of mice and rabbits. *Amer. J. Physiol.* **111,** 201.

Chang, M. C. (1955): Fertilization and normal development of follicular oocytes in the rabbit. *Science* **121,** 867.

Corker, S. S., Exley, D. and Naftolin, F. (1969): Assay of 17β-oestradiol by competitive protein binding methods. *Nature (Lond.)* **222,** 1063.

Eaton, L. W., Jr. and Hilliard, J. (1971): Estradiol-17β, progesterone and 20_α-hydroxypregn-4-en-3-one in rabbit ovarian venous plasma. I. Steroid secretion from paired ovaries with and without corpora lutea; effect of LH. *Endocrinology* **89,** 105.

Endrőczi, E. and Hilliard, J. (1965): Luteinizing hormone releasing activity in different parts of rabbit and dog brain. *Endocrinology* **71,** 667.

Everett, J. W. (1948): Progesterone and estrogen in the experimental control of ovulation time and other features of the estrous cycle in the rat. *Endocrinology* **43,** 389.

Exley, D. and Dutton, A. (1970): Peripheral plasma 17β-oestradiol concentrations during the estrous cycle of a 4-day cyclic rat. In: *3rd International Congress on Hormonal Steroids, Hamburg.* p. 232.

Fee, A. R. and Parkes, A. S. (1929): Studies on ovulation. I. The relation of the anterior pituitary body to ovulation in the rabbit. *J. Physiol. (Lond.)* **67,** 383.

Greenwald, G. S. (1961): A study of the transport of ova through the rabbit oviduct. *Fertil. and Steril.* **12,** 80.

Harper, N. J. K. (1966): Hormonal control of transport of eggs in cumulus through the ampulla of the rabbit oviduct. *Endocrinology* **78,** 568.

Hayward, J. N., Hilliard, J. and Sawyer, C. H. (1964): Time of release of pituitary gonadotrophin induced by electrical stimulation of the rabbit brain. *Endocrinology* **74,** 108.

Hilliard, J. and Sawyer, C. H. (1964): Synthesis and release of progestin by rabbit ovary *in vivo.* In: *Proceedings 1st International Congress on Hormonal Steroids.* Vol. 1. Academic Press, New York. p. 263.

Hilliard, J. and Eaton, L. W., Jr. (1971): Estradiol-17β, progesterone, and 20_α-hydroxypregn-4-en-3-one in rabbit ovarian venous plasma. II. From mating through implantation. *Endocrinology* (In press).

Hilliard, J., Endrőczi, E. and Sawyer, C. H. (1961): Stimulation of progestin release from rabbit ovary *in vivo.* *Proc. Soc. exp. Biol. (N.Y.)* **108,** 154.

Hilliard, J., Hayward, J. N. and Sawyer, C. H. (1964): Postcoital patterns of secretion of pituitary gonadotropin and ovarian progestin in the rabbit. *Endocrinology* **75,** 957.

Hilliard, J., Penardi, R. and Sawyer, C. H. (1967): A functional role for 20_α-hydroxypregn-4-en-3-one in the rabbit. *Endocrinology* **80,** 901.

Hilliard, J., Spies, H. G., Lucas, L. and Sawyer, C. H. (1968a): Effect of prolactin on progestin release and cholesterol storage by rabbit ovarian interstitium. *Endocrinology* **82,** 122.

Hilliard, J., Spies, H. G. and Sawyer, C. H. (1968b): Cholesterol storage and progestin secretion during pregnancy and pseudopregnancy in the rabbit. *Endocrinology* **82,** 157.

Hilliard, J., Schally, A. V. and Sawyer, C. H. (1971): Progesterone blockade of the ovulatory response to intrapituitary infusion of LH-RH in rabbits. *Endocrinology* **88,** 730.

Kawakami, K. and Sawyer, C. H. (1959): Neuroendocrine correlates of changes in brain activity thresholds by sex steroids and pituitary hormones. *Endocrinology* **65,** 652.

Kawakami, M., Terasawa, E., Ibuki, T. and Manaka, M. (1971): Effects of sex hormones and ovulation-blocking steroids and drugs on electrical activity of the rat brain. In: *Steroid Hormones and Brain Function.* Ed. by C. H. Sawyer and R. A. Gorski. University of California Press.

KORENMAN, S. G., PERRIN, L. E. and MCCALLUM, T. P. (1969): A radioligand binding assay system for estradiol measurements in human plasma. *J. clin. Endocr.* **29,** 879.

KREY, L. C. and EVERETT, J. W. (1971): Ovulation after estrogen treatment early in the rat estrous cycle: significance of induced progesterone secretion. *Fed. Proc.* **30,** 310. Abst. 658.

LAWTON, I. (1970): Effect of ovarian and adrenal hormones in cyclic LH release. *Physiologist* **13,** 264.

LINKIE, D. M. and NISWENDER, G. D. (1971): Serum gonadotrophins during pregnancy in the rat. *Fed. Proc.* **30,** 535.

MCLAREN, A. (1969): Mechanisms affecting embryo development. In: *The Mammalian Oviduct.* Ed. by E. S. E. Hafez and R. J. Blandau. University of Chicago Press, Chicago—London. p. 447.

NEILL, J. D., FREEMAN, M. E. and TILLSON, S. A. (1971): Control of the proestrous "surge" of prolactin and luteinizing hormone secretion by estrogens in the rat. *Fed. Proc.* **30,** 474.

RESKO, J. A. (1969): Endocrine control of adrenal progesterone secretion in the ovariectomized rat. *Science* **164,** 70.

RONDELL, P. (1970): Follicular processes in ovulation. *Fed. Proc.* **29,** 1875.

ROSS, G. T., CARGILLE, C. M., LIPSETT, M. B., RAYFORD, P. L., MARSHALL, J. T., STROTT, C. A. and RODBARD, D. (1970): Pituitary and gonadal steroids in women. *Recent Progr. Hormone Res.* **26,** 1.

SAWYER, C. H. (1970): Electrophysiological correlates of release of pituitary ovulating hormone. *Fed. Proc.* **29,** 1895.

SAWYER, C. H. and MARKEE, J. E. (1959): Oestrogen facilitation of release of pituitary ovulating hormone in the rabbit in response to vaginal stimulation. *Endocrinology* **65,** 614.

SCARAMUZZI, R. J., CALDWELL, B. V. and MOOR, R. M. (1970): Radioimmunoassay of LH and estrogen during the estrous cycle in the ewe. *Biol. Reprod.* **3,** 110.

SMITH, P. E. and WHITE, W. E. (1931): The effect of hypophysectomy on ovulation and corpus luteum formation in the rabbit. *J. Amer. med. Ass.* **97,** 1861.

WESTMAN, A. (1926): A contribution to the question of the transit of the ovum from ovary to uterus in rabbits. *Acta obstet. gynec. scand.* **5,** 1.

WESTMAN, A. and JACOBSOHN, D. (1937): Über Oestrinwirkungen auf die Corpus luteum-Function. *Acta obstet. gynec. scand.* **17,** 13.

YOUNG, W. C. (1961): The mammalian ovary. In: *Sex and Internal Secretions.* Vol. I. Ed. by W. C. Young. Williams and Wilkins, Baltimore. p. 449.

INFLUENCE OF SYNTHETIC TRF ADMINISTRATION AND HYPOTHALAMIC STIMULATION UPON THE ULTRASTRUCTURE OF THYROTROPHS

Y. SHIOTANI, M. SAKAGAMI, K. FUJIMOTO and T. BAN

Department of Anatomy
Osaka University Medical School
Osaka, Japan

It is well known that secretory activity of the anterior pituitary gland is regulated by the hypothalamus through the humoral mediator called releasing factor (RF) or inhibiting factor (IF). In this decade, many studies have been done to purify RF or IF, and Bowers et al. (1970) reported recently that porcine thyrotropin releasing factor (TRF) is (Pyro/Glu-Hiw-Pro/NH$_2$). However, precise site of RF production or storage in the hypothalamus is still obscure. In our laboratory, electron microscopic studies have been done on the anterior pituitary cells of rabbits, which were stimulated electrically in the hypothalamus, in order to clarify the nervous control of RF or IF discharge from the hypothalamus into the anterior pituitary gland (Shiotani et al. 1969).

In this paper, we would like to report some ultrastructural changes in thyrotrophs (TSH producing cells), affected by the administration of synthetic TRF or electrical stimulation in the hypothalamus.

ULTRASTRUCTURAL CHANGES IN RAT THYROTROPHS AFTER SYNTHETIC TRF ADMINISTRATION

Adult Wistar rats were injected intravenously with 50 ng, 1 µg and 100 µg of synthetic TRF and sacrificed under Nembutal anaesthesia 5, 15, 30 and 60 min later. Anterior pituitary glands were fixed with 4 per cent glutaraldehyde and 2 per cent OsO$_4$ solution successively, dehydrated in the graded series of ethanol and embedded in Epon 812. Ultrathin sections were stained with uranyl acetate and lead hydroxide, and observed by an electron microscope.

Figure 1 shows a typical thyrotroph of a normal rat. The cell is somewhat elongated or angular in shape, and contains a nucleus (Nu), some secretory granules (Sg), mitochondria (Mi), rough-surfaced endoplasmic reticulum (rER), etc. Secretory granules are of high electron density and their maximum diameter is about 100–150 mµ.

Figure 2 shows a thyrotroph of a rat, which was injected with 50 ng of synthetic TRF and sacrificed 5 min later. The Golgi apparatus (G) develops strikingly and contains some immature granules. Many mitochondria (Mi) are concentrated

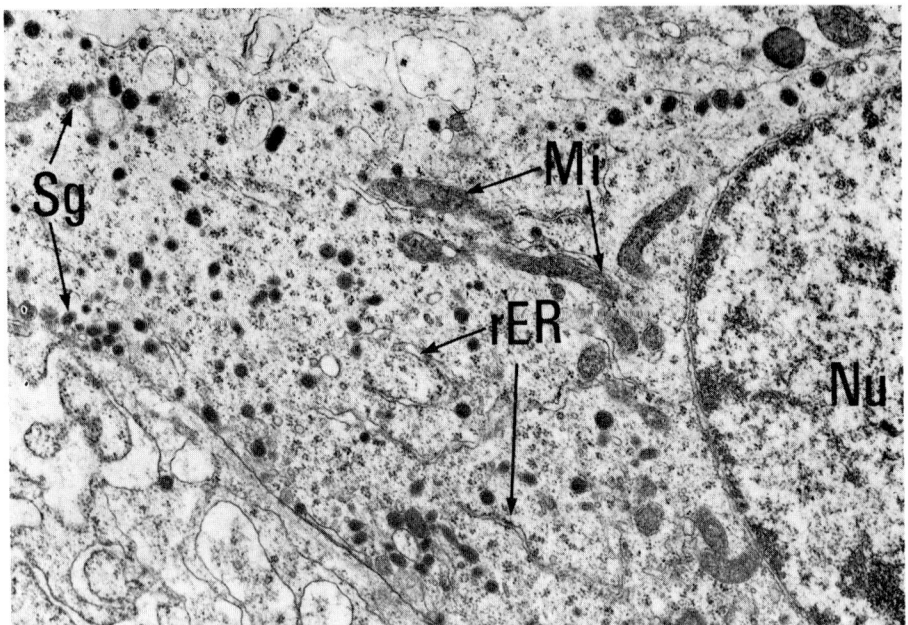

Fig. 1. Part of a thyrotroph of a normal rat. ×15,000

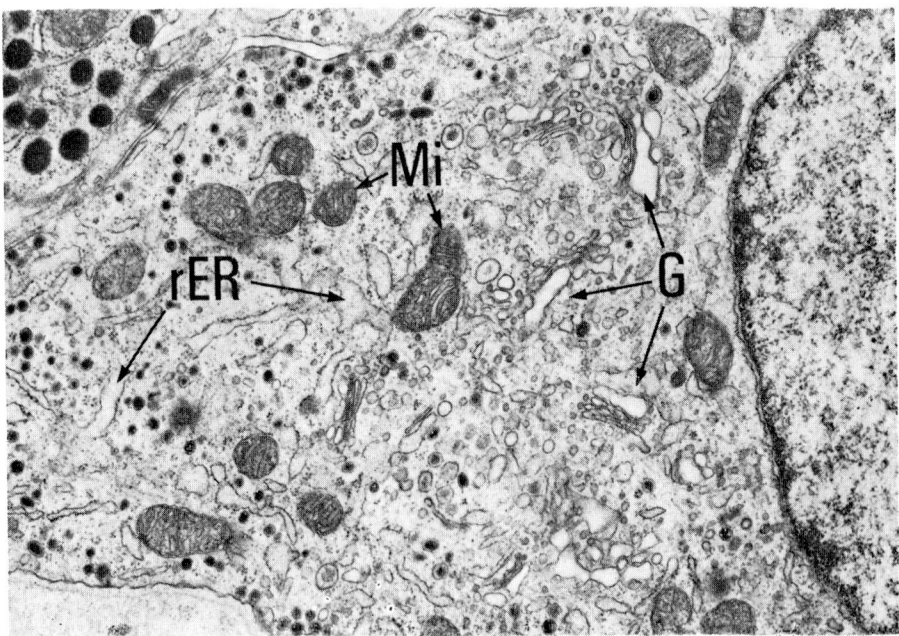

Fig. 2. Part of a thyrotroph of a rat injected with 50 ng of synthetic TRF and sacrificed 5 min later. ×15,000

around this area. The lumen of the rough-surfaced endoplasmic reticulum (rER) is dilated and some amorphous substances are observed within it.

Figure 3 shows a thyrotroph of a rat, which was injected with 1 μg of synthetic TRF and sacrificed 15 min later. The Golgi apparatus (G) develops markedly and many mitochondria (Mi) gather around it, while secretory granules (Sg) are decreased in number (degranulation).

Figure 4 shows a thyrotroph of a rat, which was injected with 100 μg, a very large dose, of synthetic TRF and sacrificed 5 min later. The rough-surfaced endoplasmic reticulum (rER) is distended extremely and looks like numerous vacuoles. The Golgi apparatus (G) develops strikingly.

Those findings observed in Figs 2, 3 and 4 would suggest an increased TSH release from thyrotrophs as well as an enhanced TSH production in thyrotrophs after synthetic TRF administration. In the other types of anterior pituitary cells we could not find any significant changes.

ULTRASTRUCTURAL CHANGES IN RABBIT THYROTROPHS INDUCED BY ELECTRICAL STIMULATION IN THE HYPOTHALAMUS

A bipolar stainless steel electrode (0.2 mm in diameter), insulated except for tips, was inserted into the hypothalamus of adult rabbits with the aid of Kurotsu-Shimizu's apparatus (Kurotsu 1953). Electrical stimulation was applied using monophasic square wave current (60 c/s, 0.5 msec, 6 V; alternately on and off for 30 sec). Immediately after stimulation, rabbits were anaesthetized with Nembutal and perfused with 4 per cent solution of glutaraldehyde in 0.1 M phosphate buffer. Pituitary glands were then removed and postfixed with 2 per cent solution of OsO_4, and prepared for electron microscopy as mentioned above.

Figure 5 shows a typical thyrotroph of a normal rabbit. The cell is angular in shape and contains a nucleus (Nu), some secretory granules (Sg), mitochondria (Mi), rough-surfaced endoplasmic reticulum (rER) and the Golgi apparatus (G). Secretory granules are of high electron density and their maximum diameter is about 100–150 mμ, similar to those in rats.

Figure 6 shows a thyrotroph of a rabbit, which was stimulated for 20 min in the dorsomedial hypothalamic nucleus, belonging to the b-sympathetic zone*. The Golgi apparatus (G) develops markedly and contains some immature granules.

Figure 7 shows a thyrotroph of a rabbit, which was stimulated for 20 min in the anterior hypothalamic nucleus, also belonging to the b-sympathetic zone. The Golgi apparatus (G) develops strikingly and many mitochondria are concentrated around it.

The findings observed in Figs 6 and 7 would suggest that hypothalamic TRF would be discharged into the portal circulation after electrical stimulation in the b-sympathetic zone and augment the secretory activity of thyrotrophs in the anterior pituitary gland.

---

* The b-sympathetic zone corresponds to the medial hypothalamic area and includes the following nuclei: nucleus supraopticus, nucleus paraventricularis, nucleus anterior, nucleus dorsomedialis, nucleus ventromedialis, nucleus posterior, nucleus premamillaris, nucleus supramamillaris and nucleus mamillaris lateralis (Ban 1964).

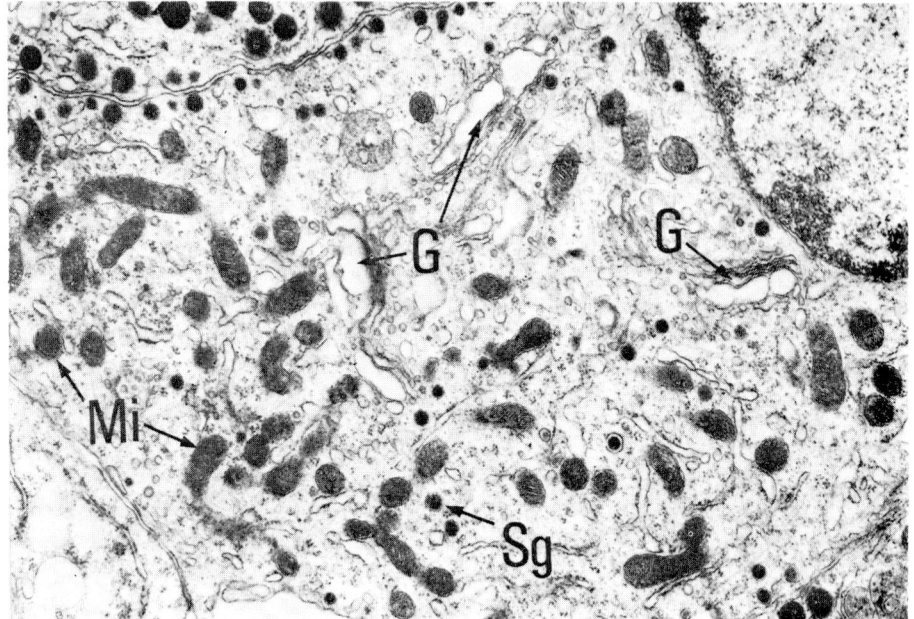

Fig. 3. Part of a thyrotroph of a rat injected with 1 µg of synthetic TRF and sacrificed 15 min later. ×15,000

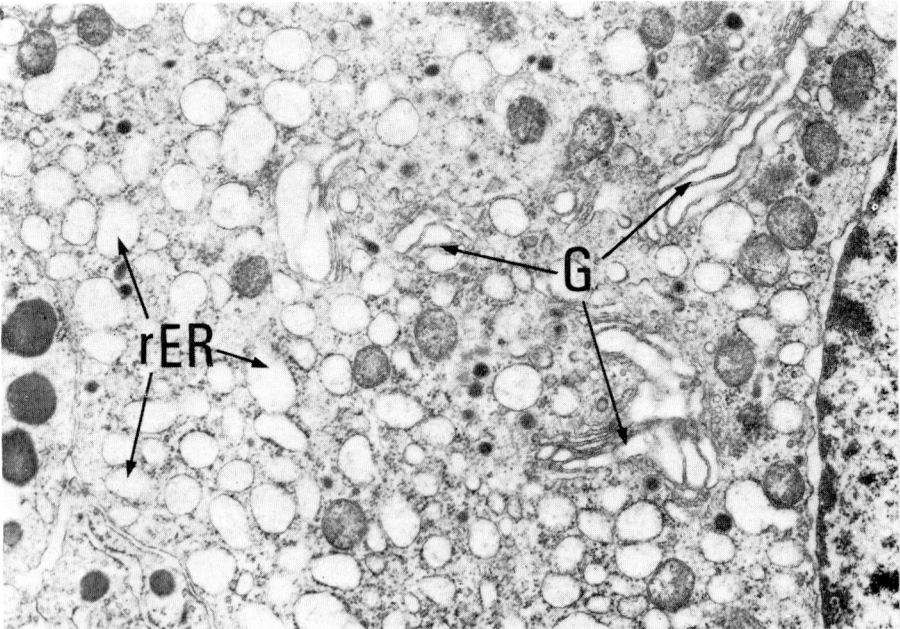

Fig. 4. Part of a thyrotroph of a rat injected with 100 µg of synthetic TRF and sacrificed 5 min later. ×15,000

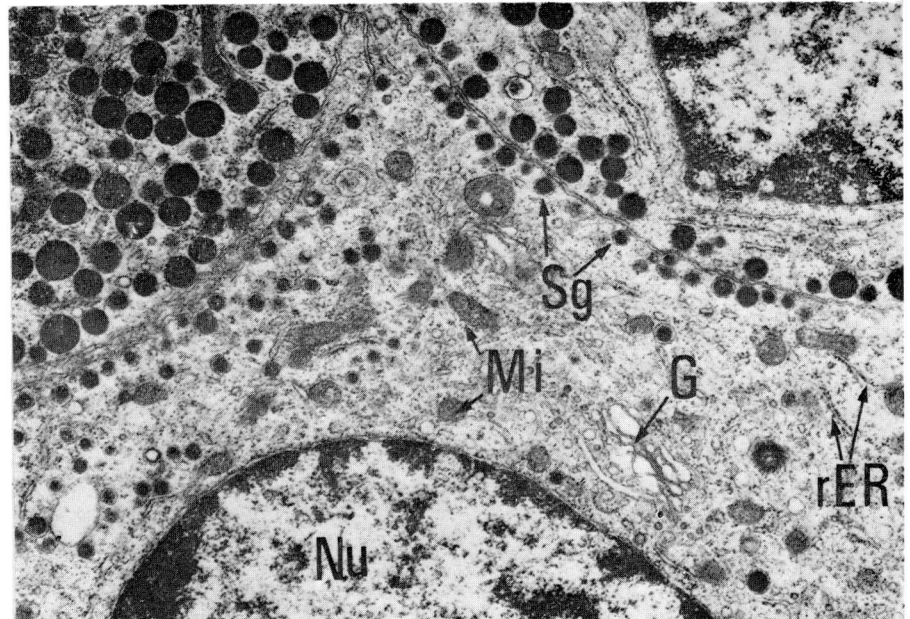

Fig. 5. Part of a thyrotroph of a normal rabbit. ×15,000

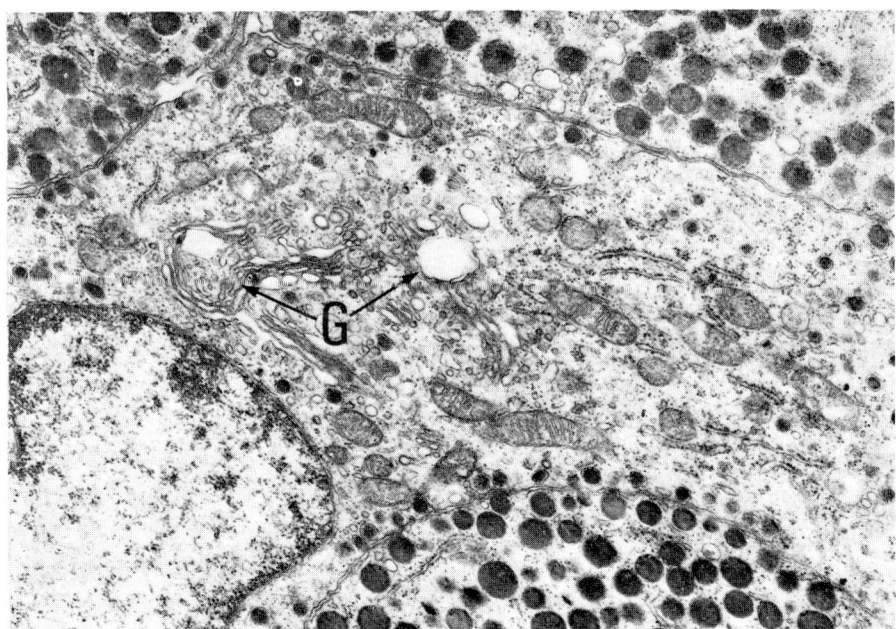

Fig. 6. Part of a thyrotroph of a rabbit stimulated electrically for 20 min in the dorsomedial hypothalamic nucleus. ×15,000

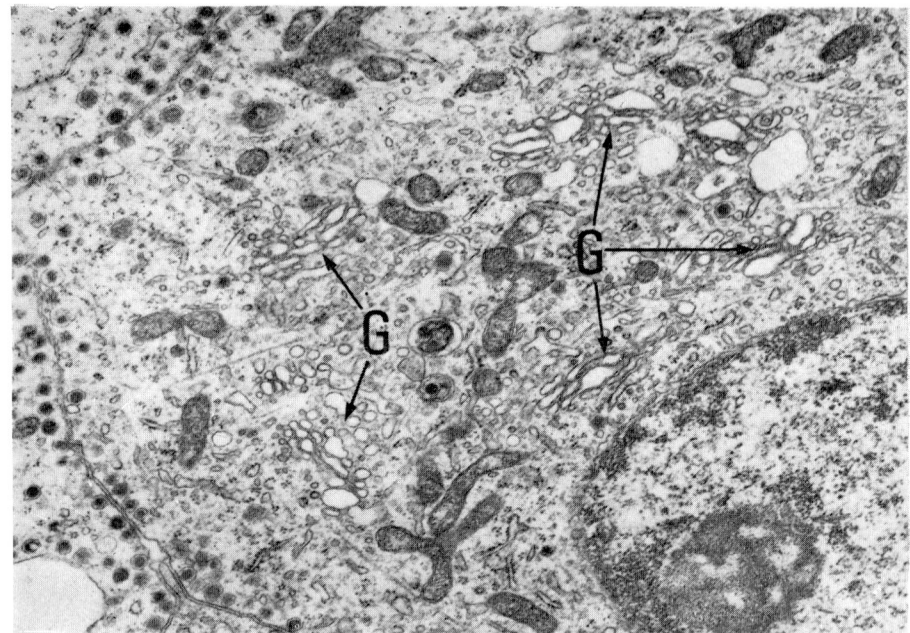

Fig. 7. Part of a thyrotroph of a rabbit stimulated electrically for 20 min in the anterior hypothalamic nucleus. ×15,000

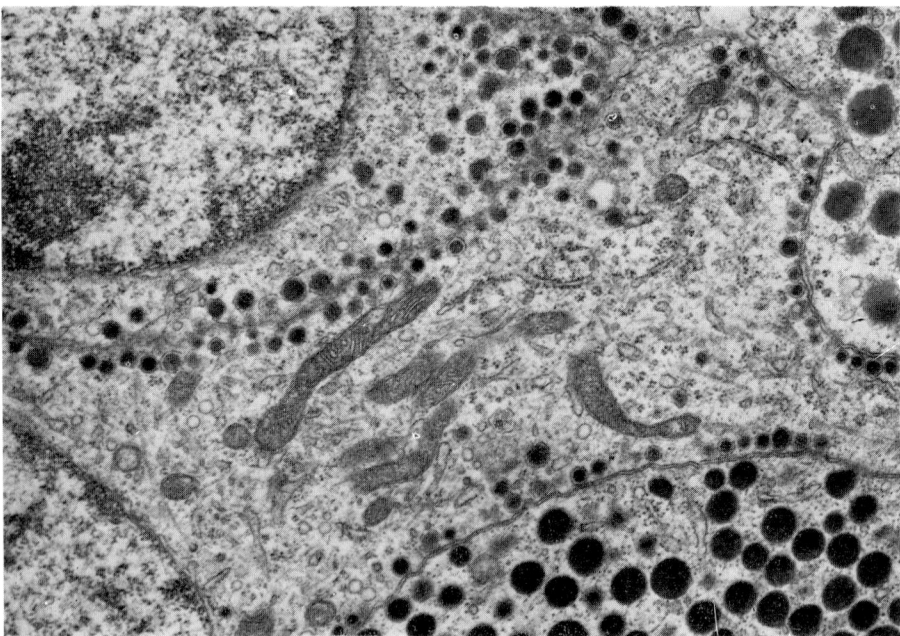

Fig. 8. Part of a thyrotroph of a rabbit stimulated electrically for 20 min in the lateral hypothalamic nucleus. ×15,000

Figure 8 shows a thyrotroph of a rabbit, which was stimulated for 20 min in the lateral hypothalamic nucleus, belonging to the c-parasympathetic zone*. The ultrastructure of the cell is not so different from that of the control animals.

This finding suggests that hypothalamic TRF would not be discharged after electrical stimulation in the c-parasympathetic zone.

SUMMARY

1. After the administration of synthetic TRF, rat thyrotrophs showed a decrease of secretory granules in number, dilatation of rER, marked development of the Golgi apparatus and concentration of mitochondria around it, as early as 5 min after injection, indicating an increased TSH release as well as an enhanced TSH production.

2. After electrical stimulation in the b-sympathetic zone, rabbit thyrotrophs showed an augmented secretory activity, due to the probable discharge of hypothalamic TRF, whereas after stimulation in the c-parasympathetic zone, thyrotrophs were not activated at all.

REFERENCES

BAN, T. (1964): The hypothalamus, especially on its fiber connections, and the septo-preoptico-hypothalamic system. *Med. J. Osaka Univ.* **15,** 1–83.

BOWERS, C. Y., SCHALLY, A. V., ENZMANN, F., BØLER, J. and FOLKERS, K. (1970): Porcine thyrotropin releasing hormone is (Pyro)Glu-His-Pro(NH$_2$). *Endocrinology* **86,** 1143–1153.

KUROTSU, T. (1953): Our experimental method for studies on hypothalamus. *Med. J. Osaka Univ.* **4,** 171–174.

SHIOTANI, Y., SAKAGAMI, M., FUJIMOTO, K. and BAN, T. (1969): Ultrastructural changes in the anterior pituitary gland induced by electrical stimulation of the hypothalamus. *Endocr. jap.* Suppl. **1,** 1–9.

---

* The c-parasympathetic zone corresponds to the lateral hypothalamic area and is composed of nucleus hypothalamicus lateralis (Ban 1964).

THE EFFECT OF OESTRADIOL ON PITUITARY–ADRENAL FUNCTION IN INTACT AND THYROIDECTOMIZED RATS

F. TALLIÁN

Department of Gynaecology and Obstetrics
Postgraduate Medical School
Budapest, Hungary

Interactions between the pituitary–adrenal and pituitary–gonadal functions as well as between those and the pituitary–thyroid axis were the subjects of many studies in recent decades. Both synergistic and antagonistic influences have been observed in animal experiments which suggested an extremely complicated regulatory process behind these events (Velardo 1957, D'Angelo and Hughes 1963, Fortier et al. 1970, etc.). Concerning the effect of oestradiol on the pituitary–adrenal axis, it is known that oestradiol administration led to the enlargement of adrenals, on the one hand, but depending on the dosages, it may enhance or inhibit the adrenal steroidogenesis under both in vivo and in vitro conditions, on the other hand (Kitay 1963, Amesbury et al. 1965, etc.).

In the present investigations we were interested to study the influence of an intrahypothalamic oestradiol implantation in combination with hydrocortisone on the compensatory adrenal and ovarian hypertrophy in the intact or thyroidectomized rats.

INFLUENCE OF THE INTRAHYPOTHALAMIC IMPLANTATION OF OESTRADIOL-17α ON THE COMPENSATORY HYPERTROPHY OF ADRENALS AND OVARY IN INTACT FEMALE RATS

Unilateral removal of the adrenal and ovary was performed in the same operation with the microcrystal implantation of either oestradiol or hydrocortisone as well as the combination of the two steroids. Sham-operated rats with the removal of the endocrine glands were implanted with equivalent amount of cholesterol. The implantation was carried out on the tip of a 0.2–0.3 mm diameter glass capillary and the average quantity of oestradiol and hydrocortisone was determined by the use of appropriate physico-chemical methods (Tallián et al. in prep.). The animals were sacrificed on the 12th postoperative day and the compensatory hypertrophy of the remaining glands was expressed in the percentage of the wet weight of the contralateral glands. The intrahypothalamic implantation was controlled in frozen sections; the majority of the implants were found in the rostral median eminence and only a few of them were located in the ventromedial and dorsal periventricular regions. The implantation of 15 µg oestradiol or its combination with 15 µg hydrocortisone led to a marked suppression of the compensatory ovarian hypertrophy. A significant decrease in the hypertrophy was found after hydrocortisone implantation alone and the combination of the two steroids suppressed the ovarian weights below the initial values (Fig. 1).

Reducing the dosis of oestradiol in the intrahypothalamic implants, it was found that 4.5 µg still produced a significant suppression of the compensatory hypertrophy but only a slight decrease in the ovarian weights had been observed as a result of hydrocortisone implantation of the same dosage alone (Fig. 2)

Intrahypothalamic implantation of the 4.5 µg oestradiol led to a marked increase in compensatory hypertrophy of adrenals and in combination with hydrocortisone partially prevented the hydrocortisone-induced blockade of the compensatory adrenal hypertrophy (Fig. 3).

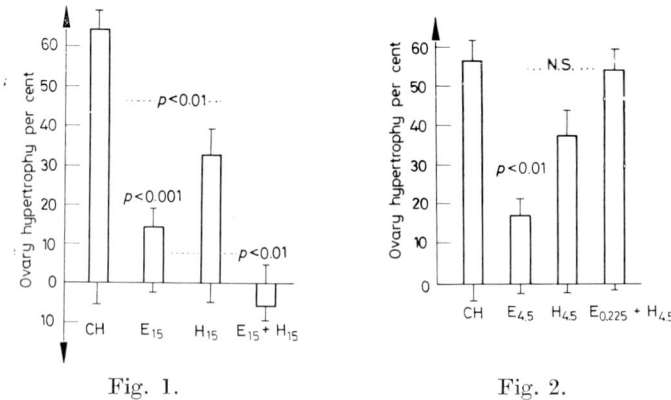

Fig. 1. Fig. 2.

Figs 1 and 2. Changes in compensatory hypertrophy of the ovary after the implantation of 15 µg, respectively 4.5 µg, oestradiol and hydrocortisone. The vertical bars on the horizontal line (as 0 line) correspond to the standard errors of the initial weights

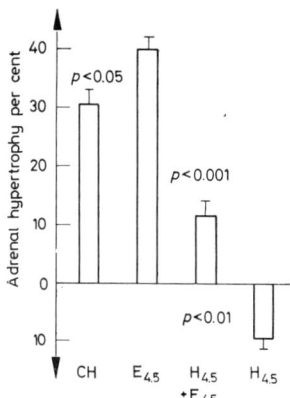

Fig. 3. Changes in adrenal hypertrophy following implantation of 4.5 µg oestradiol and hydrocortisone

INFLUENCE OF INTRAHYPOTHALAMIC OESTRADIOL IMPLANTATION ON THE COMPENSATORY ADRENAL HYPERTROPHY IN THYROIDECTOMIZED RATS

Female rats were thyroidectomized 4 weeks prior to the implantation of 15 μg oestradiol into the median eminence region and to unilateral adrenalectomy. Both the sham-operated rats with cholesterol implants and the rats with oestradiol were treated with a daily dose of 1 μg tri-iodothyronine for 12 days. The oestradiol implantation produced a marked increase in the compensatory adrenal hypertrophy both in the presence and absence of a tri-iodothyronine substitution therapy after 12 days following the adrenalectomy in thyroidectomized rats. A marked reduction in the compensatory adrenal hypertrophy of thyroidectomized rats could be prevented by the tri-iodothyronine treatment (Fig. 4).

An oestrogen-induced enlargement of the pituitary is known from earlier studies, however, the involvement of the pituitary–thyroid axis in the process remained unclear. The present investigations clearly demonstrate that the intrahypothalamic implantation of oestradiol produces a marked increase in pituitary weight both in the presence and the absence of a substitution therapy in thyroidectomized rats. These observations ruled out the possible involvement of an increased TSH-thyroid secretion in the oestrogen-induced pituitary growth (Fig. 5).

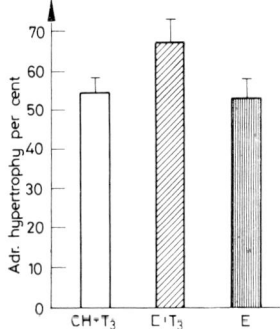
Fig. 4. Changes in compensatory hypertrophy of the adrenals of thyroidectomized rats with and without a substitution therapy of 1 μg tri-iodothyronine and with oestradiol implantation into the median eminence region

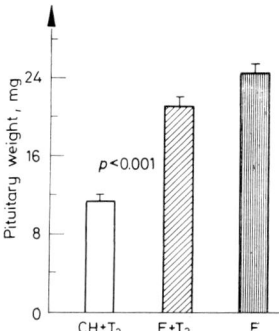
Fig. 5. Changes in the pituitary weights following implantation of cholesterol (CH), oestradiol (E) and their combination with tri-iodothyronine administration on thyroidectomized rats

CONCLUSIONS

An oestrogen-induced inhibition of hydrocortisone-mediated suppression of the compensatory ACTH secretion may be interpreted as an interference of the two steroids on common receptive sites at both the hypothalamic and the pituitary levels. The present study does not exclude the possibility that oestradiol exerted an influence on the pituitary cells without an involvement of the hypothalamic

CRF secretion, although there are data which indicate significant changes in CRF content as a result of oestradiol administration (Tallián et al. in prep.). On the other hand, a hydrocortisone-induced suppression of the compensatory ovarian hypertrophy and its synergism with oestradiol action revealed that an increased FSH release necessary for a compensatory hypertrophy of the ovary may be influenced by a nonspecific way through the pituitary–adrenal axis (Lissák and Endrőczi 1965).

Intrahypothalamic implantation of a minute amount of oestradiol is still far over the range of the physiological concentration in the circulating blood and such approach of the endocrine interrelationships must be limited for hormone actions at the hypothalamo–pituitary level which do not involve other regulatory processes taking place between the pituitary and the target organs. Thus, an increase in TSH secretion as a result of oestradiol administration plays a role in the increase of the pituitary–adrenal axis function which is mediated through an increase in plasma corticosterone binding capacity (Fortier et al. 1970). This regulation functions under physiological conditions and within a certain range of the circulating hormones. The present data dealing with a direct application of oestradiol on the pituitary target organ (or through the portal capillary with or without involvement of the secretion of releasing factors) revealed that oestradiol exerts a facilitatory influence on the pituitary ACTH secretion in the absence of an increased pituitary–thyroid function. These observations do not imply the direct effect of oestradiol on the pituitary ACTH synthesis or release and an interference between the corticosteroid-adjusted regulation of ACTH secretion and oestradiol-induced facilitation of this troph hormone may take place at the releasing factor elements of the hypothalamus.

REFERENCES

D'Angelo, S. A. (1963): Central nervous regulation of the secretion and release of thyroid stimulating hormone. In: *Advances in Neuroendocrinology*. Vol. 3. Ed. by Nalbandov, A. N. Univ. Illinois Press, Urbana. pp. 158–210.

Fortier, C., Labrie, F., Pelletier, G., Raynaud, J. P., Ducommun, P., Delgado, A., Labrie, R. and Ho-Kim, M. A. (1970): Recent studies on the feed-back control of ACTH secretion, with particular reference to the role of transcortin in pituitary-thyroid-adrenocortical interrelations. In: *Ciba Found. Symp. on Control Processes in Multicellular Organisms*. Ed. by Wolstenholme, G. E. and Knight, J. Churchill, London. pp. 178–196.

Gemzell, C. A. (1952): Increase in the formation and secretion of ACTH in rats following administration of oestradiol-monobenzoate. *Acta endocr. (Kbh.)* **11**, 221–228.

Kitay, J. I. (1963): Effects of testosterone on pituitary corticotrophine and adrenal steroid secretion in male and female rats. *Acta endocr. (Kbh.)* **43**, 601–608.

Lissák, K. and Endrőczi, E. (1965): Involvement of the limbic structures in conditioning, motivation and recent memory. In: *Symposium on Structure and Function of Limbic System*. Hakone, Japan.

Smith, E. R., Johnson, J., Weick, R. F., Levine, S. and Davidson, J. M. (1971): Inhibition of the reproductive system in immature rats by intracerebral implantation of cortisol. *Neuroendocrinology*, **8**, 94–106.

Telegdy, Gy., Schreiber, G. and Endrőczi, E. (1964): Effect of oestrogens implanted into the hypothalamus on the activity of the pituitary-adrenocortical system. *Acta physiol. Acad. Sci. hung.* **25**, 229–234.

Velardo, I. T. (1957): Steroidal aspects of pregnane inhibition of progesterone in decidual development. *Amer. J. Physiol.* **188**, 317–320.

STUDIES ON THE REGULATION OF PITUITARY-ADRENAL-THYROID AND GONADAL FUNCTIONS IN RATS WITH HYPOTHALAMIC LESIONS

L. HALMY

4th Department of Internal Medicine
Postgraduate Medical School
Budapest, Hungary

A great number of data has accumulated in the literature suggesting a leading role of the ventromedial hypothalamic region in the maintenance of pituitary function. Lesion to this hypothalamic area produces hyperphagia and obesity (Harris 1955, Szentágothai et al. 1962, Lissák and Endrőczi 1960, 1965, Hetherington and Ranson 1940, Brobeck et al. 1943, Morgane and Jacobs 1969, etc.). Though Hetherington (1943) already had pointed out that elimination of the pituitary gland did not prevent the development of hypothalamic obesity, recent observations indicate some kind of influence of the pituitary function on the syndrome and there are data showing alterations in the pituitary troph hormone secretion which seems to be accompanied by hypothalamic obesity (Morgane and Jacobs 1969, Valenstein et al. 1969). Recently, we were interested to study the possible alterations of the pituitary functions in connection with the development of hypothalamic obesity which had been produced by electrolytic lesions in the ventromedial hypothalamic area in the rats.

SEX DIFFERENCES IN THE DEVELOPMENT OF HYPOTHALAMIC OBESITY

It is known that the gain in body weight is more marked in male than in female rats after puberty. Bilateral lesion of the ventromedial nucleus produced a marked hyperphagia in both sexes and led to a characteristic obesity within a few weeks. These observations contradict the assumptions according to which male rats are more resistant to the development of hypothalamic obesity than females (Valenstein et al. 1969) (Fig. 1).

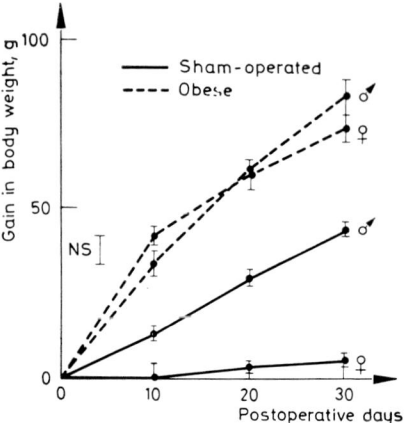

Fig. 1. Effect of ventromedial hypothalamic lesion on the body weight gain of female and male rats. Solid lines show the gain in body weight of the controls of both sexes during the course of the first 30 postoperative days

ENDOCRINE CHANGES AFTER VENTROMEDIAL HYPOTHALAMIC LESION IN OBESE RATS

Two different types of electrolytic lesion which destroyed to a different degree the ventromedial and arcuate nucleus and the periventricular region, were made in the female and male rats. The smaller lesion, called type I, destroyed only a part of the ventromedial nucleus and of the periventricular area. Type II resulted in a nearly complete damage of the ventromedial nucleus and extended into the arcuate nucleus and the median eminence area (Fig. 2).

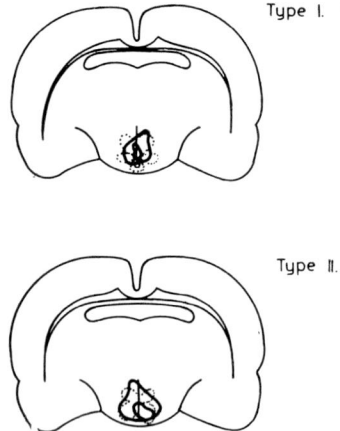

Fig. 2. The two types of lesions with their smallest and greatest extent. Type I damaged partly the ventromedial nucleus and the periventricular area. Type II destroyed the entire ventromedial nucleus and extended into the arcuate nucleus and partly into the median eminence region

Both types of lesions led to a characteristic hyperphagia and obesity, although the changes in endocrine weights showed a marked dependence on the extension of the lesions after a 14-day postoperative period. An increased food and water intake of the lesioned rats is shown in Fig. 3.

There was no difference in the adrenal and thyroid weights in the obese rats after either type of lesion (Fig. 4).

Both types of lesions produced changes in the gonadal weights, although the smaller lesions exerted only a moderate effect on the ovary and did not produce atrophy of the testicles. In contrast to these findings, type II led to a marked atrophy of the ovary and testicles as well as of the uterus, prostate and seminal vesicles (Figs 5 and 6).

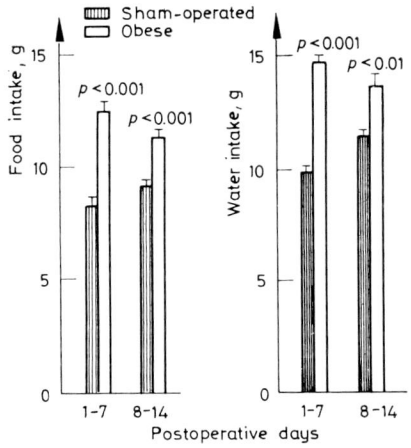

Fig. 3. Food and water intake of the lesioned and sham-operated animals expressed as an average for a 7-day period

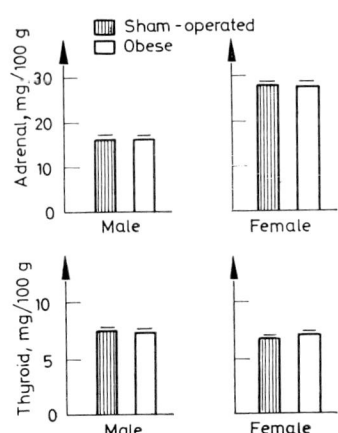

Fig. 4. The ineffectiveness of ventromedial lesion to produce changes in the thyroid and adrenal weights of the rats of both sexes

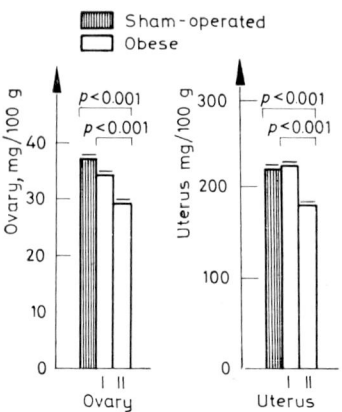

Fig. 5. Changes in the ovarian and uterine weights after types I and II lesions. Only type II lesions resulted in a significant decrease in ovarian and uterine weights

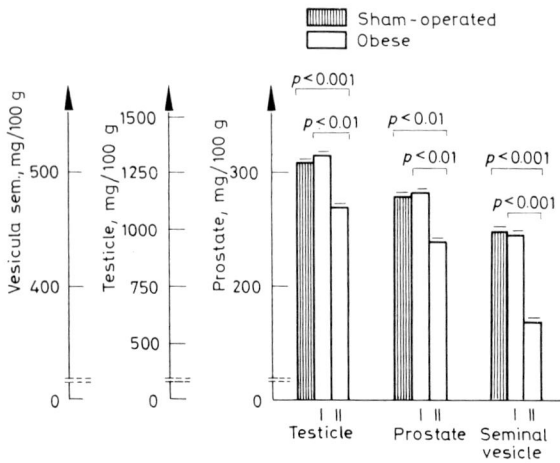

Fig. 6. The effect of ventromedial lesion on the weights of testicles and the accessory sex organs. Type II lesions led to a marked decrease in weights

COMPENSATORY HYPERTROPHY OF THE ADRENALS, OVARY AND THYROID GLAND IN HYPOTHALAMIC OBESE RATS

Female rats were used in the study and type I electrolytic lesion was performed simultaneously with the removal of the endocrine glands on the left side. The compensatory hypertrophy of the remaining glands, which were removed on the 14th postoperative day, was expressed in the percentage of the initial wet weights. Sham-operated rats were also unilaterally ectomized but instead of the electrolytic lesion only the electrode was inserted into the hypothalamus. The compensatory hypertrophy of the three glands was almost in the same range in the obese rats as in the sham-operated controls (Fig. 7).

It seems that all endocrine changes observed following hypothalamic lesions and associated with hyperphagia and obesity, are only by-products of the damages of the so-called hypophysiotropic region.

In connection with the sex differences we were unable to detect a remarkable difference between the development of obesity of the male and female rats. These observations clearly indicate that a conditioning role of the sex hormones in the development of hypothalamic obesity is unlikely. Naturally, this conclusion does not exclude the possibility that administration of sex steroids would not be able to influence the hyperphagia and obesity as we have found in recent studies (Halmy 1971). Of course, an excessive amount of sexual steroid hormones may induce changes both in the central integration of the feeding behaviour and the peripheral metabolic processes.

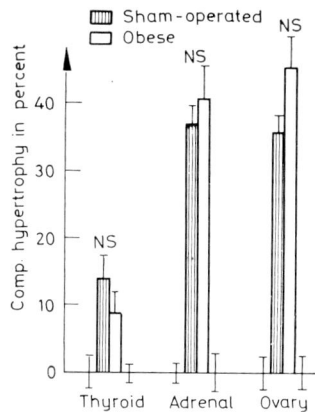

Fig. 7. Compensatory hypertrophy of the endocrine glands. Baseline corresponds to the initial weights and the bars indicate the standard errors. Both the sham-operated and the lesioned rats with obesity showed a significant compensatory hypertrophy of all three glands

REFERENCES

Cox, V. C., Kakolewsky, J. W. and Valenstein, E. S. (1969): Ventromedial hypothalamic lesions and changes in body weight and food consumption in male and female rats. *J. comp. physiol. Psychol.* **67,** 320—326.

Halmy, L. and Nyakas, Cs. (1971): Influence of ventromedical hypothalamic lesions on compensatory hypertrophy of endocrine glands. *Proc. Intern. Physiol. Sci.* **9,** 682.

Halmy, L., Nyakas, Cs. and Endrőczi, E. (1971): Compensatory hypertrophy of adrenal, ovary and thyroid glands in obese rats caused by ventromedial hypothalamic lesions. *Acta physiol. Acad. Sci. hung.* **40,** 201.

Harris, G. W. (1955): Neural Control of the Pituitary Gland. Edward Arnold Ltd., London.

Hetherington, A. W. and Ranson, S. W. (1940): Hypothalamic lesions and adiposity in the rat. *Anat. Rec.* **78,** 149—172.

Lissák, K. and Endrőczi, E. (1965): Involvement of the limbic structures in conditioning, motivation and recent memory. In: *Symposium on Structure and Function of the Limbic System.* Hakone, Japan.

Morgane, P. J. (1969): The function of the limbic and rhinic forebrain-limbic midbrain systems and reticular formation in the regulation of food and water intake. *Ann. N. Y. Acad. Sci.* **157**, 806—848.

Szentágothai, J., Flerkó, B., Mess, B. and Halász, B. (1962): Hypothalamic control of the anterior pituitary. *Acta. med. Acad. Sci. hung.*

Valenstein, E. S., Cox, V. C. and Kakolewsky, I. W. (1969): Sex differences in hyperphagia and body weight following hypothalamic damage. *Ann. N. Y. Acad. Sci.* **157**, 1030—1048.

Hormones and Brain Function, Budapest 1971, pp. 213—218 (1973)

EFFECT OF SYNTHETIC TSH-RELEASING FACTOR (TRF) AND OF SOME TRF ANALOGUES ON PITUITARY FUNCTION

H. STEINER,[1] F. PIVA, M. MOTTA, G. GAVAZZI, R. COLLU[2]
and L. MARTINI

*Department of Pharmacology
University of Milan
Milan, Italy*

Synthetic TSH-releasing factor (TRF) is by definition not contaminated with other releasing factors and acts quite specifically on its target cells, i.e. on anterior pituitary thyrotrophs. It seems, however, reasonable to make the assumption that the endocrine system, taken as a whole, may be affected in one way or another, when a very potent endocrinologically active substance like TRF modifies its equilibrium. The dynamics of TSH secretion (release and synthesis) under the influence of TRF have been recently studied in detail in our laboratory; experiments have now been performed in order to evaluate the possible actions of TRF on the pituitary–adrenocortical axis. A number of synthetic TRF analogues have also been included in this study. Their utilization proved very useful in elucidating the mode of action of TRF on both the pituitary–thyroid and the pituitary–adrenal axis.

MATERIAL AND METHODS

The TRF and its analogues used in this study were synthesized by the peptide team of Dr. R. O. Studer in research laboratories of F. Hoffmann–La Roche Co., Basle, Switzerland (Gillessen et al. 1970, 1971). As previously reported, TRF is the tripeptide L-pyro-glutamyl-L-histidyl-L-proline amide; in one analogue the L-histidine residue has been replaced by L-β-(pyrazoly-3)alanine ("Pyrala"), and in the second the pyroglutamyl-terminal has been slightly modified while leaving the ring structure intact ("P*-His-Pro"). The details of the structure modification will be published elsewhere (Gillessen et al., in preparation). The hormonal activities of these and other analogues have been recently reviewed (Gillessen et al. 1971, Steiner et al. 1971).

The effect of TRF and of its analogues on TSH release and synthesis was determined using a "pituitary depletion method" in the intact animals. Plasma levels of TSH were measured in addition to pituitary TSH stores. The validity of this

---

[1] On leave of absence from the F. Hoffmann-La Roche Co. Ltd., Basle, Switzerland, Department of Experimental Medicine.
[2] Present address: Hôpital Sainte-Justine, 3175 Côte Sainte-Cathérine, Montreal, Què., Canada.

procedure has been reviewed recently (Piva and Steiner 1971). The determination of TSH in the plasma and in the pituitaries of animals treated with TRF and its analogues was performed biologically in rats, using the modification of the McKenzie assay designed by Yamazaki et al. (1963). Corticosterone was measured fluorometrically (Guillemin et al. 1959, Fraschini et al. 1964).

RESULTS AND DISCUSSION

As indicated in Fig. 1, synthetic TRF is a potent releaser of TSH; but at the same time, this factor induces a strong resynthesis of TSH. The intracarotid injection of 10 µg of synthetic TRF is followed by a sharp increase of plasma TSH in the recipient animals. Plasma TSH levels remain elevated for at least 30 min; after this time a rapid decrease is observed. The same dose of TRF induced, at the beginning, a drop of pituitary TSH stores; however, TSH concentration in the pituitary has returned to pre-injection levels as early as 15 min after treatment, at a time when plasma TSH is still increasing.

The same separation of effects on resynthesis and release may be seen by varying the intensity of the stimulus reaching the pituitary, i.e. by injecting different doses of TRF (Fig. 2). The absolute values of pituitary TSH are not strictly comparable because in the experiments shown in Fig .1, another TSH-standard batch was used.

It has recently been observed that the analogue "Pyrala" induces TSH resynthesis and release in a manner similar to that of TRF; the only difference seems to be that when comparable doses are used, serum TSH levels return to normal more rapidly after the injection of this peptide than after TRF (Steiner, unpublished data, 1971). The other analogue "P*-His-Pro", on the other hand, induces synthesis

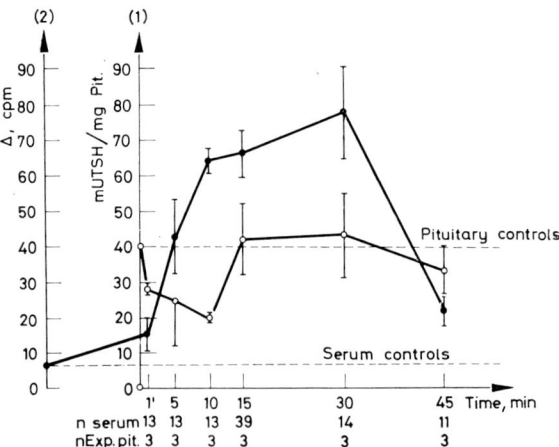

Fig. 1. Pituitary TSH levels in adult male rats (1) after intracarotid (i.c.) injection of 10 µg synthetic TSH-releasing factor as measured by bioassay and the Δ% counts per minute, cpm ^{131}I by the serum (2) of the same animals. TSH potency in pituitaries is given in terms of NIH–TSH–S5–USP standard

of TSH in the pituitary, but does not seem to release biologically measurable TSH at all (Steiner et al. 1971).

When corticosterone levels were measured in the serum of animals submitted to the stress of the surgical exposure of the carotid artery under pentobarbital anaesthesia, a significant increase was observed in all the animals killed 1 to 45 min after the intracarotid injection of saline. In animals submitted to the same stressing surgical procedure, but receiving an intracarotid injection of TRF instead of saline, the increase of plasma corticosterone measured 15 min after injection was much smaller than that observed in animals not treated with TRF (Fig. 3).

This indicates that the administration of TRF counteracts the effect the stressing procedures exert on plasma corticosterone levels. A similar observation has been reported by Sakiz and Guillemin (1965) in rats; a decrease of plasma cortisol following the injection of TRF has also been found to occur in humans (Rothenbuchner et al. 1971). It is interesting to note that the depressing effect of TRF on the stress-induced increase of plasma corticosterone levels is not seen if plasma is collected 5 min instead of 15 min after the injection. A comparison with data obtained using TRF analogues in a similar experimental scheme leads to the conclusion that the depression of stress-induced elevation of plasma corticosterone

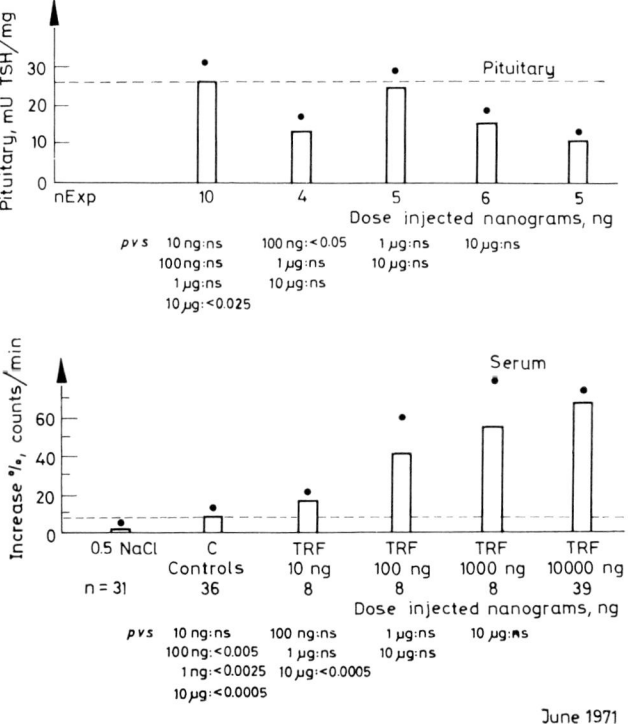

Fig. 2. TSH content in the pituitary and in the serum 15 min after i.c. injection of TRF (pH 7) in rats. Units and standard as in Fig. 1, but new batch of standard

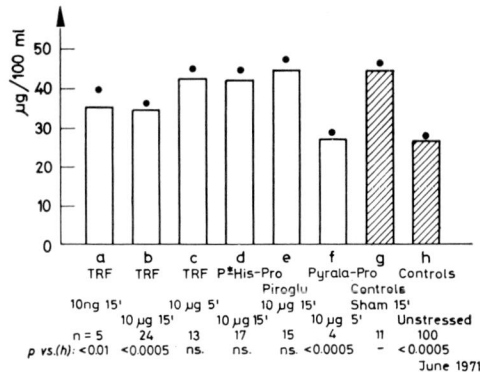

Fig. 3. Serum corticosterone levels (μg/100 ml) in pentobarbital-anaesthetized and surgically stressed male adult rats after i.c. injection of TRF and of two analogues. Fluorometric method

is not due to the increase of plasma TSH (and consequently of thyroxine) induced by TRF. The analogue "P*-His-Pro", which induces only resynthesis and not the release of TSH (and consequently does not mobilize thyroid hormones) does not depress the rise in plasma corticosterone levels. On the other hand, the other analogue "Pyrala", which induces TSH resynthesis and release, does not depress corticosterone levels 15 min after injection. Surprisingly, however, this compound induces a strong depression of the stress-induced corticosterone rise 1 and 5 min after injection (Fig. 4, Table 1). As previously stated, this "rapid" depression was not observed 5 min after injection of TRF (Fig. 3) and in the NaCl controls. The observation of a "rapid" and of a "delayed" depression of the stress-induced rise of plasma corticosterone induced respectively by "Pyrala" and by TRF can be explained only by postulating that at least 2 different mechanisms are involved in this effect on corticosterone levels. The "rapid" depression might be due to a masking of the normally assayable free corticosterone (e.g., by an increase in its protein binding, by a rapid enzymatic inactivation, by a rapid leakage from the vascular compartment, etc.). A direct effect of thyroxine mobilized by the rapidly increasing levels of TSH seems again improbable because this effect was not observed with TRF. On the other hand, the "delayed" effect on plasma cortico-

TABLE 1

The various effects of TRF and two analogues on TSH release, TSH resynthesis and depression of stress-induced corticosterone levels

	TSH release	TSH resynthesis	Corticosterone rapid depression	Corticosterone delayed depression
TRF	+	+	−	+
'P*-His-Pro"	−	+	−	−
'Pyrala"	+	+	+	−

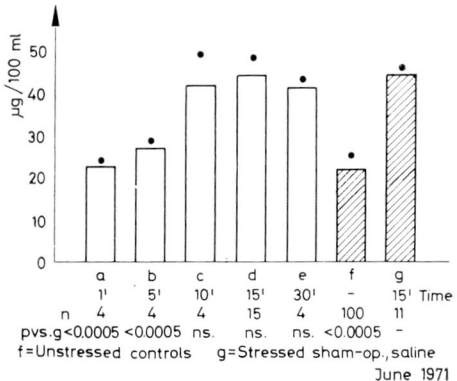

Fig. 4. Serum corticosterone levels (μg/100 ml) in pentobarbital-anaesthetized and surgically stressed male adult rats at different times after intracarotid injection of 10 μg of a TRF analogue with histidine replacement by L-β(pyrazolyl-fl)-alanine

sterone observed 15 min after the injection of TRF is probably due to a central action, i.e., to the supression of ACTH secretion. We do not believe that peripheral components might intervene in the production of such a phenomenon. One might postulate, e.g., that following injection of TRF, a shift occurs in the different functions of the pituitary: through such a mechanism, the gland might produce less ACTH when stimulated to synthesize and/or release more TSH. We do not feel, however, that the data here presented fully support this hypothesis, particularly because it has been observed that the "delayed" effect on plasma corticosterone is not induced by the two synthetic analogues of TRF, even though they exert a significant effect on the release and/or the synthesis of TSH. Another hypothesis is that TRF intervenes in regulating the production or the release of corticotropin-releasing factor at the hypothalamic level; such hypothesis would involve a strict correlation in the central nervous system of the mechanisms which control the secretion of TSH and ACTH. Such a correlation is certainly supported by the recent findings by Nicoloff et al. (1971) which indicate that glucocorticoids may depress TSH secretion both in normal subjects and in patients resistant to thyroid hormones and having high levels of plasma TSH.

It is interesting to recall that TRF seems to exert some effect also on the secretion of another pituitary product, the growth hormone (GH); such an effect, however, is completely different from the one here reported with regard to ACTH. R. Collu and H. Steiner (1971, unpublished results) have recently found that the addition of TRF to the incubation media containing rat anterior pituitary tissue in a technique described by Crighton et al. (1968) brings about the release of radio-immunoassayable GH. This observation has been confirmed by La Bella and Vivian (1971) using rat pituitaries in vitro and by Wagner and co-workers (1971) and Karlberg et al. (1971) working in vivo in humans.

SUMMARY

The dynamics of TSH release and TSH-resynthesis have been studied with synthetic TSH releasing factors (TRF) and with two of its analogues. Evidence is given that release and resynthesis are two separate phenomena. After injection of these TSH-releasing substances a rapid or a delayed depression of the serum corticosterone levels in surgically stressed animals was observed.

These and other data concerning effects on hormonal interplay after injection of TRF are discussed.

ACKNOWLEDGEMENTS

The valuable technical assistance of Miss P. Assi, Mr. Fabio Celotti and Mr. Angelo Pravettoni is gratefully acknowledged. This work was partially supported by a grant of the Ford Foundation (Grant No. 67-530).

The TSH standard is a gift from the National Institute of Health, Bethesda, Md., USA.

REFERENCES

CRIGHTON, D. B., WATANABE, S., DHARIWAL, A. P. S. and MCCANN, S. M. (1968): *Proc. Soc. exp. Biol.* (N. Y.) **128**, 537.
DAVID, M. A., FRASCHINI, F. and MARTINI, L. (1965): *Experientia (Basel)* **21**, 483.
FRASCHINI, F., MANGILI, G., MOTTA, M. and MARTINI, L. (1964): *Endocrinology* **75**, 765.
GILLESSEN, D., FELIX, A. M., LERGIER, W. and STUDER, R. O. (1970): *Helv. chim. Acta* **53**, 63.
GILLESSEN, D., PIVA, F., STEINER, H. and STUDER, R. O. (1971): *Helv. chim. Acta* **54**, 1335.
GUILLEMIN, R., CLAYTON, G. W., LIPSCOMB, H. S. and SMITH, J. D. (1959): *J. Lab. clin. Med.* **53**, 830.
KARLBERG, B., ALMQVIST, S. and WERNER, S. (1971): *Acta endocr.* (Kbh.) **67**, 288.
LA BELLA, F. S. and VIVIAN, S. R. (1971): *Endocrinology* **88**, 787.
NICOLOFF, J. T. and APPLEMAN, M. D., JR. (1971): *Endocrinology* **88**, Suppl. **131**.
PIVA, F. and STEINER, H. (1971): In: *Workshop Conference on TRH*, Basel. (In press).
ROTHENBUCHNER, G., VANHAELST, L., BIRK, J., GOLSTEIN, J., VOIGT, H. K., FEHM, H. L., LOOS, U., WINKLER, G., SCHLEYER, M., RAPTIS, S. and PFEIFFER, E. F. (1971): *Horm. Metab. Res.* **3**, 139.
SAKIZ, E. and GUILLEMIN, R. (1965): *Endocrinology* **77**, 797.
STEINER, H., MOTTA, M., PIVA, F., GILLESSEN, D. and STUDER, R. O. (1971): *Acta endocr.* (Kbh.) **67** Suppl. **155**. (In press).
WAGNER, H., HRUBESCH, M., VOSBERG, H., BÖKEL, K., BRISSE, B., JUNGE-HULSING, G. and HAUSS, W. H. (1971): *Horm. Metab. Res.* **3**, 137.
YAMAZAKI, E., SAKIZ, E. and GUILLEMIN, R. (1963): *Experientia (Basel)* **19**, 480.

EFFECT OF HYPOTHALAMIC DEAFFERENTATIONS ON PUBERTY IN THE MALE RAT

M. MOTTA, R. COLLU[1] and L. MARTINI

Department of Pharmacology
University of Milan
Milan, Italy

INTRODUCTION

Very little information is presently available on the mechanisms which regulate the onset of puberty in male animals. The present paper will summarize the results recently obtained in our laboratory, which suggest that extrahypothalamic influences may play a major role in the control of such a phenomenon.

The technique of "hypothalamic deafferentation" of Halász and Pupp (1965) was adopted for performing the experiments here to be described. As it is known, this technique permits to interrupt, totally or partially, the afferent pathways reaching the medial basal hypothalamus (MBH), and consequently represents a very useful method for studying the role played by extrahypothalamic structures in the regulation of the activity of the hypothalamic–pituitary–gonadal axis.

The effects exerted on the sexual maturation of male rats by two types of hypothalamic deafferentation (complete and frontal deafferentation, respectively) were investigated. The operations were performed on 25-day-old male rats of the Sprague–Dawley strain; for a detailed description of the techniques employed see Halász (1969). The animals were killed at 30, 35 and 50 days of age (i.e. 5, 10 and 25 days after surgery). At autopsy, body and endocrine organ weights were recorded. In addition, the plasma of the animals killed 25 days after the operations, was collected; testosterone levels were measured in these samples as well as in the plasma of appropriate controls, by gas liquid chromatography with electron capture detector according to the procedure of Kniewald et al. (1971). Sham operations were performed in some groups of rats.

RESULTS AND DISCUSSION

Table 1 shows that, at 30 and 35 days of age, the body weight of the rats with complete hypothalamic deafferentation is lower than that of intact animals of the same age. Because of this, only the relative weights of the endocrine structures are

---

[1] Fellow of the Medical Research Council of Canada. Present address: Hôpital Sainte-Justine, 3175 Côte Sainte-Catherine, Montreal, Que., Canada.

TABLE 1

Effect on body and endocrine organ weights of complete hypothalamic deafferentation performed on 25-day-old male rats (autopsy at 30 and 35 days of age)

Groups[a]	Age at autopsy days	Body weight g	Pituitary mg/100 g body weight	Testes mg/100 g body weight	Prostate mg/100 g body weight	Seminal vesicles mg/100 g body weight
Controls (25)	30	104.8 ± 1.25[b]	4.1 ± 0.29	911.8 ± 27.04	45.0 ± 1.86	25.7 ± 0.82
Complete deafferentation (13)	30	79.1 ± 0.10[c]	3.8 ± 0.06	761.6 ± 54.11[d]	29.2 ± 2.63[c]	18.2 ± 1.13[c]
Controls (38)	35	126.8 ± 1.76	4.0 ± 0.06	1,037.2 ± 18.87	44.6 ± 1.28	32.3 ± 0.91
Complete deafferentation (15)	35	96.7 ± 4.31[c]	2.7 ± 0.44[c]	437.5 ± 57.73[c]	14.0 ± 2.05[c]	12.7 ± 0.57[c]

[a] No. of rats in parentheses.
[b] Values are means ± S.E.
[c] $P \leq 0.002$ vs controls of the same age.
[d] $P \leq 0.025$ vs controls of the same age.

shown in Table 1. Following total hypothalamic deafferentation, the animals show depressed weights of the testes, of the prostate and of the seminal vesicles at both 30 and 35 days of age; the weight of the pituitaries of the operated group autopsied at 35 days of age has also been found to be significantly reduced.

No significant differences exist between the body or pituitary weights of completely deafferented animals and of intact controls, killed at 50 days of age, i.e. 25 days after surgery (Table 2). The weight of the testes, prostate and seminal vesicles are significantly depressed in the operated animals. Body and endocrine organ weights of sham-operated animals are equal to those of intact controls.

At 50 days of age, body and pituitary weights of animals bearing the frontal type of hypothalamic deafferentation are not significantly different from those of intact controls (Table 2). Testes weights, and even more prostate and seminal vesicles weights are significantly higher than those of controls.

Plasma testosterone levels of operated animals and of intact controls sacrificed at 50 days of age are shown in Fig. 1. Twenty-five days after surgery, sham-operated animals have testosterone levels not significantly different from those of intact controls; on the contrary, plasma testosterone is strikingly decreased in completely deafferented rats. Only one pool of plasma collected from 6 animals bearing the frontal type of hypothalamic deafferentation could be assayed; the level of testosterone in this sample (271.4 μg/100 ml) was found to be higher than that of intact controls (149 μg/100 ml).

The present data indicate that the transection of all neural connections to the MBH, performed in immature male rats, prevents sexual maturation; this is shown by the absence, in the operated groups, of the increase in testes and androgen-dependent structure weights, and in plasma testosterone levels, which are observed in normal animals.

It is interesting to note that, on the contrary, when only the anterior connections are severed, by a frontal type of hypothalamic deafferentation, puberty seems to be advanced; a significant hypertrophy of the testes and of the accessory glands, and an increase in plasma testosterone values has been observed in animals

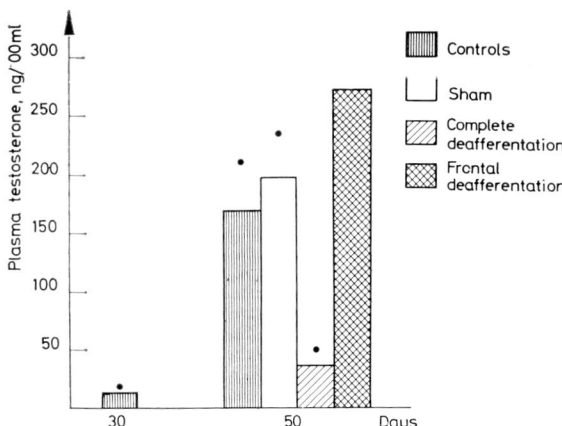

Fig. 1. Effect on plasma testosterone levels of complete and frontal hypothalamic deafferentations performed on 25-day-old male rats (autopsy at 50 days of age)

TABLE 2

Effect on body and organ weights of complete and frontal hypothalamic deafferentations performed on 25-day-old male rats (autopsy at 50 days of age)

Groups[a]	Body weight, g	Pituitary, mg/100 g body weight	Testes, mg/100 g body weight	Prostate, mg/100 g body weight	Seminal vesicles, mg/100 g body weight
Controls (20)	201.9 ± 4.39[b]	3.4 ± 0.14	1215.9 ± 3.14	58.2 ± 3.14	86.3 ± 6.00
Sham operation (19)	217.4 ± 6.06	3.5 ± 0.16	1287.5 ± 38.2	61.7 ± 2.60	96.3 ± 3.38
Complete deafferentation (12)	187.1 ± 11.60	3.8 ± 0.36	625.7 ± 100.5[c]	24.2 ± 5.94[c]	37.3 ± 10.61[c]
Frontal deafferentation (6)	180.8 ± 12.13	3.8 ± 0.21	1383.6 ± 76.8[d]	83.8 ± 9.12[c]	153.1 ± 17.98[c]

[a] No. of rats in parentheses.
[b] Values are means ± S.E.
[c] $P \leq 0.002$ vs controls.
[d] $P \leq 0.01$ vs controls.

bearing this type of operation. The present data, obtained in maturing rats, agree well with previous observations made in prepuberal guinea-pigs by Joseph et al. (1969), but show considerable differences with those reported after submitting sexually mature animals to the same types of operation. In effect, in mature animals, following a complete deafferentation of the MBH, testis weight remains normal, and only a small, non-significant reduction of prostate and seminal vesicle weights is observed (Halász and Pupp 1965, Halász 1969, Tima, personal communication). Moreover the frontal deafferentation, performed in adult male rats, induces hypertrophy of the seminal vesicles, but leaves testicular weight unmodified (Halász et al. 1967).

CONCLUSIONS

The present data suggest that extrahypothalamic influences play a significant role in modulating the secretion of pituitary gonadotropins (FSH and LH) in a way which is necessary to induce puberty in the male rat. They seem to indicate that, in the prepuberal male rat, two types of inputs reach the hypothalamic–pituitary–gonadal axis: (*i*) an inhibitory tone, transmitted by nervous pathways reaching the MBH from its frontal part; and (*ii*) stimulating impulses transported from afferent fibres which enter the MBH from the lateral and posterior regions.

ACKNOWLEDGEMENTS

The experimental work described in this paper was supported by the Department of Pharmacology of the University of Milan and by a Ford Foundation Grant, New York.

This support and the skillful technical assistance of Mr. L. Guadagni are gratefully acknowledged.

REFERENCES

HALÁSZ, B. (1969). The endocrine effects of isolation of the hypothalamus from the rest of the brain. In: *Frontiers in Neuroendocrinology*. Ed. by W. F. Ganong and L. Martini. Oxford University Press, New York. pp. 307–342.

HALÁSZ, B. and PUPP, L. (1965): Hormone secretion of the anterior pituitary gland after physical interruption of all nervous pathways to the hypophysiotrophic area. *Endocrinology* **77**, 553–562.

HALÁSZ, B. FLORSHEIM, W. H., CORCORRAN, N. L. and GORSKI, R. A. (1967): Thyrotrophic hormone secretion in rats after partial or total interruption of neural afferents to the medial basal hypothalamus. *Endocrinology* **80**, 1075–1082.

JOSEPH, S. A., KNIGGE, K. M. and VOLOSCHIN, L. (1969): Effects of isolation of the hypothalamo-pituitary unit in newborn guinea-pigs. *Neuroendocrinology* **4**, 42–50.

KNIEWALD, Z., ZANISI, M. and MARTINI, L. (1971): Studies on the biosynthesis of testosterone in the rat. *Acta endocr. (Kbh.)* **68**, 614–624.

MECHANISMS CONTROLLING PITUITARY GONADOTROPIN SECRETION IN PREPUBERAL RATS

F. FRASCHINI, R. COLLU[1] and E. E. MÜLLER

Department of Pharmacology
University of Milan
Milan, Italy

INTRODUCTION

In the last few years considerable evidence has accumulated indicating that the secretion of pituitary gonadotropins in adult animals is regulated by multiple mechanisms. The existence of an inhibitory control exerted by the pineal gland and by its principles is now generally admitted (Fraschini 1969, Reiter and Fraschini 1969, Fraschini and Martini 1970); on the other hand, it has been shown that brain catecholamines may exert a tonic stimulatory effect on the secretion of these hormones (Barraclough and Sawyer 1957, 1959, Coppola et al. 1965, Schneider and McCann 1969, Kamberi et al. 1970). The aim of the studies here to be reported was to investigate whether these two mechanisms are active also in prepuberal rats.

PINEAL PRINCIPLES

Previous results obtained in our laboratory suggest that the pineal glands exert their inhibitory effect on gonadotropin secretion in adult rats through its indole (5-hydroxytryptamine and 5-hydroxytryptophol) and methoxyindole (melatonin and 5-methoxytryptophol) derivatives; it has also been shown that these principles do not act directly on the anterior pituitary, but rather influence the central nervous system (Fraschini 1969, Fraschini and Martini 1970).

Since it is now generally accepted that both the luteinizing hormone (LH) and the follicle stimulating hormone (FSH) play an essential role in the onset of puberty (Corbin and Daniels 1967, Ramirez and Sawyer 1966, Watanabe and McCann 1969), it was decided to investigate if the administration of two pineal principles, which exert a specific inhibitory effect on the secretion of these two gonadotropins (melatonin on LH, and 5-methoxytryptophol on FSH), would interfere with the neuroendocrine processes leading to puberty in female rats.

Melatonin or 5-methoxytryptophol were injected daily into one of the lateral ventricles of the brain of different groups of prepuberal female rats; injections

---

[1] Fellow of the Medical Research Council of Canada. Present address: Hôpital Sainte-Justine, 3175 Côte Sainte-Cathérine, Montreal, Que., Canada.

were given starting from the 25th day of age, and their effect on vaginal opening time was observed. A statistically significant delay was found in the vaginal opening time of animals treated with either melatonin or methoxytryptophol (Table 1).

TABLE 1

Effect of daily intraventricular injections of melatonin or 5-methoxytryptophol on the time of vaginal opening in prepuberal female rats (means ± S.E.M.)

Treatment	No. of rats	Days to vaginal opening
Untreated controls	65	36.0 ± 0.44
Vehicle only	36	37.0 ± 0.98
Melatonin (80 µg/rat/day)	15	40.7 ± 1.30*[a]
5-Methoxytryptophol (80 µg/rat/day)	14	40.3 ± 1.00*[b]

* $P < 0.0005$ vs untreated controls.
[a] $P < 0.025$ vs saline-treated controls.
[b] $P < 0.05$ vs saline-treated controls.

These results strongly suggest that pineal methoxyindoles can play an important role in the control of sexual maturation, a physiological event which needs a balanced secretion of the two gonadotrophins; apparently when the secretion of either FSH or LH is inhibited (e.g., by the administration of its specific pineal inhibitor) puberty is delayed.

CATECHOLAMINES

In order to clarify if brain stores of catecholamines play a role in the control of gonadotrophin secretion in prepuberal animals the following approach has been used. Female rats of 20 days of age were injected with a drug which inhibits the synthesis of catecholamines; treatment was initiated immediately after the animals had been submitted to unilateral castration and was continued for 5 days. Animals were killed 24 hours after the last injection. At time of autopsy the remaining ovaries were weighed and their weights compared with those of the ovaries which were taken out at the time of unilateral ovariectomy. Uterine weight was also recorded. It was postulated that, if brain stores of catecholamines play a role in the control of gonadotrophin secretion, the remaining ovary should not show the compensatory hypertrophy which is normally found in untreated controls (D'Angelo and Kravatz 1960, Greep 1961, Benson 1968, Benson et al. 1969). Additional experiments were designed in order to establish which particular catecholamine (norepinephrine, dopamine, etc.) might be involved in this control; to this effect specific precursors of the biosynthesis of catecholamines were used.

Figure 1 shows that the administration of the inhibitor of catecholamine biosynthesis, alpha-methyl-p-tyrosine, alpha-MT, 150 mg/kg/day/i.p. (Spector et al. 1965) completely suppresses the ovarian compensatory hypertrophy which is

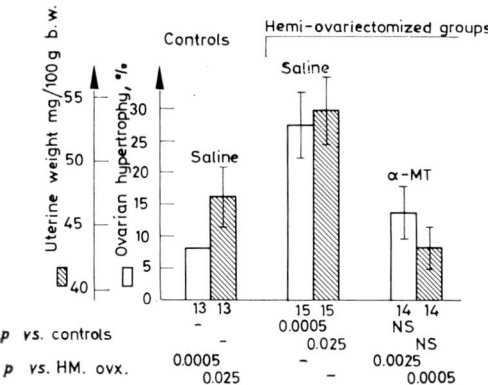

Fig. 1. Effect of α-MT treatment on ovarian compensatory hypertrophy and uterine weight of hemi-ovariectomized prepuberal rats. Vertical lines indicate standard error of the mean. Numbers below the bars indicate number of animals used

observed in saline-treated hemi-ovariectomized animals. The increase in uterine weight found in saline-treated hemi-ovariectomized animals was not present in animals receiving alpha-MT; in these animals, the weight of the uterus was even lower than that recorded in normal animals of 25 days of age.

The administration of 1-3,4 dihydroxyphenylalanine (L-dopa, 100 mg/kg/day/ i.p.), a precursor of dopamine and norepinephrine biosynthesis which brings back to normal the catecholamine stores in the brain (Corrodi et al. 1966, Andén et al. 1966), completely antagonized the effect on ovarian compensatory hypertrophy and on uterine weight of alpha-MT concurrently administered (Fig. 2).

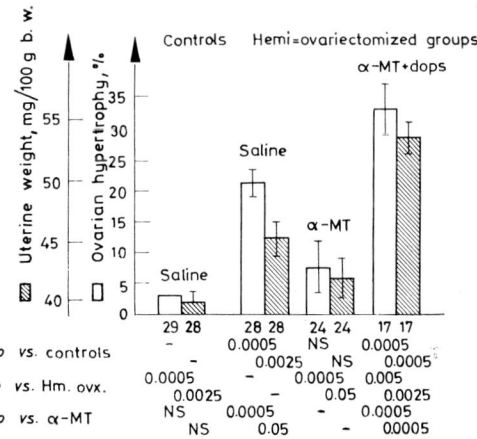

Fig. 2. Antagonism by L-dopa of the effect of α-MT treatment on ovarian compensatory hypertrophy and uterine weight of hemi-ovariectomized prepuberal rats. Results of two identical experiments were pooled. Vertical lines indicate standard error of the mean. Numbers below the bars indicate number of animals used

The possibility that the effect of alpha-MT was due to a peripheral action of the drug at the ovarian level, i.e., that the ovarian sensitivity to the action of endogenous gonadotrophins might be impaired by alpha-MT treatment, is excluded by the observation that the administration of pregnant mare serum gonadotropin (PMS, 20 IU/kg/day/s.c.) induces a comparable ovarian and uterine hypertrophy in saline- and in alpha-MT-treated animals (Fig. 3).

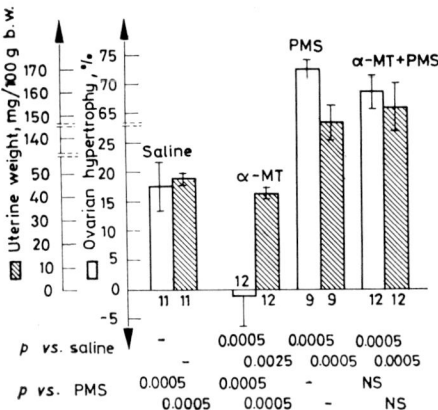

Fig. 3. Effect of α-MT treatment on the activity of exogenous pregnant mare's serum gonadotropin (PMS) in hemi-ovariectomized prepuberal rats. Vertical lines indicate standard error of the mean. Numbers below the bars indicate number of animals used

These data indicate that normal brain stores of catecholamines are necessary for ovarian compensatory hypertrophy to appear in young animals and suggest that brain catecholamines exert a stimulatory effect on the release of gonadotropins, also before puberty.

In order to clarify which catecholamine was specifically implicated in this mechanism, the following experiments were performed. L-threo-dihydroxyphenylserine (dops, 100 mg/kg/i.p./twice a day), a substance which selectively restores brain norepinephrine levels without increasing dopamine stores (Creveling et al. 1968) was injected in alpha-MT treated animals (see Fig. 4 for a detailed description of the mechanisms involved). It is apparent from the data reported in Fig. 5 that dops completely reverses the effect of alpha-MT on ovarian compensatory hypertrophy; this suggests that brain norepinephrine is probably involved in the control of gonadotrophin secretion. Experiments are under way to clarify the possible role of dopamine.

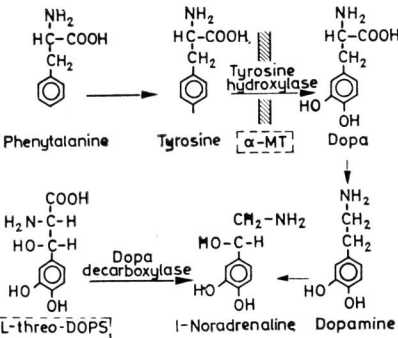

Fig. 4. Scheme of noradrenaline and dopamine biosynthesis. The steps influenced by methoxytryptamine, α-MT and L-threo-dihydroxyphenylserine (L-threo-dops) are indicated

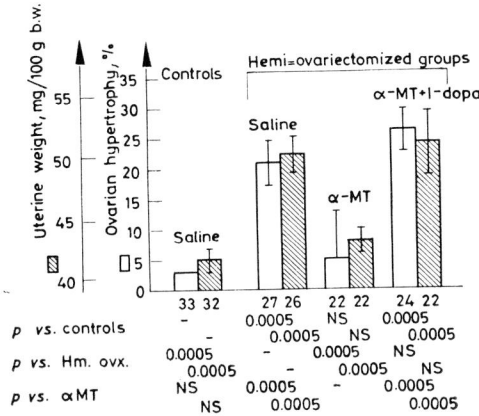

Fig. 5. Antagonism by L-threo-dihydroxyphenylserine (L-threo-dops) of the effect of α-MT treatment on ovarian compensatory hypertrophy and uterine weight of hemiovariectomized prepuberal rats. Results of two identical experiments were pooled. Vertical lines indicate standard error of the mean. Numbers below the bars indicate number of animals used

CONCLUSIONS

The data here reported suggest that the two mechanisms which control gonadotrophin secretion in mature animals exist also in prepuberal rats. It has been possible to show that (i) pineal principles exert a retarding effect on the appearance of puberty; and (ii) that normal stores of brain catecholamines are necessary for the hypothalamic–pituitary complex of prepuberal animals to respond to the stimulus of unilateral ovariectomy.

REFERENCES

Andén, N. E., Corrodi, H., Dahlström, A., Fuxe, K. and Hökfelt, T. (1966): Effects of tyrosine hydroxylase inhibition on the amine levels of central monoamine neurons. *Life Sci.* **5**, 561–568.

Barraclough, C. A. and Sawyer, C. H. (1957): Blockade of the release of pituitary ovulating hormone in the rat by chlorpromazine and reserpine: possible mechanisms of action. *Endocrinology* **61**, 341–351.

Barraclough, C. A. and Sawyer, C. H. (1959): Induction of pseudopregnancy in the rat by reserpine and chlorpromazine. *Endocrinology* **65**, 563–571.

Benson, B. (1968): On the mechanism of compensatory ovarian hypertrophy. *Anat. Rec.* **160**, 314.

Benson, B., Sorrentino, S. and Evans, S. (1969): Increase in serum FSH following unilateral ovariectomy in the rat. *Endocrinology* **84**, 369–374.

Coppola, J. A., Leonardi, R. G., Lippmann, W., Perrine, J. W. and Ringler, I. (1965): Induction of pseudopregnancy in rats by depletors of endogenous catecholamines. *Endocrinology* **77**, 485–490.

Corbin, A. and Daniels, E. L. (1967): Changes in concentration of female rat pituitary FSH and stalk-median eminence follicle stimulating hormone releasing factor with age. *Neuroendocrinology* **2**, 304–314.

Corrodi, H., Fuxe, K. and Hökfelt, T. (1966): Refillment of the catecholamine stores with 3,4-dihydroxyphenylalanine after depletion induced by inhibition of tyrosine-hydroxylase. *Life Sci.* **5**, 605–611.

Creveling, C. R., Daly, J., Tokuyama, T. and Witkop, B. (1968): The combined use of α-methyltyrosine and threo-dihydroxyphenylserine selective reduction of dopamine levels in the central nervous system. *Biochem. Pharmacol.* **17**, 65–70.

D'Angelo, A. and Kravatz, A. S. (1960): Gonadotrophic hormone function in persistent estrous rats with hypothalamic lesions. *Proc. Soc. exp. Biol. (N.Y.)* **104**, 130–133.

Fraschini, F. (1969): The pineal gland and the control of LH and FSH secretion. In: *Progress in Endocrinology*. Ed. by C. Gual. Excerpta Medica, Amsterdam. pp. 637–644.

Fraschini, F. and Martini, L. (1970): Rhythmic phenomena and pineal principles. In: *The Hypothalamus*. Ed. by L. Martini, M. Motta and F. Fraschini. Academic Press, New York. pp. 529–549.

Greep, R. O. (1961): Physiology of the anterior hypophysis in relation to reproduction. In: *Sex and Internal Secretions*. Ed. by W. C. Young and G. W. Comer. Williams and Wilkins, Baltimore. pp. 240–301.

Kamberi, I. A., Schneider, H. P. G. and McCann, S. M. (1970): Action of dopamine to induce release of FSH-releasing factor (FRF) from hypothalamic tissue "in vitro". *Endocrinology* **86**, 278–284.

Ramirez, V. and Sawyer, H. (1966): Changes in hypothalamic luteinizing hormone releasing factor (LHRF) in the female rat during puberty. *Endocrinology* **78**, 958–964.

Reiter, R. J. and Fraschini, F. (1969): Endocrine aspects of the mammalian pineal gland. *Neuroendocrinology* **5**, 219–255.

Schneider, H. P. G. and McCann, S. M. (1969): Possible role of dopamine as transmitter to promote discharge of LH-releasing factor. *Endocrinology* **85**, 121–132.

Spector, S., Sjoerdsma, A. and Udenfriend, S. (1965): Blockade of endogenous norepinephrine synthesis by α-methyl-tyrosine, an inhibitor of tyrosine hydroxylase. *J. Pharmacol. exp. Ther.* **147**, 86–95.

Watanabe, S. and McCann, S. M. (1969): Alterations in pituitary follicle-stimulating hormone (FSH) and hypothalamic FSH-releasing factor (FSH-RF) during puberty. *Proc. Soc. exp. Biol. (N.Y.)* **132**, 195–201.

THE ROLE OF PINEAL PRINCIPLES IN THE CONTROL OF ACTH SECRETION

F. PIVA[1], O. SCHIAFFINI[2], M. MOTTA and L. MARTINI

Department of Pharmacology
University of Milan
Milan, Italy

INTRODUCTION

In order to clarify whether the pineal gland and its principles play a role in the regulation of the hypothalamic–pituitary–adrenal axis several indole derivatives synthetized in the gland (melatonin, 5-hydroxytryptophol, 5-methoxytryptophol, etc.) have been injected directly into the cerebrospinal fluid of normal rats, through a cannula chronically implanted into one of the lateral ventricles of the brain. The effects of such principles on the plasma levels of corticosterone have been evaluated. The intracerebral way of administration has been selected because previous studies had indicated that the endocrine effects of pineal principles are mediated by specific receptors present in the central nervous system (Martini 1969, Fraschini and Martini 1970). Moreover, it has been repeatedly reported that indole and methoxyindole derivatives do not cross easily the blood brain barrier following systemic administrations (Wurtman et al. 1968).

METHODS

All experiments have been performed in normal adult male rats of the Sprague–Dawley strain, weighing 180 to 200 g. They were caged in standard conditions, in rooms with controlled temperature and humidity. Lights were on 14 hours per day, from 6.30 a.m. to 8.30 p.m. The rats were fed a standard pellet diet; water was given ad libitum. In all experimental animals a microcannula was introduced into one of the lateral ventricles of the brain under pentobarbital (3 mg/100 g body weight intraperitoneally) anaesthesia. A Stoelting stereotaxic apparatus was used.

In all instances the placement of intracerebral cannulae was performed two days before giving the intraventricular injections of pineal principles; these were administered without anaesthesia. All principles were dissolved in 30 lambda of

---

[1] Ford Foundation Fellow.
[2] Ford Foundation Fellow, on leave of absence from the Department of Neurobiology, Medical School, Buenos Aires, Argentina.

a 0.9 per cent saline solution containing 10 per cent of methanol. Control animals were injected intraventricularly with 30 µl of the saline–methanol mixture. Experiments were designed in a way to permit the sacrifice of all animals at the same time of the day (i.e., around noon) in order to avoid the interference of the diurnal corticosterone cycle (Critchlow et al. 1963, Mangili et al. 1966). Plasma levels of corticosterone were measured with the procedure of Guillemin et al. (1959), as modified by Fraschini et al. (1964).

RESULTS AND DISCUSSION

Figure 1 shows that intraventricular injections of melatonin, performed in animals in resting conditions, are followed in one hour by a significant drop of plasma corticosterone levels. Melatonin is effective both in the dose of 165 µg per rat and in the dose of 5 µg per rat. 5-Hydroxytryptophol and 5-methoxytryptophol are also able to inhibit the pituitary–adrenal axis of animals in resting conditions when given intraventricularly. However, they are effective only when the large dose of 165 µg per rat is used.

After showing that pineal principles may reduce plasma concentrations of corticosterone of animals in resting conditions it was of interest to study whether the most effective of these principles, melatonin, might inhibit ACTH secretion in rats exposed to an effective stressing procedure. In order to submit all animals to a stress of comparable intensity, a standard dose (400 µg/100 g body weight) of histamine was injected intravenously (Mangili et al. 1965). The scheme followed in these experiments is outlined in Table 1. Animals were first injected, through the brain cannula, with melatonin. Controls received the saline–methanol mix-

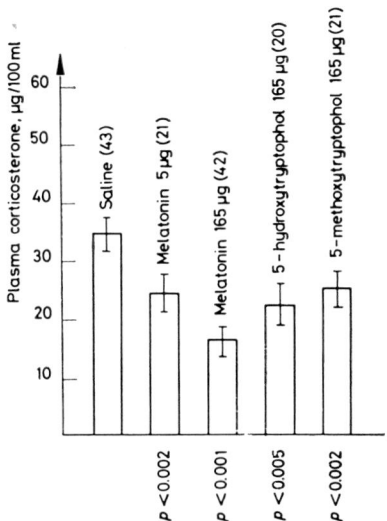

Fig. 1. Effect of intraventricular injections of pineal indoles and methoxyindoles on plasma corticosterone levels of normal male rats. No. of rats in parentheses

TABLE 1

Experimental scheme

Time (min)	Treatment	Doses	Mode of administration
0	Melatonin	5 μg and 165 μg/rat	Intraventricular
20	Pentobarbital	3 mg/100 g b. w.	Intraperitoneal
30	Histamine	400 μg/100 g b. w.	Intravenous
60	Decapitation and blood collection for measurement of plasma corticosterone		

ture intraventricularly. Thirty minutes after intraventricular administrations, histamine was injected under pentobarbital anaesthesia. As in the experiments summarized in Table 1, the animals were killed one hour after the intracerebral injections (30 minutes after exposure to histamine stress).

Table 2 shows clearly that animals treated with histamine and receiving only the vehicle intraventricularly (group indicated as Histamine) have plasma levels of corticosterone which are significantly higher than those found in the group of controls receiving saline solution intravenously and the saline–methanol mixture intraventricularly (group indicated as Saline). In animals in which histamine has been injected after the intracerebral treatment with either a low or a high dose of melatonin, plasma corticosterone concentrations do not reach the high values found in animals given the stressing drug without pineal principles. A certain degree of activation of the pituitary–adrenal axis is still present; however, the difference between the corticosterone titres of the animals receiving histamine after melatonin and those receiving histamine without melatonin protection is statistically significant.

The results of these experiments indicate that intraventricular injections of pineal principles, and particularly of melatonin, may inhibit the pituitary–adrenal axis; the inhibition brought about by melatonin seems to be a strong one since it appears also in animals submitted to an efficient stressing procedure.

TABLE 2

Effect of intraventricular injections of melatonin on histamine-induced activation of the pituitary–adrenal axis of male rats

Groups	No. of rats	Plasma corticosterone (μg/100 ml)	Significance (P)	Percent increase vs saline
Saline	48	27.67 ± 2.01^a		
Histamine 400 μg/100 g b.w.	37	46.25 ± 2.02	< 0.001 vs saline	67.15
Histamine + melatonin 5 μg	12	37.67 ± 4.96	< 0.05 vs histamine	36.14
Histamine + melatonin 165 μg	19	40.38 ± 2.67	< 0.05 vs histamine	45.93

[a] Values are means ± S.E.

Several recent data suggest that central adrenergic pathways may exert an inhibitory control on the secretion of the ACTH (Giuliani et al. 1966, Bhattacharya and Marks 1969, Van Loon et al. 1971). Because of these findings, the question was asked whether the depressing effect exerted by melatonin on the hypothalamic–pituitary–adrenal axis might be mediated through the activation of the central adrenergic pathways which inhibit ACTH secretion. To answer this question, the histamine–melatonin experiments were repeated in animals in which cerebral stores of catecholamines had been depleted by the previous administration of reserpine. The drug was given intraperitoneally, in a dose of 200 μg/100 g bodyweight, 24 hours before submitting the animals to the experimental procedure summarized in Table 1. This dose of reserpine has been shown to induce a very significant and long-lasting (up to 7 days) decrease in brain catecholamines (Carr and Moore 1968).

As shown in Table 3, histamine is still very effective as a stimulus for the pituitary–adrenal axis in animals pretreated with reserpine. This result agrees with the findings by Van Peenen and Way (1957) and by Carr and Moore (1968). In animals pretreated with reserpine, intraventricular injections of melatonin do not reduce the stressing effect of histamine (Table 3). This is the opposite of what had been previously observed in animals not pretreated with reserpine.

TABLE 3

Effect of intraventricular injections of melatonin on histamine-induced activation of the pituitary–adrenal axis of male rats pretreated with reserpine (200 μg/100 g b.w.)

Groups	No. of rats	Plasma corticosterone (μg/100 ml)	Significance (P)	Percent increase vs saline
Saline	18	22.08 ± 2.66^a		
Histamine 400 μg/100 g b.w.	23	42.28 ± 2.68	< 0.001 vs saline	92.84
Histamine + melatonin 5 μg	7	60.94 ± 4.41	< 0.001 vs histamine	175.99
Histamine + melatonin 165 μg	14	38.85 ± 4.10	NS vs histamine	75.95

[a] Values are means ±S.E.

CONCLUSIONS

1. Pineal indoles (5-hydroxytryptophol) and methoxyindoles (melatonin, 5-methoxytryptophol) are able to suppress the pituitary–adrenal axis of animals in resting conditions. This finding may be relevant with regard to the diurnal rhythm which is observed in the activity of the pituitary–adrenal axis of the rat. It is known that, in this species, plasma concentrations of corticosterone (Critchlow et al. 1963, Mangili et al. 1966) and of ACTH (Retiene et al. 1968, Retiene 1970) as well as hypothalamic stores of the corticotropin-releasing factor (David-Nelson and Brodish 1969) are significantly higher in the afternoon than in the morning. One might speculate that the increased function of the hypothalamic–pituitary–

adrenal axis observed in the afternoon is due to the reduced production of inhibiting methoxyindoles in the pineal gland, as a consequence of the suppression of the activity of the pineal enzymes N-acetyltransferase and hydroxyindole-O-methyltransferase during the light period (Klein and Weller 1970, Wurtman et al. 1968).

2. Melatonin counteracts the effect on ACTH secretion exerted by histamine, which is a potent stressful stimulus; this suggests that pineal principles might also intervene in maintaining the homeostasis of the pituitary–adrenal axis when this is disturbed by exogenous influences.

3. Melatonin loses its ability to interfere with the stimulating effect of histamine on ACTH secretion in rats deprived of brain catecholamines; this raises the possibility that the effect of melatonin on the pituitary–adrenal axis might be mediated through the activation of central adrenergic pathways normally inhibiting ACTH secretion.

4. The demonstration that melatonin influences the pituitary–adrenal axis after having been added to the cerebrospinal fluid may be taken as evidence in favour of the possibility that pineal principles are physiologically released into the cerebrospinal fluid rather than into the blood (Sheridan et al. 1969, Wurtman et al. 1968, Wurtman 1970, Fraschini and Martini 1970).

ACKNOWLEDGEMENTS

The work described in this paper was supported by a Grant of the Ford Foundation, New York. This support is gratefully acknowledged. Thanks are due to Miss Paola Assi and to Mister L. Guadagni for their skilful technical assistance.

REFERENCES

Bhattacharya, A. N. and Marks, B. H. (1969): Effects of pargyline and amphetamine upon acute stress responses in rats. *Proc. Soc. exp. Biol. (N. Y.)* **130**, 1194–1198.

Carr, L. A. and Moore, K. E. (1968): Effects of reserpine and alpha-methyltyrosine on brain catecholamines and the pituitary–adrenal response. *Neuroendocrinology* **3**, 285–302.

Critchlow, V., Liebelt, R. A., Bar-Sela, M., Mountcastle, W. and Lipscomb, H. S. (1963): Sex difference in resting pituitary–adrenal function in the rat. *Amer. J. Physiol.* **205**, 807–815.

David-Nelson, M. A. and Brodish, A. (1969): Evidence for a diurnal rhythm of corticotrophin-releasing factor (CRF) in the hypothalamus. *Endocrinology* **85**, 861–866.

Fraschini, F. and Martini, L. (1970): Rhythmic phenomena and pineal principles. In: *The Hypothalamus.* Ed. by L. Martini, M. Motta and F. Fraschini. Academic Press, New York. pp. 529–549.

Fraschini, F., Mangili, G., Motta, M. and Martini, L. (1964): Midbrain and feedback control of adrenocorticotrophin secretion. *Endocrinology* **75**, 765–769.

Giuliani, G., Motta, M. and Martini, L. (1966): Reserpine and corticotrophin secretion. *Acta endocr. (Kbh.)* **51**, 203–209.

Guillemin, R., Clayton, G. W., Lipscomb, H. S. and Smith, J. D. (1959): Fluorometric measurement of rat plasma and adrenal corticosterone concentration. *J. Lab. clin. Med.* **53**, 830–832.

Klein, D. C. and Weller, J. L. (1970): Indole metabolism in the pineal gland: a circadian rhythm in N-acetyltransferase. *Science* **169**, 1093–1094.

Mangili, G., Motta, M., Muciaccia, W. and Martini, L. (1965): Midbrain stress and ACTH secretion. *Europ. Rev. Endocr.* **1**, 247–253.

Mangili, G., Motta, M. and Martini, L. (1966): Control of adrenocorticotropic hormone secretion. In: *Neuroendocrinology*. Vol. I. Ed. by L. Martini and W. F. Ganong. Academic Press, New York. pp. 297–370.

Martini, L. (1969): Action of hormones on the central nervous system. *Gen. comp. Endocr.* Suppl. **2**, 214–226.

Retiene, K. (1970): Control of circadian periodicities in pituitary function. In: *The Hypothalamus*. Ed. by L. Martini, M. Motta and F. Fraschini. Academic Press, New York. pp. 551–568.

Retiene, K., Zimmerman, E., Schindler, W. J., Neuenschwander, J. and Lipscomb, H. S. (1968): A correlative study of endocrine rhythms in rats. *Acta endocrin. (Kbh.)* **57**, 615–622.

Sheridan, M. N., Reiter, R. J. and Jacobs, J. J. (1969): An interesting anatomical relationship between the hamster pineal gland and the ventricular system of the brain. *J. Endocr.* **45**, 131–132.

Van Loon, G. R., Scapagnini, U., Cohen, R. and Ganong, W. F. (1971): Effect of intraventricular administration of adrenergic drugs on the adrenal venous 17-hydroxycorticosteroid response to surgical stress in the dog. *Neuroendocrinology* **8**, 257–272.

Van Peenen, P. F. D. and Way, E. L. (1957): The effect of certain central nervous system depressants on pituitary–adrenal activating agents. *J. Pharmacol. exp. Ther.* **120**, 261–267.

Wurtman, R. J. (1970): The role of brain and pineal indoles in neuroendocrine mechanisms. In: *The Hypothalamus*. Ed. by L. Martini, M. Motta and F. Fraschini. Academic Press, New York. pp. 153–165.

Wurtman, R. J., Axelrod, J. and Kelly, D. E. (1968): *The Pineal*. Academic Press, New York.

EFFECT OF DEHYDROBENZPERIDOL ON PITUITARY ADRENAL FUNCTION

L. DEBRECZENI

Mohács Hospital
Mohács, Hungary

The effect of butyrophenones on central nervous processes is known from the pioneer study of Janssen et al. (1963) and the mechanism of their action was analysed by a number of investigators. Observations, both experimental and empirical, indicate that the most potent butyrophenone, dehydrobenzperidol or droperidol support the adaptation of the organism to noxious stimuli.

Concerning the psychodelic effect of dehydrobenzperidol as a neuroleptic and anti-shock agent, we were interested to study the influence of dehydrobenzperidol on the pituitary–adrenocortical function in humans and in rats. In rats we have investigated the effect of the drug in acute experiments and in a chronic treatment.

The activation of corticosteroidogenesis was measured by using the in vitro corticosteroid production of the adrenals according to Van der Vies et al. (1960) and the production rate as index of the endogenous ACTH release was expressed according to Van Gogh et al. (1963).

In the 30th min following the administration of 6 mg/kg body weight dehydrobenzperidol there was an expressive increase in the adrenal corticosteroid production as compared to the controls (Fig. 1).

Significantly increased corticosteroid production was found following a pretreatment with dehydrobenzperidol plus immobilization, and a slight difference was observed between the groups receiving electric shocks or electric shocks plus dehydrobenzperidol pretreatment (Fig. 2).

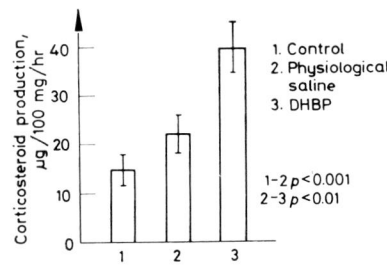

Fig. 1. Effect of DHBP on corticosteroid production

There was no further activation of pituitary–adrenocortical function by dehydrobenzperidol if it was given in combination with 200 μg/kg body weight of adrenaline.

Dehydrobenzperidol treatment for 5 days led to an increase in the adrenocortical steroid production of rats receiving electric shock 30 min following the last injection. Similarly, the dehydrobenzperidol produced an increase in the pituitary–adrenocortical response in those rats which received electric shocks for 5 day

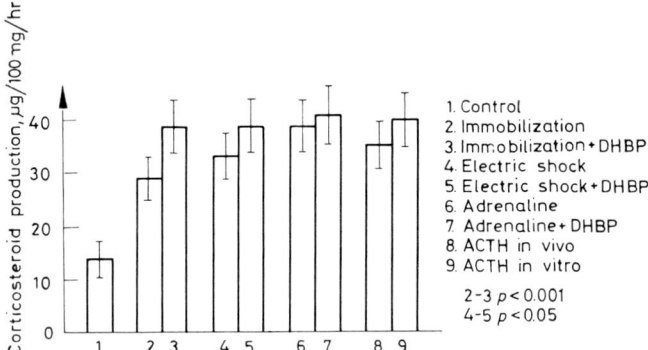

Fig. 2. Effect of DHBP on the stress-induced adrenocortical responses

(once daily) and were treated with dehydrobenzperidol 30 min prior to decapitation (Fig. 3).

Following a 30-day dehydrobenzperidol treatment there was no significant difference between the weight of the adrenals of the control and of the test animals. In the corticosteroid production a moderate increase occurred in dehydrobenzperidol treated rats as compared to the controls (Fig. 4).

Observations were made on 28 hospitalized patients. A dose of 0.17 mg/kg body weight dehydrobenzperidol was given intramuscularly. One and 3 hours later

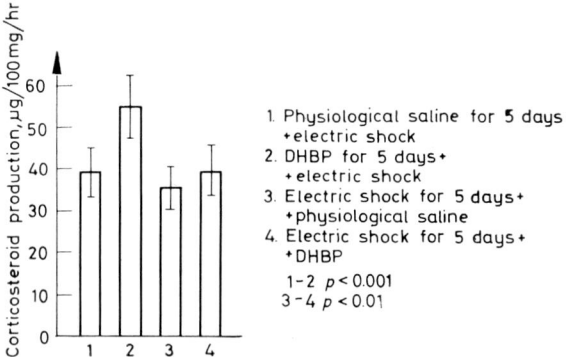

Fig. 3. Effect of DHBP on the stress-induced pituitary=adrenocortical activation

blood samples were taken and the plasma cortisol concentration was determined fluorometrically by the method of Mattingly (1962). Routine therapeutic dose of dehydrobenzperidol produced a moderate increase in plasma cortisol concentration in the first hour after injection which became more pronounced after 3 hours (Fig. 5).

Dexamethasone blockade of pituitary–adrenal function, which resulted in a suppression of plasma cortisol concentration, led to the prevention of dehydrobenzperidol-induced pituitary ACTH release (Fig. 6).

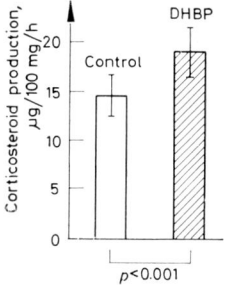

Fig. 4. Effect of prolonged DHBP treatment

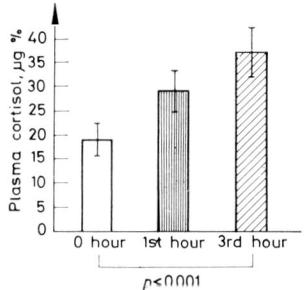

Fig. 5. Effect of DHBP on the plasma cortisol level

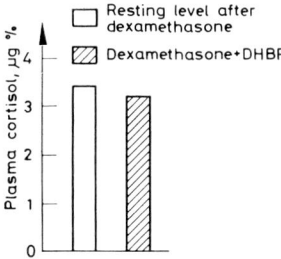

Fig. 6. Effect of DHBP on the plasma cortisol level in dexamethasone-treated patients

DISCUSSION

Administration of dehydrobenzperidol resulted in a maximal activation of the pituitary–adrenocortical function in comparison with the response following injection of a supramaximal dose of ACTH.

There are no data in the literature concerning the mechanism of the control of nervous action exerted by butyrophenones but the similarities in the action of butyrophenones and other major tranquillizers are very striking. According to a number of investigators both reserpine and chlorpromazine increase plasma corticosterone level and decrease the ACTH content in the anterior pituitary. In rats prolonged reserpine and chlorpromazine treatment resulted in a marked depletion of the pituitary ACTH content, manifested in a diminution of stress induced responses.

In the present study, dehydrobenzperidol pretreatment caused no pituitary ACTH depletion and the response of adrenals to stressors was augmented by dehydrobenzperidol both after a single injection and after a 5-day treatment. Moreover, dehydrobenzperidol induced a significant increase in the corticosteroid production of the adrenals after a 30-day treatment, too.

Our opinion is that dehydrobenzperidol influences the pituitary ACTH function in two ways: by increased release of ACTH from pituitary cells and by increased resynthesis of the tropic hormone.

A prevention of dehydrobenzperidol by a previous dexamethasone treatment suggested that dehydrobenzperidol exerted its influence at the suprapituitary level.

Dehydrobenzperidol-induced alterations in the pituitary–adrenal function seem to be in accordance with its shock-preventive action. This favourable effect cannot be limited to its influence on the pituitary–adrenocortical function. This is an important part of the complex effect of this drug influencing the central nervous system, which plays an important role in the adaptation of the organism.

REFERENCES

JANSSEN, P. A. J., NIEMEGEERS, C. J. E., SCHELLEKENS, K. H. L., VERBRUGGEN, F. J. and VAN NUETEN, J. M. (1963): The pharmacology of dehydrobenzperidol, a new potent and short acting neuroleptic agent chemically related to haloperidol. *Drug Res. (Arzneimittel-Forsch.* **13**, 205—211.

MATTINGLY, D. (1962): A simple fluorometric method for the estimation of free 11-hydroxycorticoids in human plasma. *J. clin. Path.* **15**, 374—379.

VAN DER VIES, J., BAKKER, R. F. M. and DE WIED, D. (1960): Correlated studies on plasma-free corticosterone and on andrenal steroid formation in vitro. *Acta Endocr. (Kbh.)* **34**, 513—523.

VAN GOGH, J. J., DE WIED, D. and SCHÖNBAUM, E. (1963): Adrenocorticotropic activity in the rat assessed by in vivo and in vitro indices. *Amer. J. Physiol.* **205**, 1083—1088.

SECTION III
PSYCHOPHARMACOLOGICAL AND NEUROCHEMICAL BASES OF DRUG ACTIONS

Chairman: S. V. ANICHKOV

ACTION OF NEUROTROPIC DRUGS ON THE TROPIC FUNCTIONS OF THE PITUITARY

S. V. ANICHKOV and V. E. RYZHENKOV

Department of Pharmacology
Institute of Experimental Medicine
U.S.S.R. Academy of Medical Sciences
Leningrad, U.S.S.R.

Studies of neurotropic drugs acting through the nervous system on the endocrine glands belong to that field of neuroendocrinology which may be called pharmacological neuroendocrinology. The basis of these studies lies in the acceptance of the close interactions between the central nervous system and the endocrine system (Itsenko 1946, Harris 1955, 1967, Lissák and Endrőczi 1960, Szent-ágothai et al. 1962, Schally and Kastin 1969).

When studying the action of neurotropic drugs on the adrenocorticotropic function of the pituitary two problems with respect to their clinical significance arise. (*i*) Protection of the hypothalamic centres from excessive stimulation with subsequent exhaustion of the pituitary–adrenal system and resistance decrease in the organism. This problem is particularly important in surgery. (*ii*) Stimulation of the hypothalamo–pituitary–adrenal axis to increase the adrenal cortex secretion is important in producing an increase in the resistance to inflammation, allergic agents, etc.

Protection of the hypothalamic centres controlling adrenocorticotropic function may be accomplished to a certain degree by means of various drugs which depress the central nervous system like barbiturates, chlorpromazine (Woodbury 1958, Mason 1962, Bohus and de Wied 1966). However, these drugs, possessing a wide spectrum of action, exert also an inhibitory action upon vital functions of the brain.

The blockade of central cholinoreceptors has the advantage of a more selective effect. One of the most active central m-cholinolytics is metamizyl (hydrochloride of the 2-diethylaminopropyl benzylic acid ether) synthetized in our department (Anichkov and Denisenko 1962).

We studied the action of central cholinolytics upon the hypothalamo–pituitary–adrenal system experimentally and in clinical practice. Experiments were performed on dogs under chloralose anaesthesia (85 mg/kg, intravenously). The 17-hydroxycorticosteroid (17-OHCS) level was determined by the method described by Yudaev (1961).

Figure 1 shows the rate of 17-OHCS secretion into the adrenal vein (μg per g of adrenal weight per min) under severe stress (electrical stimulation of the sciatic nerves for a two-hour period). In Fig. 1 an initial rise in corticosteroid secretion occurs which is followed by a considerable fall. At the same time the reaction of the adrenal cortex to ACTH injection (20 I.U. intravenously) was inhibited, which may be regarded as a block of the ACTH action at the adrenal cortical level. It is to be noted that the concentration of 17-OHCS in peripheral blood plasma was constantly high throughout the experiments.

If metamizyl (0.3 mg/kg) was administered 15 min prior to electrical stimulation of the sciatic nerves, the initial increase in 17-OHCS secretion was less pronounced and secretion rate was more uniform during the two-hour period of stress. Accordingly, the corticotropin-stimulating test (20 I.U. ACTH, intravenously) applied in

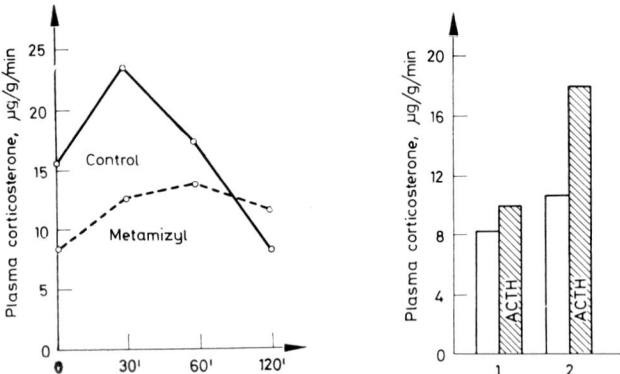

Fig. 1. Effect of central m-cholinolytic metamizyl on the 17-OHCS concentration of the adrenal vein blood in chloralose-anaesthetized dogs. 1. Sciatic nerve stimulation (50 cps, 5 msec and 6 V). 2. Effect of metamizyl (0.3 mg/kg) given 15 min prior to the sciatic stimulation. ACTH induced changes of adrenal corticosteroid secretion (20 I.U., intravenously) under the experimental conditions of 1 and 2 are shown on the right columns

these conditions showed that the secretion rate of 17-OHCS increases considerably in spite of a two-hour stimulation of the sciatic nerves (Fig. 1).

Thus, experiments have shown that the blockade of the central m-cholinoreceptors protects the hypothalamo–pituitary–adrenal system from exhaustion caused by severe nerve stimulation.

Our experiments on dogs have also shown that metamizyl (0.1 mg/kg) reduced the hypersecretion of ACTH caused by the electrical stimulation of some regions of the brain (Ryzhenkov and Sapronov 1968). The protective effect of central m-cholinolytic metamizyl was also observed in patients subjected to cardiac surgery.

Figure 2 shows the 17-OHCS level in the blood of patients under routine preoperative treatment in the surgical ward and that in patients having received moreover the metamizyl (5 mg) twice, the day before the operation and just prior to it; metamizyl was also injected for 7 days after the operation.

It is worth mentioning that changes in 17-OHCS concentration observed during surgical intervention depend not only on the trauma as such but also on the emotional tension preceding it. The question arises as to what extent do neurotropic drugs of central action protect the hypothalamo–pituitary–adrenal system from psychogenic stress.

To elucidate this point it was useful to elaborate a conditioned reflex hypersecretion of ACTH. The conditioned reflex to sound was obtained in dogs on the basis of electric irritation of their paws. As seen in Fig. 3, conditioned hypersecretion of 17-OHCS is sufficiently prevented by small doses of metamizyl (0.1 mg/kg) and adequate doses of other sedative drugs: trasentine (3 mg/kg), chlorpromazine (1.5 mg/kg), barbamyl (15 mg/kg), injected 10 min before the application of the conditioned stimuli. It must be noted that these doses are still insufficient to prevent the ACTH hypersecretion to unconditional stimuli

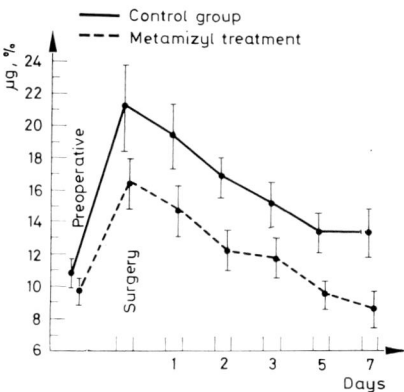

Fig. 2. Effect of metamizyl administration on the plasma cortisol concentration in human patients with surgical intervention

which was elicited by electrical shocks on the dog's paws serving as an unconditional stimulus of the conditioned reflex (Fig. 3). Moreover, by increasing the doses of these drugs, except barbamyl, we obtain a higher level of 17-OHCS (Anichkov and Ryzhenkov 1965).

Thus, our experiments as well as clinical observations show that the blockade of central m-cholinoreceptors effectively protects the hypothalamo–pituitary–adrenal system from excessive stimulation and exhaustion.

The blockade of central m-cholinoreceptors effected by metamizyl reduced also the gonadotropic activity of the pituitary (Ryzhenkov and Pavlysh 1963, Bekhtereva 1966). Metamizyl inhibits also vasopressin hypersecretion observed after electric stimulation of the supraoptic nucleus of the hypothalamus in dogs (Ryzhenkov and Sapronov 1968).

We have also studied some drugs acting upon the monoaminergic mechanisms of the brain. For this purpose we used drugs influencing the synthesis of monoamines and their storage in tissues (α-methyl-parathyrosine; α-methyl-dopa; parachlor-phenylalanine, reserpine). Experiments were performed on male albino rats (150 to 180 g of body weight). The 11-hydroxycorticosteroid level was determined in blood plasma (de Moor et al. 1960). Noradrenaline (NA) content of the brain (hypothalamic and also midbrain areas) was examined by the method of von Euler and Floding, modified by Matlina and Rachmanova (1967). For brain 5-hydroxytryptamine (5-HT) evaluation we used the method of Snyder et al. (1965).

Figure 4 shows that despite the inhibition of noradrenaline synthesis by means of α-methyl-parathyrosine (100 mg/kg during three days) the 11-OHCS concentration remained practically unaltered and the reaction of the pituitary–adrenal axis to immobilization (stretch) of the rats remains similar to that in intact animals. Parachlorophenylalanine treatment (400 mg/kg) does not prevent the activation of corticosteroid secretion in spite of the low 5-HT level in the

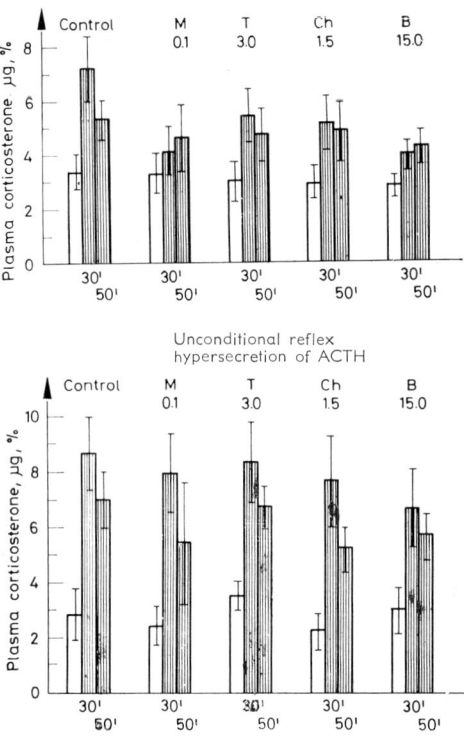

Fig. 3. Effects of neurotropic drugs on the plasma 17-OHCS response levels to the conditional and unconditional stimuli of a defensive conditional reflex in dogs.

M = metamizyl (0.1 mg/kg)
T = trasentine (3.0 mg/kg)
Ch = chlorpromazine (1.5 mg/kg)
B = barbamyl (15.0 mg/kg)

brain. Reserpine pretreatment (1 mg/kg, 18 hours before the experiment) had no effect upon the reaction of the pituitary–adrenal axis to stress stimulus. At the same time NA and 5-HT level in the rat's brain was considerably reduced (Fig. 4).

The above studies show that in spite of alterations in the brain monoaminergic mechanism activity of the hypothalamo–pituitary–adrenal system may remain unchanged. This is confirmed by our experiments on the determination of NA and 5-HT values in the brain of rats under the influence of various stimuli. It was noted that 30 min after (1) immobilization (stretch), (2) formaline (0.15 ml, 10 per cent, subcutaneously) or (3) neurotropic drug injection (aethymizol; see below) an approximately similar increase in 11-OHCS level in blood plasma was observed in rats (Fig. 5).

However, the decrease in noradrenaline content in the brain may be observed only after immobilization, while 5-HT content remained unchanged (Fig. 5). It is

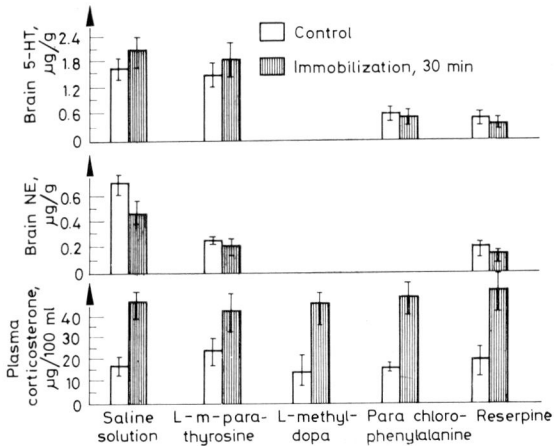

Fig. 4. Changes in the plasma corticosterone concentration and the brain monoamine content after administration of drugs which block either the synthesis or the storage of monoamines

worth noting that in rats immobilized after dexamethasone blockade (600 μg/kg) no decrease of the brain's noradrenaline content is observed; but in this group of rats the blockade of 11-OHCS secretion was only partial (Fig. 5).

These results are in agreement with the opinion that the central catecholamines do not play any significant role in the control mechanisms of the hypothalamo–pituitary–adrenal activity (Lissák and Endrőczi 1960, Smelik 1967, Schaepdryver et al. 1969).

Many neurotropic drugs are capable of inducing ACTH secretion. Among these are m- and n-cholinomimetics (Anichkov et al. 1963, Ryzhenkov 1968). Strong stimulators of ACTH secretion are the central sympathomimetics, amphetamine in particular. However, the effect of all these drugs does not alter the feedback action of corticosteroids. In this respect a rather exceptional place belongs to drugs of the so-called antiffeine group synthetized at our department (Anichkov et al. 1962). One of the most effective drugs of this group is aethymizol (bis-methylamide-1-aethylimidazol-4,5-bicarbonic acid). Aethymizol has a strong direct stimulating action on the respiratory centres, and is used as a respiratory analeptic.

Of great interest is the effect of aethymizol on the hypothalamic centres which control ACTH secretion. It increases the 17-OHCS level in the blood of guinea-pigs and dogs. Figure 6 illustrates the values of 17-OHCS in blood plasma of guinea-pigs 2 hours after aethymizol injection (20 mg/kg, intraperitoneally). In hypophysectomized animals it produced no effect; hence its action is due to the increase of ACTH secretion. Our experiments have shown that the action of aethymizol remains at a constant level during a two- to three-week period of daily injections (Anichkov and Ryzhenkov 1965). By increasing the corticosteroid level in the blood plasma, aethymizol produces an antiinflammatory effect (Ryzhenkov 1967).

The question arises, what is the mechanism of aethymizol effect. In order to obtain an answer to this question we performed a series of experiments upon rats and guinea-pigs with the purpose of studying the interaction of aethymizol and dexamethasone. Dexamethasone is known to be a synthetic analogue of hydrocortisone with markedly pronounced inhibiting action on the hypothalamic centres controlling ACTH secretion (Mangili et al. 1964). Figure 7 shows the results of these experiments. It will be seen that administration of dexamethasone

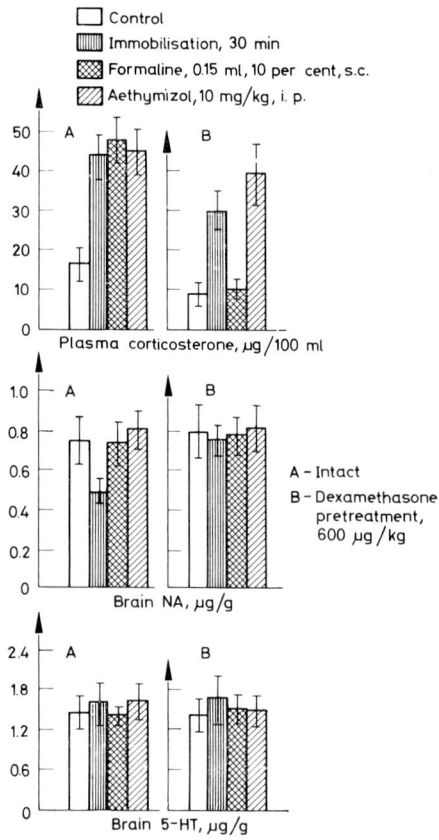

Fig. 5. Effect of aethymizol administration on the formaline- and immobilisation-induced changes in the plasma corticosterone concentration and the brain monoamine content without and with dexamethasone pretreatment

(300 µg/kg, intraperitoneally) inhibited the corticosteroid secretion. Injection of aethymizol (10 mg/kg) completely eliminated this inhibition. On the contrary, amphetamine (5 mg/kg) and placing the rats in water (for 30 sec), which also causes an increase of 11-OHCS level in the blood, proved to be incapable of eliminating the inhibiting effect of dexamethasone (Fig. 7).

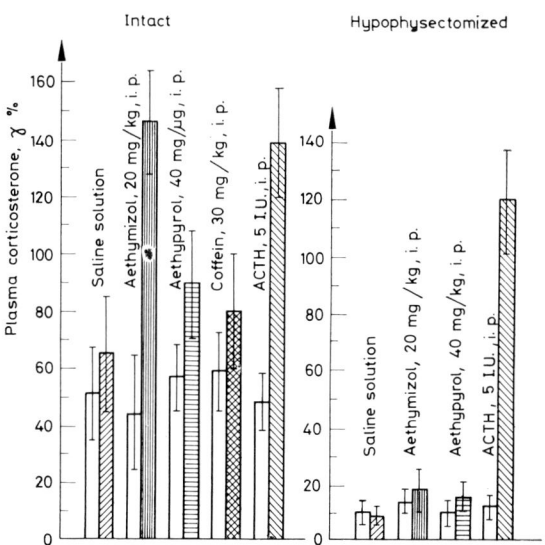

Fig. 6. Effects of aethymizol, aethypyrol, coffein and ACTH on the plasma 17-OHCS concentration in intact and hypophysectomized guinea-pigs

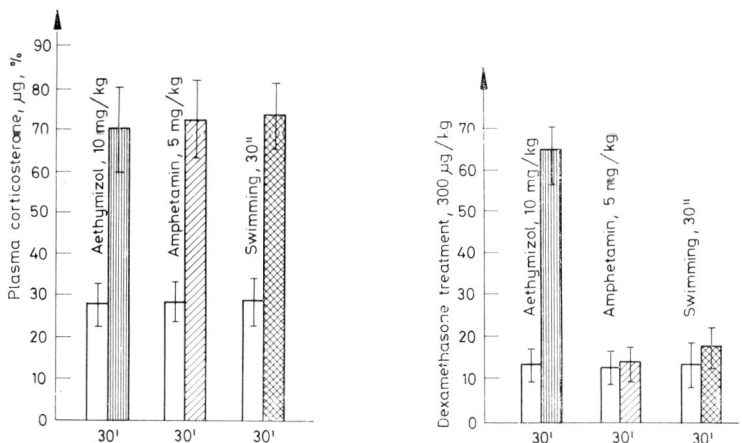

Fig. 7. Changes of plasma corticosterone concentration in rats with aethymizol and amphetamine treatment and after exposure to swimming without and with dexamethasone pretreatment

Hence aethymizol decreases the sensitivity of the hypothalamus to the inhibiting action of glucocorticoids. In other words, aethymizol adjusts the sensitivity of the hypothalamic centres to a higher level of corticosteroids.

This conclusion is confirmed by the experiments on guinea-pigs (Fig. 8). One group of the animals was injected cortisone acetate (3 mg/100 g of body weight, during 17 days). Owing to the inhibition of the hypothalamic centres controlling ACTH secretion, cortisone considerably decreased the functional ability of the

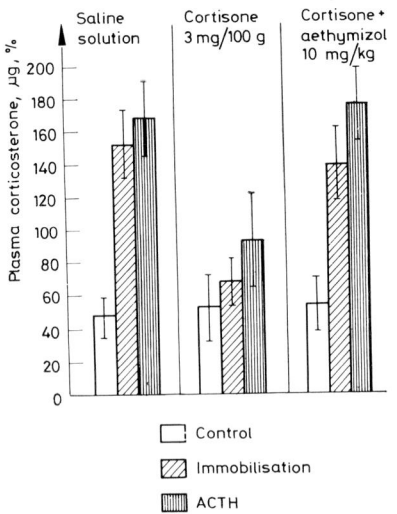

Fig. 8. Antagonistic effect of aethymizol administration on the inhibitory effect of cortisone: the plasma corticosteroid response levels to immobilisation and ACTH administration are shown without and with aethymizol administration

adrenal cortex. Even 6 days after termination of the injections of cortisone neither ACTH (5 I.U., intraperitoneally) nor immobilisation (stretch) of the guinea-pigs (5 hours) caused the usual 17-OHCS stimulating effect (Fig. 8). When aethymizol was injected simultaneously with cortisone, the sensitivity of the adrenals to ACTH and their reaction to immobilisation remained almost normal. Hence aethymizol protects the hypothalamic centres from feedback action of corticosteroids and prevents the inhibition of the hypothalamo–pituitary–adrenal system. This particular mode of action of aethymizol distinguishes it from other means of increasing the corticosteroid level in blood especially from corticosteroid therapy which inevitably inhibits the function of the adrenals.

Experimental evidence allows us to recommend aethymizol for the treatment of allergic diseases, bronchial asthma and rheumatoid arthritis in particular (Ryzhenkov et al. 1967).

REFERENCES

ANICHKOV, S. V. and DENISENKO, P. P. (1962): In: *Pharmacology of the New Sedative Drugs and their Clinical Use*. Leningrad, pp. 5—16.

ANICHKOV, S. V. and RYZHENKOV, V. E. (1965): In: *The Questions of the Surgical Pathology*. Leningrad, pp. 66—77.

ANICHKOV, S. V., CHROMOV-BORISOV, N. V., BORODKIN, YU. S. and VINOGRADOVA, N. B. (1962): In: *Pharmacology of the New Sedative Drugs and their Clinical Use*. Leningrad, pp. 151—156.

ANICHKOV, S. V., POSKALENKO, A. N. and RYZHENKOV, V. E. (1963): Action of neurotropic drugs upon ACTH secretion. *Proceedings of the 1st International Pharmacological Meeting*. Pergamon Press, Oxford and London.

BEKHTEREVA, E. P. (1966): *Farmakol. i Toksikol.* **6**, 739—742.

EULER, U. S. VON and FLODING, I. (1955): *Acta physiol. scand.* **33**, Suppl. **118**, 45.

HARRIS, G. (1955): *Neural Control of the Pituitary Gland*. Arnold, London.

HARRIS, G. (1967): In: *Biological and Clinical Aspects of the Central Nervous System*. Basel. pp. 85—102.

LISSÁK, K. and ENDRŐCZI, E. (1960): *Die neuroendokrine Steuerung der Adaptationstätigkeit*. Akadémiai Kiadó, Budapest.

MANGILI, G., MARTINI, L., MOTTA, M., MÜLLER, E. and PECILLE, A. (1964): In: *Progress in Biocybernetics*. Vol. 1, pp. 36—43.

MASON, P. (1962): Pharmacological control of the secretion of ACTH. In: *Proceedings of the 1st International Pharmacological Meeting*. Pergamon, Oxford, etc. pp. 11—24.

MOOR, P. DE, STEENO, O., RASKIN, M. and HENDRICX, X. (1960): *Acta endocr. (Kbh.)* **33**, 297.

RYZHENKOV, V. E. (1967): *Farmakol. i Toksikol.* **1**, 11—14.

RYZHENKOV, V. E. (1968): *Probl. Endokr. Gormonoter.* **5**, 67—69.

RYZHENKOV, V. E. and PAVLYSH, V. V. (1963): *Probl. Endokr. Gormonoter.* **3**, 102—104.

RYZHENKOV, V. E. and SAPRONOV, N. S. (1968): *Farmakol. i Toksikol.* **2**, 163—166.

RYZHENKOV, V. E., PITKOVSKAYA, E. N. and LIPHSHYZ, R. S. (1967): *Sovetsk. Med.* **4**, 127—131.

SCHAEPDRYVER, A. DE, PREZIOSI, P. and SCAPAGNINI, U. (1969): *Brit. J. Pharmacol.* **35**, 460.

SCHALLY, A. and KASTIN, A. (1969): *Triangel* **9**, 19—25.

SMELIK, P. W. (1967): *Neuroendocrinology* **2**, 247—254.

SNYDER, S. H., AXELROD, I. and ZWEIG, M. (1965): *Biochem. Pharmacol.* **14**, 831.

SZENTÁGOTHAI, J., FLERKÓ, B., MESS, B. and HALÁSZ, B. (1962): *Hypothalamic Control of the Anterior Pituitary. An Experimental-Morphological Study*. Akadémiai Kiadó, Budapest.

WOODBURY, D. (1958): *Pharmacol. Rev.* **10**, 275—357.

ACTION OF CENTRAL CHOLINOLYTICS AND OESTROGENS ON GONADOTROPIC RELEASE AFTER DESTRUCTION OF THE AMYGDALA IN RATS

E. P. BEKHTEREVA

Department of Pharmacology
Institute of Experimental Medicine
U.S.S.R. Academy of Medical Sciences
Leningrad, U.S.S.R.

It is known that different areas of the hypothalamus and overlying brain structures connected with them take part in the nervous regulation of gonadotropin secretion.

Recently, great attention has been drawn to brain structures representing the limbic system. Some data are available showing that structures of this system such as the hippocampus, amygdala, septum and others, take an active part in the regulation of anterior pituitary functions. The present report deals with the influence of the amygdaloid complex upon the neurohumoral regulation of the pituitary gonadotropic function. Numerous data indicate that the amygdala might be involved in the regulation of pituitary gonadotropic function (Koikegami et al. 1954, Bunn and Everett 1957, Elvers and Critchlow 1960, Eleftheriou et al. 1967, Kawakami et al. 1968, Lawton and Sawyer 1970, Bekhtereva 1970).

In the present investigations the effect of electrolytic destruction of various parts of the amygdaloid complex was studied on the action of hormones (oestradiol monobenzoate) and some neurotropic drugs like m- and n-cholinolytics, methylbenactizine (methamizyl) as well as spasmolytine on the secretion of follicle-stimulating (FSH) and luteinizing hormones (LH) from the pituitary gland.

The present experiments were carried out on mature female and male rats, which were anaesthetized with barbiturate, and the electrolytic lesion was made by the use of a stereotaxic instrument. According to the atlas of König and Klippel (1963) the lesions were made bilaterally in one of the following amygdaloid areas: in the basal amygdaloid complex, including basolateral and basomedial nuclei (ABL + ABM) and the medial nucleus of amygdala (AME).

Electrocoagulation was performed with anodic polarization of 2 mA current intensity for 10 sec through a monopolar stainless steel electrode. The localization of lesions was confirmed by histological examination. Figures 1 and 2 represent the frontal sections of the brain and different localizations of the amygdala destruction. After brain surgery the rats received injections of oestradiol monobenzoate or neurotropic drugs and were sacrificed 1, 2 or 4 weeks after the operation. Pituitary FSH level was estimated by the method of Steelman and Pohley (1953), plasma FSH level was determined by Igarashi and McCann's method (1964).

Pituitary and plasma LH levels were determined by the ovarian ascorbic acid depletion method (OAAD, Parlow 1961).

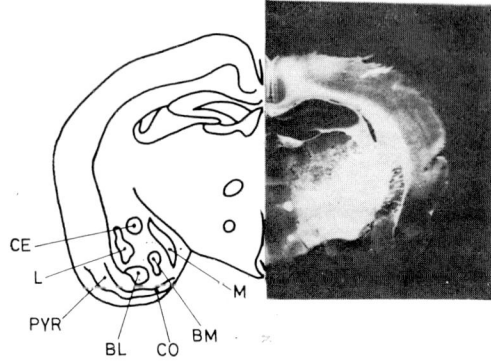

Fig. 1. Diagrammatic and photomicrographic representation of the diencephalon with location of various amygdaloid lesions (basal amygdaloid complex and medial amygdaloid nucleus. BL — basolateral amygdaloid nucleus. BM — basomedial amygdaloid nucleus. CE — central amygdaloid nucleus. L — lateral amygdaloid nucleus. M — medial amygdaloid nucleus. CO — cortical amygdaloid nucleus

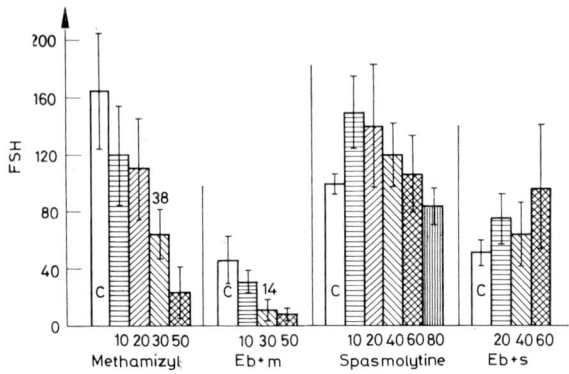

Fig. 2. The effect of different doses of m- and n-cholinolytics, methamizyl and spasmolytine on pituitary FSH (mg ovarian weight) level in intact rats. Light columns — control pituitary FSH levels. Shaded columns — pituitary FSH levels in rats, receiving the drugs

RESULTS

Administration of m-cholinolytic methylbenactizine, in large doses, exerts a marked inhibitory effect on the pituitary FSH content of intact rats and potentiates the inhibitory effect of the oestradiol monobenzoate (Fig. 2).

In smaller doses (20 mg/kg) methylbenactizine, given for 3 weeks, was not effective. n-Cholinolytic spasmolytine (trasentine) in doses of 20–40 mg/kg enhanced FSH secretion in intact rats and synthesis (Bekhtereva 1966, 1968).

In Fig. 3 the effects of the lesion of the basal portion of the amygdala on pituitary and plasma FSH levels are shown at different periods after the operation (1, 2 and 4 weeks). The pituitary FSH concentration is expressed by the changes in ovarian weight of the recipients, and the plasma FSH level in mg of mice uterus weight per 10 ml of plasma. The lesion of the basal part of the amygdaloid complex resulted in an increase in pituitary FSH content of male rats 1, 2 and 4 weeks after the destruction. In contrast to these observations the pituitary FSH level was decreased on the 3rd week when the plasma FSH activity was twice as large as in the previous period.

Destruction of the basal parts of the amygdala led to a more pronounced augmentation of the inhibitory action of central cholinolytic methylbenactizine (20 mg/kg for 10 days) on the pituitary FSH secretion than in the intact rats when the drug was given after a 4-week postoperative period.

The stimulating action of spasmolytine as a central n-cholinolytic on the pituitary secretion, which had been observed in intact animals, could not be detected after the destruction of the amygdala.

Figure 4 shows the effect of 10 µg oestradiol monobenzoate given for 5 days on the pituitary and plasma FSH levels.

Following lesioning of the amygdaloid complex of nuclei the oestradiol monobenzoate administration did not decrease the pituitary FSH content, it was even significantly higher than that of the sham-operated or untreated group. Similarly, the amygdala lesion produced an increase of plasma FSH level and prevented the inhibitory influence of oestradiol treatment.

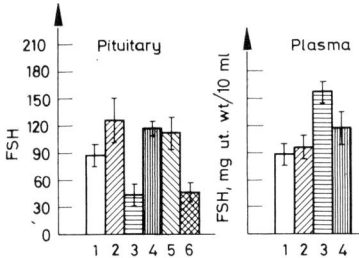
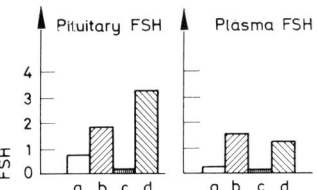

Fig. 3. See text for details. 1 — control; 2, 3, 4 — FSH levels at 1, 2, 4 weeks after the lesion of the basal amygdaloid complex (AB); 5 — lesions of the basal amygdaloid complex (4 weeks) + spasmolytine 40 mg/kg 10 d.; 6 — lesions of the basal amygdaloid complex + α-methylbenactizine 20 mg/kg 10 d

Fig. 4. Pituitary and plasma FSH $\left(\dfrac{\text{mg HMG 2IRP}}{\text{pit. or 1.5 ml plasma}}\right)$ levels after basal amygdaloid lesions and effects of oestradiol monobenzoate on FSH release. a — sham-operation; b — lesions of the basal amygdaloid complex (4 weeks); c — oestradiol monobenzoate; d — lesions of the basal amygdaloid complex + oestradiol monobenzoate

Both the pituitary and plasma LH activity showed an increase after the lesion of the basal amygdala. In contrast to these findings, the destruction of the medial amygdaloid nucleus produced a decrease in both pituitary and plasma LH concentration of femal rats (Figs 5 and 6). The LH levels are expressed in µg of standard bovine luteinizing hormone (NIH LHB-6) pituitary or ml of plasma.

Figure 5 shows the changes in the pituitary and plasma LH concentration in the sham-operated rats (*i*) after the lesion of medial amygdaloid 2 weeks (*ii*) and 4 weeks (*iii*) after surgery, and in rats with amygdala destruction and methylbenactizine treatment.

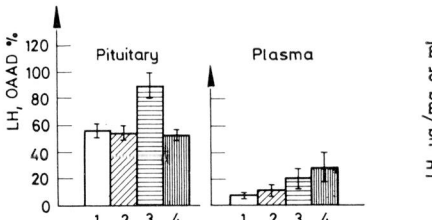
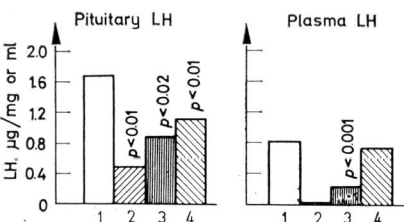

Figs 5–6. Pituitary and plasma LH levels after the lesion of basal parts of amygdala. LH levels are represented as the percentage of ovarian ascorbic acid depletion (OAAD). 1 — control; 2 — sham operation; 3 — lesions of basal parts of amygdala (2 weeks after the operation); 4 — lesions of basal parts of amygdala (4 weeks after the operation)

DISCUSSION

The observations indicate that the destruction of the basal parts of the amygdaloid complex results mainly in an increase of the pituitary FSH secretion in male and female rats and to a certain degree of the LH secretion of females. In contrast to these findings, the destruction of the medial amygdaloid nucleus was followed by a decrease of the pituitary and plasma LH concentration of female rats.

The inhibitory action of central cholinolytic α-methylbenactizine on FSH secretion was more pronounced in rats with lesion of the basal amygdaloid nuclei than in the sham-operated controls.

More pronounced inhibitory action of m-cholinolytic methamizyl on the pituitary FSH level after the lesion of the basal parts of the amygdala may be considered through its action on the hypothalamus.

A facilitatory action of spasmolytine, as a central n-cholinolytic on FSH secretion in intact animals, could not be detected after the destruction of the amygdala. These observations confirm our assumption that n-cholinolytic spasmolytine exerts its action through the limbic structures and in particular through the amygdala.

The inhibitory effect of oestradiol monobenzoate on the FSH secretion after the destruction of basal parts of the amygdala was markedly decreased in female rats. Oestradiol treatment resulted in an increase in pituitary FSH level. On the other hand, the lesioning of basal part of the amygdala decreased the inhibitory action of methylbenactizine on LH secretion. Moreover, in some cases methamizyl prevented the decrease in pituitary and plasma LH levels. It is worth mentioning that in some cases both the medial and basal portion of the amygdala were destroyed, though, the effect was the same as after the destruction at the medial portion alone.

With regard to LH secretion it is quite possible that the medial complex of the amygdaloid nuclei exerts a facilitatory influence which apparently is dominant over the inhibition of the basal portion.

Moreover, we may assume that impulses from the basal portion of the amygdala to the hypothalamus pass through the medial portion and induce the inhibition of LH secretion. Obviously, the destruction of the medial portion of the amygdala will be followed by the cessation of amygdala–hypothalamic connections received from the basal parts.

The amygdala plays a role in the susceptibility of central brain structures to the action of cholinolytics as well as to the feedback action of sex steroid hormones. An antagonistic organization within the amygdala mediates functionally different, apparently opposite effects on the hypothalamic regulation of pituitary gonadotropic hormone secretion.

REFERENCES

BEKHTEREVA, E. P. (1966): *Farmakol. i Toksikol.* **6,** 739.
BEKHTEREVA, E. P. (1968): *Bull. exp. Biol. Med.* **8,** 66.
BEKHTEREVA, E. P. (1970): *Probl. Endokr. Gormonoter.* **3,** 50–53.
BUNN, I. P. and EVERETT, I. W. (1957): *Proc. Soc. exp. Biol. (N.Y.)* **96,** 369.
ELEFTHERIOU, B. E., ZOLOVICK, A. J. and NORMAN, R. L. (1967): *J. Endocr.* **38,** 469.
ELVERS, M. and CRITCHLOW, V. W. (1960): *Amer. J. Physiol.* **198,** 381.
IGARASHI, M. and McCANN, S. M. (1964): *Endocrinology* **74,** 440.
KAWAKAMI, M., SETO, K. and YOSHIDA, K. (1968): *Jap. J. Physiol.* **3,** 356.
KOIKEGAMI, H., YAMADA, T. and USUI, K. (1954): *Folia psychiat. neurol. jap.* **8,** 7.
KÖNIG, J. F. R. and KLIPPEL, R. A. (1963): *The Rat Brain.* Williams and Wilkins, Baltimore.
LAWTON, I. E. and SAWYER, C. H. (1970): *Amer. J. Physiol.* **218,** 622–626.
PARLOW, A. T. (1961): In: *Human Gonadotropins.* Ed. by A. Albert. Springfield, p. 300.
STEELMAN, S. L. and POHLEY, F. M. (1953): *Endocrinology* **53,** 604.

THE ROLE OF BRAIN MONOAMINES IN THE SUSCEPTIBILITY TO SEIZURES BROUGHT ABOUT BY CHEMICAL AND ELECTRICAL STIMULATIONS

A. K. PFEIFER and G. UNYI

Institute of Experimental Medicine
Hungarian Academy of Sciences
Budapest, Hungary

It is well known that the brain monoamines depleting agents such as reserpine and tetrabenazine beside their tranquillizing effect increase the susceptibility to seizures induced by pentetrazol and by electrical stimulation. Both actions of the drugs are considered to be in connection with the low norepinephrine (NE), dopamine (DA) and serotonin (5-HT) content of the brain. Both the tranquillizing and convulsion facilitating effects can be reversed by monoamine oxidase inhibitors, which elevate the content of all three monoamines in the brain.

Contradictory are the data as to which monoamine from the three is responsible for the convulsion facilitating effect. Lessin and Parkes (1959) consider the low brain 5-HT level to be the cause of convulsion facilitation, while De Schaepdryver et al. (1962) reject the theory that 5-HT would have any role in the change of convulsive threshold assuming that the change of brain DA could be the cardinal alteration of the susceptibility to seizures. Truitt and Ebersberger (1962), Chen et al. (1968a, b), Jones and Roberts (1968) assume the change of brain NE level responsible for the change of convulsion threshold.

The present experiments attempt to clarify whether the convulsion facilitating effect of monoamine depletors is of universal validity, which monoamine is responsible for the effect and whether or not the convulsion facilitation and tranquillization are separable properties.

METHODS

Albino mice of both sexes, weighing 18 to 22 g each, and albino rats of the Wistar strain, weighing 120 to 150 g each, were used. The animals were grouped at random. Statistical analysis was done following variance analysis by Dunn's multiple comparison method (1961), or by Student's t test.

Cerebral norepinephrine and dopamine levels were estimated by spectrophotofluorometry according to Drujan et al. (1959). The animals were killed by decapitation, the brain was dropped in liquid N_2 and stored at $-30°C$ until tested. Four mouse brains were pooled for each test. The brain level of α-methyl-m-tyramine and metaraminol was estimated according to Shore and Alpers (1964).

The motility of mice was estimated by the method of Knoll and Vojnovszky (1960). The mice were placed into the motimeter 30 min after the administration of physiological NaCl solution or of the test substance and motility was observed for 30 min.

The susceptibility to seizures was tested in mice according to Orloff et al. (1949). A 0.5 per cent solution of pentetrazol was injected into a tail vein at a rate of 0.05 ml per 10 sec until tonic extensor convulsions had developed. Convulsive threshold is understood to mean the dose of pentetrazol required to evoke tonic extensor convulsions.

Electroshock was elicited by means of bitemporal electrodes and a Disa Multistim stimulator, with 125/sec frequency, 6 msec delay, 3 msec duration and 8.5 to 10.5 mA intensity for mice and 15 to 16 mA for rats. The duration of stimulus was 0.5 sec in the case of mice and 1.0 sec in that of rats. A tonic extensor convulsion was accepted as being a convulsion.

RESULTS AND DISCUSSION

Table 1 displays the convulsion facilitating effect of reserpine on insulin and semicarbaside convulsions and the reversal action of the MAO inhibitors iproniazid and nialamide. It has been established that neither reserpine nor nialamide and iproniazid influenced the hypoglycaemic effect of insulin or the glutamic acid decarboxylase inhibiting effect of semicarbaside. Thus, it can be assumed that the change in sensitivity to seizures is due to the altered brain monoamine content.

It is indisputable that the biochemical mechanism of convulsions brought about by pentetrazol, semicarbaside, insulin or electrical stimulation has nothing in common. So one seems to be entitled to assume that the change in brain mono-

TABLE 1

The effect of reserpine, respectively MAO inhibitors + reserpine on the insulin and semicarbaside convulsions in mice

Pretreatment	Time hours	Treatment	Number of mice with convulsion / number of experimental mice
Vehicle	—	3 U/kg insulin i.v.	10/24
5 mg/kg reserpine i.p.	2	0.9 NaCl	17/24
Vehicle	—	5 U/kg insulin i.v.	17/24
100 mg/kg iproniazid + 5 mg/kg reserpine	18 2	5 U/kg insulin i.v.	4/24
Vehicle	—	130 mg/kg semicarbaside s.c.	5/12
2.5 mg/kg reserpine i.p.	2	130 mg/kg semicarbaside s.c.	11/12
100 mg/kg nialamide i.p. 2.5 mg/kg reserpine i.p.	18 2	130 mg/kg semicarbaside s.c.	4/12

amine content — caused by reserpine — increases the susceptibility to seizures in general.

The discovery of the so-called selective catecholamine depletors gave the opportunity to investigate how the decreased brain catecholamine level, beside normal 5-HT level, influences the susceptibility to seizures. The experiments were carried out on mice and pentetrazol convulsion was used as test.

As Table 2 shows, prenylamine and guanethidine increase the susceptibility to seizures similarly to reserpine. The brain level of all the three monoamines is considerably decreased by 2.5 mg/kg reserpine, while 50 mg/kg prenylamine, respectively, 5 mg/kg guanethidine did not influence the brain 5-HT content. While prenylamine depleted both NE and DA, guanethidine decreased NE level without changing the DA content of the brain. α-Methyl-m-tyrosine (MMT) and α-methyl-m-tyramine (MMT-ine) decreased brain catecholamine, did not influence the brain 5-HT level and convulsion threshold.

In mice pretreated with MAO inhibitors all the amine depletors elevate the convulsion threshold. As Table 3 shows, tranylcypromine administered alone does not influence the susceptibility to seizures, it elevates however the NE, DA and 5-HT level of the brain. All the catecholamine depletors except guanethidine became anticonvulsive after tranylcypromine similar to reserpine. They did not change the CA level significantly. One can assume that free CA content is increased and is responsible for the anticonvulsant effect. In the case of guanethidine there is no anticonvulsive effect, but increased susceptibility to seizures does not develop either.

TABLE 2

The effect of amine depletors on the pentetrazol convulsion threshold and brain amine level in mice

Treatment	Time hours	Convulsion threshold ml/10 g pentetrazol mean ± S.D.	NA	DA	5-HT
			γ/g mean ± S.D.		
Control	—	0.199 ± 0.036 (25)	0.436 ± 0.061 (12)	0.624 ± 0.266 (18)	0.600 ± 0.185 (10)
Reserpine 2.5 mg/kg i.p.	2	0.133 ± 0.015 (10)	0.103 ± 0.074 (10)	0.294 ± 0.021 (4)	0.151 ± 0.035 (4)
Prenylamine 50 mg/kg s.c.	2	0.151 ± 0.03 (15)	0.105 ± 0.098 (9)	0.298 ± 0.155 (9)	0.618 ± 0.142 (4)
Guanethidine 5 mg/kg i.p.	2	0.162 ± 0.02 (20)	0.256 ± 0.136 (6)	0.620 ± 0.160 (4)	0.648 ± 0.025 (4)
MMT 50 mg/kg i.p.	2	0.212 ± 0.041 (10)	0.210 ± 0.140 (4)	0.216 ± 0.141 (4)	0.570 ± 0.210 (5)
MMT-ine 100 mg/kg i.p.	2	0.215 ± 0.06 (10)	0.230 ± 0.106 (5)	0.282 ± 0.106 (4)	0.585 ± 0.139 (5)

( ) Number of experiments.

TABLE 3

The effect of tranylcypromine plus amine depletors on the pentetrazol convulsion threshold and brain amine level in mice

Treatment	Time hours	Convulsion threshold ml/10 g pentetrazol mean ± S.D.	NA	DA	5-HT
				γ/g mean ± S.D.	
Control	—	0.201 ± 0.05 (15)	0.319 ± 0.112 (8)	0.554 ± 0.165 (11)	0.634 ± 0.176 (20)
5 mg/kg tranylcypromine s.c.	3	0.100 ± 0.06 (30)	0.406 ± 0.149 (9)	0.712 ± 0.022 (9)	1.332 ± 0.407 (12)
5 mg/kg tranylcypromine s.c. 2.5 mg/kg reserpine s.c.	3 2	0.372 ± 0.110 (15)	0.349 ± 0.132 (5)	0.583 ± 0.236 (6)	1.423 ± 0.385 (6)
5 mg/kg tranylcypromine s.c. 50 mg/kg prenylamine s.c.	3 2	0.403 ± 0.132 (18)	0.246 ± 0.081 (5)	0.595 ± 0.235 (9)	1.249 ± 0.379 (6)
5 mg/kg tranylcypromine s.c. 50 mg/kg MMT i.p.	3 2	0.348 ± 0.09 (10)	0.431 ± 0.158 (6)	0.647 ± 0.124 (8)	1.568 ± 0.276 (6)
5 mg/kg tranylcypromine s.c. 100 mg/kg MMT-ine i.p.	3 2	0.374 ± 0.08 (10)	0.402 ± 0.160 (6)	0.424 ± 0.207 (6)	1.572 ± 0.226 (6)
5 mg/kg tranylcypromine s.c. 5 mg/kg guanethidine i.p.	3 2	0.231 ± 0.061 (20)	0.424 ± 0.153 (20)	0.651 ± 0.180 (10)	1.120 ± 0.252 (3)

( ) Number of experiments.

When mice are pretreated 16 hours before tranylcypromine with 100 mg/kg prenylamine, reserpine, prenylamine and MMT do not influence the convulsion threshold (Table 4). The 5-HT level is just as high as without prenylamine pretreatment, the CA level is below the control. A fact, which seems also to emphasize the role of CA in the susceptibility to seizures.

As it has been demonstrated the specific catecholamine depletor MMT did not influence the convulsive threshold. The displayed experiments were made two hours after the administration of MMT. Table 5 shows the time curve of pentetrazol convulsion threshold, the amount of missing NE + DA and the MMT-ine + metaraminol level of the mouse brain. It is well known that MMT-ine and metaraminol are formed from MMT in brain and presuming that these methyl analogues of the physiologic mediator substances dislocate the CA from their storages, this would be the cause of the depleting effect of MMT. As it can be seen, two hours after the administration of MMT the decrease in convulsive threshold is not significant, the amount of missing CA-s is considerable and the

TABLE 4

The effect of tranylcypromine plus amine depletors on pentetrazol convulsion threshold and brain amines with prenylamine pretreated mice

Treatment	Time hours	Convulsion threshold ml/10g pentetrazol mean ± S.D.	NA	DA	5-HT
				γ/g mean ± S.D.	
100 mg/kg prenylamine s.c.	16				
5 mg/kg tranyl-cypromine s.c.	3	0.251 ± 0.091 (10)	0.268 ± 0.103 (6)	0.140 ± 0.028 (5)	1.153 ± 0.429 (7)
2.5 mg/kg reserpine i.p.	2				
100 mg/kg prenylamine s.c.	16				
5 mg/kg tranyl-cypromine s.c.	3	0.224 ± 0.03 (10)	0.257 ± 0.088 (5)	0.256 ± 0.147 (5)	0.914 ± 0.150 (5)
50 mg/kg prenylamine i.p.	2				
100 mg/kg prenylamine s.c.	16				
5 mg/kg tranyl-cypromine s.c.	3	0.239 ± 0.028 (10)	0.219 ± 0.057 (6)	0.264 ± 0.180 (6)	0.965 ± 0.213 (5)
50 mg/kg MMT i.p.	2				

( ) Number of experiments.

brain level of the methyl analogues is very high. After 4 and 18 hours the decrease of convulsive threshold is significant. After 4 hours the amount of missing NE + DA is more than after two hours and the level of MMT-ine and metaraminol is slightly lower. After 18 hours the CA depletion is the same as after two hours, but the brain content of methyl analogues is about one quarter of the measured amount after two hours.

These results correspond with those of Carlsson and Lindquist (1962), who demonstrated that MMT had no tranquillizing effect beside its strong CA depleting action. They assumed that the tranquillization did not take place because the formed metaraminol and MMT-ine are acting as false transmitters. In their experiments the amount of methyl analogues of the physiological mediators agreed roughly with the missing amount of CA-s in the brain.

The present results indicate that in case of susceptibility to seizures the methylated amines take over the function of CA, too.

In summary, all the investigated drugs facilitate convulsions beside low brain NE and DA and unaltered 5-HT level. The demonstrated results with guanethidine emphasize the role of NE lowering solely the brain NE content.

Experiments on adrenalectomized rats underline also the role of CA against 5-HT in the susceptibility to seizures. Table 6 shows that the convulsive threshold of the adrenalectomized rats does not differ from that of the intact animals. There is no change in the brain NE level, but the brain 5-HT content is about 50 per

TABLE 5

The effect of MMT on pentetrazol convulsion threshold, and on the NA and DA level in mice

Time hours	50 mg/kg MMT i.p.			
	Increase in susceptibility to seizures %	Missing		Metaraminol + MMT-ine mp Mol/g
		NA p Mol/g	DA p Mol/g	
2	17	1.254	2.450	8.10
		3.704		
4	35	1.923	4.418	6.20
		6.314		
18	32	1.526	2.098	2.41
		3.624		

TABLE 6

The effect of reserpine on the ES threshold and on the brain NA and 5-HT level in intact and adrenalectomized rats

Treatment	Control			Adrenalectomized		
	Convulsion threshold mA	NA	5-HT	Convulsion threshold mA	NA	5-HT
		γ/g mean $\pm$ S.E.			γ/g mean $\pm$ S.E.	
—	14.5	0.270 ± 0.019	0.690 ± 0.101	15.5	0.248 ± 0.031	0.313 ± 0.086*
0.15 mg/kg reserpine i.p.	13.3	0.213 ± 0.02	0.630 ± 0.111	11.3	0.162 ± 0.017	0.285 ± 0.070

* $p < 0.01$.

cent of the controls; 0.15 mg/kg reserpine does not influence the convulsive threshold and brain amine level in the intact animals, but it decreases the convulsive threshold and NE level significantly without influencing the 5-HT level in adrenalectomized rats.

These results indicate that the decreased brain 5-HT content in the adrenalectomized rats does not induce any change in the susceptibility to seizures, but the reduced NE level, produced by reserpine, decreases the convulsive threshold.

A series of experiments with reserpine and α-methyl dopa (MD) indicate also the importance of NE in the susceptibility to seizures and make probable the separation of the convulsion facilitating and tranquillizing effect.

As Table 7 shows, MD inhibits the convulsion facilitating effect and the brain NE depleting effect of reserpine, without influencing narcosis potentiation, decreased motility and 5-HT depletion.

TABLE 7

The effect of reserpine, alpha-methyl dopa, respectively, reserpine and alphamethyl dopa on the convulsion threshold, hexobarbital (50 mg/kg i.v.) sleeping time, spontaneous motility and brain NA and 5-HT content in mice

Treatment	Time	Convulsion threshold ml/10 g pentetrazol mean ± S.E.	Hexobarbital sleeping time sec mean ± S.E.	Motimeter value in 30 min mean ± S.E.	NA γ/g mean ± S.E.	5-HT γ/g mean ± S.E.
0.9% NaCl	—	0.219±0.007	165±10	186±15	0.282±0.012	0.745±0.071
2.5 mg/kg reserpine i.p.	2	0.141±0.025*	423±105*	30± 7*	0.090±0.017*	0.299±0.042*
400 mg/kg α-methyl dopa i.p	4	0.222±0.050	3.417±514*	23± 7*	0.180±0.019*	0.282±0.047*
α-methyl dopa reserpine	4 / 2	0.232±0.053	3.227±439*	13± 5*	0.317±0.031	0.258±0.031*

* $p < 0.01$.

It may be concluded that reserpine loses the convulsion facilitating effect when brain NE is restored to normal and only 5-HT content is low, but the narcosis potentiating and motility decreasing effects persist. This and further experiments suggest that the convulsion facilitating and tranquillizing effects of reserpine are separable.

Table 8 displays that all the investigated amphetamine derivatives inhibit the convulsion facilitating effect of reserpine in mice, testing either with the intravenous pentetrazol method, or with ES. Reserpine suspends the hypermotility produced by amphetamine derivatives — except for amphetamine, moreover a slightly decreased motility can be observed and in the case of trifluormethyl derivative the tranquillizing action of reserpine comes to force completely. This is another fact, which supports the possibility that the tranquillizing and convulsion facilitating effects are independent.

Among the amphetamine derivatives p-chloro-amphetamine has perhaps the strongest anti-reserpine effect regarding the susceptibility to seizure. Experiments were performed to study the effect of the compound on amine depletion produced by reserpine. As Table 9 shows, p-chloro-amphetamine does not influence the amine depletion caused by reserpine. On the other hand, it decreases significantly the NE and DA depleting effect of MMT. The CA depleting effect of MMT is considered to be a displacing action by the formed methylated amines. Perhaps it may be sup-

TABLE 8

The effect of amphetamine and its derivatives on the pentetrazol and ES threshold and on the motility in mice pretreated with reserpine. Reserpine, respectively, amphetamine and its derivatives were administered two, respectively, half an hour before the experiments

Pretreatment	Treatment	ml/10 g pentetrazol mean ± S.E.	ES number of mice with convulsion / number of experimental mice	Motimeter value in 30 min mean ± S.E.
0.9% NaCl	0.9% NaCl	0.183 ± 0.012	15/16 (10.5 mA)	228 ± 26
Reserpine 2.5 mg/kg i.p.	0.9% NaCl	0.092 ± 0.003	16/16 (8.5 mA)	8 ± 1.5
Reserpine 2.5 mg/kg i.p.	amphetamine 50 μM/kg s.c.	0.126 ± 0.012	14/16 (8.5 mA)	800 ± 137
Reserpine 2.5 mg/kg i.p.	methamphetamine 50 μM/kg s.c.	0.161 ± 0.012	10/16 (8.5 mA)	168 ± 41
Reserpine mg/kg i.p.	p-Cl-amphetamine 50 μM/kg s.c.	0.183 ± 0.015	8/16 (8.5 mA)	145 ± 36
Reserpine mg/kg i.p.	trifluoromethylamphet- amine 75 μM/kg s.c.	0.160 ± 0.02	12/12 (8.5 mA)	20 ± 6

TABLE 9

The effect of reserpine and MMT on the pentetrazol convulsion threshold and on brain amine content in control and in p-chloro-amphetamine-treated mice. The (±) p-chloro-amphetamine (10 mg/kg i.p.) was administered 4 hours before the experiments. Reserpine (2.5 mg/kg/i.p.) and MMT (50 mg/kg i.p.) were applied two hours after p-chloro-amphetamine

Treatment	Pretreatment: 0.9% NaCl				Pretreatment: p-Cl-amphetamine			
	brain			Convulsion threshold ml/10g pentetrazol	brain			Convulsion threshold ml/10g pentetrazol
	NA γ/g	DA γ/g	5-HT γ/g		NA γ/g	DA γ/g	5-HT γ/g	
Control	0.445 ± 0.08 (13)	0.997 ± 0.20 (13)	0.565 ± 0.06 (4)	0.177 ± 0.044 (50)	0.514 ± 0.10 (13)	1.044 ± 0.19 (12)	0.551 ± 0.10 (4)	0.237 ± 0.073 (20)
Reserpine	0.087 ± 0.03 (5)	0.134 ± 0.04 (5)	0.199 ± 0.02 (4)	0.118 ± 0.029 (20)	0.149 ± 0.07 (5)	0.178 ± 0.09 (5)	0.152 ± 0.02 (4)	0.304 ± 0.081 (20)
MMT	0.179 ± 0.05 (8)	0.332 ± 0.07 (8)		0.161 ± 0.043 (20)	0.376 ± 0.14 (7)	0.598 ± 0.04 (8)		0.331 ± 0.057 (15)

posed that the p-chloro-amphetamine inhibits the bindings of the methylated amines, competing with the binding site. Considering that in case of reserpine the convulsion facilitation is hampered by p-chloro-amphetamine beside low brain amine content it may be supposed that amphetamine derivatives act directly and are able to substitute CA in the susceptibility to seizure. Our findings may support the theory that the rat brain synaptic vesicles — the storage sites of CA — take up amphetamine and p-chloro-amphetamine in in vivo experiments (Pfeifer et al. 1969).

Experiments with reserpine and semicarbaside underline also the role of NE in the susceptibility to seizures. The experiments were made on rats, NE and DA were estimated in various parts of the brain. The brain was dissected to cortex, hypothalamus, corpus striatum, midbrain and cerebellum according to Glowinski and Iwersen (1966).

Figure 1 shows that 0.25 mg/kg reserpine and 25 mg/kg semicarbaside facilitate convulsions induced by electrical stimulation. When the two drugs were administered together a potentiation of effect could be demonstrated.

Determining the DA content of several regions of the brain it was found that in the applied dosage neither reserpine, nor semicarbaside alone or together influenced the DA content. On the other hand, reserpine and semicarbaside applied together decreased the NE content in all parts of the brain and in the whole brain, too. Neither reserpine nor semicarbaside administered alone influenced the NA content (Fig. 2).

These results indicate that in the change of susceptibility to seizures the change in NE content is of crucial importance rather than the change in DA level.

Indisputable is the fact that separately applied reserpine and semicarbaside facilitate ES without influencing NA level. It can be presumed perhaps that in case of reserpine such a low dose might reduce NE level in one or another brain area, but the method is not sensitive enough to show it. In case of semicarbaside one must count with its glutaminic acid decarboxylase inhibiting activity and consequently with the change of gamma-aminobutyric acid turnover.

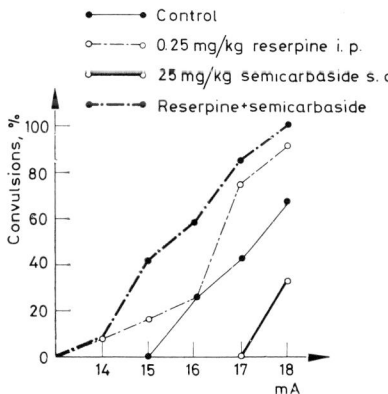

Fig. 1. Effect of reserpine and semicarbaside on the ES threshold in rats. The compounds were administered two hours before the experiments

To approach the role of monoamines in the susceptibility to seizures from another side, the influence of the specific 5-HT depletors and antiserotonin drugs on the convulsive threshold has been investigated.

p-Chloro-amphetamine, besides its amphetamine-like properties, is a selective 5-HT depletor. It decreases the brain 5-HT level in rats and guinea-pigs considerably without influencing the CA content. The compound is ineffective in mice (Pletscher et al. 1964, Fuller et al. 1965).

Figure 3 shows the influence of p-chloro-amphetamine on pentetrazol convulsion threshold and on brain 5-HT content in mice and rats. The compound has an

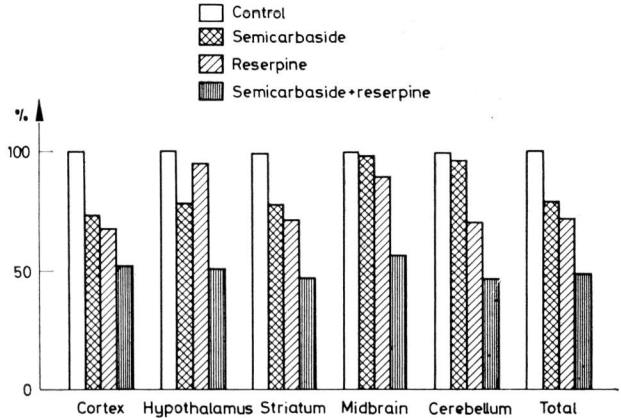

Fig. 2. Effect of reserpine and semicarbazide on the brain NE content in rats.
$S^2 = 0.026$

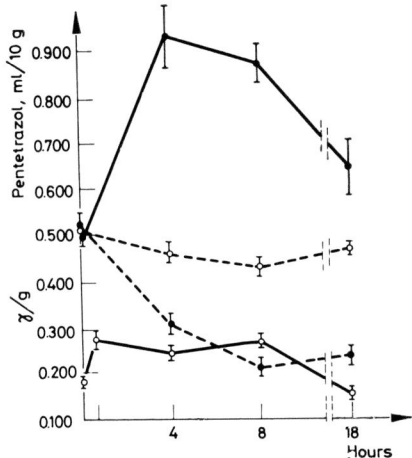

Fig. 3. The effect of 10 mg/kg ($\pm$)-p-chloro-amphetamine on the pentetrazol convulsion threshold and on brain 5-HT level. ○———○ convulsion threshold in mice, ●———● convulsion threshold in rats, ○------○ 5-HT level in mice, ●-----● 5-HT level in rats

anticonvulsant effect in both species, decreases the brain 5-HT level significantly in rats, but not in mice. The maximal anticonvulsive action in rats is between 4 and 8 hours, the convulsive threshold is again normal after 18 hours. The decrease in brain 5-HT level reaches its maximum about 8 hours later and remains at this low level after 18 hours, too.

These results support the theory that the change in brain 5-HT has no influence on the susceptibility to seizures. p-Chloro-amphetamine is anticonvulsive both in mice and rats, while in one of the two species the brain 5-HT content is low and in the other species it is normal.

p-Chloro-phenylalanine (p-ClPhe) decreases brain 5-HT content by 90 per cent. The effect starts about 8–16 hours after administration, reaches its maximum after 3 days in rats. The site of action is the inhibition of tryptophane hydroxylase (Koe and Weissman 1966). Koe and Weissman (1968) demonstrated that the compound decreased the electroshock (ES) threshold after 24 hours in rats. The experiments displayed in Fig. 4 confirm this and show that the compound facilitates the ES in rats after 48 and 72 hours, too. After 6 days the facilitating effect decreases considerably and after 10 days the convulsion threshold is not different from the control. These results indicate that there are connections between the convulsion facilitating and brain 5-HT level decreasing effect, because according to Koe and Weissman (1968) the brain 5-HT level is only 60 per cent of the control even after 10 days.

The afore-said makes the role of 5-HT in the convulsion facilitating effect of p-chloro-phenylalanine unlikely since 5-HTP does not eliminate it (Fig. 5).

According to Koe and Weissma (1966) p-chloro-phenylalanine decreases brain 5-HT in mice only when the drug is administered on three consecutive days. We showed that the drug did not influence ES in mice either after a single or after three

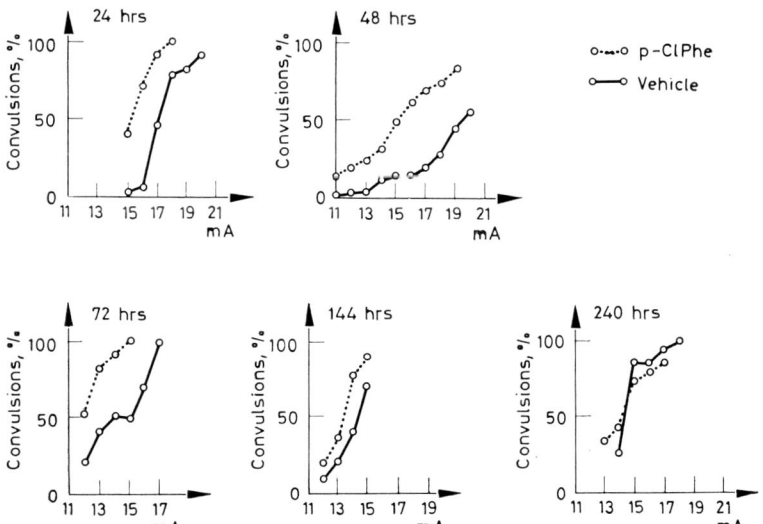

Fig. 4. The effect of p-Cl-phenylalanine (300 mg/kg orally) on the ES threshold in rats

doses. On the other hand, both ways of administration elevated the convulsion threshold in mice considerably after 48 and 72 hours (Fig. 6).

We consider that these results indicate that though specific 5-HT depletors influence the susceptibility to seizures, this effect is independent of the change in brain 5-HT content. It seems to be very probable that the drugs act directly on the susceptibility to seizures.

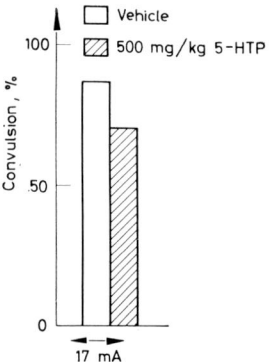

Fig. 5. The effect of 5-HTP on the ES threshold with p-Cl-phenylalanine (300 mg/kg orally) pretreated (48 hours) rats. $p < 0.1$

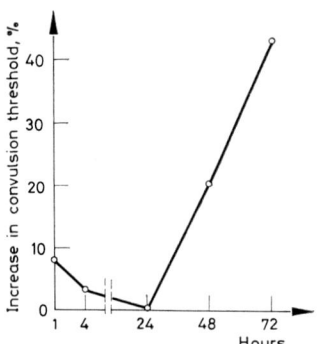

Fig. 6. The effect of p-Cl-phenylalanine (300 mg/kg orally) on the pentetrazol convulsion threshold in mice

In order to gain further information about the possible role 5-HT may play in the susceptibility to seizures the effect of antiserotonin compounds has been investigated.

As Fig. 7 shows, methysergid and cyproheptadine decrease the sensitivity to pentetrazol convulsion in mice considerably, while LSD is ineffective.

These results indicate that the anticonvulsive effect of methysergid and cyproheptadine is independent of their antiserotonin action.

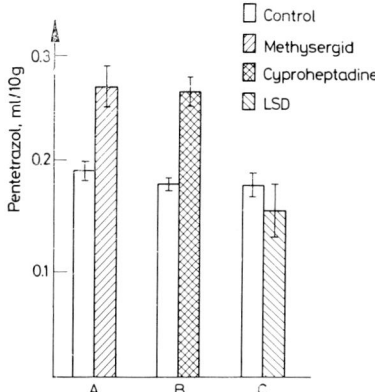

Fig. 7. The effect of methysergid (5 mg/kg i.p.), cyproheptadine (0.1 mg/kg i.p.) and LSD (1 mg/kg i.p.) on the pentetrazol convulsion threshold in mice. The drugs were administered two hours before the experiments

SUMMARY

For the study of the role of monoamines in the susceptibility to seizures it was necessary to investigate whether the convulsion facilitating effect of reserpine could be extended to other types of convulsions such as pentetrazol and electrically induced seizures. It was proved that reserpine facilitates insulin and semicarbaside convulsions, too. The facilitation can be connected with the brain monoamine depleting effect of reserpine because it can be reversed by MAO inhibitors.

The presented experiments indicate that decreased brain CA level means increased, while elevated CA level a decreased susceptibility to seizures. All the investigated selective CA depletors (prenylamine, MMT and guanethidine) facilitate seizures and the effect can be reversed by MAO inhibitors. It seems to be probable that NE is the responsible factor as indicated by the following proofs:

1. Guanethidine decreases only brain NE level, without influencing DA level.
2. α-Methyl dopa suspends the convulsion facilitating and NE depleting effect of reserpine, without influencing 5-HT depletion.
3. The brain of adrenalectomized rats has the normal amount of NE, but only 50 per cent of 5-HT: the convulsion threshold is unchanged. A low dose of reserpine, which does not influence the amine level and convulsion threshold in control animals decreases the NE level and convulsion threshold in adrenalectomized rats.
4. Low doses of reserpine and semicarbaside administered together increase the susceptibility to seizures, decrease brain NE level and do not influence DA level.

Amphetamine and its derivatives are able to substitute the function of CA regarding the sensitivity to seizures. They suspend the convulsion facilitating effect of reserpine without influencing amine depletion.

The change in brain 5-HT content has no role in the change to susceptibility to seizures. However, the selective 5-HT depletors alter the susceptibility to seizures, this is the per se effect of the molecule: p-chloro-amphetamine is anticonvulsive while p-chloro-phenylalanine facilitates seizures in rats.

The tranquillizing and convulsion facilitating effects of reserpine can be separated; α-methyl dopa inhibits the convulsion facilitating effect of reserpine, but does not influence the tranquillizing action. Trifluormethyl amphetamine inhibits the convulsion facilitating effect of reserpine, while tranquillization takes place fully.

REFERENCES

CARLSSON, A. and LINDQUIST, M. (1962): In vivo decarboxylation of α-methyl-dopa and α-methylmetatyrosine. *Acta physiol. scand.* **54**, 87–94.

CHEN, G., ENSOR, C. R. and BOHNER, B. (1968a): Studies of drug effects on electrically induced extensor seizures and clinical implications. *Arch. int. Pharmacodyn.* **172**, 183–218.

CHEN, G., ENSOR, C. R. and BOHNER, B. (1968b): Drug effects on the disposition of active biogenic amines in the CNS. *Life Sci.* **7**, 1063–1074.

DE SCHAEPDRYVER, A. F., PIETTE, Y. and DELAUNOIS, A. L. (1962): Brain amines and electroshock threshold. *Arch. int. Pharmacodyn.* **140**, 358–367.

DRUJAN, B. D., SOURKES, T. L., LAYNE, D. S. and MURPHY, G. F. (1959): The differential determination of catecholamines in urine. *Canad. J. Biochem.* **37**, 1153–1159.

DUNN, O. J. (1961): Multiple comparison among means. *J. Amer. statist. Ass.* **56**, 52–64.

FULLER, R. W., HINES, C. W. and MILLS, J. (1965): Lowering of brain serotonin level by chloramphetamine. *Biochem. Pharmacol.* **14**, 483–488.

GLOWINSKI, J. and IVERSEN, L. L. (1966): Regional studies of catecholamines in the rat brain. I. The disposition of (^{3}H)-norepinephrine, (^{3}H)-dopamine and (^{3}H)-dopa in various regions of the brain. *J. Neurochem.* **13**, 655–669.

JONES, B. J. and ROBERTS, D. J. (1968): The effects of intracerebroventricularly administered noradnamine and other sympathomimetic amines upon leptazol convulsions in mice. *Brit. J. Pharmacol.* **34**, 27–31.

KNOLL, J. and VOJNOVSZKY, B. (1960): Motiméter, új érzékeny készülék kis állatok mozgásának mérésére (Motimeter, a new sensitive apparatus for measuring the movements of small animals). *Magy. Tud. Akad. Biol. Orv. Tud. Oszt. Közl.* **11**, 313–328.

KOE, B. K. and WEISSMAN, A. (1966): P-chlorophenylamine: a specific depletor of brain serotonin. *J. Pharmacol. exp. Ther.* **154**, 499–516.

KOE, B. K. and WEISSMAN, A. (1968): The pharmacology of para-chlorophenylamine, a selective depletor of serotonin stores. In: *Advances in Pharmacology.* Vol. 6. Ed. by S. Garattini and P. A. Shore. Academic Press, New York. pp. 29–47.

LESSIN, A. W. and PARKES, M. W. (1959): The effects of reserpine and other agents upon leptazol convulsions in mice. *Brit. J. Pharmacol.* **14**, 108–111.

ORLOFF, J. J., WILLIAMS, H. L. and PFEIFFER, C. C. (1949): Timed intravenous infusion of metrazol and strychnine for testing anticonvulsant drugs. *Proc. Soc. exp. Biol.* (N. Y.) **70**, 254–257.

PFEIFER, A. K., CSÁKY, L., FODOR, M., GYÖRGY, L. and ÖKRÖS, I. (1969): The subcellular distribution of (+)-amphetamine and (±)-p-chloroamphetamine in the rat brain as influenced by reserpine. *J. Pharm. Pharmacol.* **21**, 687–689.

PLETSCHER, A., BARTHOLINI, G., BRUDERE, H., BURKARD, W. P. and GEY, K. F. (1964): Chlorinated arylalkylamines affecting the cerebral metabolism of 5-hydroxytryptamine. *J. Pharmacol. exp. Ther.* **145**, 344–450.

SHORE, P. A. and ALPERS, H. S. (1964): Fluorometric estimation of metaraminol and related compounds. *Life Sci.* **3**, 551–554.

TRUITT, E. B., JR. and EBERSBERGER, E. M. (1962): Decarboxylase inhibitors affect convulsion thresholds to hexafluorodiethyl ether. *Science* **135**, 105–106.

ANALGESIA, TOLERANCE AND DRUG DEPENDENCE

K. KELEMEN

Department of Pharmacology
Semmelweis University of Medicine
Budapest, Hungary

Pain is a peculiar function with many psychic, neural and endocrine aspects. It is the most common reason for patients to come to a doctor, and in spite of the rapidly expanding possibilities of causal therapy, symptomatic pain relief has still remained one of the main tasks of medical practice. In addition, as a result of rapid drug development, the majority of drugs prescribed, especially those for causal therapy, have been produced in the last two decades, while the analgetics most widely used like morphine, codeine, acetylsalicylic acid, aminopyrine, phenacetin were all developed before this century. Unfortunately, these analgetics do not owe their steady use to some ideal properties but to the mere fact that none of the many products of a world-wide intensive research has met better the requirements of the "ideal agent". An ideal agent would be effective against either mild or severe pain, it would be free from respiratory depressant and other side effects and it would be non-addicting. Of the drugs used neither the so-called "major" nor the "minor" analgetics fulfil these criteria. The minor, or antipyretic analgetics are effective only against mild pain and evoke serious side effects. Because of the danger of bone-marrow depression and agranulocytosis aminopyrine is not used anymore in many countries. There is a world-wide tendency to withdraw phenacetin, too, since it damages haemoglobin in the circulating erythrocytes. Even the seemingly most harmless salicylates cause such a damage in the gastric mucosa that had they been discovered nowadays, they would not have had much chance to stand up to the regulations for new drugs in this or many other countries (de Stevens 1965). The situation is not more favourable in case of major, or narcotic analgetics, either. Although compounds some thousand times more effective than morphine had been synthetized it seems that addictive properties and respiratory depressant side effects cannot be separated from the major analgetic activity, even if different chemical structures are involved (Schaumann 1956). Discovery of the analgetic action of morphine antagonists means a somewhat more promising way, for psychic dependence, compulsive drug abuse do not seem to be concomitant with these drugs. Their practical use, however, is limited by a peculiar psychotomimetic, dysphoric effect (Kelemen 1968, Lewis et al. 1971).

At our Department several aspects of the pharmacology of analgetics are investigated and some practical results have also been obtained. Two particular problems shall be dealt with in the following.

1. It was found by Knoll that an appropriate substitution of the so far scarcely exploited homopyrimidazol structure resulted in a strong analgetic activity (Knoll 1969, Knoll et al. 1969, Knoll et al. 1971d). Out of some 100 compounds examined, the agent named MZ-144 (Fig. 1) proved to be the most promising. Recently it has been clinically used under the name "Probon". Several reports on the pharmacology and therapeutic use of the drug have been published (Knoll et al. 1971a, b, Fürst et al. 1969, 1970, Graber et al., Selley and Eckhardt). As far as the classification is concerned homopyrimidazol analgetics cannot be included either in the category of minor or major analgetics. Based on their pharmacological properties they can be considered as an intermediary group between these two categories. As shown in Fig. 2, morphine proved to be fully effective in all of the 5 tests applied, while aminopyrine exerted full effect only in one case, partial effect was noticed in two tests, and no effect could be detected in two further tests.

Homopyrimidazols, however, were fully effective in four and partially effective in one test. This classification is further supported by the comparative data of Table 1; considering the analgetic activity, homopyrimidazols have an intermediate position between minor and major analgetics, regarding potentiation of general anaesthesia they recall the major analgetics, whereas due to the lack of dysphoric action, tolerance and respiratory depression and the presence of a mild antiphlogistic activity they are similar to minor analgetics. The results of a

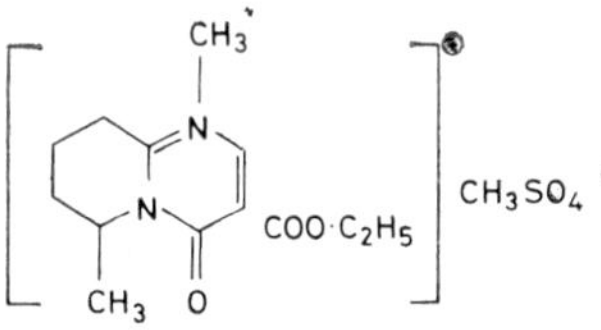

Fig. 1. 1,6-dimethyl-2-carbethoxy-4-oxo-6,7,8,9-tetrahydro-homopyrimidazol methyl-sulphate (compound MZ-144, Probon®)

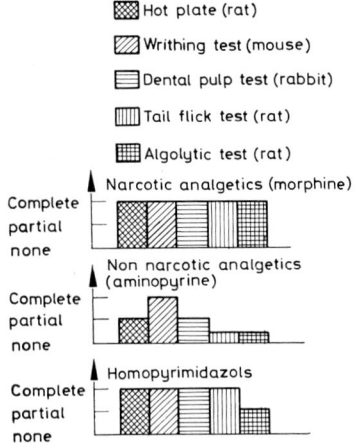

Fig. 2. Spectrum of analgetic activity of narcotic, non-narcotic and homopyrimidazol analgetics

TABLE 1

Comparison of some pharmacological effects of narcotic
and non-narcotic analgetics with homopyrimidazols

Effect	Major analgetics	Minor analgetics	MZ-144
Analgetic effect	+++	+	++
Dysphoric effect	+++	0	0
Potentiation of anaesthesia	+++	0	+++
Tolerance	+++	0	0
Nalorphine antagonism	+++	0	0
Respiratory depression	+++	0	0
Antiphlogistic effect	0	++	+

+++ Very strong; ++ Strong; + Weak; 0 No effect.

double blind clinical pharmacological study on 440 patients corresponded with those of the experimental data.

In the course of chronic treatment with MZ-144 no tolerance developed. As shown in Fig. 3, dose–response curves plotted after chronic treatment of 10 weeks and 6 months, respectively, did not differ significantly from the curve obtained in untreated animals. Similarly, the effect of morphine was not influenced either by pretreatment with MZ-144 (Fig. 4). The same correlation can be observed in the case of morphine pretreatment, too. As demonstrated in Fig. 5, in the state of tolerance to morphine, when the dose–response curve of morphine is shifted

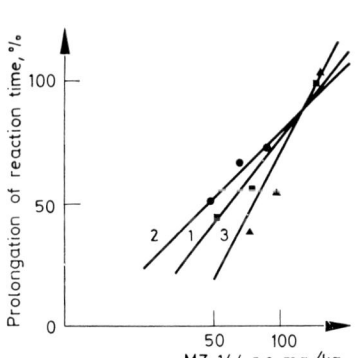

Fig. 3. The effect of pretreatment with MZ-144 on the s.c. dose-response curve of MZ-144 in the rat, measured by the hot plate test. (1) Untreated animals; (2) pretreated with MZ-144 (400 mg/kg/day) orally for 10 weeks, (3) pretreated with MZ-144 (400 mg/kg/day) orally, for 6 months. (From Knoll et al. Orvostudomány 20, 371, 1969)

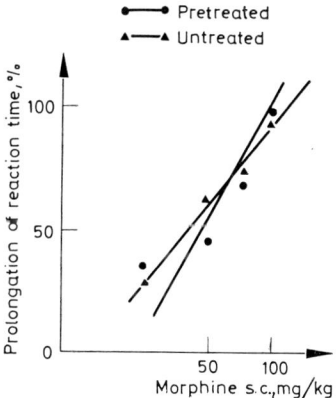

Fig. 4. The effect of pretreatment with MZ-144 (400 mg/kg/day orally, over six months) on the s.c. dose–response curve of morphine in the rat, measured by the hot plate test. (From Knoll et al. Orvostudomány 20, 371, 1969)

to the right, i.e. its action is decreased, the effect of MZ-144 remains the same as in untreated animals.

A further feature of Probon which distinguishes it from minor analgetics is that it strongly potentiates the analgetic effect of morphine. Figure 6 represents the combined effect of MZ-144 and morphine measured by the hot plate. MZ-144 causes a dose-dependent shift to the left in the dose–response curve of morphine. As it is evident from Fig. 7, there is a strong potentiation of the analgetic effect of morphine by MZ-144 even in the state of morphine tolerance. The original morphine effect has significantly decreased after a 10-week treatment with morphine, but it could be strongly increased again by MZ-144. Clinical results were the same. Figure 8 shows the abrupt increase of morphine requirement in the course of regular treatment in patients with inoperable tumours. Though Probon (MZ-144) is not able to substitute morphine itself, but increases its analgetic effect so that in a combined administration only a slight increase of the morphine dose is necessary.

Homopyrimidazols can be regarded as a new, promising group of analgetics. When administered alone they exert a stronger analgetic effect than the minor analgetics, without any objective side effect. In case of combined administration

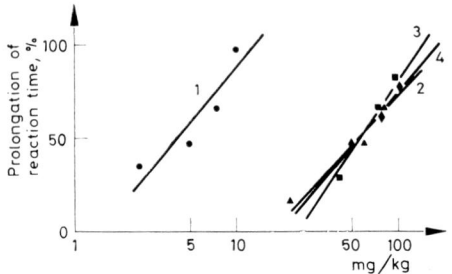

Fig. 5. The analgetic effect of MZ-144 and morphine as measured by the hot plate method in rats made tolerant to morphine. Tolerance developed according to the method of Ungar and Cohen (1966). (1) s.c. dose–response curve of morphine in untreated animals, (2) s.c. dose–response curve of morphine in animals pretreated with morphine, (3) s.c. dose–response curve of MZ-144 in untreated animals, (4) s.c. dose–response curve of MZ-144 in animals pretreated with morphine (From Knoll et al. *Orvostudomány* 20, 371, 1969)

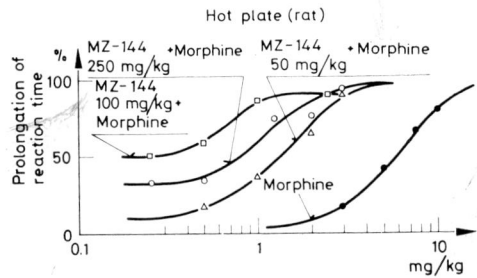

Fig. 6. Potentiation of the analgetic effect of morphine (s.c.) by different oral doses of MZ-144 in the rat

with morphine they potentiate the effect of the latter so that the significant elevation of morphine dose can be avoided in the course of chronic treatment.

2. The other problem concerns the investigation of new analgetics obtained by the modification of the morphine structure. This type of research has a long history. Much is known about the structure–activity relationship but all efforts hitherto done supported the idea that increase of the analgetic activity is inevitably accompanied by the increase of addiction liability. At this Department we have studied the pharmacology of new morphine derivatives synthetized in the course of a stereochemical study (Bognár and Makleit 1968, 1969a, b, Makleit and Bognár 1968, 1969). The most interesting compound of this group, 6-deoxy-6-azido-dihydroisomorphine, as shown in Fig. 9, is peculiarly differing in its steric structure from morphine.

Results of the pharmacological analysis performed by Knoll's group have been published only in preliminary form (Fürst and Knoll 1968, 1971, Fürst et al. 1971).

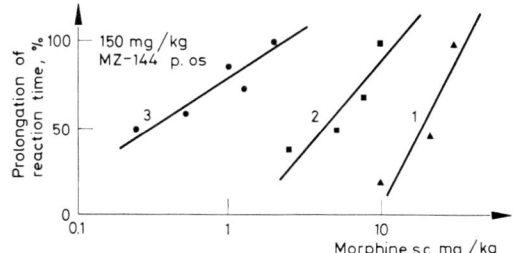

Fig. 7. The analgetic effect of MZ-144 as measured by the hot plate test in rats made tolerant to morphine. (1) s.c. dose–response curve of morphine in rats treated 300 times with daily s.c. dose of 10 mg/kg morphine, (2) s.c. dose–response curve of morphine in untreated controls, (3) the effect of 150 mg/kg MZ-144 (orally) on the s.c. dose–response curve of morphine in rats treated 300 times with a daily dose of 10 mg/kg morphine. (From Knoll et al. Orvostudomány, 20, 371, 1969)

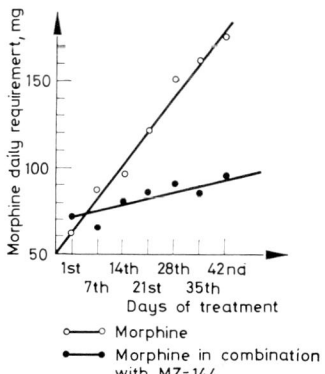

Fig. 8. Effect of MZ-144 on the increase of daily morphine requirement of patients with inoperable tumours

277

Efficacy and toxicity of the compound compared with that of morphine is shown in Table 2. It can be seen that this compound is a 270 times stronger analgetic than morphine, however, its toxicity is only 40 times higher. This results in a much wider safety margin. Since acute toxicity of morphine derivatives is connected with respiratory paralysis, the wider safety margin refers to a possible dissociation of analgetic activity and respiratory depression.

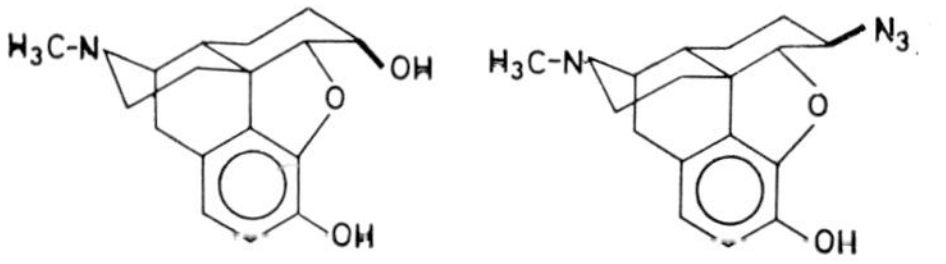

Fig. 9. Chemical structure of morphine (left) and 6-deoxy-6-azido-dihydroisomorphine (right). Note the difference in position of the substituent at C-6 in relation to the cyclohexene ring

An even more important fact is with this isomorphine derivative that a dissociation seems to be present also between the analgetic activity and the phenomenon of tolerance and dependence.

Tolerance to morphine is easy to measure in rats: as a result of chronic treatment the effective analgetic dose of morphine keeps growing and the actual degree of tolerance may be quantitatively expressed by the "dose ratio", i.e. the ratio between ED_{50} values in treated and control animals. Dynamics of dose ratio changes depend also on the mode of chronic analgetic treatment. As shown in Table 3, when

TABLE 2

Toxicity and analgetic efficacy of 6-deoxy-6-azido-dihydroisomorphine in comparison with morphine

Compound	LD 50 mg/kg			ED_{50} hot plate s.c.	T.I. s.c.
	i.v.	s.c.	oral		
6-deoxy-6-azido-dihydro-isomorphine	8.1	13.0	62.0	23 $\mu g/kg$	565
Morphine	360.0	520.0	1,200.0	6.2 mg/kg	84

TABLE 3

Changes in the "dose ratio" of morphine depending on the mode of chronic treatment

	Dose ratio (5th–6th weeks of treatment)
Constant dose of morphine (10 mg/kg per day)	3.0
Increasing dose of morphine	10.0

the rats were treated once a day with the ED_{95} of morphine, between the 5th and 6th week of treatment, dose ratio reached a value of 3.0. However, if the dose was increased every other day, the dose ratio increased up to 10 during the same period of time. Various degrees of tolerance developed to azidoisomorphine in the course of various chronic administrations but in the majority of cases this tolerance spontaneously regressed during continuous treatment. Table 4 demonstrates the temporary changes of dose ratio when animals were given constant doses. Chronic treatment with increasing doses resulted either in a morphine-type tolerance or in a regression similar to that shown in Table 4. Parallel to this phenomenon regression of cross tolerance to morphine has been consequently observed. Regression of tolerance is quite unusual with morphine derivatives.

Tolerance is only one side of addiction and from the practical point of view a much more important question is whether dependence develops.[1] In animal experiments first of all the development of physical dependence can be measured evaluating the abstinence symptoms which occur on the interruption of the treatment or on the administration of morphine antagonists. Using the method of Ettles and Lister (1963) in Buckett's (1964) modification, it was found that rats, pretreated with morphine according to the scheme of these authors, responded to the morphine antagonist nalorphine with a violent abstinence syndrome, while in the rats treated with azidoisomorphine dependence of only a slight degree developed (Fig. 10). It is also characteristic that abstinence syndrome in morphine-dependent rats was effectively suppressed by morphine but hardly with azidoisomorphine (Fig. 11).

Monkeys are considered the best test objects for studying dependence on narcotic analgetics because the abstinence syndrome of these animals is very similar to that of humans, therefore, such a study allows a reliable extrapolation to man. Using the method of Seevers and Deneau (1963) ten monkeys (*Rhesus macacus*)

TABLE 4

Temporary changes in the "dose ratio" of 6-deoxy-6-azido-dihydroisomorphine in the course of a continuous treatment with a constant dose (50 μg/kg, i.e. ED_{95}, once daily)

Weeks	DR (hot plate)
2nd	5.2
3rd	6.2
4th	3.5
.	.
.	.
.	.
14th	1.8

[1] As defined by WHO, dependence on morphine is an adaptive state characterized by severe disturbances of neuromuscular, autonomic and endocrine systems when administration of the drug is abruptly suspended, or its action is counteracted by a specific antagonist (WHO, 1964).

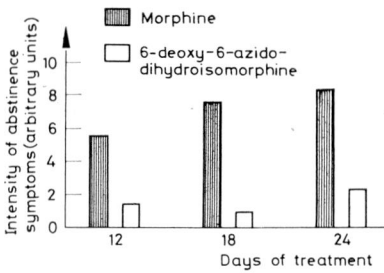

Fig. 10. Abstinence syndrome precipitated by nalorphine (10 mg/kg s.c. instead of the subsequent dose of morphine or 6-deoxy-6-azido-dihydroisomorphine). Abstinence syndrome was scored for 30 min according to the schedule of Buckett (1964)

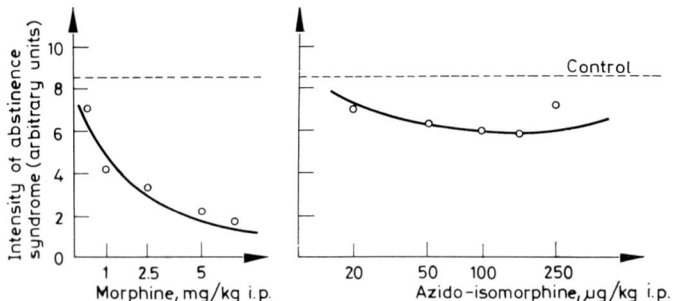

Fig. 11. Suppression of abstinence syndrome in morphine-dependent rats by morphine (right) and 6-deoxy-6-azido-dihydroisomorphine (left). Control (broken lines) — intensity of abstinence symptoms precipitated by 10 mg/kg of nalorphine, without suppressing agent. Abstinence syndrome was scored for 30 min according to the schedule of Buckett (1964)

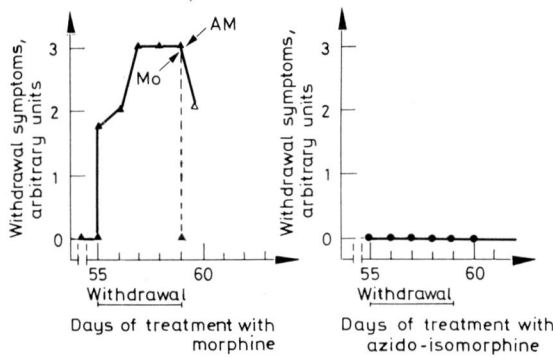

Fig. 12. Withdrawal of chronically given morphine (right) and 6-deoxy-6-azido-dihydroisomorphine (left), respectively, in monkeys. Treatment and evaluation of withdrawal symptoms according to the schedule of Seevers and Deneau (1963). Withdrawal symptoms of morphine were effectively suppressed by morphine (Mo) but only to a minor degree by 6-deoxy-6-azido-dihydroisomorphine (AM), while withdrawal of the latter did not cause any behavioural changes

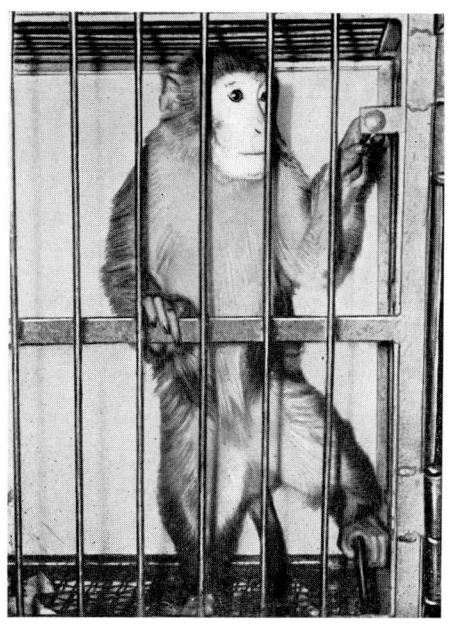
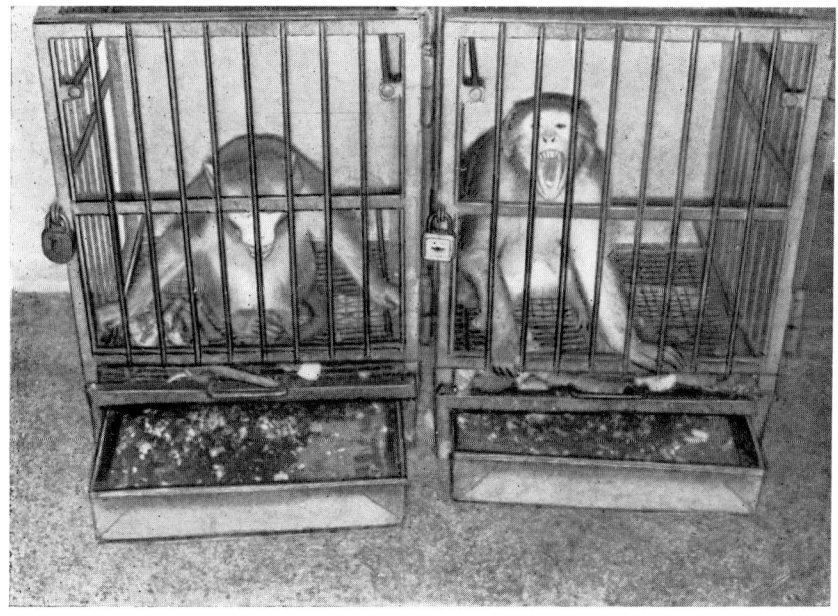

Fig. 13. Above: normal behaviour of a monkey, deprived of its daily dose of 6-deoxy-6-azido-dihydroisomorphine. Below: withdrawal symptoms in monkeys deprived of their daily dose of morphine

were treated with morphine and azidoisomorphine, respectively, and their behaviour was observed after withdrawal of the drugs. As it is shown in Fig. 12, according to expectation morphine evoked a strong physical dependence while withdrawal of chronically given azidoisomorphine did not cause any behavioural changes in the monkeys. Figure 13 illustrates the difference between the two drugs; above, the monkey of apparently normal behaviour is deprived of its daily dose of azidoisomorphine; below, the abnormal posture of the animals is one of the characteristic features of morphine withdrawal. So far we have no data about the effect of this drug on humans.

Anyway, the apparently most difficult problem of analgesia, the development of tolerance and dependence may be favourably influenced in two separate ways: (i) the combined use of narcotic analgetics with homopyrimidazol analgetics and (ii) a suitable stereochemical change in the structure of morphine.

REFERENCES

BOGNÁR, R. and MAKLEIT, S. (1968): Conversions of tosyl and mesyl derivatives of th morphine group. Aminomorphides and aminocodides. *Acta chim. Acad. Sci. hung.* **58,** 203—205.

BOGNÁR, R., MAKLEIT, S. and MILE, T. (1969a): Conversions of tosyl and mesyl derivatives of the morphine group. Synthesis of acetylmercapto and mercapto derivatives. *Acta chim. Acad. Sci. hung.* **59,** 161—164.

BOGNÁR, R., MAKLEIT, S. and MILE, T. (1969b): Conversions of tosyl and mesyl derivatives of the morphine group. Preparation of "azido- and aminomorphides". *Acta chim. Acad. Sci. hung.* **59,** 379—385.

BUCKETT, W. R. (1964): A new test for morphine-like physical dependence (addiction liability) in rats. *Psychopharmacologia* **6,** 410—416.

ETTLES, M. and LISTER, R. E. 1963. cit. by Buckett (1964): The assessment of withdrawal symptom in narcotic dependent rats. *Communication to the British Pharmacological Society.* Dublin 1963.

FÜRST, S. and KNOLL, J. (1968): Újabb adatok a morfintolerancia kérdéséhez (Recent data to the question of morphine tolerance). *Herba Hung.* **7,** 53.

FÜRST, S. and KNOLL, J. (1970): Homopyrimidazols and tolerance to narcotic analgetics. In: *7th Congress of the Collegium Internationale Neuropsychopharmacologicum.* Abstracts, Prague, p. 145.

FÜRST, S. and KNOLL, J. (1971): A new approach to dependence and tolerance. Pharmacology of azidomorphine derivatives. *Acta physiol. Acad. Sci. hung.* (In press).

FÜRST, S., SZENTMIKLÓSI, P., KELEMEN, K. and KNOLL, J. (1969): A detailed analysis of the analgetic action of MZ-108, a new homopyrimidazol derivative. In: *5th Hungarian Conference for Therapy and Pharmacological Research.* Budapest. Abstracts, p. 83.

FÜRST, S., MÉSZÁROS, Z. and KNOLL, J. (1970): Pharmacology of MZ-144, new homopyrimidazol derivative. *Acta physiol. Acad. Sci. hung.* **37,** 189.

FÜRST, S., KELEMEN, K. and KNOLL, J. (1971): Comparative pharmacology of azidomorphine derivatives. *Acta physiol. Acad. Sci. hung.* (In press.)

GRABER, H. and VARGA, E.: The effect of MZ-144 (Probon®) on the respiratory acidosis of aged patients. *Clin. Pharmacol. Ther.* (In press.)

GRABER, H., SZENTMIKLÓSI, P. and KREPUSKA, J.: Clinical evaluation of the analgetic action of Probon®. *Clin. Pharmacol. Ther.* (In press.)

KELEMEN, K. (1968): Új szempontok az analgetikus morfin antagonisták farmakológiájában (Recent aspects in the pharmacology of analgetic morphine antagonists). *Orvostudomány* **19,** 369—374.

KNOLL, J. (1969): Homopyrimidazols, a new group of analgesics. In: *5th Hungarian Conference for Therapy and Pharmacological Research.* Budapest, Abstracts. 1968.

KNOLL, J., MÉSZÁROS, Z. and FÜRST, S. (1969): Homopyrimidazols, a new group of analgesics, with unique spectrum of activity. In: *4th International Congress of Pharmacology*, Basel, Abstracts, p. 455.

KNOLL, J., FÜRST, S. and MÉSZÁROS, Z. (1971a): The pharmacology of 1,6-dimethyl-3-carbetoxy-4-oxo-6,7,8,9-tetrahydrohomopyrimidazol-methylsulphate (MZ-144), a new potent, non-narcotic analgesic. Toxicity and analgesic effect of MZ-144 compared to narcotic and non-narcotic analgesics. *Arzneimittel Forsch.* **21,** 719—727.

KNOLL, J., FÜRST, S. and MÉSZÁROS, Z. (1971b): The pharmacology of 1,6-dimethyl-3-carbetoxy-4-oxo-6,7,8,9-tetrahydrohomopyrimidazol-methylsulphate (MZ-144), a new potent, non-narcotic analgesic. Analysis of the central and peripheric effects. *Arzneimittel Forsch.* **29,** 727—733.

KNOLL, J., MAGYAR, K. and BÁNFI, D. (1971c): The pharmacology of 1,6-dimethyl-3-carbetoxy-4-oxo-6,7,8,9-tetrahydrohomopyrimidazol-methylsulphate (MZ-144), a new potent, non-narcotic analgesic. The fate of MZ-144 within the organism. *Arzneimittel Forsch.* **21,** 733—738.

KNOLL, J., MÉSZÁROS, Z., SZENTMIKLÓSI, P. and FÜRST, S. (1971d): The pharmacology of 1,6-dimethyl-3-carbetoxy-4-oxo-6,7,8,9-tetrahydrohomopyrimidazol-methylsulphate (MZ-144), a new potent, non-narcotic analgesic. Some basic correlations between the chemical structure and activity of homopyrimidazol analgesics. Selection of MZ-144. *Arzneimittel Forsch.* **21,** 717—719.

LEWIS, J. W., BENTLEY, K. W. and COWAN, A. (1971): Narcotic analgesics and antagonists. *Ann. Rev. Pharmacol.* **11,** 241—270.

MAKLEIT, S. and BOGNÁR, R. (1968): Amino-morfidok és amino-kodidok előállításának és térkémiájának vizsgálatáról (Study of the production and stereochemistry of amine morphides and amine codides). *Kémiai Közl.* **30,** 289—295.

MAKLEIT, S. and BOGNÁR, R. (1969): Conversions of tosyl and mesyl derivatives of the morphine group. A new method for the preparation of isocodeine and dihydroisocodeine. *Acta chim. Acad. Sci. hung.* **59,** 387—388.

Report of WHO Scientific Group (1964): *Wld Hlth Org. techn. Rep. Ser.* 273.

SCHAUMANN, O. (1956): Some new aspects of the action of morphine-like analgesics. *Brit. med. J.* **2,** 1091—1093.

SEEVERS, M. H. and DENEAU, G. A. (1963): Physiological aspects of tolerance and physical dependence. In: *Physiological Pharmacology*. Vol. 1. Ed. by W. S. Root and H. Hofmann. Academic Press, New York. pp. 565—640.

SELLEY, C. and ECKHARDT, S.: Clinical study of the morphine-potentiating effect of MZ-144 in oncologic patients. (In press.)

DESTEVENS, G. (Ed.) (1965): *Analgetics.* Academic Press, New York. pp. 475.

UNGAR, G. and COHEN, M. (1966): Induction of morphine tolerance by material extracted from brain of tolerant animals. *Int. J. Neuropharmacol.* **5,** 183—192.

BRAIN MONOAMINERGIC MECHANISMS AND HYPOTHALAMIC–PITUITARY–ADRENAL ACTIVITY

V. E. RYZHENKOV

Department of Pharmacology
Institute of Experimental Medicine
U.S.S.R. Academy of Medical Sciences
Leningrad, U.S.S.R.

The interest in brain monoaminergic mechanisms in the control of anterior pituitary functions has considerably increased. The present paper discusses the results of investigation of the activity of hypothalamic–pituitary–adrenal system after pharmacologically induced changes in brain monoaminergic mechanisms. For this purpose, drugs blocking central m- and n-cholinoreceptors and agents changing the catecholamine synthesis and their storage in tissues were used.

In our chronic experiments on dogs the blockade of central m-cholinoreceptors produced by methyl-benactisine (metamizyl) decreased ACTH secretion caused by the stimulation of the premamillary area of the hypothalamus, frontal cortex or by the injection of acetylcholine into the carotid arteries. The blockade of central n-cholinoreceptors was not effective. Central cholinolytics as well as chlorpromazine did not alter ACTH secretion in dogs caused by pain stimuli; but these substances strongly inhibited ACTH secretion caused by conditioned reflectory activation.

Our experiments on rats have shown that the blockade of noradrenaline synthesis by α-methyl-parathyrosine and inhibition of serotonin synthesis by means of parachlorophenylalanine do not change significantly ACTH secretion after immobilization and pain stimulation. However, by the blockade of noradrenaline synthesis ACTH secretion becomes inhibited in response to a weak stimulus (rats placed in water for 30 sec). After depletion of catecholamines and serotonin by means of reserpine, the pituitary–adrenal system is markedly activated in response to the stimuli applied.

The precursor of catecholamine synthesis, L-dopa, increases the degree of ACTH secretion when rats are immobilized and at the same time it prevents the reduction of noradrenaline content in brain which is usually observed after immobilization.

The data here presented show that in spite of the considerable change in brain monoaminergic mechanisms, activity of the hypothalamic–pituitary–adrenal system may be strongly pronounced. This is confirmed by our experiments concerning determination of noradrenaline and serotonin content in brain of rats under the influence of various stimuli. It was noted that 30 min after the immobilization of rats or after injections of the neurotropic drug aethymizol [(bis-methylamid)1-ethyl-imidazol-4,5-bicarbonic acid] and/or formalin, an approximately similar increase in 11-OHCS content in blood plasma was observed. However, a marked decrease in noradrenaline content in brain may be observed only after immobilization, while the serotonin content is not changed. Immobilization of rats after dexamethasone blockade did not cause a decrease in noradrenaline content of the brain. But in this instance there was an incomplete blockade of 11-OHCS secretion.

In conclusion, it must be noted that the activation of hypothalamic–pituitary–adrenal system is not limited strictly by any brain monoaminergic mechanism.

Hormones and Brain Function, Budapest 1971, pp. 287–292 (1973)

INFLUENCE OF SOME NEUROTROPIC DRUGS ON THE HYPOTHALAMO-PITUITARY-ADRENAL SYSTEM AFTER DEXAMETHASONE BLOCKADE

N. S. SAPRONOV

Department of Pharmacology
Institute of Experimental Medicine
U.S.S.R. Academy of Medical Sciences
Leningrad, U.S.S.R.

Interest in the mechanisms of neural control of the hypothalamo–pituitary–adrenal system has not declined. The virtual absence of nervous connections between the hypothalamus and the anterior pituitary prompted the assumption that humoral mechanism would be responsible for the increased ACTH secretion observed after stress. A transmitter substance originating in the hypothalamus and released into the portal vessels of the pituitary (Harris 1955) could act directly and in a relatively high concentration on the anterior pituitary cells.

In the last years rather convincing evidence as to the existence of such a corticotrophin-releasing factor (CRF) has been collected (Guillemin and Schally 1961, Porter 1969, Sayers et al. 1958). Some authors connect the release of CRF with a change in the brain 5-OH-tryptamine level (Naumenko 1968, Rosecrans 1970, Schreiberg and Dunaeva 1970), others explain the activation of the hypothalamo–pituitary–adrenal system by the participation of central adrenergic structures (Fuxe 1964, Schalyapina and Rakitskaya 1971, Schedrina 1971).

The present work is only a part of the research carried out at the Department of Pharmacology of the Institute for Experimental Medicine of the Academy of Sciences and is devoted to the analysis of the properties and the mechanism of action of central neurotropic drugs on the endocrine functions. In different series of experiments the influence of drugs affecting the central transmitter mechanisms on the hypothalamo–pituitary–adrenal system has been studied.

METHODS

For the experiments male albino rats, weighing between 180 and 200 g, were used. The animals were kept under the same conditions and were fed a standard diet. Each experimental group consisted of 10 to 15 rats. The investigations were performed on intact animals and the hypothalamo–pituitary–adrenal system was inhibited by dexamethasone pretreatment (300 μg/kg 2 hours before drug injection).

It is known that dexamethasone has a more potent depressive action on the central control of ACTH secretion than other corticosteroids. Data of some authors show that dexamethasone in appropriate doses can block the response of the pituitary–adrenal–cortical system to a number of stimuli (Mangilli et al. 1964, Martini et al. 1966, Ryzhenkov 1970, Yates 1967).

In certain experiments dexamethasone was administered twice: first, 1 day prior to drug injection in a dose of 600 µg/kg and second, 2 hours before it in a dose of 300 µg/kg.

The drugs investigated were injected intraperitoneally in the following doses: norepinephrine 0.25 µg/kg, amphetamine 5 to 10 mg/kg, arecoline 10 mg/kg, physostigmine 0.3 to 2 mg/kg, 5-OH-tryptamine 5 mg/kg, 5-OH-tryptophane 250 mg/kg, histamine 10 mg/kg, histidine 300 mg/kg. The substances were injected into the third ventricle or into the anterior pituitary in doses 10 to 30 times less than used in case of intraperitoneal administration and in 0.005—0.010 ml volume of physiological saline solution. The control animals were injected with the equal volume of 0.9 per cent NaCl intraperitoneally or bidistilled water intraventricularly.

Injections into the brain ventricle were made through steel canules (425 µ) inserted previously by the stereotaxic method according to the coordinates described by Szentágothai and co-workers. Into the pituitary the drugs were injected by means of the special apparatus designed for transauricular hypophysectomy (Fedotov and Bagramyan 1968).

Thirty and 90 minutes after the injection of the drugs studied, the rats were decapitated and the blood was collected. The level of 11-hydroxycorticosteroids (11-OHCS) in the blood plasma was determined by the fluorometric method of de Moor et al. (1960). The concentration of corticosteroids reflected the state of the hypothalamo–pituitary–adrenal system. Because of the diurnal variations in the plasma steroid levels all experiments were performed between 9 a.m. and 1 p.m.

RESULTS AND DISCUSSION

Behavioural responses to injections of substances investigated were as follows: in animals arecoline caused tremor and salivation for 5 to 6 minutes; after the injection of amphetamine some excitation and stereotypical movements were noticed. These responses increased when the dose was elevated. The injections of 5-OH-tryptamine led to stupor and impulsive breathing. After histamine injection the rats became restless with irregular breathing. The same responses were observed following the injection of these drugs into the brain ventricle. Less pronounced behavioural responses were observed in the animals after treatment with the precursors of transmitters. These facts indicate that, judged by the behavioural responses, the substances studied were used in effective doses.

As Figs 1 and 2 indicate all drugs investigated possess an obvious stimulating action on the hypothalamo–pituitary–adrenal system. The effect is observed both in case of intraperitoneal and intravenous drug injections. In evaluating these results it should be considered that, on the basis of the data obtained under our conditions, it is possible to assume that the activation of the hypothalamo–pituitary–adrenal system by these substances is mediated through the hypothalamo–pituitary connections. This assumption is confirmed particularly by the experiments when the drugs were administered directly into the pituitary. The results of these experiments shown in Fig. 3 indicate that there is no substantial difference in blood plasma corticosteroid level between the control and experimental animals. In this respect the data obtained are in agreement with those of Krieger and Krieger (1970a, b). These investigators have shown that injections of norepinephrine, Carbachol or serotonin into the pituitary of a cat were not accompanied by the response of the activation of the adrenal cortex.

In our further experiments rats were treated with dexamethasone (300 μg/kg intraperitoneally). Two to 3 hours after dexamethasone injection the blood plasma concentration of corticosteroids decreased about twofold as compared to the intact animals (Figs 1 and 2). This fact points to the inhibition of the hypothalamo–pituitary–adrenal system by dexamethasone. It should be noted that dexa-

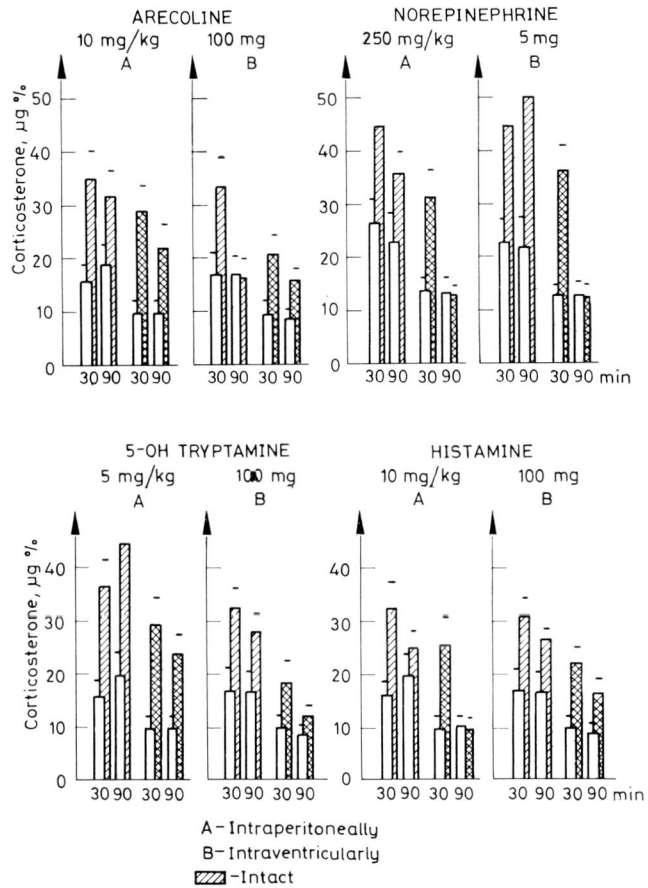

Fig. 1. Plasma 11-OHCS levels in rats after the injections of monoamines. Light columns are controls, shaded and dark columns are animals after the injection of drugs. Numbers at the bottom of columns indicate the time after administration of the substances studied

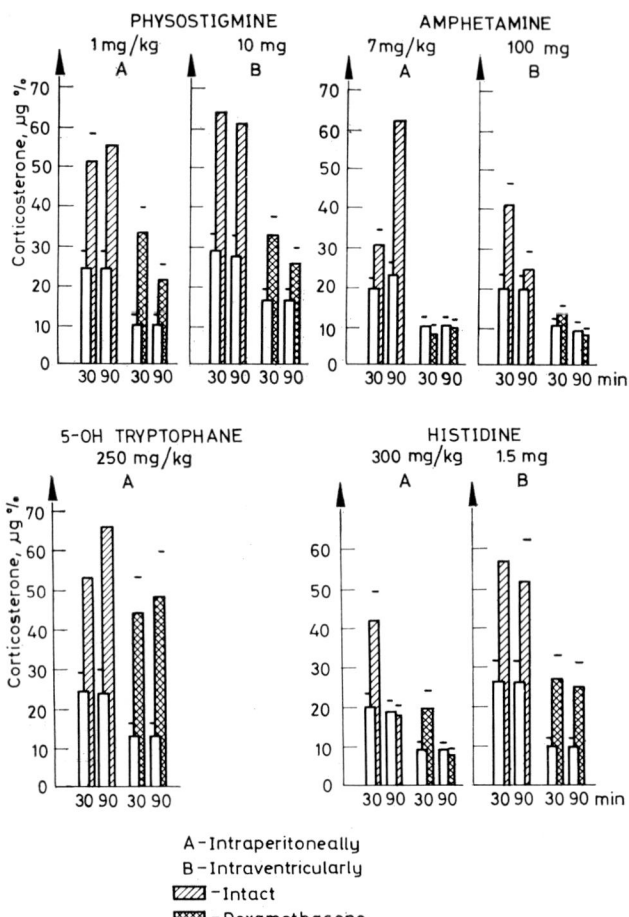

Fig. 2. Plasma 11-OHCS levels in rats after injections of precursors. Legend same as in Fig. 1

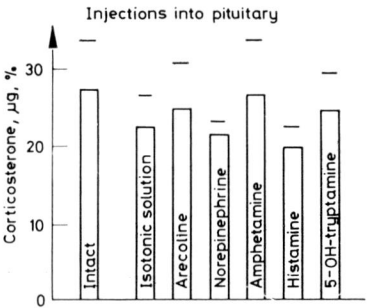

Fig. 3. Plasma 11-OHCS levels in rats after the injections of some neurotropic drugs directly into the pituitary

methasone in appropriate doses blocks the response of the adrenal cortex to a painful stimulus (10 per cent formaline solution, 0.15 ml subcutaneously).

These experiments have shown that dexamethasone in the dose applied diminished the stimulating action of the drugs studied. The results demonstrate that dexamethasone decreases the stimulating effect of precursors to a much greater extent as compared to the transmitters and the action of amphetamine is blocked completely. The last finding is in agreement with the data of some investigators who had shown that the stimulating effect of amphetamine on the above-mentioned system was not observed in animals treated with prednisolone (Ohler and Sevy 1956, Smelik and de Wied 1958).

When increasing the dose of dexamethasone up to 1 mg/kg, the response of the adrenal cortex to arecoline, norepinephrine, 5-OH-tryptamine or histamine was not observed (Fig. 4).

Our experiments show that activation of the hypothalamo–pituitary–adrenal system may be caused by the excitation of central adrenergic, cholinergic, serotoninergic, or histaminergic receptors. One can believe that the responses of the above system are not strictly determined by any of the brain monoaminergic mechanisms. The response of the hypothalamo–pituitary–adrenal system to the drugs studied does not appear after an appropriate dexamethasone blockade.

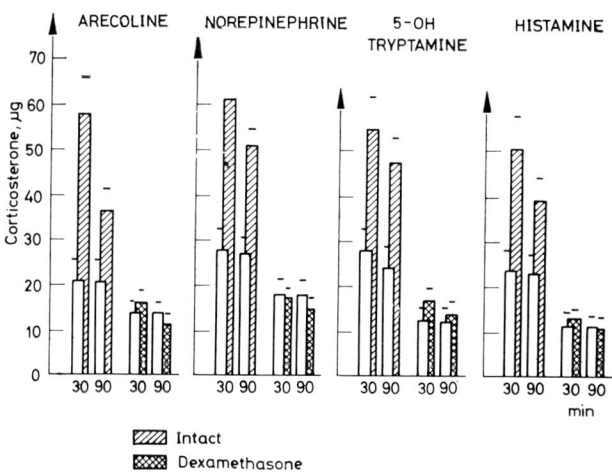

Fig. 4. Influence of dexamethasone (increasing up to 1 mg/kg) on the stimulating effect of some transmitters. Legend same as in Figs 1 and 2

REFERENCES

Fedotov, V. P. and Bagramyan, E. R. (1968): *Probl. Endokr. Gormonoter.* **4,** 114.
Fuxe, K. (1964): *Z. Zellforsch.* **61,** 710.
Guillemin, R. and Schally, A. V. (1961): *Acta neuroveg. (Wien)* **23,** 58.
Harris, G. W. (1955): *Neural Control of the Pituitary Gland.* Arnold, London.
Krieger, D. T. and Krieger, H. P. (1970a): *Endocrinology* **87,** 179.
Krieger, H. P. and Krieger, D. T. (1970b): *Amer. J. Physiol.* **218,** 1632.

Mangilli, G., Martini, L., Motta, M., Müller, E. and Pecile, A. (1964): *Progress in Biocybernetics* **1**, 36.
Martini, L., Guiliani, G. and Motta, M. (1966): *Acta endocr. (Kbh.)* **5**, 497.
Moor, P. de, Steeno, O., Raskin, M. and Hendricx, X. (1960): *Acta endocr. (Kbh.)* **33**, 297.
Naumenko, E. V. (1968): *Brain Res.* **11**, 1.
Ohler, E. and Sevy, R. (1956): *Endocrinology* **59**, 347.
Porter, J. C. (1969): *Endocrinology* **84**, 1398.
Rosecrans, J. A. (1970): *Arch. int. Pharmacodyn.* **187**, 349.
Ryzhenkov, V. E. (1970): Meeting of Pribalt.-Leningrad-Finland Pharmacological Societies, Tartu, p. 24.
Sayers, G., Redgate, E. S. and Royce, R. C. (1958): *Ann. Rev. Physiol.* **20**, 243.
Schalyapina, V. G. and Rakitskaya, V. V. (1971): *Problemy endocrinol.* **2**, 107.
Schedrina, R. N. (1971): *Problemy endocrinol.* **1**, 58.
Schreiberg, G. L. and Dunaeva, L. P. (1970): *Rep. Acad. Sci. U.S.S.R.* **194**, 1237.
Smelik, P. and Wied, D. de (1958): *Experientia (Basel)* **14**, 17.
Szentágothai, J., Flerkó, B., Mess, B. and Halász, B. (1965): *Hypothalamic Control of the Anterior Pituitary. An Experimental-Morphological Study.* Akadémiai Kiadó, Budapest.
Yates, F. E. (1967): In: *The Adrenal Cortex.* Ed. by A. Eisenstein. Little, Brown and Co., Boston. p. 33.

EFFECT OF CHRONIC ETHANOL ADMINISTRATION ON ADENYL CYCLASE AND CYCLIC 3',5'-NUCLEOTIDE PHOSPHODIESTERASE ACTIVITIES OF MOUSE BRAIN*

K. KURIYAMA and M. A. ISRAEL

Division of Neuropharmacology and Neurochemistry
Department of Psychiatry
State University of New York
Downstate Medical Center
Brooklyn, N.Y., U.S.A.

Adenosine 3',5'-monophosphate (cyclic AMP) has been implicated as an intracellular mediator of the action of a large number of amine and polypeptide hormones (Robison et al. 1968).

Previous studies in this laboratory and by other investigators indicated that biochemical changes observed in brain following chronic ethanol administration may involve an alteration of the endocrine system (Ellis 1966, Kuriyama et al. 1971a, b). Of particular interest is the possibility that although the steady-state level of biogenic amines in brain is not altered by ethanol administration (Häggendal and Lindqvist 1961, Kuriyama et al. 1971 b), the sensitivity of the cyclic AMP system to various neurohormones may be affected.

In this study, we have examined in chronically ethanol-treated mice both the levels of adenyl cyclase and cyclic 3',5'-nucleotide phosphodiesterase (phosphodiesterase) activity and the sensitivity of adenyl cyclase to the in vitro addition of norepinephrine and histamine.

METHODS

Female Swiss albino mice weighing 25–28 g were chronically administered ethanol as previously described (Freund 1969). The liquid diet consisted of 61% commercial Metrecal, 6% (w/v) ethanol or isocaloric sucrose, and distilled water. Daily intake of the liquid diet in ethanol-treated mice was measured and exactly the same amount of liquid diet containing sucrose isocaloric to the ethanol intake in experimental mice was given to the control mice. The daily dose of ethanol was 26–33 mg/g body weight. The average blood ethanol level in treated mice was 2.9–3.1 mg/ml at the time of sacrifice.

Adenyl cyclase activity in a homogenate of cerebral cortex prepared in 0.32 M sucrose was measured by the separation of cyclic ^{3}H–AMP formed from ^{3}H–ATP as described by Krishna et al. (1968). The recovery of a known amount of cyclic ^{3}H–AMP was used to correct all experimental results. The basic reaction mixture

---

* Supported in part by grants MH 18663 and MH-16477 from the National Institute of Mental Health.

contained Tris-HCl (pH 7.3): 40 mM, $MgSO_4$: 3.3 mM, theophylline: 10 mM, tris ATP: 2 mM (including 0.125 mM of ^{3}H-ATP (S. A. 7.93 C/mM)) and 1–2 mg protein of enzyme preparation.

The formation of cyclic AMP in slices of cerebral cortex was measured by a modification of the method of Shimizu et al. (1969). Following the pulse-labelling of adenosine-5'-triphosphate in slices of brain with (8-^{14}C) adenine, the slices from both ethanol-treated and control animals were incubated in a media containing a neurohormone. Following 4 minutes incubation the reaction was stopped by the addition of 10 μM cyclic AMP followed immediately by boiling for 3 minutes and homogenization. This homogenate was brought to near dryness by a cool air blower and the residue was suspended and centrifuged. Total radioactivity was determined by a liquid scintillation procedure and cyclic ^{14}C-AMP was isolated from other labelled nucleotides in an aliquot of the supernatant as described by Krishna et al. (1968). The results of these experiments are expressed as the percentage of cyclic ^{14}C-AMP converted from the total ^{14}C-adenine present in the tissue following pulse labelling and as $\mu\mu$M cyclic AMP formed per g wet weight per minute.

Cyclic nucleotide phosphodiesterase activity was determined by the method of Butcher and Sutherland (1962) as modified by Weiss (1971). Inorganic phosphate liberated was assayed by the method of Martin and Doty (1949) as modified by Swanson et al. (1964).

Protein content was determined by the method of Lowry et al. (1951) and ethanol levels in blood serum were measured by an enzymatic procedure (Bonnischen 1963) after deproteinizing with perchloric acid.

RESULTS AND CONCLUSION

Continuous oral ethanol administration for 2 weeks induced a significant increase of adenyl cyclase activity in cerebral cortex (Table 1). In addition, cyclic ^{14}C–AMP formation in slices pulse labelled with ^{14}C-adenine showed a significant

TABLE 1

Effect of chronic ethanol administration on cyclic AMP formation in mouse cerebral cortex

	Slice		Homogenate
	% Conversion	Cyclic ^{14}C-AMP formed ($\mu\mu$M/g w.w./min)	Adenyl cyclase activity ($\mu\mu$M/mg protein/min)
Control	0.35 ± 0.08	412 ± 13	176 ± 20
Ethanol-treated	0.60 ± 0.02 (+71)*	835 ± 124 (+102)*	253 ± 22 (+44)*

* $P < 0.01$

Both control and ethanol-treated animals were fed by liquid diets for 2 weeks. Incubation, homogenate 30°C; 7 min; Slice 37°C, 4 min.

Results in this Table indicate mean ± S.D. obtained from 4 separate experiments and numbers in parentheses indicate percent changes compared with respective controls.

increase in ethanol-treated mice. Similar increases were found 1 and 3 weeks after continuous administration of ethanol. In contrast, phosphodiesterase activity in cerebral cortex was not changed by chronic ethanol administration (Table 2).

It has been reported that cyclic AMP formation measured in homogenate and slice preparations of brain is stimulated by the in vitro addition of various amines (Robison et al. 1968, Shimizu et al. 1969). In this study the addition of norepinephrine (0.1 mM) and histamine (0.1 mM) to slices and homogenate of mouse cerebral cortex also significantly increased the formation of cyclic AMP (Table 3). However, in homogenates of cerebral cortex from ethanol-treated mice, adenyl cyclase activity was not stimulated by the addition of either amine although the stimulation by fluoride remained. Decreased sensitivity of cyclic AMP formation to the stimulation by norepinephrine and histamine in ethanol-treated animals was also observed in preparations of brain slice (Table 3).

TABLE 2

Effect of chronic ethanol administration on cyclic nucleotide phosphodiesterase activity of mouse brain

Duration of feeding	Phosphodiesterase activity* (μM/mg protein/min)	
	Control	Ethanol-treated
1 Week	57.6 ± 2.9	59.2 ± 4.0 (+2.8)
2 Weeks	59.7 ± 10.7	56.6 ± 6.5 (−5.2)

Incubation; 37° C, 6 min.
* Mean ±S.D. obtained from 5 separate experiments. Numbers in parentheses indicate percent changes compared with respective controls.

TABLE 3

Effect of various drugs on cyclic AMP formation in cerebral cortex from control and ethanol-treated mice

Drug	Slice (% conversion)		Homogenate ($\mu\mu$M/mg protein/min)	
	Control	Ethanol-treated	Control	Ethanol-treated
None	0.35 ± 0.08	0.60 ± 0.02	176 ± 20	253 ± 22
dl-norepinephrine: 0.1 mM	0.68 ± 0.04* (+94)	0.77 ± 0.23 (+28)	280 ± 24* (+64)	260 ± 42 (+3)
Histamine: 0.1 mM	0.56 ± 0.05* (+60)	0.78 ± 0.07* (+30)	130 ± 36** (+31)	242 ± 40 (−5)
Fluoride: 10 mM	—	—	387 ± 68* (+120)	405 ± 59* (+60)

* $P < 0.01$, ** $P < 0.05$ compared with value for same preparation without drug addition.
For experimental conditions see Table 1.
Mean ± S.D. obtained from 4 separate experiments.

These results suggest that alterations in cyclic AMP metabolism and its responsiveness to neurohormones may mediate the effects of chronic ethanol administration on the central nervous system.

REFERENCES

Bonnischen, R. (1963): In: *Method of Enzymatic Analysis*. Ed. by H. U. Bergmeyer. Academic Press, New York. p. 285.
Butcher, R. W. and Sutherland, E. W. (1962): *J. biol. Chem.* **237**, 1244.
Ellis, F. W. (1966): *J. Pharmacol. exp. Ther.* **153**, 121.
Freund, G. (1969): *Arch. Neurol. (Chic.)* **21**, 315.
Häggendal, J. and Lindqvist, M. (1961): *Acta pharmacol. (Kbh.)* **18**, 278.
Krishna, G., Weiss, B. and Brodie, B. B. (1968): *J. Pharmacol. exp. Ther.* **163**, 379.
Kuriyama, K., Sze, P. Y. and Rauscher, G. E. (1971a): *Life Sci.* **10**, 181.
Kuriyama, K., Rauscher, G. E. and Sze, P. Y. (1971b): *Brain Res.* **26**, 450.
Lowry, O. H., Rosebrough, N. J., Farr, A. L. and Randall, R. J. (1951): *J. biol. Chem.* **193**, 265.
Martin, J. B. and Doty, D. M. (1949): *Analyt. Chem.* **21**, 965.
Robison, G., Butcher, R. W. and Sutherland, E. W. (1968): *Ann. Rev. Biochem.* **37**, 149.
Shimizu, H., Daly, J. W. and Creveling, C. R. (1969): *J. Neurochem.* **16**, 1609.
Swanson, P. D., Bradford, H. F. and McIlwain, H. (1964): *Biochem. J.* **92**, 235.
Weiss, B. (1971): *J. Neurochem.* **18**, 469.

L-DOPA: ITS ACTION ON SEXUAL BEHAVIOUR AND BRAIN MONOAMINES OF THE RAT*

M. HYYPPÄ, P. LEHTINEN and U. K. RINNE

Department of Anatomy
Department of Psychology
Department of Neurology
University of Turku
Turku, Finland

Among many side-effects following (L-3,4-dihydroxyphenylalanine) treatment short-lasting aphrodisiac action has in some cases been found in male and female parkinsonian patients (Hyyppä et al. 1970, Calne and Sandler 1970, Jenkins and Groh 1970). Whether this phenomenon is directly due to the action of L-dopa treatment has not been confirmed exactly. However, plenty of neuroendocrinologic data about the role of dopamine (DA), as well as of other monoamines in the hypothalamic regulatory function of gonadotrophic hormones (Fuxe and Hökfelt 1969, McCann 1970) make possible to understand the action of L-dopa on the sexual functions. Firstly, L-dopa might increase the content of DA in the regions which are important in mediating sexual behaviour and/or gonadotrophin secretion. Secondly, L-dopa treatment might act through the metabolism of other monoamines in those brain regions.

It has been shown that serotonin (5-HT), in particular, affects gonadotrophin secretion (O'Steen 1965, Kordon 1969, Brown 1971) and sexual behaviour (Meyerson 1964). On the other hand, pineal indole amines may modify gonadotrophin secretion (Fraschini et al. 1971). Recent findings (Tagliamonte et al. 1969, Ahlenius et al. 1971) suggest that indole amines may decrease and primary catecholamines increase sexual activity in rats. Bearing this in mind, it is of interest to note that L-dopa can lower 5-HT content in the whole brain of the rat when given with an aromatic amino acid decarboxylase inhibitor (Ro 4–4602) which cannot penetrate through the blood brain barrier (Bartholini et al. 1968, Butcher and Engel 1969).

In the present paper we have first studied the incorporation of radioactive L-dopa in order to get information about its localization in the central nervous system. Then we analysed the hypothalamic, striatal and pineal contents of DA, noradrenaline (NA), 5-HT, and the degradation compound of 5-HT, 5-hydroxy indole acetic acid (5-HIAA) as well as the sexual behaviour of male rats after treatment with L-dopa, with or without Ro 4–4602. In these experiments we tried to get further information about the metabolism and possible aphrodisiac action of L-dopa.

* Supported by grants from the Sigrid Juselius Foundation and the National Research Council for Medical Sciences, Finland.

METHODS

The test animals used in this study were male and female albino mice and rats which were fed a basic standard pellet diet of constant composition. Food and tap water were available ad libitum. Rats were kept in a room where humidity, light–dark cycles and temperature were controlled.

RADIOAUTOGRAPHY

Peripheral decarboxylase inhibitor (Ro 4–4602, F. Hoffmann-La Roche & Co· Ltd., Switzerland) 50 mg/kg i.p. and 25 minutes later, DL–3 (3,4-dihydroxyphenylalanine-2-^{14}C; 52 mCi/mM, The Radiochemical Centre, Amersham, Bucks., England) (5 μCi) in 40 mg/kg of cold L-dopa (Ro 5–4759/B–4, F. Hoffmann-La Roche & Co. Ltd., Switzerland) i.v. were injected in volumes of 0.2 ml into five adult mice and into four 4-day-old rats. The animals were killed at intervals of 10, 30, 60 and 240 minutes after the last injection. Whole body radioautograms were made according to Ullberg's method as modified by Rajaniemi and Niemi (1971).

CHEMICAL ASSAYS

L-dopa was injected in a dose of 100 mg/kg i.p. into 12 female and 9 male adult rats. Saline in similar volume (0.2 ml) was injected into 9 female and 8 male control rats. The animals were killed after 75 minutes and the hypothalamus, striatum and pineal gland were immediately used for monoamine assays.

In another experiment, 20 female rats were given Ro 4–4602 (50 mg/kg) i.p. and 25 minutes later the treatment with L-dopa was given, as described above, to 11 of these rats. The others were kept as controls, and all the animals were killed 75 minutes after the last injection. The method of Maickel and his coworkers (1968) was used for determining NA and 5-HT. DA was analysed by a modification of Chang's method (1964). All three monoamines were measured in one sample which consisted of extracts pooled from three pieces of the above. The pineal extract used was taken from the pineal gland of 9–12 animals. In part of the experiments 5-HIAA was also determined according to Curzon and Green (1970). Results were not corrected for losses in recovery. Recoveries were 80 per cent for NA, 92 per cent for 5-HT, 97 per cent for 5-HIAA, and over 100 per cent for DA. Statistical analyses were performed by Student's t-test.

BEHAVIOURAL TEST

Thirty inexperienced male rats, 6 months old, were used in this study. They were kept as described earlier, except that the light–dark cycle was reversed. After preliminary studies the following dosage schedule and time-table for L-dopa injections were used: 10 rats were injected daily with 100 mg/kg of L-dopa and 50 mg/kg of Ro 4–4602 i.p. divided into four doses at two and a half-hour intervals. Rats were treated for three and a half days. Ten control rats were injected with the same volume (0.3 ml) of Ro 4–4602 only.

For testing the sexual behaviour a satiation test was used. Tests were performed during the dark phase of the light–dark cycle. They were started 25 minutes after the last injection. The subject was given an adaptation time of 15 minutes in the observation cage. Then a receptive female rat was placed in the cage. The test was terminated when the male had failed to mount the female within 30 minutes of the last ejaculation, or when there was an interval of 60 minutes between successive ejaculations. The parameters indicating sexual activity were chosen according to Larsson (1966) and they are seen in Table 2. Statistical analyses were performed according to the two-tailed Mann-Whitney U-test.

RESULTS

Whole body radioautography showed that the radioactivity concentrated equally in mice and newborn rats in the hypothalamus and in the striatum of brain. The pancreas and kidney were strongly labelled, as well. In 30 to 60 minutes the activity seemed to be maximal, disappearing rapidly thereafter (Fig. 1a, b).

Chemical determinations (Table 1) showed that L-dopa treatment increased the DA content of the hypothalamus and striatum threefold, and that of the pineal gland fourfold. It had no effect on the NA content nor any significant effect on the 5-HT content. No significant differences were observed between male and female animals. When animals were given Ro 4–4602 before the L-dopa injection, the DA content increased markedly, but now the 5-HT content decreased significantly in all regions. NA level remained again unaffected. The content of 5-HIAA increased somewhat (Fig. 2). The most marked changes in 5-HT concentration were found in the pineal gland.

Among the animals tested for their sexual behaviour, 9 experimental and 9 control rats ejaculated during the test period. For them the average number of ejaculations was 5 for L-dopa + Ro 4–4602 group with a range of 2–8, and 6 for the control group with a range of 1–9. These groups did not differ statistically significantly. The results obtained from the recorded parameters of sexual behaviour were calculated separately for each of the first four series of copulations, and for the combined results of the first four series (Table 2). Of these data only one, the postejaculation interval in the third series of copulations showed significant

TABLE 1

Concentration of DA, NA and 5-HT ($\mu g/g \pm$ S.D.) after L-dopa treatment

		Hypothalamus	Striatum	Pineal gland
1. DA	Control	1.42 ± 0.65 (6)	2.41 ± 2.15 (6)	9 ng/gland
	L-dopa	4.85 ± 2.42 (7)[a]	6.12 ± 3.16 (7)[b]	38 ng/gland
2. NA	Control	1.71 ± 0.36 (7)	0.63 ± 0.30 (7)	0–2 ng/gland
	L-dopa	1.37 ± 0.31 (7)	0.38 ± 0.38 (7)	3 ng/gland
3. 5-HT	Control	1.43 ± 0.24 (6)	1.30 ± 0.62 (6)	50 ng/gland
	L-dopa	1.96 ± 0.77 (7)	1.44 ± 0.43 (7)	54 ng/gland

[a] $P < 0.01$; [b] $P < 0.05$.

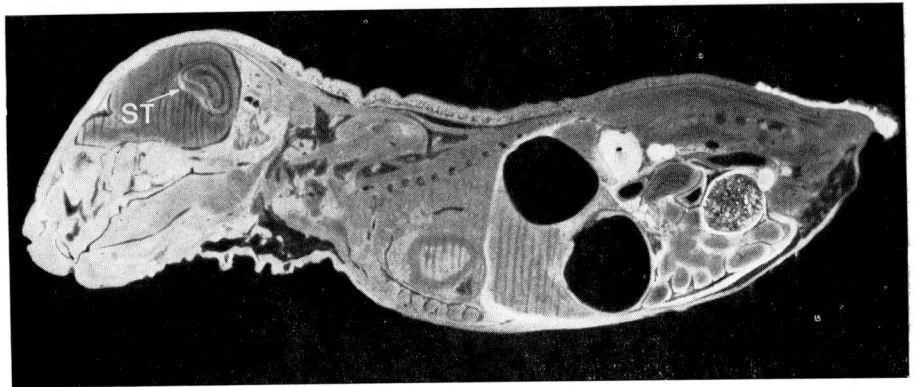

a)

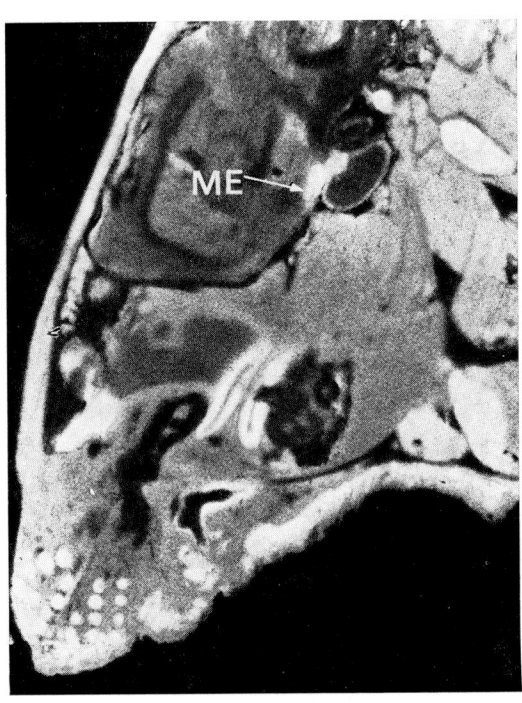

b)

Fig. 1. Whole body radioautograms. Ro 4–4602 (50 mg/kg) was given i.p. 55 minutes before killing and ^{14}C-DL-dopa (5 μCi in 40 mg/kg of cold L-dopa) was given i.v. to a 4-day-old rat (a) and adult mouse (b) 30 minutes before killing. Incorporation in the central nervous system is seen in the striatum (ST) and median eminence (ME)

difference statistically in the experimental and control groups. It was longer in the experimental group. The median of mounts together with intromissions in the whole test was 100 for the L-dopa treated animals and 144 for the controls. The difference was statistically significant at the 0.05 level. The time needed for final ejaculation before exhaustion was 85 and 116 minutes for the experimental and control groups, respectively, but the difference was not statistically significant.

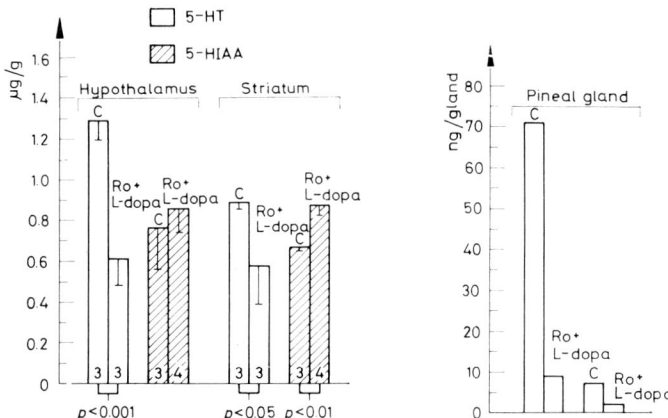

Fig. 2. Concentration of 5-HT and 5-HIAA ($\mu g/g \pm$ S.D.) after Ro 4–4602 + L-dopa treatment in the hypothalamus, striatum and pineal gland

TABLE 2

Sexual behaviour of male rats injected with L-dopa and peripheral decarboxylase inhibitor or with the inhibitor only

	L-DOPA + Ro 4-4602 (8) Mean	Ro 4-4602 (8) Mean
Number of mounts before ejaculation	5.25	5.50
Number of intromissions before ejaculation	7.00	7.25
Ejaculation latency (minutes and seconds)	5.46	8.56
Average intercopulation interval (minutes and seconds)	0.56	1.06
Post-ejaculation interval (minutes and seconds)	8.28	8.58

Scores for the tests do not include scores for the animals (2 + 2) which failed to ejaculate at least four times. Means are calculated from the average of the individual rats' performances in the first four series of copulations.

DISCUSSION

It has been shown earlier that after the injection of radioactive L-dopa, cerebral accumulation is observed mostly in the caudate nucleus and hypothalamus (Bartholini and Pletscher 1968). This observation, made by using the liquid scintillation technique, has been confirmed in the present paper by using whole body radioautography. Similar findings have been made by Van Rossum and coworkers (1969) in Mongolian gebril. This provides an opportunity to study further the possible role of L-dopa metabolism in those regions. The marked accumulation of L-dopa in striatum, found also in this study, provides the theoretical basis for the use of L-dopa in the treatment of Parkinson's disease. This has been widely discussed in literature (Hornykiewicz 1966, Calne and Sandler 1970). In the present study the clarification of the biological background for the possible aphrodisiac action of L-dopa was emphasized. Therefore, hypothalamic, as well as pineal monoamines were measured.

The hypothalamus is thought to play some role in the mediation of sexual behaviour (Dörner and Staudt 1969, Orthner 1968) and in the regulation of gonadotrophin release (Szentágothai et al. 1968). There is also evidence that the hypothalamic DA is necessary for gonadotrophin release (Kamberi et al. 1970, McCann 1970). The opposite has also been suggested, viz., that DA inhibits the release of gonadotrophins (Fuxe and Hökfelt 1969). In the present study it was found that L-dopa also increases the pineal DA level from the control. Thus, L-dopa affects at least the DA metabolism in both regions which are considered to be important for gonadotrophin secretion.

As regards NA, our results are in agreement with recent findings which show that the exogenously administered L-dopa is mainly converted to DA and its degradation compounds, only a minor proportion undergoing betahydroxylation to NA and its further metabolites (Bartholini and Pletscher 1968, Calne and Sandler 1970, Wurtman et al. 1970). Similar results have been obtained by Rinne et al. (1971) in Parkinson's disease. In the present study it was possible to see that L-dopa, when given in conjunction with the peripheral decarboxylase inhibitor, decreases the 5-HT content in the hypothalamus, pineal gland and striatum. This finding has earlier been made by others using whole brain (Bartholini et al. 1968, Butcher and Engel 1969). It is important to notice that the concentration of 5-HT has decreased in the regions which are important in the regulation of sexual functions. The reason for this decline is not clear, and it might be due to a combination of several mechanisms.

Recently it has been found that 5-HT may have an excitatory role in the control of follicle-stimulating hormone secretion (Brown 1971) and an inhibitory role in the ovulatory surge of the luteinizing hormone (O'Steen 1965). These effects may be mediated through pineal melatonin which can change the metabolism of the hypothalamic 5-HT as has been demonstrated by Wurtman and his coworkers (Antón-Tay et al. 1968). It is known that the pineal indole amines exert an inhibitory effect on the reproductive system (Wurtman et al. 1968, Fraschini et al. 1971).

Our results indicate that L-dopa after Ro 4-4602 can reduce the 5-HT content in the hypothalamus and pineal gland. Thus, it seems possible that treatment with L-dopa and Ro 4-4602 may affect gonadotrophin secretion and/or sexual behaviour. However, we do not have any direct evidence of the action of L-dopa on the gonadotrophins though we have seen some peculiar "menstrual bleedings" in postmenopausal female parkinsonian patients after L-dopa treatment (Hyyppä et al. 1970). We have measured the gonadotrophin contents after the treatment with L-dopa in parkinsonian patients and in the rat, but the results are not yet available. In any case we were able to show similar changes as in the present experiments in brain monoamines and their metabolites in autopsy material of parkinsonian patients treated with L-dopa (Rinne et al. 1971).

In order to get direct data about the action of L-dopa on sexual behaviour we tested male rats by the satiation method. The treatment, however, has no clear effect on the sexual activity of rats, in spite of some slight changes which we have thought to be unspecific. Some animal experiments using other drugs, which have previously been published, led us to expect that L-dopa would increase sexual behaviour, e.g., the results obtained by Tagliamonte and his coworkers (1969) and Ahlenius et al. (1971) with p-cholorophenylalanine together with pargyline. In our experiment L-dopa with Ro 4–4602 shift the balance between the brain monoamines in the same direction as do p-chlorophenylalanine together with pargyline. The content of DA and 5-HIAA increased, that of 5-HT decreased. Tagliamonte and his coworkers interpreted their results to show that the primary catecholamines increase and 5-HT decreases the sexual activity of male rats (Tagliamonte et al. 1969). However, with the same dosage and time schedule of injection using p-cholorophenylalanine and pargyline before satiation tests, Whalen and Luttge (1970) could not detect any effect on the heterosexual behaviour of male rats. Thus, as regards sexual behaviour, our observations support the findings of Whalen and Luttge (1970).

The variations in the contents of monoamines in the areas studied here seem to be of no direct importance to sexual behaviour. However, if we accept the theory about the role of the relative balance of brain monoamines in the mediation of sexual behaviour, it is possible that our negative finding obtained from behavioural tests is caused by a failure to set an optimal dosage and time schedule for L-dopa injections. On the other hand, if we consider the action of L-dopa on the sexual behaviour of man, it could perhaps be better understood by using psychodynamic rather than biochemical concepts.

ACKNOWLEDGEMENT

L-dopa, ^{14}C-DL-dopa and Ro 4–4602 were kindly made availabe by F. Hoffmann-La Roche and Co. Ltd., Switzerland.

REFERENCES

AHLENIUS, S., ERIKSSON, H., LARSSON, K., MODIGH, K. and SÖDERSTEN, P. (1971): *Psychopharmacologia (Berl.)* **20**, 383.
ANTÓN-TAY, F., CHOU, C., ANTON, S. and WURTMAN, R. J. (1968): *Science* **162**, 277.
BARTHOLINI, G. and PLETSCHER, A. (1968): *J. Pharmacol. exp. Ther.* **161**, 14.
BARTHOLINI, G., DAPRADA, M. and PLETSCHER, A. (1968): *J. Pharm. Pharmacol.* **20**, 228.
BROWN, P. S. (1971): *Neuroendocrinology* **7**, 183.
BUTCHER, L. L. and ENGEL, J. (1969): *Brain Res.* **15**, 233.

Calne, D. B. and Sandler, M. (1970): *Nature (Lond.)* **226**, 21.
Carlsson, A. (1964): *Acta neuroveg. (Wien)* **26**, 484.
Chang, C. C. (1964): *Int. J. Neuropharmacol.* **3**, 643.
Curzon, G. and Green, A. R. (1970): *Brit. J. Pharmacol.* **39**, 653.
Dörner, G. and Staudt, J. (1969): *Neuroendocrinology* **5**, 103.
Fraschini, F., Collu, R. and Martini, L. (1971): In: *The Pineal Gland*. Ciba Foundation Symposium. Churchill-Livingstone, London. p. 259.
Fuxe, K. and Hökfelt, T. (1969): In: *Frontiers in Neuroendocrinology*. Ed. by W. F. Ganong and L. Martini. Oxford Univ. Press, New York. p. 47.
Hornykiewicz, O. (1966): *Pharmacol. Rev.* **18**, 925.
Hyyppä, M., Rinne, U. K. and Sonninen, V. (1970): *Acta neurol. scand.* **46**, Suppl. 43, 223.
Jenkins, R. B. and Groh, R. H. (1970): *Lancet II*, 177.
Kamberi, I. A., Mical, R. S. and Porter, J. C. (1970): *Endocrinology* **87**, 1.
Kordon, C. (1969): *Neuroendocrinology* **4**, 129.
Larsson, K. (1966): *Physiol. Behav.* **1**, 255.
Maickel, R. P., Cox, R. H. Jr., Saillant, J. and Miller, F. P. (1968): *Int. J. Neuropharmacol.* **7**, 275.
McCann, S. M. (1970): *Fed. Proc.* **29**, 1888.
Meyerson, B. J. (1964): *Acta physiol. scand.* **63**, Suppl. **241**.
Orthner, H. (1968): In: *Die Sexualität des Menschen. Handbuch der medizinischen Sexualforschung*. Ed. by H. Giese. Ferdinand Enke, Stuttgart. p. 446.
O'Steen, W. K. (1965): *Endocrinology* **77**, 937.
Rajaniemi, H. and Niemi, M. (1971): (In preparation).
Rinne, U. K., Sonninen, V. and Hyyppä, M. (1971): *Life Sci.* **10**, 549.
Szentágothai, J., Flerkó, B., Mess, B. and Halász, B. (1968): *Hypothalamic Control of the Anterior Pituitary*. Akadémiai Kiadó, Budapest.
Tagliamonte, A., Tagliamonte, P., Gessa, G. L. and Brodie, B. B. (1969): *Science* **166**, 1433.
Van Rossum, J., Wijffels, C. and Rijntjes, N. (1969): *Europ. J. Pharmacol.* **7**, 337.
Whalen, R. E. and Luttge, W. G. (1970): *Science* **169**, 1000.
Wurtman, R. J., Chou, C. and Rose, C. (1970): *J. Pharmacol. exp. Ther.* **174**, 351.

SEXUAL BEHAVIOUR AFTER NEONATAL RESERPINE AND pCPA TREATMENT WITH COMMENT ABOUT HYPOTHALAMIC INDOLE AMINES IN THE RAT*

P. LEHTINEN, M. HYYPPÄ, P. LAMPINEN and U. K. RINNE

Department of Psychology
Department of Anatomy
Department of Neurology
University of Turku
Turku, Finland

When reserpine, which is a depletor of monoamines, has been given during the assumed period for the sexual differentiation of rat brain, delay of the vaginal opening and continued or prolonged dioestrous phases in the vaginal oestrous cycles of adult female rats have been reported (Carraro et al. 1965, Nagy et al. 1967, Martini et al. 1968, Hyyppä 1969). On the other hand, many workers have not found alterations in the vaginal oestrous cycles after neonatal reserpine treatment (Kikuyma 1961, Arai and Gorski 1968, Simmons and Lusk 1969, Björklund et al. 1969).

In male rats neonatally injected reserpine inhibits the development of the male pattern of gonadotrophin secretion (Kawashima 1964). It can reduce the growth rate of testes and accessory sex glands without affecting the body weight measured at 30 and 60 days of age (Hyyppä 1969).

Hypothalamic monoamine levels are reduced until puberty in neonatally reserpinized female and male rats (Hyyppä and Rinne 1971).

Sexual behaviour of neonatally reserpinized female rats has also been studied (Zucker and Feder 1966). In the present work, however, no alterations were seen either in the cyclicity of sexual behaviour or in sexual responses to oestrogen–progesterone injections after ovariectomy.

Since in our laboratory, reserpine was found to have effects on sexual functions of female rats as well as marked effects on hypothalamic monoamines, as described above (Hyyppä 1969, Hyyppä and Rinne 1971), we repeated the experiment of Zucker and Feder (1966) with some modifications. We also studied the sexual behaviour of male rats after neonatal reserpine treatment, which seemed to be of interest especially in the light of the observations made by Kawashima (1964) and in our laboratory (Hyyppä 1969).

It has been shown by Ladosky and Gaziri (1970) that the 5-HT concentration of the brain may be related to the process of sexual differentiation of the brain, since it is modified by the same procedures that induce masculinization. We set out to further clarify the significance of 5-HT concentration and, in particular, of the metabolism of 5-HT in both sexes. The role of serotonin in the development

* Supported by grants from Sigrid Juselius Foundation and the National Research Council for Medical Sciences, Finland.

of mechanisms mediating sexual behaviour was studied here by giving female and male rats neonatal injections of pCPA (p-chlorophenylalanine), which is a rather specific tryptophanhydroxylase inhibitor (Koe and Weissman 1966). In females, in addition to sexual behaviour, the times of vaginal opening and vaginal cyclicity were observed.

MATERIAL AND METHODS

Female and male albino rats of a local strain (originally Sprague–Dawley) were used in these experiments. They were maintained as described in our previous paper (Hyyppä and Rinne 1971).

BEHAVIOURAL TESTS

The reserpine treatment consisted of a single 50 μg injection of reserpine per rat on the 4th day after birth and the pCPA treatment of 20 mg/kg injections on the 2nd and 3rd and 100 mg/kg on the 5th and 6th days. All the injections were intraperitoneal. Control animals from the same litters received injections of the same volume of saline. The vaginal opening times of the pCPA treated female rats were recorded. The vaginal cycles of both the reserpinized and pCPA treated females were observed without behavioural tests.

At the beginning of the behavioural tests the animals were approximately 5 months old. For testing the spontaneous feminine sexual behaviour of the reserpine and pCPA treated females, sexual behaviour and vaginal cycles were observed for 11 consecutive days. In each test the mounts of the control vasectomized male and the lordosis response of the experimental female were recorded. The receptivity quotient, i.e. the ratio of lordosis responses to mounts multiplied by 100, was calculated, and the occurrence of ear wiggling, typical of intense oestrous behaviour, was observed. The reserpine treated animals were observed for 10 minutes each day, the pCPA treated animals were allowed 10 mounts by the male.

After ovariectomy the females were tested for hormone-induced sexual behaviour. The hormone doses for the reserpine treated females were 10 μg/kg, 100 μg/kg and 500 μg/kg of oestrogen benzoate 48 and 24 hours and 0.5 mg/animal of progesterone 6–8 hours before each weekly test. For the pCPA treated females the doses were 150 μg/kg, 50 μg/kg and 10 μg/kg of oestradiol benzoate and 0.5 mg/animal of progesterone, respectively. Thereafter the pCPA treated females were also tested for male sexual behaviour with receptive females. For this purpose they were given 1 mg of testosterone propionate daily. The tests were made on the 10th, 14th, 21st and 27th days after the beginning of the injections. The tests lasted 10 minutes. Items recorded were the mount and intromission latencies as well as the frequencies of these.

The reserpine and pCPA treated male rats were tested for spontaneous masculine sexual behaviour when approximately 7 months old. The items recorded and test procedure were the same as described earlier in this congress (Hyyppä and Rinne 1971), with the exception of testing time. In this study, the test was terminated after the first intromission after ejaculation or after 30 minutes if no ejaculation occurred. The reserpine treated rats received two, the pCPA treated animals three tests.

The pCPA treated males were also tested for feminine sexual behaviour after castration and therapy with female sex hormones. For the three tests they received 150 µg/kg of oestrogen benzoate 24 and 48 hours and 0.5 mg/animal of progesterone 6–8 hours before each weekly test.

They were allowed 5 mounts by a control male. Statistical analyses were made by the t, Mann-Whitney U and X^2 two-tailed tests.

CHEMICAL ASSAYS

Serotonin (5-HT) and 5-hydroxy indole acetic acid (5-HIAA) contents were measured in the hypothalami, pineal glands and the rest of the forebrains of newborn female and male rats according to Maickel et al. (1968) and Curzon and Green (1970). Some of these rats were treated with pargyline (75 mg/kg) 60 minutes before killing and 5-HT turnover approximations were calculated according to Neff and Tozer (1968). A group of these animals was masculinized with 11 mg of testosterone enanthate on the 2nd day of life.

RESULTS

Vaginal opening in the pCPA treated females occurred at the age of 52.7 ± 8.7 (mean $\pm$ S.D.) and that of the controls, at the age of 41.3 ± 3.1. The difference is significant at the 0.01 level according to the t test. The vaginal cycles were quite normal. The cycles of the reserpine treated females had prolonged periods of dioestrus in this series of experimental animals as in our earlier experiments (Hyyppä 1969). According to these studies vaginal opening was delayed after neonatal reserpine treatment (Hyyppä 1969).

BEHAVIOURAL TESTS

Reserpine treated females

The results regarding the spontaneous sexual behaviour of the neonatally reserpinized females are seen in Tables 1 and 2. The receptivity quotients of the reserpinized females were reduced to a statistically significant degree. When the behavioural and vaginal cycles were compared it was seen that fewer reserpinized than control animals had coincident cycles. Some of the reserpinized and none of the controls had prolonged oestrous behaviour, i.e. the lordosis response occurred on more than two consecutive days. The vaginal cycle was not prolonged accordingly. There were no statistically significant differences in the sexual behaviour after ovariectomy and replacement therapy with oestrogen and progesterone.

TABLE 1

Spontaneous oestrous behaviour during 11 consecutive daily tests in female rats injected neonatally with reserpine

	Reserpinized (26)	p	Controls (18)
Average number of days per animal when at least one lordosis response occurred	2	NS[c]	3
Mean of receptivity quotients[a]	64	< 0.05[b]	96
Tests positive for ear wiggling (%)	59	NS[c]	75

[a] Only those tests are included in which lordosis response occurred at least once.
[b] By Mann-Whitney U test.
[c] By X^2 test.

TABLE 2

Relations of behavioural and hormonal oestrous cycles during 11 consecutive daily tests in female rats injected neonatally with reserpine[a]

	Reserpinized (26)	p[b]	Controls (18)
Regular hormonal and behavioural oestrous cycle (%)	23	< 0.05	56
Prolonged hormonal dioestrus and coinciding oestrous behaviour (%)	27	NS	17
Prolonged behavioural oestrus without coinciding hormonal oestrus (%)	19	$0.05 < p < 0.10$	0
Hormonal oestrus without coinciding hormonal oestrus (%)	12	NS	17
Behavioural oestrus without coinciding hormonal oestrus (%)	19	NS	11

[a] The cycle was considered irregular whenever the smears indicated dioestrus on more than 4 following days. The vaginal and behavioural oestrous cycles were considered to coincide whenever the lordosis response occurred within a margin of one day from preoestrus, oestrus or no oestrus.
[b] By X^2 test.

pCPA treated females

For the pCPA treated females the only differences in feminine sexual behaviour, spontaneous and induced, were in the number of animals showing ear wiggling, which was reduced in the experimental animals.

In the masculine sexual behaviour of the pCPA treated females there were no statistically significant differences, although the difference between the mount latencies approached statistical significance, $0.05 < p < 0.10$. The average of the mount latencies was 0.08 for the pCPA treated and 0.12 for the controls. The medians of the frequency of mounts was 23 for the pCPA treated and 20 for the controls; and of the frequency of intromissions were 2.5 and 1.5, respectively. None of the animals showed ejaculation behaviour.

Reserpine treated males

The results for the mating tests of the males are shown in Table 3. It is seen that the number of intromissions needed to reach ejaculation was reduced in these animals.

TABLE 3

Sexual behaviour of male rats injected neonatally with reserpine
Averages above mean values of two tests[a]

	Reserpinized (8)	p^b	Controls (8)
Mount frequency	3.5	NS	3.8
Intromission frequency	8.5	< 0.05	15.0
Intromission latency (min and sec)	0.41	NS	1.08
Ejaculation latency (min and sec)	8.07	NS	11.22
Postejaculation interval (min and sec)	5.20	NS	5.01
Average intercopulation interval (min and sec)	1.00	NS	0.41

[a] Of the reserpinized rats 5 ejaculated in the first test and 7 in the second. All of the control rats ejaculated in both tests. Only tests in which ejaculation occurred are included.
[b] By Mann-Whitney U test.

pCPA treated males

All the recorded items of the masculine sexual behaviour were changed in the pCPA treated males as it is seen in Table 4. In the feminine sexual behaviour of the pCPA treated males there were no alterations. Fifty-three per cent of the experimental and 40 per cent of the control animals showed lordosis in at least one of the three tests. The average receptivity quotients were 40 and 45, respectively.

TABLE 4

Masculine sexual behaviour of male rats injected neonatally with pCPA
Medians of three tests[a]

	pCPA (15)	p^b	Controls (16)
Mount frequency	4	< 0.002	7
Intromission frequency	8	< 0.02	13.5
Intromission latency (sec)	0.10	< 0.002	0.24
Ejaculation latency (min and sec)	4.37	< 0.002	13.16
Postejaculation interval (min and sec)	4.45	< 0.002	5.54
Average intercopulation interval (min and sec)	0.26	< 0.002	1.06

The pCPA treated animals ejaculated in each of the three tests. Of the control animals 11 ejaculated in the first test, all of them ejaculated in the second test and 15 ejaculated in the third test.

[a] Only tests in which ejaculation occurred are included.
[b] By Mann-Whitney U test.

CHEMICAL ASSAYS

Results concerning the effect of early injected reserpine have been presented earlier (Hyyppä and Rinne 1971 — Fig. 1). Our whole study on hypothalamic 5-HT metabolism in newborn rats is not yet completed. According to the preliminary data, no differences between the sexes in 4- and 6-day-old rats were seen in the hypothalamic, pineal or forebrain contents of 5-HT and 5-HIAA. At the age of 20 days pargyline treatment increased the 5-HT content more in female than in male rats (Table 5). When testosterone enanthate was used as a masculinizing agent in female rats no sexual differences were seen in the hypothalamic and forebrain 5-HT metabolism at the age of 16 days (Table 6).

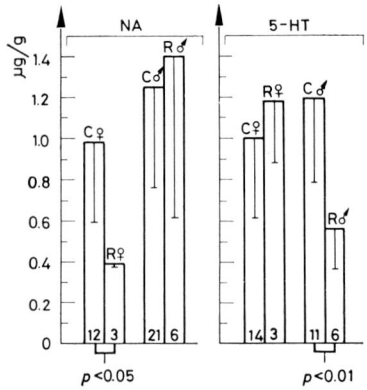

Fig. 1. Hypothalamic monoamines in 30-day-old rats after neonatal reserpinization

TABLE 5

The hypothalamic, forebrain 5-HT and 5-HIAA contents in 20-day-old rats after pargyline (75 mg/kg) treatment

		Hypothalamus	Forebrain
5-HT (μg/g)	Male	1.28 ± 0.24 (4)[a]	0.42 ± 0.09 (8)
	Female	2.00 ± 0.38 (2)	0.45 ± 0.04 (4)
5-HIAA (μg/g)	Male	0.40 ± 0.43 (4)	0.15 ± 0.02 (7)
	Female	0.36 ± 0.11 (2)	0.17 ± 0.02 (4)

Mean $\pm$ S.D.
[a] Difference between sexes: $p < 0.01$.

TABLE 6

5-HT metabolism after pargyline in the hypothalamus and forebrain of 16-day-old masculinized female and male rats

	Female		Male	
	Hypothalamus	Forebrain	Hypothalamus	Forebrain
5-HT accumulation (μg/g/1 hr)^a	0.59	0.13	0.63	0.20
k (5-HIAA decline)^b	0.66	0.77	0.87	0.62
5-HT turn-over rate (μg/g/1 hr)^c	0.57	0.32	0.63	0.25
5-HT turn-over time (hr)^d	1.5	0.9	1.5	1.0

^{a} Increase of 5-HT concentration 60 minutes after 75 mg/kg pargyline.
^{b} Decline constant calculated as the log decline of 5-HIAA after pargyline.
^{c} k × steady state level of 5-HIAA.
^{d} $\dfrac{\text{steady state level of 5-HT}}{\text{k × steady state level of 5-HIAA}}$.

DISCUSSION

BEHAVIOURAL TESTS

Reserpine treated rats

In this study we were able to repeat our earlier observations about the effect on the vaginal cycle of a single neonatal injection of reserpine, i.e. the prolongation of vaginal dioestrous phases in the cycles. The experimental animals did not, however, have prolonged vaginal dioestrus in the behavioural tests as compared to controls. This is probably due to the fact that also part of the controls had prolonged vaginal oestrus as compared with behavioural dioestrus, possibly caused by pseudopregnancy. This is a known effect after sterile mating (Adler and Zoloth 1970). Nevertheless, normal vaginal and behavioural cycles were encountered less frequently in reserpinized than in control animals. Prolonged oestrous behaviour was seen only in reserpinized females, although the difference only approached statistical significance. The reduction in the reserpinized animals of receptivity quotients in spontaneous sexual behaviour suggests a decrease in the intensity of sexual behaviour after neonatal reserpine treatment. In hormone induced sexual behaviour there were no statistically significant differences.

Altogether, our results are contrary to the observations of Zucker and Feder (1966) as regards spontaneous sexual behaviour. The reason is difficult to explain, but we want to point to some earlier studies, where, contrary to our findings, reserpine did not affect vaginal cyclicity (Kikuyma 1961, Arai and Gorski 1968, Björklund et al. 1969, Simmons and Lusk 1969).

In male rats the reduction in the number of intromissions needed to reach ejaculation is the same effect that has been found in adult male rats after reserpine treatment, but in the latter case the effect was only temporary (Soulairac and Soulairac 1961, 1962, Soulairac 1963, Dewsbury and Davis 1970, Dewsbury 1971). On the other hand, according to Bloch and Davidson (1968), a decline in intromission frequency may result from a variety of factors, including both stressful stimuli and testosterone withdrawal. Both of these interpretations may apply to our data, if we consider that the findings of Kawashima (1964) and Hyyppä (1969) reflect diminished secretion of androgens.

pCPA treated rats

The most interesting result for the action of pCPA on the females is the fact that it altered the vaginal opening time but not the vaginal cyclicity. Neither the feminine nor the masculine sexual behaviour of female rats was essentially changed afterwards.

In contrast to the females, the sexual behaviour of the males seems to be very much altered after neonatal pCPA treatment. All the alterations point to increased sexual activity (Larsson 1966) but the treatment has affected only masculine behaviour, the feminine behaviour of these rats remained unchanged.

CHEMICAL ASSAYS

We have shown earlier that a neonatal single injection of reserpine can lower some monoamine contents in the hypothalamus for the prepuberal period (Hyyppä and Rinne 1971). Among these monoamines 5-HT is thought to be related to the sexual differentiation of rat brain (Ladosky and Gaziri 1970). It has been shown that the 5-HT concentration of the brain rose more rapidly in female than in male rats on the 12th day. It was possible to prevent 5-HT levels when the females were injected with testosterone propionate on the day of birth. By comparison, males castrated at birth had brain 5-HT levels comparable to those of intact females and significantly higher than those of intact littermates (Ladosky and Gaziri 1970). Because we do not consider monoamine analyses in the whole brain sufficiently informative, we measured indole amine metabolism separately in the hypothalamus, pineal gland and forebrain of newborn rats. There were no sexual differences in the 5-HT and 5-HIAA levels in 4- and 6-day-old rats. However, when using pargyline as a monoamine oxidase inhibitor we found significantly lower hypothalamic 5-HT but not 5-HIAA concentrations in 20-day-old male than female rats. When we studied masculinized females we found quite similar hypothalamic and forebrain 5-HT concentrations and 5-HT turnover approximations in masculinized female and male rats. These observations are in agreement with the results obtained by Ladosky and Gaziri (1970).

Because our results for 5-HT metabolism in newborn rats are of preliminary nature we do not want to speculate as to the possible interaction between serotoninergic transmission systems in the separate brain regions with regard to the development of sexual behaviour. However, it seems quite possible that pCPA has its effects through these links. We hope to get evidence about this hypothesis by studying 5-HT metabolism in conjunction with behavioural tests after pCPA in newborn rats.

REFERENCES

ADLER, N. T. and ZOLOTH, S. R. (1970): *Science* **168**, 1480—1482.
ARAI, Y. and GORSKI, R. A. (1968): *Endocrinology* **82**, 1005—1009.
BJÖRKLUND, A., FALCK, B. and NOBIN, A. (1969): *Endocrinology* **85**, 788—790.
BLOCH, G. J. and DAVIDSON, J. M. (1968): *Physiol. Behav.* **3**, 461—465.
CARRARO, A., CORBIN, A., FRASCHINI, F. and MARTINI, L. (1965): *J. Endocr.* **32**, 387—393.
CURZON, G. and GREEN, A. R. (1970): *Brit. J. Pharmacol.* **39**, 653.
DEWSBURY, D. A. (1971): *Psychol. Sci.* **22**, 177—179.
DEWSBURY, D. A. and DAVIS, H. N. (1970): *Physiol. Behav.* **5**, 1331—1333.
HYYPPÄ, M. (1969): Monistepalvelu. Thesis. Turku.
HYYPPÄ, M. and RINNE, U. K. (1971): *Acta endocr. (Kbh.)* **66**, 317—324.
KAWASHIMA, S. (1964): *Annot. Zool. Jap.* **37**, 79—85.
KIKUYMA, S. (1961): *Annot. Zool. Jap.* **34**, 111—116.
KOE, B. K. and WEISSMAN, A. (1966): *J. Pharmacol. exp. Ther.* **154**, 361.
LADOSKY, W. and GAZIRI, L. C. J. (1970): *Neuroendocrinology* **6**, 168.
LARSSON, K. (1966): *Physiol. Behav.* **1**, 255.
MAICKEL, R. P., COX, R. H. JR., SAILLANT, J. and MILLER, F. P. (1968): *Int. J. Neuropharmacol.* **7**, 275.
MARTINI, L., CARRARO, A., CAVIEZEL, F. and FOCHI, M. (1968): In: *Pharmacology of Reproduction.* Ed. by E. Diczfalusy. Pergamon Press, Oxford, etc. p. 13.
NAGY, E., DONHOFFER, A. and FLERKÓ, B. (1967): Proceedings of the 3rd Meeting of the Hungarian Society of Endocrinology. Budapest.
NEFF, N. H. and TOZER, T. N. (1968): *Adv. Pharmacol.* **6A**, 97.
SIMMONS, J. E. and LUSK, M. (1969): *Acta endocr. (Kbh.)* **61**, 302—305
SOULAIRAC, M. L. (1963): *Ann. endocr. (Paris)* **24**, Suppl. **1**, 1—98.
SOULAIRAC, A. and SOULAIRAC, M. L. (1961): *C.R. Soc. Biol. (Paris)* **155**, 1010—1013.
SOULAIRAC, A. and SOULAIRAC, M. L. (1962): *Ann. endocr. (Paris)* **23**, 281—292.
ZUCKER, I. and FEDER, H. H. (1966): *J. Endocr.* **35**, 423—424.

A COMPARISON OF CHLORPROMAZINE-INDUCED EXTRAPYRAMIDAL SYNDROME IN MALE AND FEMALE RATS

J. F. MISLOW[1] and A. J. FRIEDHOFF

Department of Psychiatry and Neurology
New York University Medical Center
School of Medicine
New York, N.Y., U.S.A.

INTRODUCTION

One of the most intriguing observations on the effects of drugs used for the treatment of psychotic disorders is the relationship between the therapeutic effects of these drugs and their ability to produce parkinsonian-like extrapyramidal syndrome in man. It has been pointed out (Friedhoff 1969) that all effective antipsychotic drugs have the potential for producing a parkinsonian-like reaction in man. Effective drugs of divergent chemical structure which are used for the treatment of psychoses such as the phenothiazines, butyrophenones, and the rauwolfia alkaloids all have this potential. Within a given class, drugs which do not readily produce extrapyramidal disturbance are also ineffective antipsychotic agents. Among the phenothiazines, e.g., phenergan is one such drug with a low extrapyramidal disturbing potential. But again this compound is not an effective antipsychotic agent. Although not all patients receiving antipsychotic drugs develop clinical manifestations of Parkinsonism, it has been shown (Alpert 1967) through the use of a sensitive device for measuring resting finger tremor, that patients receiving effective doses of these drugs all have subclinical manifestations of extrapyramidal disturbance.

Of equal interest is the observation that all anti-Parkinson drugs have the potential for producing psychotic reactions. It has been reported that L-dopa, one of the newer treatments for Parkinsonism, can produce an incidence of serious psychiatric disturbance as high as 20 per cent (Duvoisin 1970). In recent years, it has been demonstrated that an important factor in the pathogenesis of Parkinsonism disorder is the alteration in the dopaminergic neural transmission in the extrapyramidal nuclei (Hornykiewicz 1966). Thus, attention has been focused on this catecholamine system, both as a mediator of extrapyramidal control and as a possible center of pathology in certain psychotic disorders.

The appearance of a parkinsonian-like disorder as a sequel of treatment with antipsychotic drugs has been discussed by a number of authors (Friedhoff and Alpert 1960, Gailitis et al. 1960, Haase 1959, Heilizer 1959, May and Voegel 1956,

---

[1] Present address: Department of Anatomy, Rutgers Medical School, New Brunswick, New Jersey, U.S.A.

Paulson 1959). While the dose of the drug, duration of treatment, manner of administration, and the sex of the patient are important factors affecting the occurrence of extrapyramidal signs (EPS), none of these factors is, in itself, decisive. The reaction is dependent on the individual, and certain patients are affected only with extreme doses (Heilizer 1960). However, Freyhan (1957, 1959) reports that female patients treated with phenothiazines develop EPS at a much higher rate than males treated with equivalent doses. This finding is in contrast to the occurrence of endogenous Parkinsonism which is usually more prevalent in males after the age of forty. Although the site of action of chlorpromazine is as yet undecided, Freyhan's finding suggests that there is an important link between the subcortical motor and the neuroendocrine systems.

In addition to the extrapyramidal effects, the phenothiazines may also produce other side effects. In humans, they have been reported to result in aberrations of mammary gland function (Rahill 1957), in alterations of the menstrual cycle (Kulcsár et al. 1957), to interfere with the *Rana pipiens* chorionic gonadotrophin pregnancy test (Brillhart 1959) and to affect endocrine regulation in other ways (CoTui et al. 1960, Fotherby et al. 1959, Gold et al. 1960, Suzuki et al. 1956).

Similarly, rats treated with chlorpromazine have shown alterations in the estrous cycle (Dasgupta and Hausler 1955, Barraclough and Sawyer 1957), in formation of pseudopregnancy (Shelesnyak 1954, Khan and Bernstorf 1964), and in milk secretion (Ben-David et al. 1965; Benson, 1960, Talwalker 1960). Khazen et al. (1968 on p. 271) suggest that the mammotropic activity only occurs with phenothiazines containing ring systems "which by their structural arrangement render them similar to the steroids", and that this similarity might explain their hypothalamotropic effect.

It has been reported that those drugs which evoke EPS in humans can also produce catalepsy, which is presumably of extrapyramidal origin, in animals including the rat (Baruk et al. 1956, Brady 1959; Essig and Carter 1957, Fink and Swinyard 1960, Irwin and Govier 1957, Taeschler and Cerletti 1959). There is a high correlation between the dose of phenothiazine necessary to produce EPS in humans and that dose which results in catalepsy in rats.

A catalepsy test has been described and modified by a number of investigators. Courvoisier et al. (1953, 1957) noted that at doses of 10–15 mg/kg, rats exhibited a full cataleptic response at six to seven hours. Their criterion for catalepsy was that of the original workers, de Jong and Baruk, with bulbocapnine; i.e., "fixity, negativism and passivity". Tedeschi et al. (1959) have modified this technique using oral administration of the drug, with the cataleptic response apparent at 10–25 mg/kg. The onset of catalepsy occurred three hours after drug administration, persisted for approximately three hours and was no longer evident seven hours after treatment. The animals were considered to be cataleptic if they remained immobile for a period of five seconds or more after their paws were placed on four #7 rubber stoppers. This phenomenon is generally associated with immobility, moldability of the extremities, absence of curiosity, widespread stance of the forelimbs and hindlimbs and apparent loss of contact with the environment, without loss of the consciousness or ataxia.

The object of the present study was to determine whether there is a difference in the incidence and character of catalepsy in phenothiazine-treated male rats as compared with female rats.

MATERIALS AND METHODS

All male and female albino rats used in these experiments were of the Wistar strain from Blue Spruce farms. The animals were caged in a thermostatically-controlled room and maintained on a standard diet of Wayne Lab Blox and water ad libitum. The phenothiazine employed in the experiment was chlorpromazine ("Thorazine", Smith, Kline and French Laboratories) in the pediatric suspension form of 10 mg/5 ml. Chlorpromazine was administered directly into the stomach of each rat by means of a #8 rubber catheter tube attached to a syringe filled with the medication. In order to determine the presence of catalepsy, each rat was removed from its cage, gentled and then placed with each paw on one of our rubber stoppers arranged in approximately 4" × 2" rectangle. Using a stop-watch, the time was determined from the moment all four paws were in position until the animal walked off the stoppers. Each animal was positioned twice and an average time, in seconds, was calculated. In a preliminary study with 5 male and 6 female rats, it was ascertained that a satisfactory dose for discriminating cataleptic responses was 20 mg/kg. It was also found that no untreated rats remained on the stoppers for more than 4 seconds. The cataleptic response, therefore, was defined as one in which a rat remained on the stoppers for more than 5 seconds.

INTACT ANIMALS

Male and female groups

Thirteen male and thirteen female rats, each approximately 160 g, were divided into two groups: Group A contained 7 animals of each sex and Group B contained 6 animals of each sex. The two different groups were treated on alternated days to test the reproducibility of the cataleptic response. As there was no statistically significant difference found between these two groups, the experimental data were combined.

First drug administration, Run I

Each animal was marked, weighed and then tested on the stoppers prior to treatment, thereby acting as its own control. Chlorpromazine was administered by the oral catheter intubation as previously described. Each animal was given a 20 mg/kg dose of the commercial 10 mg/5 cc suspension: e.g., 1 cc suspension for a 100 g rat. Three hours after treatment, each animal was timed twice with a stop-watch and the average duration on the stoppers was calculated. Subsequent hourly tests were conducted until seven hours after medication, at which time the reaction generally declined.

Second drug administration, Run II

At 160 g, the male animals were about seven weeks old and the females about nine weeks old. As sexual maturity in the male rat occurs from 50–60 days (Carworth Farms, Inc. 1961), the males were retested two weeks later for comparison with the nine-week-old females. The female rats were also retested to determine if a second drug administration altered their reaction.

In the first drug administration, one of the male animals from Group B was eliminated due to loss of medication; therefore, twelve males and thirteen females were used in Run I.

Two weeks later, in Run II, thirteen male and ten female rats received a second phenothiazine dose of 20 mg/kg. Two females from Group A and one female from Group B died during the two-week interval.

CASTRATE MALE AND OOPHORECTOMIZED FEMALE ANIMALS

Five castrate male and six oophorectomized female rats were obtained five days after surgery from Blue Spruce farms. At the time of their operations, they weighed approximately 150 g. Drug administration and test technique on these gonadectomized animals were performed exactly as for the intact animals.

Run I, the first drug dose study, was performed 9 days postoperatively and the second dose study, Run II, was carried out two weeks later on the same animals which were then 24 days postoperative.

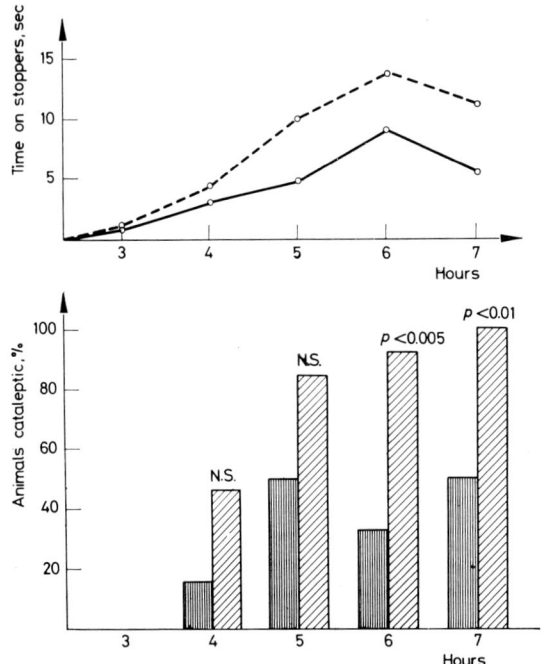

Fig. 1. Intact male rats vs intact female rats. Group comparison of the cataleptic response to the first oral administration of 20 mg/kg of chlorpromazine (Run I). Top: mean time, in sec, on the stoppers at hourly intervals after medication. Males (solid line); females (broken line). Bottom: Percent of animals having a positive cataleptic response, i.e. remain on the stoppers 5 sec or more. Males (dark bars); females (light bars)

RESULTS

INTACT ANIMALS

In Fig. 1, the results of the first drug administration are displayed. Three hours after the first medication, none of the animals were cataleptic. At four hours, two of the twelve males and six of the thirteen females gave a positive response. At five hours, the incidence was six males and eleven females; at seven hours, the cataleptic reaction had occurred in six males (50 per cent) and all of the thirteen females (100 per cent), which was the highest incidence recorded (Fig. 1). The average maximum time on the corks occurred 6.2 hours after medication for all the males and 6.07 hours for all the females. Using the non-parametric Fisher–Yates test for significant difference (Siegel 1956) the p value for difference in male and female cataleptic incidence was determined to be 0.005 at six hours and 0.01 at seven hours.

The Run II values, i.e. the same rats treated two weeks later, are presented in Fig. 2. Three hours after medication, none of the thirteen males, but one of the ten females was cataleptic. The incidence in the females increased rapidly until 5 hours, when all (100 per cent) had a positive reaction which persisted for the rest

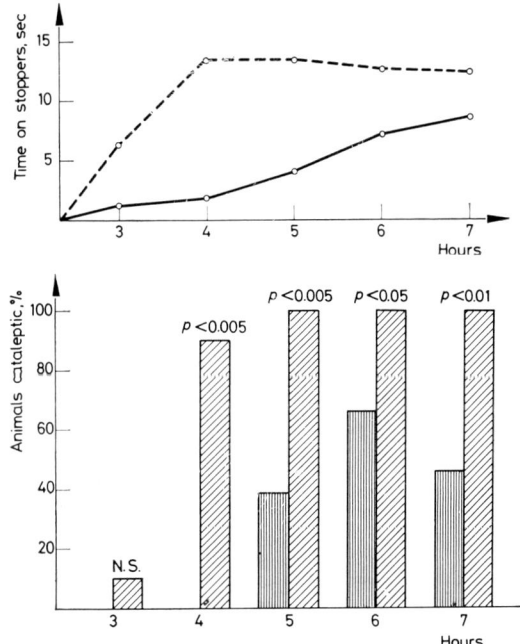

Fig. 2. Intact male rats vs intact female rats. Group comparison of the cataleptic response to the second 20 mg/kg oral dose of chlorpromazine administered two weeks after the first dose (Run II). Top: mean time, in sec, on the stoppers at hourly intervals after medication. Males (solid line); females (broken line). Bottom: Percent of animals having a positive, cataleptic response, i.e. remain on the stoppers 5 sec or more. Males (dark bars); females (light bars)

of the test period. At this time, only five males had a positive response, but the total rose to eight animals (66.7 per cent) at six hours and began to decline to six males (46.2 per cent) by seven hours. The average maximum time on the corks for the female rats occurred about two hours earlier than for the male rats (*see* top of Fig. 2).

Those female rats which survived the two-week interval, became cataleptic earlier in the test period and had a longer average duration on the corks than in the first dose study (Run I).

It should be mentioned that all animals that became cataleptic at any time during the test period generally maintained that response throughout the test period; i.e., an animal would not suddenly become cataleptic and recover abruptly, but rather would follow a gradually increasing curve which would taper off at about seven hours after medication.

Once again there is a significant difference in the incidence of catalepsy between intact male and female phenothiazine-treated rats. In addition, the Run II animals that gave a positive reaction after the second medication, were the same animals which had responded to the first drug dose (Run I), indicating an individual susceptibility.

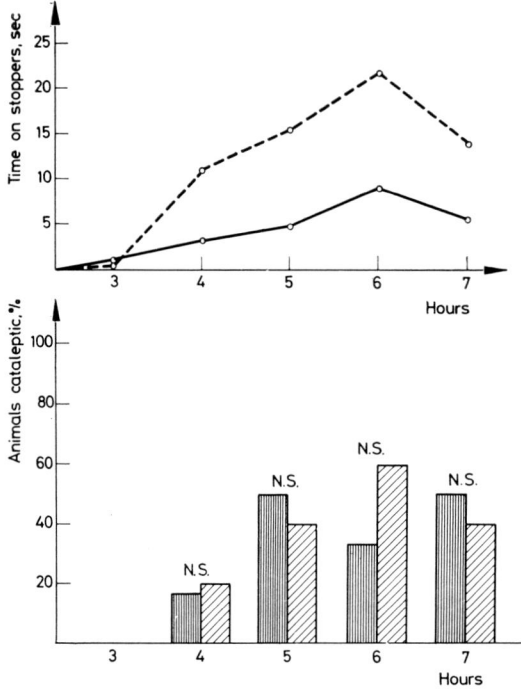

Fig. 3. Intact male rats vs castrate male rats. Group comparison of the cataleptic response to the first oral administration of 20 mg/kg of chlorpromazine (Run I). Top: mean time, in sec, on the stoppers at hourly intervals after medication. Intact males (solid line); castrate males (broken line). Bottom: percent of animals having a positive cataleptic response, i.e. remain on the stoppers 5 sec or more. Intact males (dark bars); castrate males (light bars)

CASTRATED ANIMALS

Three of the five castrate males (60 per cent) and two of the six oophorectomized females (33.3 per cent) became cataleptic after their first dose of chlorpromazine (Figs 3 and 5). At the peak time of reaction, which was about six hours after medication, the castrate male mean duration on the corks was 21.63 seconds ± ± S.E. 16.24, while the mean female duration was only 3.18 seconds ± S.E. 1.81.

When these same operated animals received the drug again two weeks later, a total of three males (60 per cent) and three females (50 per cent) became cataleptic (Figs 4 and 6). The male peak time of response occurred sooner after the second dose (5.6 hours after medication), while the female peak was at 6.4 hours after medication. Although the duration on the stoppers was longer for the castrate males than for the oophorectomized females, there was no statistically significant difference between these two groups of gonadectomized animals in the occurrence of phenothiazine-induced catalepsy.

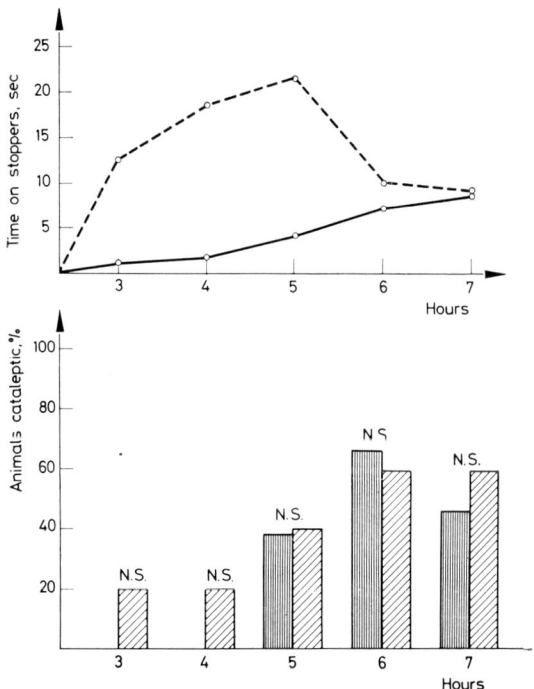

Fig. 4. Intact male rats vs castrate male rats. Group comparison of the cataleptic response to the second 20 mg/kg oral dose of chlorpromazine administered 2 weeks after the first dose (Run II). Top: mean time, in sec, on the stoppers at hourly intervals after medication. Intact males (solid line); castrate males (broken line). Bottom: percent of animals having a positive cataleptic response, i.e. remain on the stoppers for 5 sec or more. Intact males (dark bars); castrate males (light bars)

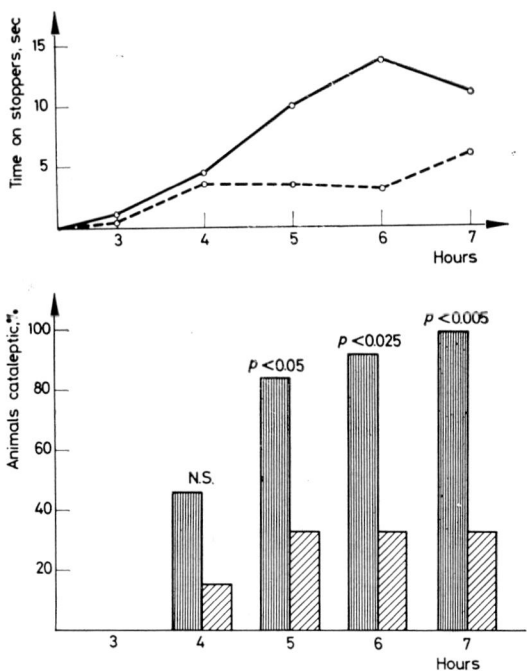

Fig. 5. Intact female rats vs oophorectomized female rats. Group comparison of the cataleptic response to the first 20 mg/kg oral dose of chlorpromazine (Run I). Top: mean time, in sec, on the stoppers at hourly intervals after medication. Intact females (solid line); oophorectomized females (broken line). Bottom: percent of animals having a positive cataleptic response, i.e., remain on the stoppers 5 sec or more. Intact females (dark bars); oophorectomized females (light bars)

DISCUSSION

An analysis of data from these experiments demonstrates that intact females have a higher incidence of phenothiazine-induced catalepsy than do intact male rats treated with the same dose per body weight. It is possible that the dose per unit weight might not provide an equivalent dose at the biological site of action in animals of different weights. Thus, e.g., if chlorpromazine is soluble in fat, then the male rat may be receiving a higher actual dose than the sexually mature female rat, which has a greater percentage of subcutaneous fat per body weight (Velardo 1958). Several findings in this study militate against this possibility.

Run I females tested a second time, after an average increase in weight of 17.4 g, showed no difference in response to the medication as compared to the first trial. During this two-week interval, it is assumed that a change in the percentage of their body fat occurred. Furthermore, castrate males did not demonstrate the intact female response to chlorpromazine treatment, even though their weight gain occurred in a female pattern rather than in an intact male pattern.

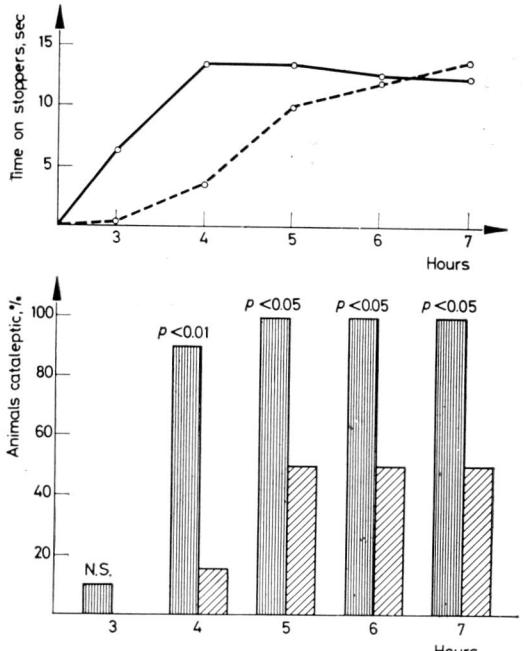

Fig. 6. Intact female rats vs oophorectomized female rats. Group comparison of the cataleptic response to the second 20 mg/kg oral dose of chlorpromazine (Run II), administered 2 weeks after the first dose. Top: mean time, in sec, on the stoppers at hourly intervals after medication. Intact females (solid line); oophorectomized females (broken line). Bottom: percent of animals having a positive cataleptic response, i.e. remain on the stoppers 5 sec or more. Intact females (dark bars); oophorectomized females (light bars)

While the castrate males did not differ significantly from the intact male insofar as the incidence of the cataleptic reaction is concerned, they seemed to have a longer duration on the corks (top of Figs 3 and 4). The two controls of weight and age factors indicated that sexual maturation and body fat distribution had little, if any, effect upon the sexual dimorphism of this reaction. The incidence of drug-induced catalepsy in the castrate male was similar to that seen in the intact male. Therefore, the higher incidence of catalepsy in females does not appear to result from a protective effect of male hormones in male rats.

There was no significant difference between the intact males and oophorectomized females, although the incidence increased slightly in both groups after the second medication. In Run I, 50 per cent of the males as compared to 33.3 per cent of the ovariectomized females became cataleptic; in Run II, the incidence increased to 66.7 per cent for the males and 50 per cent for the ovariectomized females. Comparison of the normal female groups with the castrate male groups revealed that the significant difference between the two sexes in response to the drug was not altered by castration of males.

The most striking difference in the cataleptic response in these experiments was found when the intact females (high incidence) were compared to the oophorectomized female rats (low incidence).

While 100 per cent of the intact females reacted to the medication, only 33.3 per cent of the ovariectomized females exhibited a positive cataleptic response. This difference was statistically significant. In addition, the operated females remained a shorter time on the corks, as illustrated in the top of Figs 5 and 6.

The data presented in this paper suggest that:

1. The action of phenothiazine induced catalepsy is influenced by the level of circulating steroid.
2. Since gonadal ablation provides a dramatic alteration in the female incidence, the female sex hormones appear to predispose the animal to a drug-induced catalepsy.
3. Since the rat estrous cycle is primarily estrogenic, it seems likely that estrogen is responsible for the female susceptibility to these extrapyramidal symptoms.

If chlorpromazine achieves its therapeutic effect by altering the catecholamine transmission in the brain, it is not unreasonable to suppose that these alterations occur not only in the extrapyramidal nuclei, but also in other areas of the brain where high concentrations of catecholamines occur, such as in the hypothalamus. Of particular interest to this investigation are the tubero-infundibular neurons implicated in the regulation of gonadotropic function which Fuxe and Hökfelt (1966) identified as rich in dopamine. The catecholamine levels of these neurons vary with the state of gonadotropic activity, i.e. increased amine levels probably indicated increased activity (Fuxe et al. 1967, Lichtensteiger 1969, Stefano and Donoso 1967). This may correspond to the relatively high secretion of estrogen (or LH-RF) which occurs at proestrus (Schneider and McCann 1969).

Changes in amine levels (or turnover) may be the cause as well as the consequence of changes in endocrine activity such as occur during proestrus. On the other hand, changes in neural activity in the central monoamine neurons probably occur in different hormonal states (Antón-Tay and Wurtmann 1968, Lichtensteiger et al. 1969). It is not surprising, therefore, that medication which causes variations in catecholamine content will also effect changes related to the control of the gonadotropic function via the hypothalamic tuberal neurons.

Alternative explanations of these findings may be that the effect of female sex hormones mediates by lowering the threshold of the extrapyramidal neurons, or that estrogen acts to increase the penetration of chlorpromazine into the brain by altering the blood-brain-barrier.

Additional studies are underway in our laboratories in order to elucidate the mechanism in further detail.

REFERENCES

ALPERT, M. (1967): The parameters of physiological and pathological tremor. In: *Proceedings of the 1st NIMH Workshop on Tardive Dyskinesia*, St. Louis, Mo., Jan.

ANTÓN-TAY, F. and WURTMAN, R. J. (1968): Norepinephrine: Turnover in rat brain after gonadectomy. *Science* **159**, 1245.

BARRACLOUGH, C. A. and SAWYER, C. H. (1957): Blockage of the release of pituitary ovulating hormone in the rat by chlorpromazine and reserpine: possible mechanisms of action. *Endocrinology* **61**, 341—351.

BARUK, M., LAUNAY, J. and BERGES, J. (1956): Physiologie psychiatrique expérimentale de la chlorpromazine chez les animaux et ses applications thérapeutiques chez l'homme. *Encéphale* **45**, 1258—1263.

BEN-DAVID, M., DIKSTEIN, S. and SULMAN, F. G. (1965): Production of lactation by non-sedative phenothiazine derivatives. *Proc. Soc. exp. Biol. (N. Y).* **118**, 265—270.

BENSON, G. K. (1960): Further studies on the effects of tranquilizing drugs on mammary involution in the rat. *Proc. Soc. exp. Biol. (N. Y.)* **103**, 132—137.

BRILLHART, J. R. (1959): Tranquilizer interference in the *Rana pipiens* chorionic gonadotropin test. *Obstet. and Gynec.* **14**, 581—587.

BRADY, J. (1959): Comparative psychopharmacology: Animal experimental studies on effect of drugs on behavior. In: *Psychopharmacology, Problems of Evaluation*. Ed. by J. O. Cole and R. Gerard. Nat. Acad. Sci., Nat. Res. Council, Wash. D.C. pp. 46—63.

Carworth Farms, Inc. Personal Communication. New City, Rockland County, New York, 1961.

COTUI, F., BRINITZER, W., ORR, A. and ORR, E. (1960): The effect of chlorpromazine and reserpine on adreno-cortical function. *Psychiat. Quart.* **34**, 47—61.

COURVOISIER, S., FOURNEL, J., DUCROT, R., KOLSKY, M. and KOETSCHET, P. (1953): Propriétés pharmacodynamiques du chlorhydrate de chloro-3-(dimethylamine-3'-propyl)10 phenothiazine. *Arch. int. Pharmacodyn.* **92**, 305—361.

COURVOISIER, S., DUCROT, R. and JULOU, L. (1957): New experimental aspects of the central activity of the phenothiazine derivatives. In: *Psychotropic Drugs*. Ed. by S. Garattini and V. Ghetti. E. L. Seevier, Princeton, N.J. pp. 373—391.

DASGUPTA, S. R. and HAUSLER, H. F. (1955): The effect of chlorpromazine on the induced continuous estrus of ovariectomized rats. *Bull. Calcutta Sch. trop. Med.* **3**, 113—114.

DUVOISIN, R. (1970): Behavioral abnormalities occurring in Parkinsonism during treatment with levodopa. In: *9th Annual Meeting of American College of Neuropsychopharmacology*, San Juan.

ESSIG, G. F. and CARTER, W. W. (1957): Convulsions and bizarre behavior in monkeys receiving chlorpromazine. *Proc. Soc. exp. Biol. (N. Y.)* **95**, 726.

FINK, G. B. and SWINYARD, E. A. (1960): Effect of psychopharmacologic agents on experimentally induced seizures in mice. *J. Amer. pharm. Ass.* **49**, 510—513.

FOTHERBY, K., FORREST, A. D. and LAVERTY, S. G. (1959): The effect of chlorpromazine on adrenocortical function. *Acta endocr. (Kbh.)* **32**, 425—436.

FREYHAN, F. A. (1957): Psychomotility and Parkinsonism in treatment with neuroleptic drugs. *Arch. Neurol. Psychiat. (Chic.)* **78**, 465—472.

FREYHAN, F. A. (1959): Selection of patients from the clinical point of view. In: *Psychopharmacology. Problems of Evaluation*. Ed. by J. O. Cole and R. W. Gerard. Nat. Acad. Sci., Nat. Res. Council, Wash. D.C. pp. 372—389.

FRIEDHOFF, A. J. (1969): Methylation processes in schizophrenia. In: *Schizophrenia. Current Concepts and Research*. Ed. by D. V. Siva Sankar. PJD Publications. Hicksville, N.Y. pp. 552—556.

FRIEDHOFF, A. J. and ALPERT, M. (1960): The effect of chlorpromazine on the variability of motor task performances in schizophrenia. *J. nerv. ment. Dis.* **130**, 110—116.

FUXE, K. and HÖKFELT, T. (1966): Further evidence for the existence of tuberoinfundibular dopamine neurons. *Acta physiol. scand.* **66**, 245—246.

FUXE, K., HÖKFELT, T. and NILSSON, O. (1967): Activity changes in the tuberoinfundibular neurons of the rat during various states of the reproductive cycle. *Life Sci.* **6**, 2057—2061.

GAILITIS, J., KNOWLES, R. and LONGOBARD, A. (1960): Alarming neuromuscular reactions due to prochlorperazine. *Ann. intern. Med.* **52**, 538—543.

GOLD, E. M., DIRAIMONDO, V. C., KENT, J. R. and FORSHAM, P. H. (1960): Comparative effects of certain non-narcotic central nervous system analgesics and muscle relaxants on pituitary adrenocortical system. In: *Non-Narcotic Drugs for the Relief of Pain and their Mechanisms of Action. Ann. N.Y. Acad. Sci.* **86**, 178—190.

HAASE, H. J. (1959): The role of drug induced extrapyramidal syndromes. In: *Psychopharmacology Frontiers*. Ed. by N. S. Kline. Little, Brown and Co., New York. pp. 197—208.

HEILIZER, F. (1959): The effects of chlorpromazine upon psychomotor and psychiatric behavior of chronic schizophrenic patients. *J. nerv. ment. Dis.* **128**, 358—364.

HEILIZER, F. (1960): A critical review of some published experiments with chlorpromazine in schizophrenic, neurotic and normal humans. *J. chron. Dis.* **11**, 102—148.

HORNYKIEWICZ, O. (1966): Dopamine (3-hydroxytryptamine) and brain function. *Pharmacol. Rev.* **18**, 925—964.

IRWIN, S. and GOVIER, W. M. (1957): Chlorpromazine, a new tranquilizer: comparison with chlorpromazine in the mouse, rat, cat, dog and monkey. *J. Pharmacol. exp. Ther.* **119**, 154—155 (Abstract).

KHAN, M. Y. and BERNSTORF, E. C. (1964): Effect of chlorpromazine and reserpine upon pituitary function. *Exp. Med. Surg.* **22**, 363—378.

KHAZEN, K., MISHKINSKY, J., BEN-DAVID, M. and SULMAN, F. G. (1968): Structure-activity relationship of mammotropic phenothiazine derivatives. *Arch. int. Pharmacodyn.* **171**, 251—273.

KULCSÁR, S., POLISHUK, W. and RUBIN, L. (1957): Aspects endocriniens du traitement à la chlorpromazine. *Presse méd.* **65**, 1288—1290.

LICHTENSTEIGER, W. (1969): Cyclic variations of catecholamine content in hypothalamic nerve cells during the estrous cycle of the rat, with a concomitant study of the substantia nigra. *J. Pharmacol. exp. Ther.* **165**, 204—215.

LICHTENSTEIGER, W., KORPELA, K., LANGEMANN, H. and KELLER, P. J. (1969): The influence of ovariectomy, estrogen and progesterone on the catecholamine content of hypothalamic nerve cells in the rat. *Brain Res.* **16**, 199—214.

MAY, R. H. and VOEGEL, G. E. (1956): Parkinsonism reactions following chlorpromazine and reserpine. *Arch. Neurol. Psychiat. (Chic.)* **75**, 522—524.

PAULSON, G. (1959): Phenothiazine toxicity, extrapyramidal seizures and oculogyric crises. *J. ment. Sci.* **105**, 798—802.

RAHILL, M. A. (1957): Mammary gland changes during chlorpromazine therapy. *Brit. med. J.* **2**, 906.

SCHNEIDER, H. P. G. and MCCANN, S. M. (1969): Possible role of dopamine as transmitter to promote discharge of LH-releasing factor. *Endocrinology* **85**, 121—132.

SHELESNYAK, M. C. (1954): Comparative effectiveness of antihistamines in suppression of the decidual cell reaction in the pseudopregnant rat. *Endocrinology* **54**, 396—401.

SIEGEL, S. (1956): In: *Nonparametric Statistics for the Behavioral Sciences*. Ed. by C. T. Morgan. McGraw-Hill Book Co., New York, N.Y. pp. 256—270.

STEFANO, F. J. E. and DONOSO, A. O. (1967): Norepinephrine levels in the rat hypothalamus during the estrous cycle. *Endocrinology* **81**, 1405—1406.

SUZUKI, M., KAMIO, K., YASUDA, M., AKIYAMA, S., MITANI, K., OYAMA, T., SATO, K. and YAMASHITA, T. (1956): The effect of chlorpromazine on the function of the endocrine organs. *Endocrin. jap.* **3**, 67—72.

TAESCHLER, M. and CERLETTI, A. (1959): Effets de quelques dérivés de la phenothiazine sur des réactions matrices et émotionnelles du rat. *J. Physiol. (Paris)* **51**, 873—878.

TALWALKER, P. K. (1960): Initiation and maintenance of milk secretion in the rat following chlorpromazine administration. *Fed. Proc.* **19**, 157.

TEDESCHI, D. H., TEDESCHI, R. E., COOK, L., MATTIS, P. and FELLOWS, E. J. (1959): The neuropharmacology of triflooperazine: a potent psychotherapeutic agent. *Arch. int. Pharmacodyn.* **122**, 129—143.

VELARDO, J. T. (Ed.) (1958): In: *The Endocrinology of Reproduction*. Oxford University Press, New York. pp. 340.

SECTION IV

HORMONAL INFLUENCES ON BRAIN FUNCTIONS

Chairman: D. H. FORD

ACCUMULATION OF ³H-LYSINE IN LIMBIC AND BRAINSTEM STRUCTURES

D. H. FORD and R. K. RHINES

Department of Anatomy
State University of New York
Downstate Medical Center
Brooklyn, N.Y., U.S.A.

The current literature is filled with numerous references concerning the effect of stimulation or lesion placement in limbic or brainstem regions on the function of the neuroendocrine system. Both anatomical and physiological evidence (Colvin et al. 1968, Hayward 1970, Innes and Michal 1970, Kawakami et al. 1968, Mietkiewski and Miskowiak 1969, Komisaruk et al. 1967, Shimada and Gorbman 1970, Terasawa and Timiras 1968, Martini 1969) suggest a functional interrelationship between these two components of the CNS which in turn may influence the hypothalamic release of factors regulating the anterior pituitary gland. With our interests in protein synthesis in the CNS (Ford 1967, Ford and Rhines 1969a, b, Ford and Rhines 1970a, b), particularly in relation to accumulation of amino acids in different types of neurons, we thought it would be of interest to compare amino acid accumulations in neurons and brain regions associated with limbic, neurosecretory and brainstem areas as compared to other regions of the CNS.

The components which one may readily evaluate are limited to those regions of the brain which can be reasonably well separated from other areas and to cells which are fairly large and which occur in relatively discrete aggregates. Thus, one may dissect from the brain portions of the hippocampal cortex, the supraoptic nucleus and preoptic areas, as well as many regions not associated with the limbic–brainstem–neuroendocrine systems. Further, neurons of the hippocampal cortex and supraoptic nucleus may also be readily dissected from their surrounding neuropil. In the brainstem, the reticular nuclei are perhaps the most significant in relation to the systems concerned here. However, the cells are either too small or too widely scattered to be dissected. Further, the midbrain is so heterogenous that uptake studies in blocks of tissues would be uninterpretable. However, the cells of the red nucleus are both closely aggregated and large and thus readily dissectable. Thus, the following study will deal with the accumulation of ³H-lysine into area 6 of the cerebral premotor cortex, hippocampal cortex, spinal cord, grey matter, preoptic area and for comparison muscle and plasma. The cell types which will be compared will be the pyramidal cells of the hippocampus, the supraoptic neurons and the parvo and magnocellular elements of the red nucleus. These latter cells may be considered as relating to an entirely unrelated system inasmuch as their primary projections are into the spinal cord where they will excite motoneurons and the static γ neurons innervating flexor muscles or they may be involved in the thalamic relay back to the motor cortex.

Thus, what will be compared is neurons of the limbic and neurosecretory systems and neurons which are unrelated to the limbic–neurosecretory components of the brain which may be considered to be a part of the motor system.

Inasmuch as the procedure used involves a prolonged period of formalin fixation after the tissues have been removed from the animals, essentially all unbound amino acids have diffused out of the tissues. As a result, the remaining radioactivity in the tissue after injecting the rats with a labeled amino acid is associated with molecules which are either incorporated into or bound to proteins.

MATERIALS AND METHODS

Male rats were used throughout the experiment. They were maintained in separate cages in a quiet room for 2 weeks prior to injection with labeled amino acid. During this period they received water and laboratory chow ad libitum. The day prior to injection with labeled amino acid, the animals were anesthetized with 20 per cent ethanol and a permanent polyethylene cannula was implanted in the left external jugular vein. The rats were allowed to recover and 24 hours later were injected via the cannula while unanesthetized with a dose of 3.2 μg of ^{3}H-DL-lysine/kg. The animals were then sacrificed 1/2, 1, 2 or 4 hours later after withdrawing a sample of blood to obtain a plasma fraction. The brains and spinal cords were rapidly removed and fixed in 10 per cent neutral formalin for a period of over 1 month to allow leaching of free amino acid from the tissue. Duplicate samples of premotor cortex, spinal cord, grey matter, hippocampus, preoptic area and plasma were prepared for dry oxidation in Schöniger flasks and the radioactivity determined by a liquid scintillation counting procedure. Duplicate samples of hippocampal pyramidal cells and supraoptic nucleus cells were also prepared for oxidation, there being 400 cells per sample. Cells of the red nucleus are not so numerous, so only single samples were prepared for oxidation and scintillation counting. [Data from a previous investigation provided information relative to the percent of the radioactivity present in neurons (86 per cent) which would be in the form of lysine.] Inasmuch as the weights of the various types of neurons were determined as well (for procedure see Ford and Cohan, 1968), the final data was expressed in terms of ng of lysine/g of tissue and analysed for significance by a simple 2-way analysis of variance.

RESULTS

Figure 1 illustrates the appearance of the various types of neurons which can be dissected from the surrounding neuropil in formalin-fixed brain preparations. Note that the cells are essentially free of glia, although there is some glial material present in the preparation.

Figure 2 illustrates the relative accumulation of lysine in various areas of brain and muscle in comparison to plasma. One may first note that not all the areas

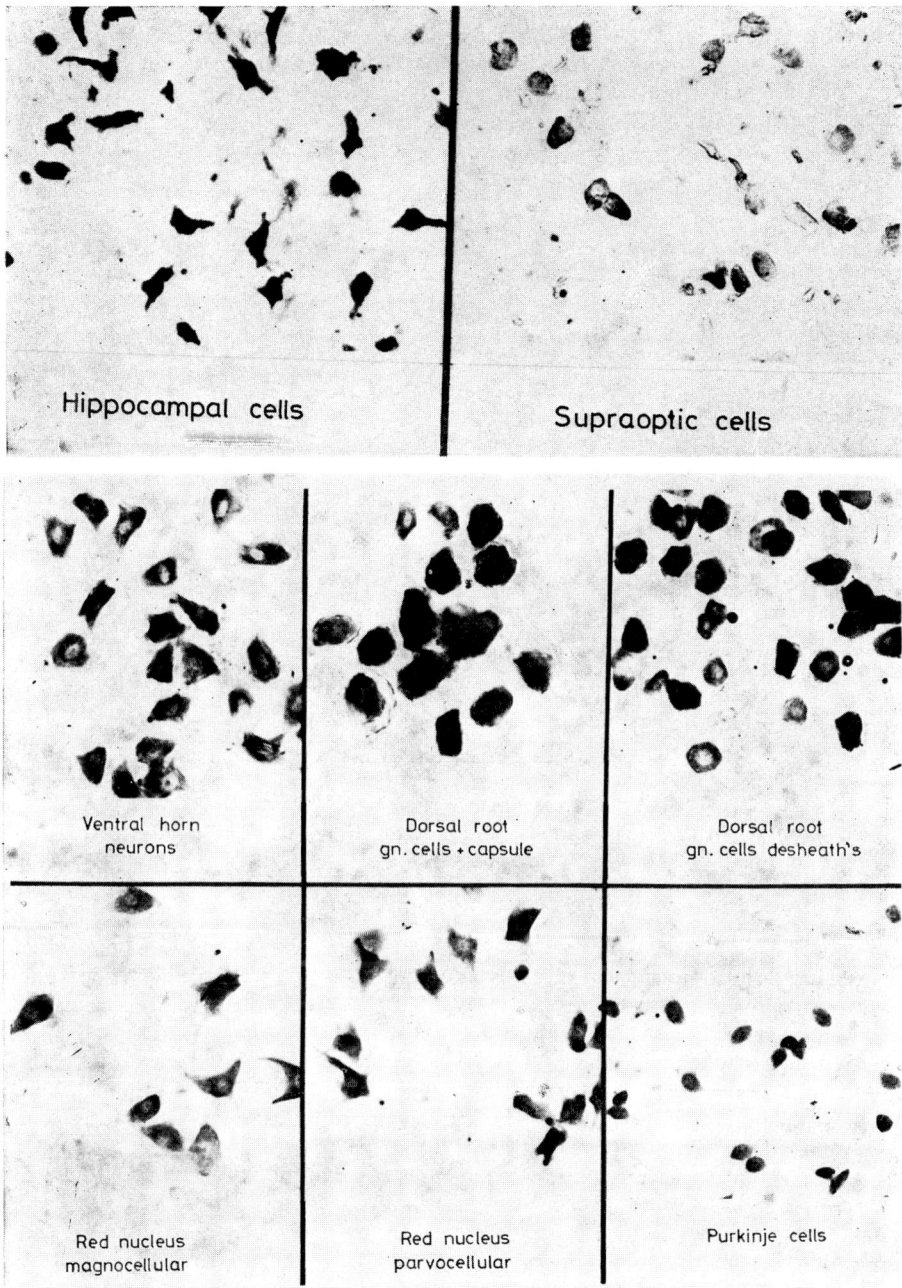

Fig. 1. A photographic depiction of various types of neurons dissected from the formalin-fixed CNS of the rat. Magnification: ×400

of brain grey matter have similar levels of lysine accumulation. Area 6 of the cerebral cortex had significantly higher levels of lysine accumulation ($p < 0.001$) than did the hippocampus, preoptic area or spinal grey matter, while the spinal grey, preoptic area and hippocampus were essentially similar in uptake. One might further conclude from this Figure that there is a relative barrier effect to accumulation in the brain, because plasma levels of ^3H activity were significantly

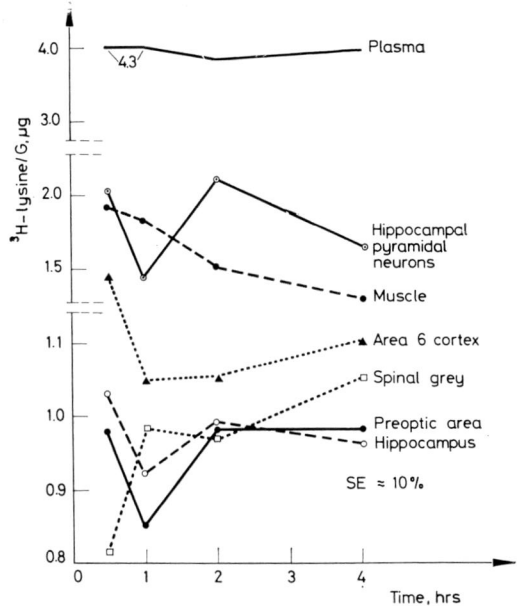

Fig. 2. A graphic illustration of the amount of ^3H-lysine accumulated in plasma, muscle and various areas of the brain at various time intervals after intravenous injection of ^3H-DL-lysine

higher than brain. However, muscle lysine uptake, which was significantly higher than occurred in blocks of brain tissue was also less than plasma levels. Further, as will appear with cells of the red nucleus, other neurons of the CNS will have levels of amino acid accumulation which exceed those of plasma. Also note in this Figure that the level of lysine accumulation in hippocampal pyramidal cells is significantly higher than that observed for whole hippocampus, for cerebral cortex, spinal cord grey, preoptic area or for muscle.

Figure 3 compares the accumulation levels of lysine in the 4 types of neurons investigated. Both supraoptic cells and hippocampal pyramids have levels of accumulation below that of plasma. However, it should be borne in mind that the activity in the plasma represents both free and bound lysine, while that in the neurons is representative of only the bound pool of amino acid. Further, the supraoptic neurons show a positive gradient for uptake in relation to plasma. The cells of the red nucleus significantly exceeded all other cell types and brain regions in their accumulation of lysine. It is also to be noted that the cells of the parvocellular component of the red nucleus have a significantly higher lysine accumulation/g than occurs with the phylogenetically older magnocellular elements. Both showed a very high accumulation in the first 30 minutes, which then decreased significantly and finally increased again. It is interesting to note that the uptake in cells of parvocellular component is more comparable to the uptake

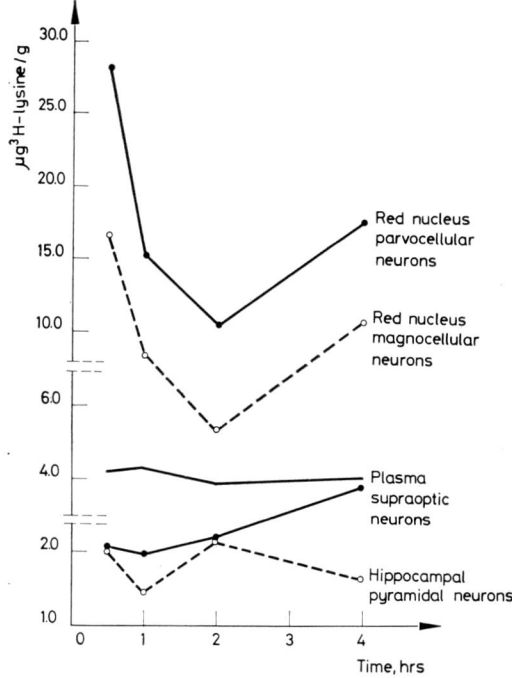

Fig. 3. A graphic illustration of the amount of ^{3}H-lysine accumulated in limbic (hippocampal) and neurosecretory (supraoptic) neurons and neurons of the red nucleus as compared to plasma at various time intervals after intravenous injection of ^{3}H-DL-lysine

observed in Purkinje cells of the cerebellar system dissected from the same animals. Comparison of the four cell types in relation to accumulation of lysine reveals that each cell type has a characteristic pattern of uptake which is significantly different from the other cell types. This presumably is related to intrinsically different rates of protein synthesis between the different cell types and hints of intrinsically different metabolic turnover rates for cells of the limbic, neurosecretory and cerebello–rubrospinal systems.

The lower uptakes in the supraoptic and hippocampal neurons as compared to the red nucleus may reflect either lower rates of uptake or greater turnover rates with a subsequent dilution of labeled amino acid in the cells by non-labeled amino acid.

SUMMARY

In summary, the comparison of uptake of ^{3}H-lysine into various functionally different regions of the CNS reveals that a non-limbic area such as the premotor cortex of the rat accumulated levels of lysine higher than occurred in limbic regions, such as the hippocampus and preoptic area, while the spinal cord uptake was similar. Further, as in previous studies, neurons demonstrated higher levels of uptake than did the regional areas from which they came. When neurons were compared it was observed that neurons not associated with the limbic system or hypothalamus had markedly higher levels of amino acid uptake and that each nerve type could be characterized as having its own particular pattern or rate of amino acid stimulation.

REFERENCES

COLVIN, G. B., WHITMOYER, D. I., LISK, R. D., WALTER, D. O. and SAWYER, C. H. (1968): Changes in sleep–wakefulness in female rats during circadian and estrous cycles. *Brain Res.* **7**, 173–181.

FORD, D. H. (1967): Changes in brain accumulation of amino acids and adenine associated with changes in the physiologic state. In: *Progress in Brain Research*, vol. 29. Ed. by A. Lajtha and D. H. Ford. Elsevier, Amsterdam.

FORD, D. H. and COHAN, G. (1968): Changes in weight and volume of rat spinal cord motor neurons with increasing age. *Acta anat. (Basel)* **71**, 311–319.

FORD, D. H. and RHINES, R. K. (1969a): (^{3}H) Lysine accumulation in motoneurons in rats of different age compared with the accumulation in other tissues. *Acta neurol. scand.* **45**, 41–52.

FORD, D. H. and RHINES, R. K. (1969b): ^{3}H-lysine accumulation in spinal cord grey matter and ventral horn motoneurons in the rat as related to age and neuronal cytoplasmic volume. *Acta neurol. scand.* **45**, 529–539.

FORD, D. H. and RHINES, R. K. (1970a): Accumulation of (^{3}H) lysine in various types of neurons in male rats. *J. Neurol. Sci.* **10**, 179–183.

FORD, D. H. and RHINES, R. K. (1970b): Accumulation of ^{14}C by ventral horn and dorsal root ganglion neurons after intravenous injection of (^{14}C)GABA. *J. Neurol. Sci.* **10**, 331–337.

HAYWARD, J. N. (1970): Central neural regulation of antidiuretic hormone release and unit activity in the supraoptic nucleus of the behaving rhesus monkey. *Amer. J. Anat.* **129**, 203–206.

INNES, D. I. and MICHAL, E. K. (1970): Effects of progesterone and oestrogen on the electrical activity of the limbic system. *J. exp. Zool.* **175**, 487–492.

KAWAKAMI, M., SETO, K. and YOSHIDA, K. (1968): Influences of the limbic structure on biosynthesis of ovarian steroids in rabbits. *Jap. J. Physiol.* **18**, 356–372.

KOMISARUK, B. R., MCDONALD, P. G., WHITMOYER, D. I. and SAWYER, C. H. (1967): Effects of progesterone and sensory stimulation on EEG and neuronal activity in the rat. *Exp. Neurol.* **19**, 494–507.

MARTINI, L. (1969): Action of hormones on the central nervous system. *Gen. comp. Endocr.* Suppl. **2**, 214–226.

MIETKIEWSKI, K. and MISKOWIAK, B. (1969): Histologic and histochemical changes induced by cyproterone (antiandrogen) in the supraoptic nucleus of the hypothalamus in rats. *Folia Morphol. (Warszawa)* **28**, 316–325.

SHIMADA, H. and GORBMAN, A. (1970): Long lasting changes in RNA synthesis in the forebrains of female rats treated with testosterone soon after birth. *Biochem. biophys. Res. Commun.* **38**, 423–430.

TERASAWA, E. and TIMIRAS, P. S. (1968): Electrical activity during the estrous cycle of the rat: cyclic changes in limbic structures. *Endocrinology* **83**, 207–216.

FACILITATORY AND INHIBITORY MESENCEPHALIC INFLUENCE ON GONADOTROPIN RELEASE

S. TALEISNIK and H. F. CARRER

Instituto de Investigación Médica
Mercedes y Martín Ferreyra
Córdoba, Argentina

It is well known that the maintenance of a basic level of gonadotropin secretion by the anterior pituitary depends on its connection with the hypothalamus. This neural structure contains neurons which elaborate chemical agents that regulate pituitary hormone secretion after reaching the gland by the portal vessels. Although the hypothalamus is recognized to have autonomic activity and is capable of maintaining a tonic release of gonadotropin even when disconnected from the rest of the brain (Halász and Gorski 1967), a number of stimuli can affect its activity. The most clear evidence in this respect is provided by coitus in the so-called reflex ovulators. Many other internal as well as external stimuli of different modalities are known to exert a modulating influence on the endocrine function. These signals, of diverse origin, reach the hypothalamic neurons by different routes being the neural information transformed into a chemical one before influencing the anterior pituitary. The pool of hypothalamic neurons which secrete the releasing and inhibitory factors thus form the final common pathway for the pituitary gland.

The limbic system has been demonstrated to influence gonadotropin secretion, the stimuli arriving from the amygdala being facilitatory and those of the hippocampus inhibitory (Koikegami et al. 1954, Bunn and Everett 1957, Shealy and Peele 1957, Velasco and Taleisnik 1969a, b). Much less information had been provided about the influence exerted by the midbrain although obviously many of the sensory modalities which affect gonadotropin secretion are conveyed by pathways which in some way are related to that structure. A dual role of the midbrain has been described for the control of corticotropin hormone release (Mangili et al. 1966, Fortier 1966) but even in that case the lack of specific organized systems is evident. In the literature there exists very little information concerning the influence of the midbrain on gonadotropin secretion and some of it shows contradictory results (Critchlow 1958, Pekary et al. 1967, Benedetti et al. 1965). In the present communication the results on this subject obtained in our laboratory, part of which have already been published (Carrer and Taleisnik 1970), are discussed.

METHODS

In this work the effect of electrochemical stimulation on ovulation and secretion of LH and FSH was investigated in rats. A direct current of 1 mA for 10 sec was passed through a unipolar stainless steel electrode. This procedure was shown (Everett and Radford 1961) to produce an electrolytic deposition of iron which is effective in activating neuronal cell bodies as well as fibre tracts. Both facilitatory and inhibitory influences on gonadotropin secretion were observed after mesencephalic stimulation.

FACILITATORY INFLUENCES ON GONADOTROPIN SECRETION

We have demonstrated (Carrer and Taleisnik 1970) that bilateral electrochemical stimulation of the mesencephalic reticular formation at the level of the ventral tegmental nucleus, lateral and inferior to the periaqueductal grey substance, induced ovulation in rats made persistently oestrous by continuous illumination (Fig. 1). Normally these animals failed to ovulate spontaneously. Stimulation at the same level in the midline also induced ovulation although less effectively than that more laterally located. Several other mesencephalic regions were stimulated but no ovulatory response was obtained.

Stimulation of the dorsal tegmentum at the site from which ovulatory response was obtained was also effective in inducing the release of LH in ovariectomized rats (Carrer and Taleisnik 1970). The elevated levels of LH in the spayed animals were lowered by the injection of 20 μg oestradiol benzoate 3 days before stimulation. Fifteen minutes after the stimulus was applied a rise in serum LH was observed, however, after 1 hour the values returned to normal. Similar effect

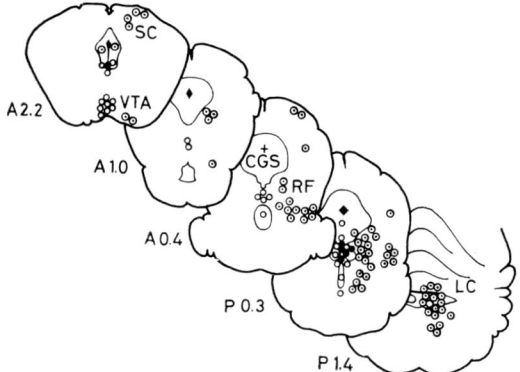

Fig. 1. Ovulatory response provoked by electrochemical stimulation in rats in persistent oestrus induced by continuous illumination. Schematic drawing of serial frontal sections; solid circles indicate sites where stimulation evoked an ovulatory response, open circles site where stimulation did not induce ovulation. Double concentric circles = bilateral stimulation; single circles = unilateral stimulation. CGS = central grey substance. LC = locus coeruleus. RF = reticular formation. SC = superior colliculus. VTA = ventral tegmental area (Taken from Carrer and Taleisnik 1970)

resulted from the stimulation of castrated–oestrogen-primed male rats. No effect on serum FSH levels were observed after stimulations were applied to spayed–oestrogen-primed rats.

We were also interested to find out as to what extent the limbic system is involved in the response evoked by the stimulation of the dorsal tegmental area. Therefore, stimulations of the mesencephalic ovulating area were applied to animals in which the afferents from the amygdala and hippocampus had been completely transected or selectively interrupted by cutting the stria terminalis (ST) or the fornix (FX) (Fig. 2). Rats with long-term complete transection of the limbic afferents to the hypophysiotropic area (a horizontal circular cut placed at the upper part of the preoptic area interrupts the fibres of the ST and FX system; designed as preoptic area-roof section because of its position) showed a significant decrease in the ovulatory response after stimulation as compared with the intact rats. Transections of the ST were also effective in preventing the ovulatory response. On the contrary, interruption of the fornix was followed by a normal response. These results indicate that the amygdala is in some way involved in the gonadotropic facilitatory response to mesencephalic stimulation. Previous studies have demonstrated that the amygdala has a facilitatory effect on gonadotropin secretion and that the ST is the route by which the stimulus from the amygdala reaches the hypothalamus (Velasco and Taleisnik 1969a). It is not yet clear whether the observed effect is due to the activation of the amygdala by the dorsolateral mesencephalic stimulation or to a tonic facilitatory action of this structure on the preoptic–hypophysiotropic system. However, the fact that stimulation of the midbrain tegmentum was shown to be capable of modifying the activity of amygdaloid units (Machne and Segundo 1956) gives strong support to the first of these two possibilities.

The effect of lesions at the mesencephalic area from which ovulatory response is evoked was studied. In rats lesioned in the morning of pro-oestrus the expected ovulation was found to be normal. Neither was there any effect on ovulation by

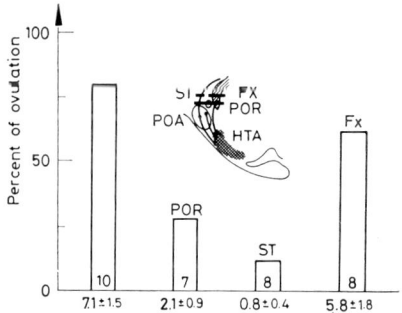

Fig. 2. Effect of interruption of limbic afferents to the hypothalamus on the ovulatory response induced by electrochemical stimulation of the dorsal tegmental area of rats with spontaneous ovulation blocked by continuous illumination. Stimulation was applied to intact rats and to animals with long-term section of the stria terminalis (ST), the fornix (FX) or at the preoptic area-roof (POR). The figures at the foot of the columns indicate the number of stimulated rats. Figures for eggs/rat are means ±S.E. POA = preoptic area. HTA = hypophysiotropic area. The horizontal bars show the number of eggs per rat

long-term lesions. Furthermore, animals with long-term lesions showed normal oestrous cycles indicating that this area is not required for maintaining the sequence of events that leads to the cyclic ovulatory discharge of gonadotropin. These results are in contrast with the findings showing that transection of the ST in the morning of pro-oestrus blocked the expected ovulation (Velasco and Taleisnik, in press).

INHIBITORY INFLUENCE ON GONADOTROPIN SECRETION

1. Effect on the phasic release

The effect of mesencephalic stimulation on spontaneous ovulation was studied. The animals were stimulated on the day of pro-oestrus before the critical period of the preovulatory release of gonadotropin and were searched for ova the following day. When stimulation was applied to the paramedian region of the mesencephalon, namely to the ventral tegmental area (VTA), the medial raphe nucleus or the periaqueductal grey, blockade of ovulation was obtained (Fig. 3). The response occurred after midline stimulation but bilateral stimulation of the VTA placed as far as 1.5 mm from the midline was equally effective. Unilateral stimulations in the midline, dorsal to the medial raphe nucleus or bilateral stimulations lateral to this nucleus were ineffective in blocking ovulation. Likewise, stimulations in the superior colliculus, the lateral reticular formation, mamillary bodies or the interpeduncular nucleus failed to block ovulation (Fig. 3). That the inhibitory effect on ovulation was not due to the lesion produced by electrochemical stimu-

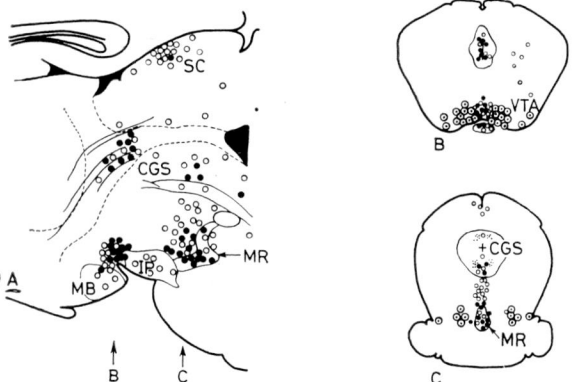

Fig. 3. Effect of mesencephalic stimulation on spontaneous ovulation in pro-oestrous rats. A, Schematic drawing of a parasagittal brain section showing midline stimulation. B and C, frontal sections at levels indicated by the corresponding arrows in A. The circles mark the location of the electrode tip. Solid circles indicate blockade of ovulation, open circles sites where ovulation was not blocked. Double concentric circles indicate bilateral stimulation, single circles unilateral stimulation. CGS = central grey substance; IP = interpeduncular nucleus. MB = mamillary bodies, MR = medial raphe nucleus, SC = superior colliculus, VTA = ventral tegmental area (Taken from Carrer and Taleisnik 1970)

lation was demonstrated by the fact that lesions in the VTA made with cathodic current, which does not deposit iron, did not block ovulatory response.

The effect of stimulation of the VTA on the release of LH and FSH was also studied. Two types of animals with high levels of serum LH were used: rats on the day of pro-oestrus primed with progesterone and spayed rats in which the serum LH levels were first lowered by the administration of 20 µg oestradiol benzoate and 3 days later raised again by the injection of progesterone. Three hours after stimulation of the VTA a significant decrease in serum LH was observed in both types of animals (Fig. 4). Sham stimulations or stimuli applied to the dorsal tegmental area or superior colliculus were without effect. In order to discard the possibility that this effect could be due to the suppression of some activating structure because of the lesion that this type of stimulus produces rather than to the activation of an inhibition, pro-oestrus–progesterone-primed rats were stimulated with a cathodic current which produces a lesion similar to the anodic one but without deposition of iron. Such procedure failed to induce any change in serum LH concentration (Fig. 4).

Serum FSH levels were also reported to be decreased after VTA stimulation in spayed rats primed with oestrogen and progesterone but the difference was significant statistically (Carrer and Taleisnik 1970).

We were interested to know about the neural pathways through which the inhibitory stimuli on gonadotropin secretion are transmitted from the mesencephalon to the hypothalamus. In an attempt to trace out the circuits which may be associated with such stimuli we have studied the influence on gonadotropin secretion of either stimulating or transecting the ascending pathways from the mesencephalon.

Midline stimulations along the course of the dorsal longitudinal fasciculus (DLF) in rats on the day of pro-oestrus resulted in the blockade of ovulation (Fig. 5). Stimulations placed from the level of the interstitial nucleus up to the caudal hypothalamus where the DLF becomes part of the periventricular system were equally effective in blocking ovulation.

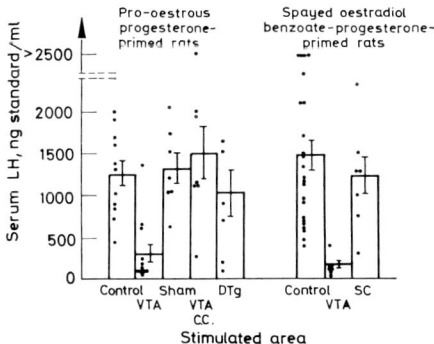

Fig. 4. Serum luteinizing hormone (LH) levels of rats after electrochemical stimulation. Each point represents one animal. The bars represent means and the vertical lines the S. E. VTA = ventral tegmental area. C. C. = cathodic current. DTg = dorsal tegmentum, SC = superior colliculus. Sham = insertion of electrode only
(Taken from Carrer and Taleisnik 1970)

Also bilateral stimulations of the medial forebrain bundle (MFB) at the level where it traverses the hypothalamic area blocked ovulation, whereas those placed at the level of the lateral preoptic area were ineffective (Fig. 6). Unilateral stimulation of the MFB also failed to affect ovulation. Several other areas of the brain were stimulated without any effect (Figs 5 and 6).

In the following experiment the effect of interrupting the course of these pathways on the transmission of the inhibitory impulses resulting from stimulation of mesencephalic structures was studied.

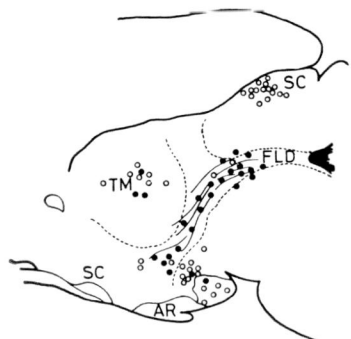

Fig. 5. Schematic drawing of a parasagittal brain section showing the location of the electrode tip from midline stimulations on spontaneous ovulation of pro-oestrous rats. Dots indicate blockade of ovulation, circles sites where stimulation failed to block ovulation. AR = arcuate nucleus. TM = thalamus. FLD = dorsal longitudinal fasciculus. SC = superior colliculus

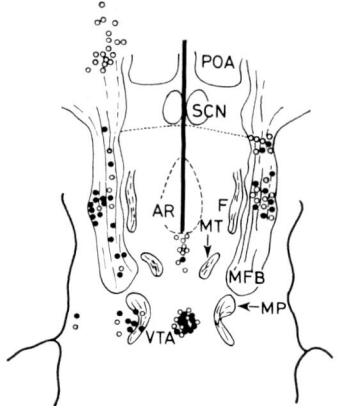

Fig. 6. Schematic drawing of a horizontal brain section at the level of the medial forebrain bundle (MFB) course. Dots on the midline and at the right show the sites of the electrode tip from unilateral stimulations. Dots on the left refer to bilateral stimulation. Circles indicate ineffective stimulation sites. VTA = ventral tegmental area. MP = mamillo-peduncular tract. MT = mamillo-thalamic tract. SCN = suprachiasmatic nucleus. POA = preoptic area. F = fornix. AR = arcuate nucleus

Figure 7 shows that the blockade of ovulation resulting from VTA electrochemical stimulation is prevented by the transection of either the DLF or the MFB showing the importance of these pathways in the conduction of the inhibitory stimuli to the hypothalamus. The fact that VTA stimulation requires the integrity of both routes to induce blockade of ovulation is interpreted as reflecting summated neuronal impulses on the hypothalamus. The blocking effect on ovulation was also suppressed by interrupting the course of the CHT, a result which suggests that the hippocampus is involved. In fact it has been demonstrated that stimulation of the hippocampus has an inhibitory effect on the release of gonadotropin, which can be suppressed by the transection of the CHT (Velasco and Taleisnik 1969b).

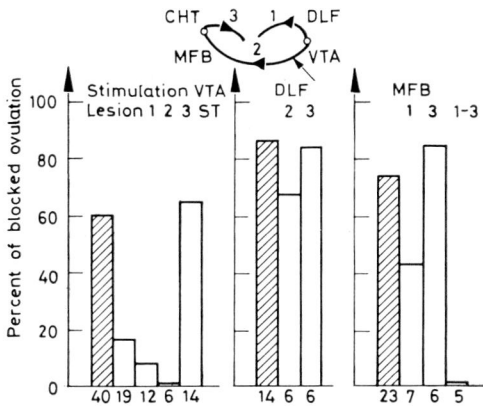

Fig. 7. Effect of interrupting the neural pathways to the hypothalamus on the inhibition of ovulation. Rats on the day of pro-oestrus were electrochemically stimulated in the ventral tegmental area (VTA), dorsal longitudinal fasciculus (DLF) or the medial forebrain bundle (MFB). Shaded bars represent intact animals; 1 refers to animals with transection of the DLF; 2 to that of MFB and 3 to that of the medial corticohypothalamic tract (CHT). Figures at the foot of the columns indicate number of animals

On the other hand, the blockade of ovulation after stimulation of the DLF was not prevented by the transection of the MFB or the CHT indicating that these pathways are not required for the effect to occur.

Moreover, the effect of stimulation of the MFB was not prevented by the transection of either the DLF or the CHT showing that the inhibitory stimuli can reach the hypothalamus by any one of these two pathways. However, when both tracts were transected simultaneously the blockade of ovulation was prevented. These results indicate that the inhibitory impulses resulting from the stimulation of the MFB cannot reach the hypothalamus once the CHT and the DLF have been interrupted and suggest that there are no fibres from the MFB to the hypophysiotropic area either through the lateral hypothalamus or mediated by the preoptic area.

2. Effect on the tonic release of LH

The effect of mesencephalic stimulation on serum LH concentration was also studied in ovariectomized rats. In these animals the serum levels of the hormone are elevated due to the removal of the negative feedback effect of the ovarian steroids. Stimulation of VTA or DLF did not affect significantly the elevated levels (Fig. 8). However, since these results could depend on a decrease in CNS excitability, due to the removal of the ovaries, stimulations were applied to spayed animals 24 hours after they had been injected with 0.5 µg oestradiol benzoate. Oestrogen was shown to increase the excitability of the CNS (Wooley and Timiras 1962), to lower the thresholds for electrical stimulation (Kawakami

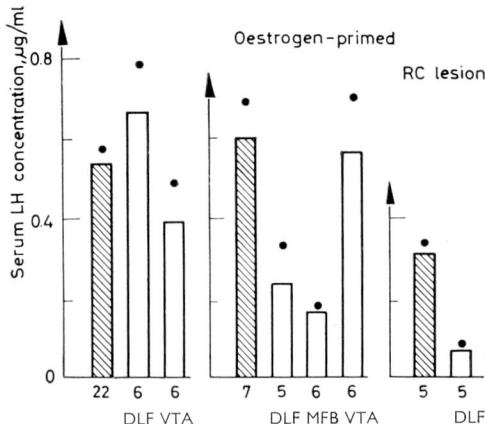

Fig. 8. Effect of stimulation of efferent pathways from the mesencephalon on the tonic release of LH. Long-term ovariectomized rats were used. Primed animals were injected with 0.5 µg oestradiol benzoate 24 hours before stimulation. The dorsal longitudinal fasciculus (DLF), medial forebrain bundle (MFB) or ventral tegmental area (VTA) were stimulated in the afternoon and blood was drawn 3 hours later. Serum LH concentration was compared with values of non-stimulated animals (shaded bars). Each column is the mean value and points are SE. Figures at the foot of the columns are number of animals. RC = animals with retrochiasmatic lesions

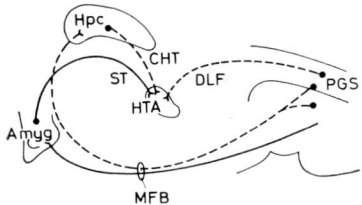

Fig. 9. Schematic drawing of neural systems affecting gonadotropin secretion. Continuous lines indicate the facilitatory system and the broken lines the inhibitory system. PGS = periaqueductal grey substance. MFB = medial forebrain bundle. DLF = dorsal longitudinal fasciculus. CHT = medial cortico-hypothalamic tract. ST = stria terminalis. HTA = hypophysiotropic area. Amyg = amygdala. Hpc = = hippocampus

and Sawyer 1959) and to increase the amplitude of the evoked potentials in the hypothalamus in response to stimulation of the reticular formation (Endrőczi et al. 1968). Stimulation of DLF or MFB in these spayed, oestrogen-primed rats resulted in a significant decrease in serum LH concentration 3 hours later (Fig. 8). Likewise hippocampal stimulation was shown to decrease plasma LH levels of ovariectomized–oestrogen-primed rats while the same stimulus was ineffective in non-injected animals (Velasco and Taleisnik 1969b). Since the hypothalamus, disconnected from the CNS, is capable of maintaining a tonic release of LH (Halász and Gorski 1967, Taleisnik et al. 1970), the blockade of such release in the above experiments should be considered as reflecting a direct action of the stimuli on the neurons secreting LH-RF and not by the inhibition of the incoming fibres which activate them. Further support to this content was provided by the experiments in animals in which the preoptic area and hypothalamic connections were interrupted by a retrochiasmatic lesion. Stimulation of DLF in such animals also resulted in a decrease in serum LH concentration (Fig. 8) indicating that the impulses transmitted by this fasciculus are affecting the hypophysiotropic area directly and not through the preoptic area.

CONCLUSIONS

The data presented show that both facilitatory and inhibitory influences on gonadotropin secretion can be evoked by stimulation of the midbrain. A similar effect was also described for ACTH secretion (Mangili et al. 1966, Fortier 1966). Furthermore, stimulation of the midbrain was shown to inhibit some neurons and to activate others of the supraoptic nucleus (Brooks et al. 1962), the hypothalamic ventromedial nucleus (Tsubokawa and Sutin 1963) and the posterior hypothalamus (Dafny and Feldman 1969). The foregoing account strongly suggests that the dual effect on gonadotropin secretion depends on the action of two systems.

Facilitatory effects on gonadotropin secretion were obtained by stimulating an area of the dorsal tegmentum located lateral and inferior to the periaqueductal grey substance. This area seems to be related to an ascending noradrenergic pathway since lesions at this level have been shown to produce decrease in norepinephrine content in telencephalic structures (Andén et al. 1966). The fibres of this pathway arise from neurons located in the lower brainstem (Dahlström and Fuxe 1964).

The facilitatory effect seems to depend on the activation of the amygdala as shown by the fact that transection of the ST abolished the ovulatory response which follows mesencephalic stimulation. Previous studies have demonstrated that ovulation induced by amygdaloid stimulation is prevented by interrupting the course of ST (Velasco and Taleisnik 1969a).

The contention that the mesencephalon projects to the amygdala finds support in several evidences. Stimulation of the midbrain tegmentum was found to modify the activity of amygdaloid units (Machne and Segundo 1956) and histochemical fluorescence studies reveal that a large number of norepinephrine-containing fibres ascend in the MFB and synapse in the amygdala (Andén et al. 1966). Furthermore, stimulation of the MFB caused release of norepinephrine from the amygdala (Stein and Wise 1969).

However, the possibility has not been completely discarded that the gonadotropin release after midbrain stimulation depends also on impulses arriving into the preoptic area or the hypothalamus in view of the fact that noradrenergic ascending fibres have been traced up to these areas (Andén et al. 1966).

The system which inhibits gonadotropin release is related to the paramedian region of the mesencephalon and corresponds to what Nauta has designed as the limbic midbrain area (Nauta 1958). This region extends rostrally from the ventral tegmental area, through the medial raphe nucleus up to the central grey substance in its more caudal aspect. From there the stimuli can reach the hypothalamus either directly by the DLF or by way of the MFB–hippocampus–CHT system.

The ascending fibres of the DLF which arise in the central grey substance project to various regions of the hypothalamus (Ban 1964, Guillery 1957). The current studies indicate that stimulation of this bundle inhibits LH secretion by acting on the hypothalamus and strongly suggest a direct action on the neurons which secrete LH-releasing factor. Electrophysiological studies in turn have demonstrated that evoked potentials can be recorded from the tuberal region of the hypothalamus after stimulation of the central grey substance (Beyer 1962).

The involvement of the hippocampus in the inhibition of gonadotropin secretion after midbrain stimulation is inferred from the fact that the blockade of ovulation was prevented by transecting the CHT since it has been demonstrated that interruption of the course of this tract avoids the blockade of spontaneous ovulation produced by hippocampal stimulation (Velasco and Taleisnik 1969b). Support for this view comes also from the fact that stimulation of the VTA elicited responses in the hippocampus (Green and Adey 1956).

Anatomical studies have demonstrated that the midbrain is linked with the hippocampus by the MFB, a bidirectional pathway which permits reciprocal influences between these two structures thus integrating the limbic forebrain–midbrain circuit of Nauta (1958).

It is of interest to note that the paramedian region of the mesencephalon contains numerous 5-HT cells (Andén et al. 1966). They give rise to ascending fibres most of which enter the MFB. After lesioning that bundle a decrease in brain levels of 5-HT was observed (Andén et al. 1966, Heller and Moore 1965). Furthermore, stimulation of the midbrain raphe nuclei was shown to increase 5-HT turnover (Dahlström and Fuxe 1964) and 5-hydroxy indole acetic acid content, a metabolic product of 5-HT (Gumulka et al. 1969) in forebrain. This facts may suggest that inhibition of gonadotropin secretion depends on the release of 5-HT. Support for this contention is the fact that implants of 5-HT into the 3rd ventricle blocked LH release (Eccleston et al. 1968).

These two antagonistic systems subserve the transmission from the periphery to the hypothalamus of most of the sensory stimuli affecting gonadotropin secretion. Their lower pole at the midbrain acts not only as a central station for the distribution of the flow of afferent impulses to the hypothalamus or to the limbic system but also modulates the magnitude of sensory inputs according to the information received from upper neural structures and the prevailing hormonal background.

ACKNOWLEDGEMENTS

This work was supported by grants M 70.23.C from the Population Council and from the Consejo Nacional de Investigaciones Científicas y Técnicas de Argentina.

REFERENCES

ANDÉN, N.-E., DAHLSTRÖM, A., FUXE, K., LARSSON, K., OLSON, L. and UNGERSTEDT, U. (1966): *Acta physiol. scand.* **67**, 313.
BAN, T. (1964): *Med. J. Osaka Univ.* **15**, 1.
BENEDETTI, W. L., APPELTAUER, L. C., REISSENWEBER, N. S., DOMINGUEZ, R., GRIÑO, R. and SAS, J. (1965): *Acta physiol. lat.-amer.* **15**, 218.
BEYER, C., TINDAL, J. J. and SAWYER, C. H. (1962): *Exp. Neurol.* **6**, 435.
BROOKS, C. McC., USHIYAMA, J. and LANGE, G. (1962): *Amer. J. Physiol.* **202**, 487.
BUNN, J. P. and EVERETT, J. W. (1957): *Proc. Soc. exp. Biol. (N. Y.)* **96**, 369.
CARRER, H. F. and TALEISNIK, S. (1970): *J. Endocr.* **48**, 527.
CRITCHLOW, V. (1958): *Endocrinology* **63**, 596.
DAFNY, N. and FELDMAN, S. (1969): *Electroenceph. clin. Neurophysiol.* **26**, 578.
DAHLSTRÖM, A. and FUXE, K. (1964): *Acta physiol. scand.* **62**, Suppl. **232**.
ECCLESTON, D., PADJEN, A. and RANDIC, M. (1968): *J. Physiol. (Lond.)* **201**, 228.
ENDRŐCZI, E., BABICHEV, V., HARTMANN, G. and KORÁNYI, L. (1968): *Endocr. Exp.* **2**, 1.
EVERETT, J. W. and RADFORD, H. M. (1961): *Proc. Soc. exp. Biol. (N. Y.)* **108**, 604.
FORTIER, C. (1966): In: *The Anterior Pituitary Gland.* Vol. 2. Ed. by G. W. Harris and B. T. Donovan. Univ. of California Press, Los Angeles. p. 195.
GREEN, J. D. and ADEY, W. R. (1956): *Electroenceph. clin. Neurophysiol.* **8**, 245.
GUILLERY, R. W. (1957): *J. Anat. (Lond.)* **91**, 91.
GUMULKA, W., SAMANIN, R., GARATTINI, S. and VALZELLI, L. (1969): *J. Pharmacol.* **8**, 830.
HALÁSZ, B. and GORSKI, R. A. (1967): *Endocrinology* **80**, 608.
HELLER, A. and MOORE, R. Y. (1965): *J. Pharmacol. exp. Ther.* **150**, 1.
KAWAKAMI, M. and SAWYER, C. H. (1959): *Endocrinology* **65**, 625.
KOIKEGAMI, H., YAMADA, T. and USUI, K. (1954): *Folia psychiat. neurol. jap.* **8**, 7.
MACHNE, X. and SEGUNDO, J. P. (1956): *J. Neurophysiol.* **19**, 232.
MANGILI, G., MOTTA, M. and MARTINI, L. (1966): In: *Neuroendocrinology.* Vol. 1. Ed. by L. Martini and W. F. Ganong. Academic Press, Los Angeles. p. 297.
NAUTA, W. J. H. (1958): *Brain* **81**, 319.
PEKARY, A. E., DAVIDSON, J. M. and ZONDEK, B. (1967): *Endocrinology* **80**, 365.
SHEALY, C. W. and PEELE, T. L. (1957): *J. Neurophysiol.* **20**, 125.
STEIN, L. and WISE, C. D. (1969): *J. comp. physiol. Psychol.* **67**, 189.
TALEISNIK, S., VELASCO, M. E. and ASTRADA, J. J. (1970): *J. Endocr.* **46**, 1.
TALEISNIK, S., CALIGARIS, L. and ASTRADA, J. J. (1971): In: *Proceedings of the IIIrd International Congress on Hormonal Steroids.* Excerpta Medica. (In press).
TSUBOKAWA, T. and SUTIN, J. (1963): *Electroenceph. clin. Neurophysiol.* **15**, 804.
VELASCO, M. E. and TALEISNIK, S. (1969a): *Endocrinology* **84**, 132.
VELASCO, M. E. and TALEISNIK, S. (1969b): *Endocrinology* **85**, 1154.
VELASCO, M. E. and TALEISNIK, S. (1972): *J. Endocr.* (In press).
WOOLEY, D. E. and TIMIRAS, P. S. (1962): *Endocrinology* **70**, 196.

CORRELATED CHANGES IN GONADOTROPIN RELEASE AND ELECTRICAL ACTIVITY OF THE HYPOTHALAMUS INDUCED BY ELECTRICAL STIMULATION OF THE HIPPOCAMPUS IN IMMATURE AND MATURE RATS

M. KAWAKAMI, E. TERASAWA, F. KIMURA and K. KUBO

2nd Department of Physiology
Yokohama City University School of Medicine
Yokohama, Japan

For the past forty years, attention has been focussed on the limbic structure implicated in gonadal function and sexual behaviour. Klüver and Bucy (1937), Schreiner and Kling (1953) and Green et al. (1957) demonstrated hypersexual behaviour in the monkey and cat with ablations of the pyriform cortex or amygdala, and MacLean (1957a, b) reported intensive grooming and penile erection following the after-discharges induced by electrical stimulation of the hippocampus in the rat, cat and monkey.

Furthermore, it was shown that electrical stimulation of the amygdala led to ovulation in the rabbit (Koikegami et al. 1954) and in the light-induced constant oestrous rat (Bunn and Everett 1959), while stimulation of the hippocampus blocked spontaneous ovulation in the rat (Velasco and Taleisnik 1969) and slightly facilitated the induction of ovulation in the rabbit (Kawakami et al. 1966a, Kawakami et al. 1967). Bilateral lesions of the hippocampus or amygdala in the adult rat altered the oestrous cycle (Koikegami et al. 1960, Koikegami 1964) and destruction of the amygdala in the immature rat induced precocious puberty (Elwers and Critchlow 1960, 1961), while destruction of the hippocampus delayed onset of puberty (Riss 1958, Riss et al. 1963). It was also found that limbic structures played a role in the feedback control of gonadal hormone, as indicated by the experiments of sex steroid implantation or electrophysiological studies (Kawakami et al. 1967, Kawakami and Saito 1967, Kawakami and Terasawa 1967, Stumpf 1968, Davidson 1969, Kawakami et al. 1970a, Terasawa and Timiras 1968, Terasawa and Sawyer 1969b, Sawyer 1970, Kawakami and Kubo 1971).

Recently, Halász and Köves demonstrated in their brilliant work of neural deafferentation that the neural trigger for ovulation is located in the medial preoptic area, i.e. animals in which this region was deafferented both anteriorly and rostrally ovulated, while ovulation was blocked in rats with a frontal cut behind the optic chiasma. The animals with preoptic deafferentation had, however, irregular cycles suggesting that other structures of the brain are involved in the regulation of pituitary–gonadotropic function (Köves and Halász 1970). However, the functional significance of each part of the limbic areas is not yet clearly defined. Therefore, a study has been made to elucidate the nature of limbic function, especially the manner of modulating control of the hypothalamo–pituitary–gonadal system by means of electrophysiological methods and radioimmunoassay.

MATERIAL AND METHODS

Wistar female rats weighing 180 to 250 g were maintained in a room illuminated from 5 a.m. to 7 p.m. Vaginal smears were taken every morning, and at least 2 consecutive 4-day cycles were determined from the beginning of the experiments.

Several kinds of electrodes were used for this experiment. For the electrical stimulation, concentric bipolar electrodes made of stainless steel were employed. The electrodes consisted of an insulated inner wire with the exception of a tip of 0.1 mm (0.13 mm in diameter) which served as the cathode and an outer barrel (0.15 mm exposed surface) which served as the anode. For the recording of the MUA, the macro-micro electrodes (tip diameter was 20 to 40 μ) made of No. 00 stainless steel insect pins with stainless steel attachments (diameter 100 μ) and insulated with epoxilite, were used. For the recording of single unit activity, tungsten electrodes which were electro-polished in a sodium nitrate saturated solution to reduce the tip to less than 1 μ in diameter and coated by epoxilite, were used.

Throughout the experiments, several kinds of electrodes were inserted stereotaxically into the brain according to the atlas of Albe-Fessard et al. (1966) and that of Sherwood and Timiras (1968).

Recordings of MUA were performed acutely or chronically. In the acute experiment, animals were anaesthetized with urethane (1.2 g/kg body weight) or pentobarbital (30 mg/kg body weight), and macro-micro electrodes were inserted into several regions in the brain, and recordings were made by polygraph connected to a preamplifier, an oscilloscope, rectifier and RC integrator (Sanei Co.). In the chronic experiment, electrodes were fixed by dental cement after the insertion of electrodes under pentobarbital anaesthesia, and soldered to an ITT Cannon plug for the leads to a preamplifier. Unanaesthetized and unrestrained recordings were performed when in the animal the oestrous cycle was restored after the electrode implantation.

Recording of single unit activity was made as follows: the animals were anaesthetized with urethane (1.2 g/kg body weight) from 9 a.m. to 10 a.m. and placed in a stereotaxic apparatus. After the insertion of the recording electrodes for EEG and unit discharges, and electrodes for the electrical stimulation, the skull window was covered with agar-saline solution. Micro electrodes were connected to a push–pull cathode follower preamplifier (Nihon Kohden Co.). The output was fed into a polygraph for continuous writing, directly on paper, of unit discharges. Electrocorticogram was recorded simultaneously, to compare the changes in unit activity with those in the EEG pattern.

The parameters of electrical stimulation were as follows: prepuberal animals were stimulated for 30 min (30 sec on and 30 sec off for each 1 min) with 100 μA of monophasic square wave pulses of 0.1 msec duration at a frequency of 100 c/s on the day following implantation. Thirty minutes after stimulation, the animals were anaesthetized with ether, and blood and APG samples were collected.

In the mature female rats the train pulses of square wave for the electrical stimulation were delivered for 30 min. The parameters of the MPO stimulation were 50 to 500 μA at 100 c/s, with 0.5 msec given for 30 sec on/off periods, and that of the HPC were 20 to 100 μA at 100 c/s, with 0.1 msec given for 30 sec on/off periods.

Animals for measurement of gonadotropin were prepared as follows: in the acute preparation the electrodes were inserted under the pentobarbital anaesthesia (sodium pentobarbital, Abbott 30 mg/kg body weight, was injected 15 min before 2 p.m. in the MPO stimulated animals and 30 min before starting the stimulation in the HPC stimulated animals) and electrical stimulation was performed through the concentric bipolar electrodes. Animals were sacrificed at various times after the stimulation. In the chronic preparation the concentric electrodes were implanted into the HPC under pentobarbital anaesthesia preceding the stimulation. Unanaesthetized and unrestrained animals were stimulated when the oestrous cycle was restored, and sacrificed at various times after the stimulation under ether anaesthesia. In the immature rats, the electrodes were implanted into several regions of the brain one day before sacrifice (27 and 28 days of age). Blood samples were collected by incision of the femoral vein, then the head was guillotined and APG was quickly removed. APG was weighed and homogenized with 2.0 ml of phosphate buffered saline. All samples were stored at $-20°C$ until the assay started.

The assay procedure of LH, FSH and prolactin was based on the methods described by Niswender et al. (1968).

Ovulation was determined microscopically by the presence of ova in oviducts the next morning following treatment.

Histological sections were made to determine the sites of electrodes used in stimulation and recording.

Abbreviations: AMYG: amygdala, APG: anterior pituitary gland, ARC: arcuate nucleus, HPC: hippocampus, IC: internal capsule, LPO: lateral preoptic area, ME: median eminence, MPO: medial preoptic area, MUA: multiple unit activity, NAC: nucleus accumbens, OC: optic chiasma, SC: suprachiasmatic nucleus, SO: supraoptic nucleus, SEPT: septum, Sup. Coll.: superior colliculus, TDB: nucleus diagonal bundle of Broca, Olf.: olfactory tract, VMH: ventromedial hypothalamic nucleus

RESULTS

ELECTRICAL ACTIVITY IN THE MPO AND THE ARC INDUCED BY ELECTRICAL STIMULATION OF THE LIMBIC STRUCTURES

Changes in electrical activity in the MPO and the ARC were observed in relation to the release of gonadotropin, when electrical stimulation was applied to several parts of the limbic–forebrain area under pentobarbital or urethane anaesthesia.

1. Single and multiple unit activity in the ARC during oestrous cycle.

The spontaneous firing patterns in the ARC neurones differed from those in the neurones of the limbic structures and the midbrain reticular formation. The former showed a low frequency (0.2 to 4 c/s) and a tendency to make a burst, and the latter showed a high frequency (5 to 10 c/s). The burst in the ARC lasted for about 3 to 7 min which was followed by a silent interval of 15 to 20 min alternately. During the burst, the firing rate of the ARC neurones increased its frequency and reached about 10 c/s. There was no significant relationship between the firing pattern of the ARC neurones and the EEG patterns of the frontal cortex. The appearance of bursts in the spontaneous single unit discharges in the ARC was most frequently observed between noon and 4 p.m. throughout the 4-day oestrous cycle, particularly in the afternoon of pro-oestrus (Fig. 1). It was rather indistinct on the days of oestrus, dioestrus I and dioestrus II. The firing rate of spontaneous discharges was consistently low throughout the cycle, except on the day of dioestrus I when the rate of discharges increased.

An increase of unit firing in the ARC was induced by electrical stimulation of the MPO on the days of pro-oestrus, oestrus, dioestrus I and dioestrus II. However, the firing rate in the medial part of the VMH and in the transient zone between the ARC and the VMH decreased by stimulation of the MPO throughout the oestrous cycle (Fig. 2).

Threshold current to increase the firing rate of the ARC discharges which was induced by the MPO stimulation, was lowest (i.e. 40 μA) on the day of pro-oestrus and highest (i.e. more than 80 μA) on the day of dioestrus I as shown in Fig. 3. The facilitation of threshold current of the ARC discharges on the day of pro-oestrus through the day of oestrus might depend on the circulatory level of oestrogen, e.g., the threshold current was lower in the ovariectomized-oestrogen primed rats (oestradiol benzoate in sesame oil, 5 μg $\times$ 2, subcutaneously) than that of ovariectomized-nontreated rats.

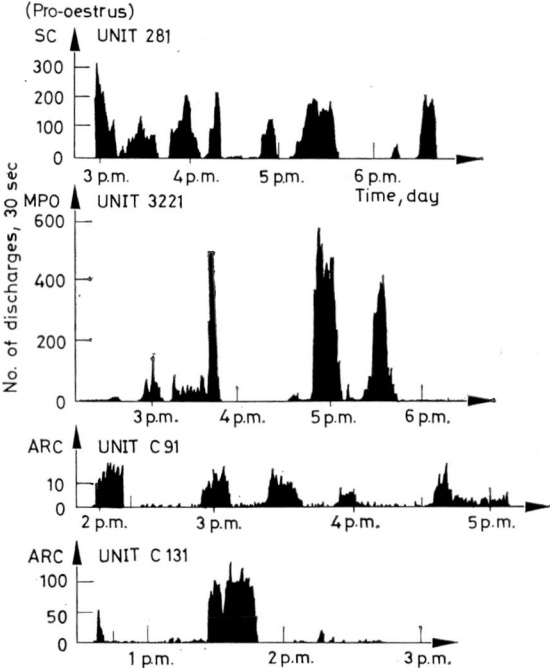

Fig. 1. Spontaneous firing rate of the single unit activity in the SC, MPO and ARC under urethane anaesthesia on the day of pro-oestrus. Ordinate indicates the number of discharges per 30 sec, and abscissa the time of day (Kawakami, M., Saito, H. and Sakuma, Y., unpublished data)

When stimulation of the MPO induced ovulation, which was checked on the following morning, the elevation of MUA in the ARC was observed in the stimulated rats, both on the days of pro-oestrus and dioestrus II. That is, on the day of pro-oestrus a remarkable elevation occurred during the stimulation and lasted for 2 hours after stimulation, in contrast to the changes occurring prominently for 2 to 4 hours after stimulation on the day of dioestrus II. However, this elevation of MUA was not observed after stimulation, when the stimulus could not induce ovulation, even though a slight elevation was observed during and shortly after stimulation.

Electrical stimulation of MPO or TDB, also, induced an increase in the firing rate of the unit discharges in the ARC for about 2 hours, when ovulation was observed the following day.

2. Effects of electrical stimulation of the SEPT on single and multiple unit activity in the MPO and the ARC.

On the day of pro-oestrus stimulation of the medial part of the SEPT induced elevation of MUA in MPO and ARC, while stimulation of the lateral part of the SEPT depressed MUA in the ARC and the MPO for more than 2 hours (Fig. 4). Stimulation of the medial SEPT induced ovulation in the pentobarbital anaesthe-

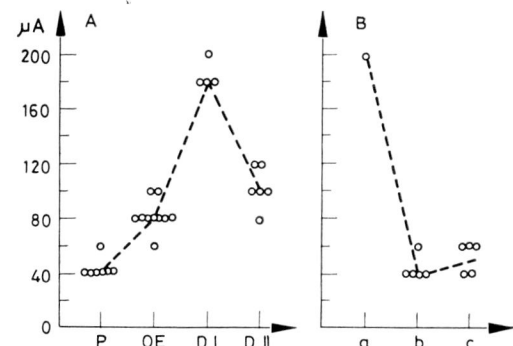

Fig. 2. Threshold current of MPO stimulation inducing facilitation of ARC unit firing in the cyclic (P = pro-oestrus, OE: oestrus, DI = dioestrus I and DII = dioestrus II) and ovariectomized (a, b, and c) rats. a = non-treated ovariectomized, b = oestrogen (oestradiol 5 μg ×2 s.c.) primed ovariectomized, c = oestrogen (oestradiol 5 μg × 2 s.c.) and progesterone (1 mg, s.c.)-primed ovariectomized

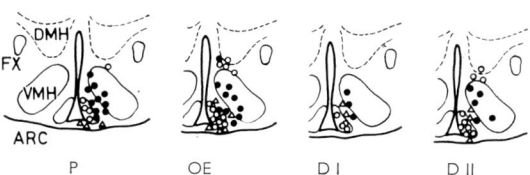

Fig. 3. Schematic illustration of the effect of MPO stimulation on unit firing in the medial basal hypothalamic region in the cyclic rats (P = pro-oestrus, OE = oestrus, DI = dioestrus I and DII = dioestrus II). (○) increase, (●) decrease or (△) no changes of unit firing were induced by MPO stimulation

tized animals during the critical period, whereas stimulation of the lateral SEPT failed to induce it. Stimulation of the medial part of the SEPT induced an increase in the firing rate of the MPO neurones with a latency of about 2.5 msec (Fig. 5).

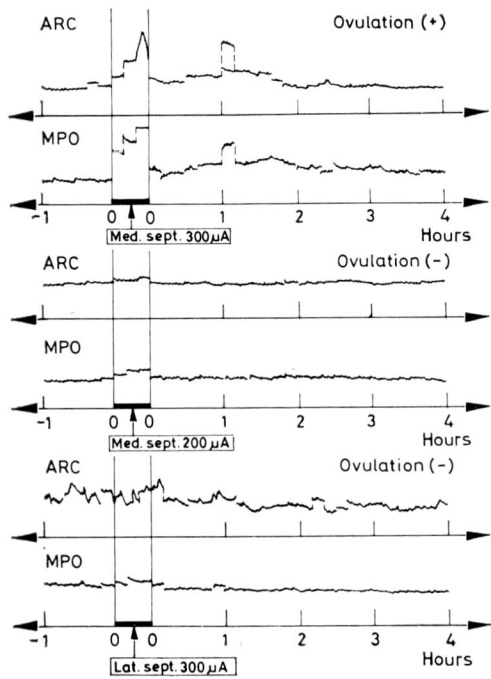

Fig. 4. Effect of electrical stimulation of SEPT on MUA in ARC and MPO. Elevation was observed during and after SEPT stimulation, when it induced ovulation on the following day

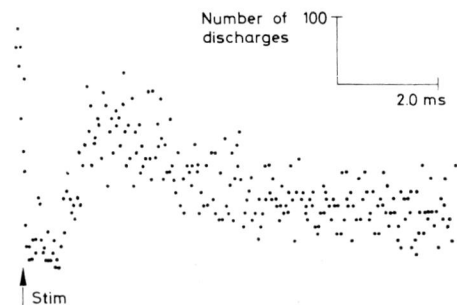

Fig. 5. Post-stimulus histogram showing the facilitatory effect of the medial part of SEPT stimulation on the MPO unit discharges in the pro-oestrous rat. The photograph was taken by the superposition of three trials of electrical stimulation, which was 50 μA of square wave at 100 c/s, with 0.1 msec given for 5 sec. The unit discharges increased with a latency of about 2.5 msec

3. Effects of electrical stimulation of the AMYG on single and multiple unit activity in MPO and ARC.

Electrical stimulation of the medial part of the AMYG caused elevation of MUA and an increase in unit firing rate in the medial part of SEPT, MP and ARC. Stimulation of this region was also effective in inducing ovulation in the pentobarbital anaesthetized rats, which blocked spontaneous ovulation on the day of pro-oestrus (Fig. 6).

4. Effects of electrical stimulation of the HPC on single and multiple unit activity in the MPO, ARC and their adjacent area.

On the day of pro-oestrus HPC (CA_2 and CA_3) stimulation with 100 c/s frequency induced relatively complicated changes of MUA in the ARC. That is, MUA in the ARC clearly diminished in 8 out of 18 rats, elevated slightly in 2 rats, and showed no changes in the remaining 8 rats. In the case of diminished MUA, the depression started during stimulation and lasted for several hours. Additionally, HPC stimulation depressed the marked elevation of MUA in the ARC that was induced by MPO stimulation in 4 out of 5 rats (Fig. 7). The HPC stimulation blocked ovulation which had been induced by MPO stimulation and blocked

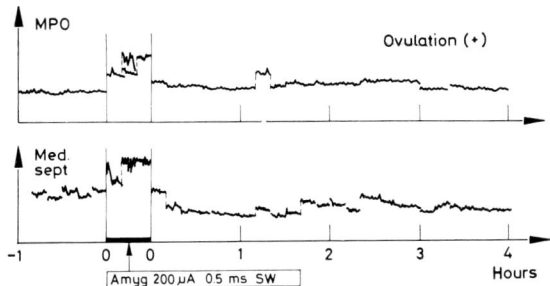

Fig. 6. Effect of electrical stimulation of medial AMYG on the MUA in MPO and the medial SEPT. The elevation of MUA was observed in both regions during the stimulation of AMYG

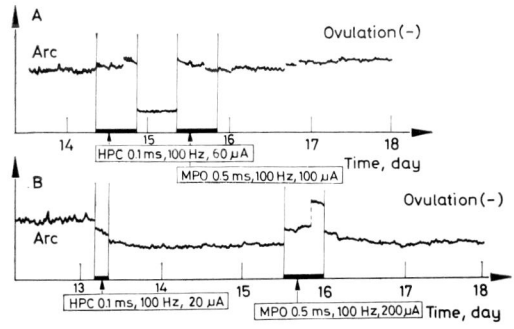

Fig. 7. Effect of electrical stimulation of HPC and MPO on MUA. HPC stimulation depressed MUA in the ARC for more than 2.5 hours and MPO stimulation following HPC stimulation elevated it to the control level, but not higher. Ovulation was not observed on the following morning

spontaneous ovulation as well. Simultaneous stimulation to HPC (60 μA) and MPO (100 μA) caused a slight elevation of MUA in the ARC–ME, and blocked ovulation. Sham stimulation to HPC followed by MPO stimulation markedly elevated the level of MUA in the ARC–ME and induced ovulation. HPC stimulation also decreased MUA in TDB in 5 out of 7 rats and stimulation of the lateral SEPT did not change MUA in the MPO in all 7 rats examined.

In contrast to the results of high frequency stimulation, MUA in ARC, MPO and TDB increased, when the electrical stimulation was delivered with 8 c/s or 60 c/s (Fig. 8). Thus, effects of electrical stimulation in the HPC (CA_2 and CA_3) seemed to depend on frequency component of the stimuli. These differences in the effects followed by the frequency component could not be observed when electrodes were in the fimbria, i.e., HPC stimulation lowered MUA level in ARC at 100 c/s and elevated it at 8 c/s. In contrast, when the electrode tip was located in the fimbria, MUA level in the ARC diminished transiently during the stimulation either with 8 c/s or 100 c/s, and then returned to the control level, sometimes reaching a higher level than the control level.

Furthermore, when HPC (CA_2 and CA_3) was stimulated at low frequency, MUA in the ARC showed a different response depending upon the timing of stimulation. Stimulation of low frequency (8 c/s) in the early afternoon increased MUA in the ARC, while the same stimulation in the late afternoon or night did not produce any changes or rather slightly decreased it. Stimulation of high frequency (100 c/s) did not cause such reversed effects.

On the day of pro-oestrus, HPC (CA_2 and CA_3) stimulation with 100 c/s at lower current (40 μA) inhibited the unit firing rate in the medial and dorsal parts

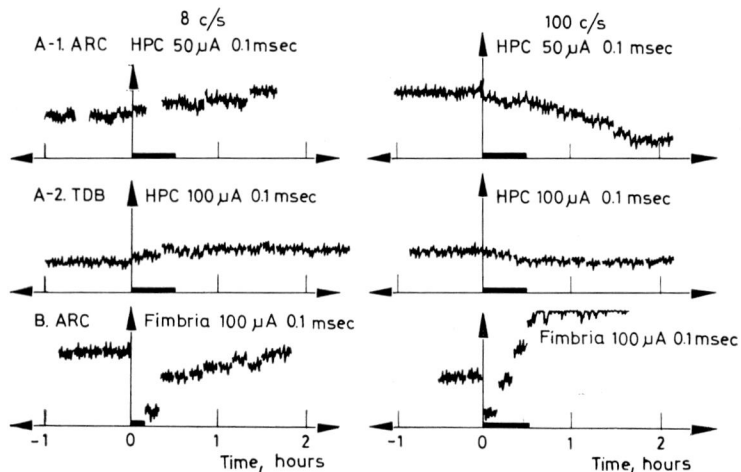

Fig. 8. Effect of electrical stimulation to HPC and the fimbria on MUA changes in ARC or TDB. HPC stimulation with low frequency induces elevation of MUA in ARC, while with high frequency it depresses it (A-1). HPC stimulation with low frequency elevates MUA in TDB, while with high frequency it diminishes it (A-2). Stimulation to the fimbria induces biphasic responses, depression followed by elevation, in ARC either with high or low frequency (B) (Kawakami, M., Konda, N. and Shinohara, Y., unpublished data)

of the ARC and facilitated it in the laterobasal part of the ARC, as shown in Fig. 9. On the day of dioestrus II, HPC stimulation did not change unit discharge in the ARC and MPO with higher current of stimulation (80 µA).

5. Effects of sex steroids on electrical activity in the limbic structures.

It was already found that the effect of sex steroids on the electrical activity of the hypothalamus differed depending on the timing of administration of the steroids, either in castrated or cyclic rats (Kawakami et al. 1970b). Such timing difference was also observed in MUA of the limbic structures as follows:

Oestrogen. When oestrogen (oestradiol benzoate in sesame oil, 25 µg per whole body, subcutaneously) was administered at 10 a.m., MUA in the medial part of AMYG showed a remarkable decrease within 3.5 hours, and remained at that level for more than 16 hours. When it was administered at 6 p.m., MUA elevated only slightly (Fig. 10).

When oestrogen was administered at 10 a.m., MUA in the dorsal HPC showed a decrease 5 hours after the injection. The decreased levels lasted for more than 16 hours. When the injection was made at 6 p.m., MUA started to increase within 1 hour, and remained at a constant level for more than 8 hours (Fig. 10).

The pattern of MUA response in HPC or AMYG to exogenous oestrogen was almost similar to that of MPO. However, it is characteristic that the latency of response in the HPC and AMYG was shorter than that in the hypothalamic areas.

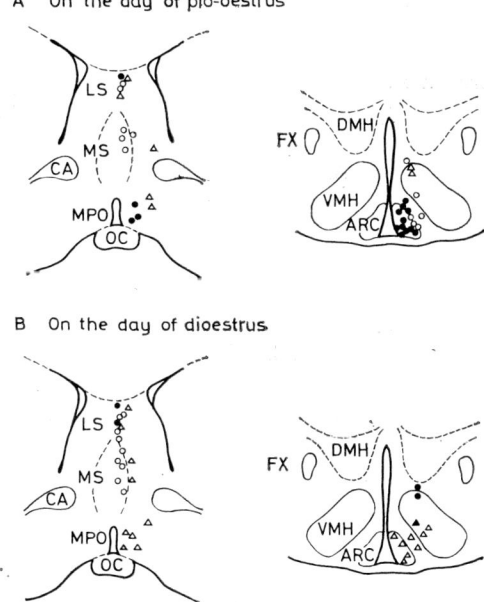

Fig. 9. Schematic illustration of the effect of dorsal HPC (CA_2 and CA_3) stimulation on unit firing of SEPT, MPO and medial basal hypothalamic region on the day of pro-oestrus (A) and dioestrus II (B): (○) increase, (●) decrease or (△) no change of unit firing were induced by HPC stimulation

Progestin. Administration of progesterone (progesterone propionate in sesame oil, 5 mg per whole body, subcutaneously), either at 10 a.m. or at 6 p.m., failed to induce any change of MUA in the medial part of AMYG.

When progesterone was administered at 7 p.m., MUA in the HPC increased slightly about 2 hours after the injection, and remained at the level for approximately 8.5 hours. When it was administered at 6 p.m., MUA started to increase about 3.5 hours after the injection, and remained elevated for more than 14 hours. Response of MUA in the HPC to progesterone was similar to that in the ARC.

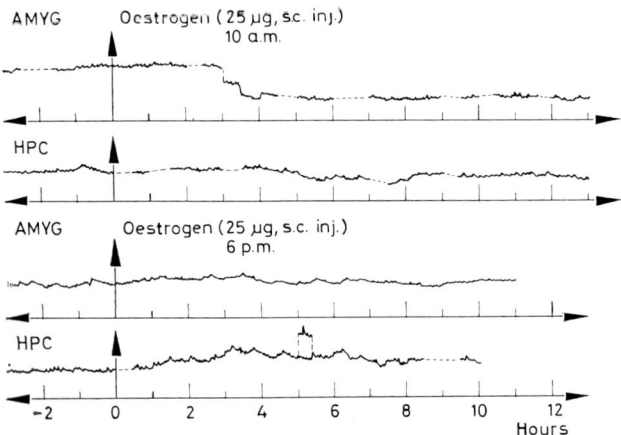

Fig. 10. Effect of oestrogen on MUA in the AMYG and HPC. When 25 μg of oestrogen was administered subcutaneously at 10 a.m. to ovariectomized rats, MUA in the AMYG decreased 3 hours after the administration for more than 16 hours and MUA in the HPC also decreased after 5 hours for more than 16 hours. When it was administered at 6 p.m. MUA in the AMYG decreased slightly but the MUA in the HPC increased 1 hour after the administration

EFFECTS OF ELECTRICAL STIMULATION OF THE LIMBIC–HYPOTHALAMIC REGION ON GONADOTROPIN RELEASE

Effects of electrical stimulation of the brain on gonadotropin release in the immature rats

Electrical stimulation was applied to the TDB, MPO, AMYG and HPC of immature rats.

1. LH and FSH concentration in the APG. There was no significance between the control group and the sham-operated group either in LH or in FSH concentration of APG. Electrical stimulation of MPO, TDB, AMYG (medial part) and HPC (CA_2 and CA_3) increased APG concentration of LH and FSH. The ARC stimulation induced an increase of LH and FSH when animals were killed

at 0 min, however, neither LH nor FSH increased when they were killed 30 min after the stimulation (Figs 11 and 12).

2. Serum LH and FSH. TDB stimulation was effective to increase serum level of LH, while stimulation of HPC increased serum level of FSH when animals were killed 30 min after the stimulation. An elevation of serum LH and FSH was observed by stimulation of both ARC and MPO, when animals were killed 0 min after the stimulation. AMYG stimulation seemed to slightly increase serum FSH, though it was statistically insignificant. Serum level of FSH was depressed by stimulation of the MPO (Figs 13 and 14).

Thus, electrical stimulation of AMYG and HPC was highly effective to synthesize and release pituitary FSH in the prepuberal animals, in contrast to the fact that stimulation of these areas did only increase pituitary LH.

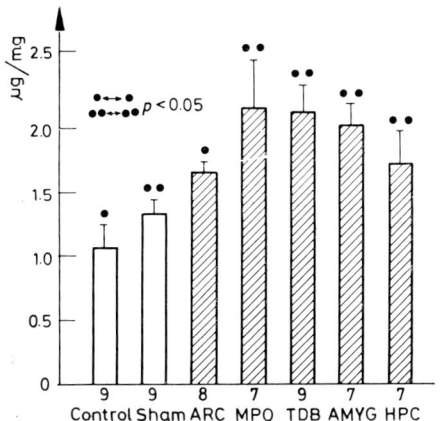

Fig. 11. Effect of electrical stimulation of several regions in the brain on pituitary content of LH in prepuberal rats. MPO, TDB, AMYG and HPC stimulated groups were significantly higher than the sham stimulated group. The ARC stimulated group was significantly higher than the control groups

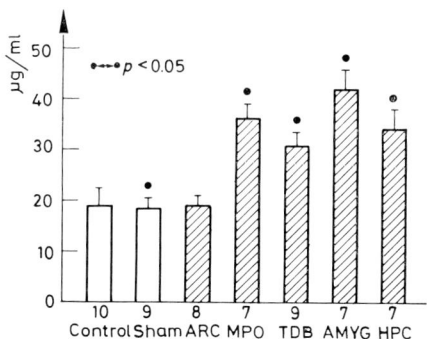

Fig. 12. Effect of electrical stimulation of several regions in the brain on pituitary FSH (μg/mg) in prepuberal rats. The stimulation of MPO, TDB, AMYG and HPC increased it

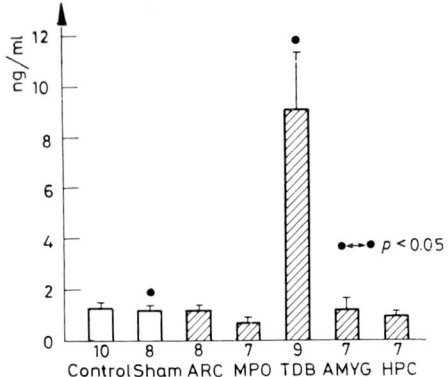

Fig. 13. Effect of electrical stimulation of the brain on serum LH in prepuberal rats. The TDB stimulated group was significantly higher than the sham stimulated group

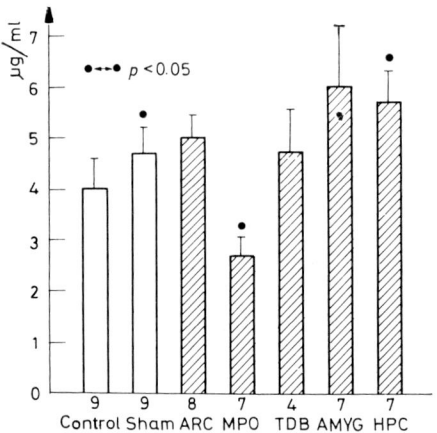

Fig. 14. Effect of electrical stimulation of the brain on serum FSH in the prepuberal rats. The HPC stimulated group was significantly higher and MPO stimulated group was significantly lower when compared with the sham stimulated group

Effects of electrical stimulation of HPC on gonadotropin release in the mature rats

Radioimmunoassay experiments in mature rats were performed during the winter and spring (December 1970–May 1971). Stimulation with 60 μA at 100 c/s or 8 c/s was delivered through the chronically implanted electrodes. Blood samples were taken 0 or 30 min after the stimulation. Experiments were performed between 10 a.m. and 2 p.m. on each day of the oestrous cycle.

Electrical stimulation of HPC at 100 c/s did not induce any change in the basal level of LH throughout the oestrous cycle (Fig. 15). Serum level of FSH increased immediately after the stimulation on the day of oestrus, while on the day of dioestrus II it decreased significantly (Fig. 16). Stimulation on the days of dioestrus I and pro-oestrus did not induce changes in serum FSH. However, stimulation with 8 c/s on the day of pro-oestrus induced a decrease of serum FSH. The HPC stimulation on the day of pro-oestrus inhibited the serum level of prolactin. This inhibitory effect was stronger when HPC was stimulated with a frequency of 8 c/s (Fig. 17). A decrease in serum prolactin after stimulation was also observed on the day of oestrus.

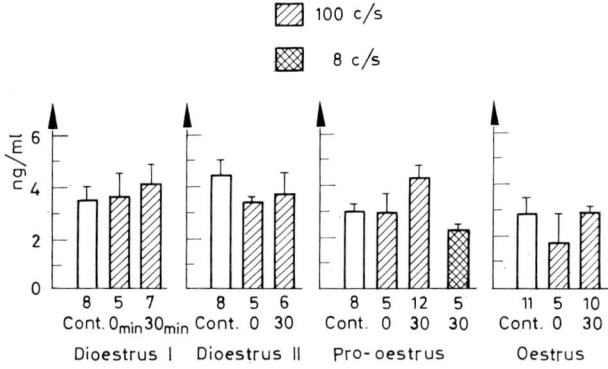

Fig. 15. Effect of electrical stimulation of the dorsal hippocampus on the serum level of LH in chronic experiment. The stimulation either with 100 c/s or 8 c/s induced no significant change on the basal level of LH throughout the oestrous cycle

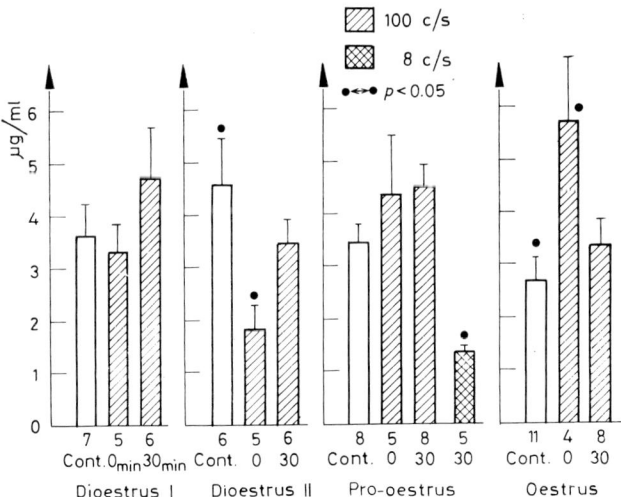

Fig. 16. Effect of electrical stimulation of the dorsal hippocampus on the serum level of FSH in chronic experiment. Stimulation with 100 c/s in the oestrus increased the release of FSH and decreased in dioestrus II. In pro-oestrus 8 c/s of stimulation decreased FSH content in serum

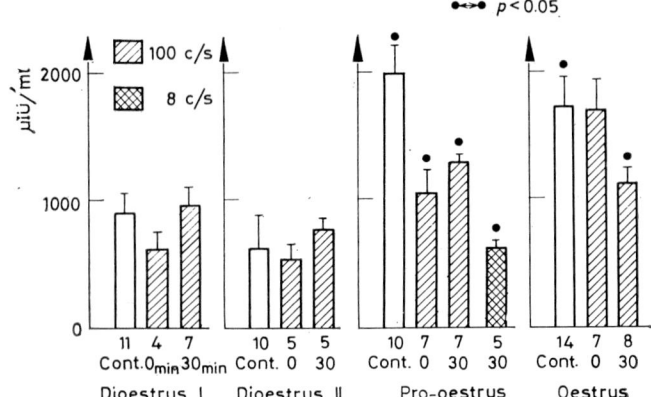

Fig. 17. Effect of electrical stimulation of the dorsal hippocampus on the serum level of prolactin in chronic experiment. Prolactin level was decreased by the stimulation either with 100 c/s or 8 c/s in pro-oestrus and oestrus

Effect of electrical stimulation of HPC with MPO stimulation on gonadotropin release in mature rats

Experimental animals were grouped in the following way: Group A, control rats under pentobarbital anaesthesia killed between 2 p.m. and 4 p.m. Group B, MPO stimulated rats. Blood samples were taken 0, 30, 60 and 120 min after the stimulation and killed immediately after blood sampling. Group B', ovulation was examined the following morning. Group C, HPC stimulation was applied simultaneously with MPO stimulation. Group D, HPC stimulation was applied 2 hours preceding MPO stimulation, which was performed between 2 p.m. and 4 p.m. The animals of dioestrus II and pro-oestrus were examined in this group. Group E, HPC stimulation was applied 4 hours preceding MPO stimulation, which was performed between 2 p.m. and 4 p.m. The animals of dioestrus II and pro-oestrus were examined in this group. Groups D' and E', ovulation was examined on the following morning, under the same condition as in the groups D and E.

1. Effect of electrical stimulation of the MPO on induction of ovulation.

The threshold current to induce ovulation by the MPO stimulation was 50 to 100 μA in the afternoon of pro-oestrus and about 500 μA in the afternoon of dioestrus II.

2. Effect of electrical stimulation of the MPO on LH and FSH release.

Electrical stimulation of the MPO induced LH release throughout the oestrous cycle, though the time of release differed on the day of pro-oestrus from that on the remaining days of the cycle, i.e. on the day of pro-oestrus, the increased level of serum LH reached the maximum 30 min later and returned to the control level after 60 min, while on the remaining days of the cycle, it reached the maximum at 60 min and did not return to the control level even 120 min after electrical stimulation. Electrical stimulation of MPO induced increase of serum FSH on the days of dioestrus II and pro-oestrus but not on the days of oestrus and dioestrus I.

3. Effect of electrical stimulation of HPC on blocking ovulation.

On the day of pro-oestrus, simultaneous stimulation of HPC and MPO blocked ovulation under pentobarbital anaesthesia. The threshold current of HPC stimulation to block ovulation (which had been induced by 100 μA of electrical stimulation of the MPO) was 40 μA with 100 c/s and 0.1 msec duration. This inhibitory effect of HPC on the release of ovulatory hormone lasted more than 4 hours after stimulation made at the threshold current. The simultaneous stimulation of HPC and MPO blocked ovulation on the day of dioestrus II.

4. Effect of electrical stimulation of HPC with MPO stimulation on APG content of LH and FSH.

HPC stimulation inhibited the rise of pituitary content of LH, which was induced by electrical stimulation of MPO throughout the oestrous cycle as shown in Fig. 18. While the inhibitory action of HPC with a current of 60 μA was stronger than that of MPO with 100 μA on the day of pro-oestrus, the action of HPC was almost equivalent to MPO with a current of 500 μA on the days of oestrus, dioestrus I and dioestrus II.

Simultaneous stimulation of HPC and MPO increased APG concentration of FSH each day throughout the oestrous cycle, while MPO stimulation induced an increase in FSH only on the days of dioestrus II and pro-oestrus (Fig. 19). Since HPC stimulation increased pituitary FSH each day of the cycle (Fig. 20), HPC itself may have an ability to increase FSH in APG. There was no significant difference in the effect of the frequency component between 100 c/s and 60 c/s, i.e. both 100 c/s and 60 c/s of stimulation to HPC either with or without MPO stimulation increased APG content of FSH (Fig. 20).

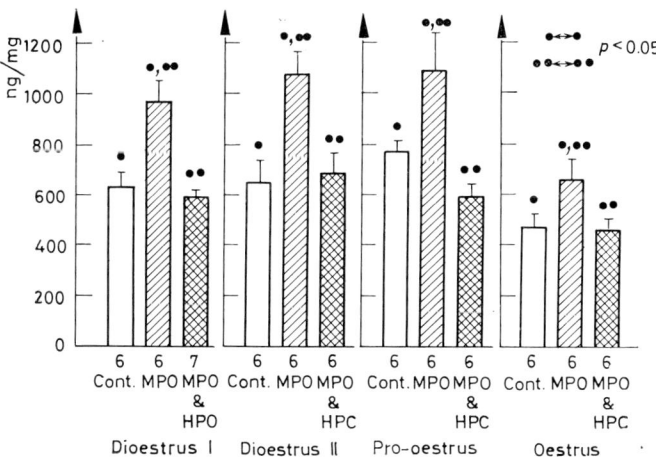

Fig. 18. Effect of electrical stimulation of HPC with MPO stimulation on LH in the pituitary gland (ng/mg) during oestrous cycle. MPO stimulation elevated it throughout the oestrous cycle, while simultaneous stimulation of MPO and HPC inhibited an increase of LH which was induced by MPO stimulation alone

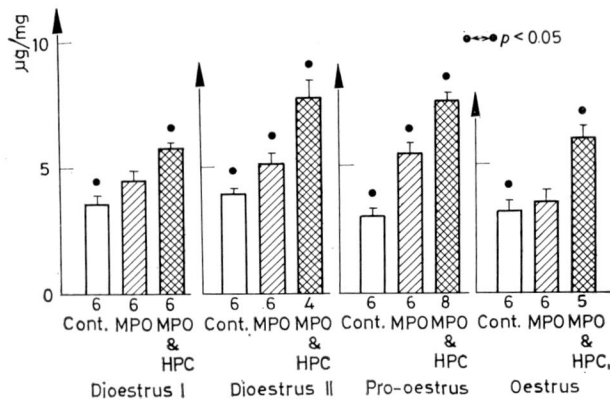

Fig. 19. Effect of electrical stimulation of the HPC with the MPO stimulation on FSH in the pituitary gland ($\mu g/mg$) during oestrous cycle. Simultaneous stimulation of HPC and MPO was highly effective to induce the elevation of pituitary FSH throughout the oestrous cycle

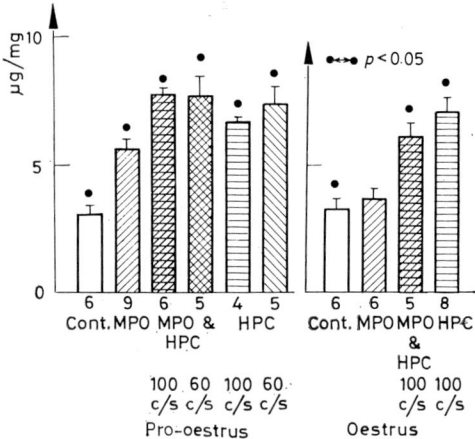

Fig. 20. Comparison with the effect of electrical stimulation of the HPC with the frequency of 60 c/s or 100 c/s on the days of pro-oestrus and oestrus. HPC stimulation induced the elevation of pituitary FSH either with or without MPO stimulation. There was no difference between the effects followed by the stimulation with 100 c/s and that with 60 c/s

5. Effect of electrical stimulation of HPC with MPO stimulation on serum LH.

Throughout the cycle, HPC stimulation inhibited LH increase, which was induced by MPO stimulation. With simultaneous HPC and MPO stimulation serum LH is significantly lower than that with MPO stimulation alone and it is the same as the control level. Furthermore, MPO stimulation was still ineffective to induce LH release not only 2 hours but even 4 hours after HPC stimulation (Fig. 21).

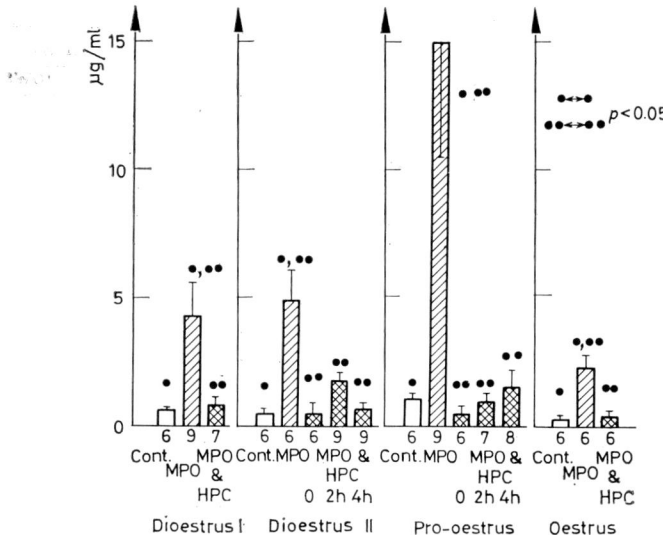

Fig. 21. Effect of electrical stimulation of HPC and MPO on serum LH. Simultaneous stimulation of HPC and MPO (MPO and HPC) inhibited the MPO induced elevation in serum LH each day throughout the oestrous cycle. HPC stimulation inhibited the MPO induced LH elevation, even when MPO was stimulated with a latency of 2 hours (MPO and HPC · 2 h) and 4 hours (MPO and HPC · 4 h)

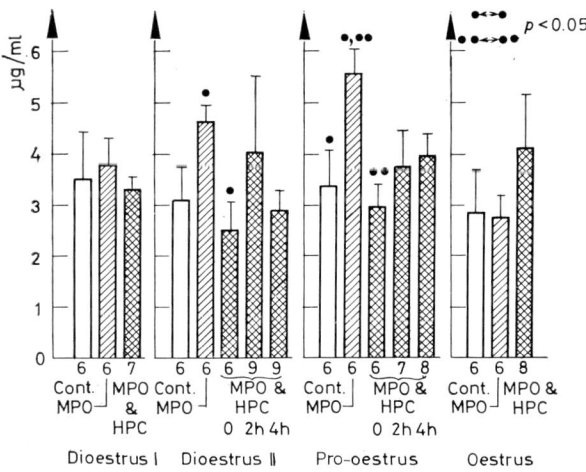

Fig. 22. Effect of electrical stimulation of MPO and HPC on serum FSH. Increase of serum FSH, that was induced by MPO stimulation on the day of pro-oestrus, was inhibited by HPC stimulation when both stimuli were applied simultaneously

6. Effect of electrical stimulation of HPC with MPO stimulation on serum FSH.

Electrical stimulation of HPC inhibited the release of FSH, which was induced by MPO stimulation on the days of dioestrus II and pro-oestrus. However, on the day of oestrus HPC and MPO stimulation increased serum FSH, yet this elevation was not observed in MPO stimulation alone. On the day of dioestrus I HPC stimulation did not induce changes in serum FSH either with or without MPO stimulation (Fig. 22).

DISCUSSION

Since Hohlweg and Junkmann (1932) postulated the existence of a sex centre in the hypothalamus, there is no doubt that the function of the anterior pituitary is under the control of the central nervous system. Today, it is generally believed that there are two "tonic and phasic" centres in the hypothalamus concerned with the maintenance and release of gonadotropin. Basal secretion of gonadotropic hormones is controlled by the medial basal hypothalamus, as shown by the results that a gross lesion of the median eminence and the adjacent area of the tuberal region leads to gonadal atrophy and to reduction of the pituitary LH and FSH in several species of animals (Dey 1943, Flerkó 1953, Bogdanove 1957, Flerkó and Bárdos 1959, D'Angelo 1959, Taleisnik and McCann 1961) and that the hypophysiotropic area in the medial basal hypothalamus can only maintain the normal structure and function of the anterior pituitary gland (Flerkó 1963, Halász and Pupp, 1965, Halász et al. 1965, Szentágothai et al. 1968). That the cyclic secretion of gonadotropic hormones is controlled by the anterior and preoptic area of the hypothalamus is proved by the facts that a lesion of these areas in the rat induces continuous vaginal oestrus (Dey 1941, Hillarp 1949, Greer 1953, Flerkó 1954, D'Angelo and Kravatz 1960, Flerkó and Bárdos 1960), and that the electrical and electrochemical stimulation of the medial preoptic–septal complex replaces neural surge in the rat which blocks spontaneous discharge of ovulatory hormone with pentobarbital anaesthesia (Everett and Radford 1961, Gorski and Barraclough 1963, Everett 1964, Everett et al. 1964, Terasawa and Sawyer 1969a, Kawakami and Terasawa 1970, Cramer and Barraclough 1971). In the anterior preoptic area a feedback centre for ovarian steroids exists controlling the cyclic discharge of gonadotropic hormones (Flerkó 1957, Flerkó and Bárdos 1961, Barraclough et al. 1964, Redmond 1968, Davidson 1969, Terasawa and Sawyer 1970).

It has been elucidated by several authors that the neurones in the anterior preoptic area involved in LH release may pass through the basal hypothalamus. Everett (1964) by means of electrochemical stimulation, Halász and Gorski (1967) by means of neural deafferentiation, and Tejasen and Everett (1967) by applying electrochemical stimulation to the deafferented rats demonstrated the fact that a diffuse afferentation from the preoptic septal complex might enter into the basal hypothalamus with point-to-point relationship. Furthermore, the activation of ARC–ME region was observed in the MUA changes, when electrochemical or electrical stimulation was applied to the MPO in inducing ovulation (Terasawa and Sawyer 1969b, Kawakami et al. 1971c). An increase in the unitary discharges was followed by MPO stimulation in the ARC (Fig. 1). Based on this confirmation, the neural pathway from the outside of preoptic area was examined in this paper.

Electrical stimulation of the medial part of SEPT induced elevation of MUA in the MPO, SC and ARC, when ovulation was observed the following morning (Fig. 4). Stimulation of the medial part of SEPT increased the firing rate of single unit activity in the MPO (Fig. 5). However, stimulation of the lateral part of SEPT neither induced elevation of MUA in the MPO and ARC nor was it followed by ovulation (Fig. 4). Elevations of MUA in the MPO, SC and ARC were also induced by the stimulation of the medial part of AMYG, at least when ovulation was observed in the following morning (Fig. 6). The release of LH by electrochemical stimulation to the amygdala was observed in the pentobarbital anaesthetized rat on the day of pro-oestrus (Lawton and Sawyer 1970). Therefore, activation of MPO and ARC which is induced by the stimulation of the SEPT or AMYG, seems to be related to the release of ovulatory hormone. In other words, adequate stimulus to the SEPT and AMYG inducing ovulation is eventually conducted into the basal hypothalamus through the preoptic area. Anatomical pathway from the AMYG to the preoptic area was quoted by Gloor (1955a, b) and Leonard and Scott (1971), and from the SEPT to the MPO was suggested by Andy and his co-workers (Andy and Stephan 1964, Andy and Koshino 1967).

Velasco and Taleisnik (1969) observed that the electrochemical stimulation of HPC inhibited the spontaneous ovulation as well as ovulation which was induced by the MPO stimulation. Electrical stimulation of HPC (CA_2 and CA_3) with high frequency depressed the elevation of MUA in the ARC as well as ovulation, that was induced by MPO stimulation under pentobarbital anaesthesia on the day of pro-oestrus (Fig. 7). Electrical stimulation of HPC depressed MUA in the ARC in some rats but not in all cases, and decreased the firing rate of single unit activity in the medial and dorsal part of the ARC (Fig. 9). Therefore, it is possible that hippocampal excitation causes some kind of an inhibitory influence on the hypothalamus responsible for the release of ovulatory hormone. The inhibitory effect of HPC stimulation with high frequency on MUA in the ARC was observed only when the electrodes were in the cell layer (CA_2 and CA_3) but not in the fimbria (Fig. 8), which mostly contain efferent fibres (Green 1960, Andy et al. 1962). This fact suggests that the effect of stimuli to HPC is integrated in the cell layer itself and sends its integrated information into the efferent pathway.

The frequency characteristics of HPC stimulation of MUA changes were observed, such as 100 c/s of stimulation depressed MUA in the ARC, while 60 c/s or 8 c/s elevated it (Fig. 8). As to the influence of HPC stimulation on the pituitary–adrenocortical system, Lissák and Endrőczi (1961, 1962) demonstrated that stimulation to the dorsal HPC with low frequencies induced the inhibition of ACTH release elicited by painful stimuli, but the application of high frequencies resulted in an increase of corticosteroid output. In this experiment, the frequency characteristics of HPC stimulation to the release of LH could not be observed, whereas that to the release of FSH or prolactin was observed (Figs 15 and 16).

The elevation of serum level of LH was inhibited, when HPC was electrically stimulated either simultaneously or preceding the stimulation of MPO throughout the oestrous cycle. This inhibitory action lasted at least for 4 hours (Fig. 21). This fact was also observed by Velasco and Taleisnik using electrochemical stimulation on the day of pro-oestrus (1969). HPC stimulation depressed APG content of LH with MPO stimulation, while it did not alter it in the absence of MPO stimulation (Fig. 18). Thus, in adult rats HPC seems to prevent the release of LH, as well as the synthesis of LH, when it is activated by MPO stimulation. In immature rats LH content of APG increased after stimulation of HPC alone, but not the serum level of LH (Figs 11 and 14).

The inhibitory action of HPC seems to appear at the certain set point of LH release, e.g. stimulation of HPC alone induced neither an increase nor a decrease in the basal level of serum LH (Fig. 15). Unappreciable release of LH by HPC stimulation was also observed by Clemens et al. (1971). However, electrical stimulation of HPC inhibited the increase in serum and APG levels of LH, which was induced by MPO stimulation. In other words, HPC stimulation could reveal its inhibitory influence on some nervous structure responsible for the synthesis and release of LH, when it is activated spontaneously or artificially by MPO stimulation. The effect of HPC stimulation is contrary to MPO stimulation, which induces elevation of LH constantly each day of the oestrous cycle, whenever stimuli are applied. Thus, HPC may have an influence on some neural factors in the hypothalamus responsible for the release of pituitary hormones, and its direct effect on the pituitary gland seems to be unlikely.

Electrical stimulation of HPC increased APG content of FSH throughout the oestrous cycle (Fig. 19), and it increased serum level of FSH on the day of oestrus (Fig. 16). Recently, constant vaginal cornification has been observed by us after the electrical stimulation of HPC (Kimura and Kawakami 1968). Stimulation of the ventral HPC induced constant oestrus, when it was applied on the days of oestrus, dioestrus I and dioestrus II. Stimulation of the dorsal HPC led to prolonged vaginal cornification following the day of oestrus, when the rats were stimulated on the days of oestrus or dioestrus II. The ovaries contained many well-developed follicles and some corpora lutea from the previous cycles. This fact suggested that HPC stimulation inhibited the neural surge of the ovulatory hormone and facilitated the release of FSH. Ablation of HPC induced irregularity of periodical appearance of vaginal cornification (Koikegami et al. 1960) or prolonged dioestrus which was intermitted by oestrus (Rodrigues 1959). The bilateral lesions of dorsal fornix interrupted the constant vaginal cornification induced by constant illumination (Kawakami et al. 1968). HPC stimulation could induce the acceleration of incorporative rate of ^{14}C-1-acetate into oestradiol and oestrone in ovarian homogenates throughout the oestrous cycle (Seto et al. unpublished observation). Furthermore, the stimulation increased FSH in serum and in APG of prepuberal rats. Therefore, it seems that the synthesis and the release of FSH are regulated, at least partially, by HPC during oestrous cycle and at the onset of puberty.

The circulatory level of FSH during oestrous cycle was reported by Goldman and Mahesh (1968). HPC stimulation induced an increase in serum FSH on the day of oestrus, when it was relatively low during the cycle, and a decrease on the day of dioestrus II, when it was relatively high. In this respect, the function of HPC appears at a certain set point for FSH release and may exert both facilitatory and inhibitory influence on the plasma FSH level.

Two separated neural systems controlling LH and FSH secretion were suggested by Flerkó and his co-workers (Flerkó 1963, Flerkó and Bárdos 1961). Recently, this hypothesis was supported by the studies using radioimmunoassay according to which there was a preoptic–tuberal pathway for the release of LH and distinct but overlapping AHA–tuberal pathway involved in the release of

FSH (Kalra et al. 1971) and that there were two neural networks distinguished by the electrochemical stimulation of the SEPT and MPO, in which the stimulation induced a significant difference in latency for the onset of hormone secretion (Clemens et al. 1971). The present experiment supports this assumption, and further, suggests the existence of completely separated pathways for the regulation of LH and FSH release and synthesis outside the hypothalamus.

In the present experiment we have demonstrated the results of HPC stimulation under both acute and chronic conditions. During the experiments we noticed that the serum level of FSH clearly rose on the day of oestrus in chronic experiment, while in acute experiment serum FSH did not change. Neill (1970) demonstrated that the serum level of prolactin was affected by the process of blood sampling whether they used ether or pentobarbital anaesthesia, and, whether incision was made on the femoral vein or the abdominal aorta. In other words, stressful condition altered the serum level of prolactin. In fact, there are several findings that the vaginal cycles were disturbed by the stressful environment in rats (Dordom and Timiras 1952, Takasugi 1956, Machida 1970, Terasawa and Sakuma, unpublished observation). Furthermore, under the stressful condition the central nervous system, which is the least involved in the ACTH control, altered its function. As to HPC, it increased ACTH release following the stimulation under non-stressful condition and inhibited it under stressful condition (Kawakami et al. 1971a, b). This fact may indicate that the effect of electrical stimulation on gonadotropin release also changes depending on the environmental conditions.

Although the lesion in the anterior hypothalamus (Donovan and van der Werff Ten Bosch 1956, 1959, 1965, Gellert and Ganong 1960, Schiavi 1964) in premature rats led to the precocious maturation in gonadal activity, and complete or anterior deafferentation of the basal hypothalamus hastened the onset of puberty. Ramaley and Gorski (1967) suggest that the neural influences for sexual maturation may come from outside of this area. HPC lesion produced delayed puberty and gonadal atrophy (Riss et al. 1963), whereas lesions of the AMYG and stria terminalis resulted in precocious puberty (Elwers and Critchlow 1960, 1961), and stimulation of the AMYG induced delayed puberty (Bar-Sela and Critchlow 1966). In premature rats, electrical stimulation of both HPC and AMYG increased APG content of either LH or FSH (Fig. 10) and induced the release of FSH (Fig. 10), while stimulation of MPO increased the content of LH and FSH in APG but not in the serum (Figs 11 and 12). TDB stimulation induced the elevation of LH in serum, and HPC stimulation increased serum FSH (Figs 11 and 12). Related experiment of our laboratory showed that the electrical stimulation of HPC as well as AMYG, MPO and ARC increased the incorporation of ^{14}C-1-acetate into progesterone and 20α-OH-en-4-pregn-3-one in ovarian homogenates, but only the stimulation of HPC and ARC accelerated the incorporation of ^{14}C-1-acetate into oestradiol and oestrone (Seto et al., unpublished observation). Therefore, in prepuberal animals the limbic forebrain area, especially HPC, is more involved in the control of synthesis and release of gonadotropin than the hypothalamus, i.e., the maturation of these areas in the brain may promote the onset of puberty. In fact, the anatomical maturation of the limbic areas rears that of the hypothalamus and occurs sometimes before weaning (Jacobson 1963, Altman and Das 1965, Timiras et al. 1968). Therefore, when HPC neurones mature functionally at the age near the onset of puberty, the secretion of FSH may start under the control of HPC. Small amount of FSH induced secretion of oestrogen, which feeds back to the brain's releasing further secretion of FSH. The role of oestrogen at the onset of puberty was reported by Ramirez and Sawyer (1965). After puberty the limbic structures, especially HPC, may be resetted to make a cyclic release of the ovulatory hormone, and may obtain the function of inhibition to keep the push–pull regulation with pituitary–ovarian axis.

HPC seems to be capable of changing its functional manner to the opposite direction under certain humoral environments: (*i*) HPC stimulation inhibits the release of FSH on the day of dioestrus II, when serum level is high, while it enhances the release of FSH on the day of oestrus, when serum level is low. (*ii*) HPC stimulation increases APG content of LH in prepuberal rats, while it inhibits the effect of MPO stimulation which increases LH content in the APG of adult rats. (*iii*) HPC stimulation during non-stressful condition facilitates ACTH secretion, while the same stimulation during stressful condition inhibits it (Kawakami et al. 1971a, b). These responses may be specific in HPC stimulation. MPO stimulation increases pituitary LH both in immature rats or in adult rats, and the stimulation increases serum and APG content of LH each day during oestrous cycle (Kawakami and Terasawa 1970, Kawakami et al. 1971c). Thus, MPO induces the release of LH constantly, whenever it is stimulated. In case of the ARC, the electrical stimulation increases serum LH and FSH both in pro-oestrous rats (Kalra et al. 1971, Clemens et al. 1971) and immature rats, and enhances ACTH secretion during both non-stressful and stressful conditions (Kawakami et al. 1971a, b). This is a one-way function in the basal hypothalamus releasing the pituitary hormones. The medial basal hypothalamus partially including the anterior hypothalamus contained LRF, FRF and PIF (McCann 1962, Nikitovitch-Winer 1962, Talwalker et al. 1963, Campbell et al. 1964, McCann et al. 1968) and the stimulation to these areas is highly effective to release LH, FSH and prolactin (Everett 1961, Everett and Quinn 1966, Kawakami and Terasawa 1970, Kalra et al. 1971). Recently, Kalra and McCann (1971) reported that MPO stimulation induced increase in LH–RF in the basal hypothalamus. Therefore, either facilitation or inhibition of pituitary gonadotropin might be induced by the activation of the basal hypothalamus, which can be called a final common pathway. Although we would not deny the concept that there is a cyclic centre in the preoptic anterior hypothalamus and a tonic centre in the medial basal hypothalamus involved in gonadotropin release, we would, moreover, postulate that the HPC may really be a cyclic centre superimposing the hypothalamus including MPO, which behaves in a tonic manner.

SUMMARY

The manner of modulation controlling the hypothalamo–pituitary–gonadal system played by the hippocampus (HPC) was studied by means of electrophysiological methods and radioimmunoassay in mature and immature female rats.

1. Electrical stimulation (100 c/s of square wave with a 0.5 msec pulse duration and a 200 μA of current applied for 30 min with 30 sec on/off) of the medial part

of amygdala (AMYG) induced elevation of the multiple unit activity (MUA) in the medial part of septum (SEPT), medial preoptic area (MPO) and the arcuate nucleus of hypothalamus (ARC), when it was effective in inducing ovulation under pentobarbital anaesthesia on the day of pro-oestrus.

2. High frequency stimulation (100 c/s, 0.1 msec of square wave pulses, 60 μA of current intensity) of the HPC (CA_2 and CA_3) lowered the MUA in the ARC (half of the cases examined), in the lateral part of SEPT (all cases), and in the diagonal bundle of Broca (TDB, 5 out of 7), but not in the MPO. HPC stimulation inhibited the elevation of MUA in the ARC that was induced by MPO stimulation (100 c/s, a 0.5 msec of pulse duration and a 100 μA of current). Simultaneous stimulation of HPC and MPO elevated MUA in the ARC slightly. HPC stimulation blocked MPO-induced ovulation. With low (8 c/s) or moderate (60 c/s) frequency, HPC stimulation increased MUA in the ARC, MPO and TDB. Electrical stimulation of the fimbria increased MUA in the ARC both at high or low frequencies. Thus, the effects of HPC stimulation seemed to be integrated in HPC itself and depended on the frequency component.

3. In prepuberal rats, the electrical stimulation of MPO, TDB, AMYG and HPC increased both LH and FSH content in the anterior pituitary gland (APG). Alone, HPC stimulation elevated the serum level of FSH, and TDB stimulation increased serum LH among the stimulated regions.

4. In mature rats, electrical stimulation with high frequency did not cause any change in the basal level of serum LH, while it inhibited the elevation of LH in both serum and APG level, that was induced by MPO stimulation. However, HPC stimulation induced an increase in serum FSH on the day of oestrus and decreased it on the day of dioestrus II. These changes of serum FSH were observed in the chronic experiment, but not in the acute experiment. Furthermore, stimulation of HPC either with or without MPO stimulation elevated APG content of FSH throughout the oestrous cycle. Serum level of prolactin decreased following HPC stimulation on the day of pro-oestrus in the chronic experiment. Low frequency stimulation to HPC showed remarkable inhibitory effects on serum FSH and prolactin. Significant differences in the effects of HPC stimulation with high or moderate frequencies could not be observed in all measured hormones.

Therefore, we arrived at the following conclusions: (*i*) There is a stimulating pathway for LH secretion in the medial AMYG, medial SEPT, TDB, MPO and ARC. (*ii*) HPC is capable of inhibiting the neural neurohormonal surge of LH on the day of pro-oestrus, whereas, (*iii*) it facilitates FSH secretion on the day of oestrus. (*iv*) HPC plays its role at the onset of puberty when an increase of FSH is needed. (*v*) HPC alters its function in an opposite direction following the changes of humoral environment, during oestrous cycle. Thus, HPC may participate in the gonadotropin secretion dominating the hypothalamus.

ACKNOWLEDGEMENTS

The authors express their appreciation to Drs K. Wakabayashi, K. Seto, T. Yanase, M. Manaka, Y. Sakuma, N. Konda, and Y. Shinohara for their helpful assistance in this experiment and to Dr. D. E. Rayson and Mrs. A. H. Shaw for their valuable advices to English expression. The work was supported by a grant from the Ministry of Education, Japan.

Following materials were kindly provided by the Endocrinology Study Section, National Institutes of Health, U.S.A.

Purified LH-NIAMD-Rat LH-1-1 (biological potency was approximately $1.0 \times$ NIH-LH-Sl by OAAD assay), NIAMD-Rat FSH-1-1 (biological potency was approximately $100 \times$ NIH-FSH-Sl by HCG-Augmentation assay), NIAMD-Rat Prolactin-1-1 (biological potency was approximately 30 International Units per mg by crop sac assay) were used for the radioionidation of LH, FSH and Prolactin.

NIAMD-Rat LH-RP-1 (biological potency was $0.03 \times$ NIH-LH-Sl by OAAD assay), NIAMD-Rat FSH-RP-1 (biological potency was $2.1 \times$ NIH-FSH-Sl by HCG-Augmentation assay) and NIAMD-Rat Prolactin-RP-1 (biological potency was approximately 11 International Units/mg by mouse deciduoma assay) were used for the standard preparations. NIAMD-Anti-Rat LH-Serum-1, NIAMD-Anti-Rat FSH-Serum-1 and NIAMD-Anti-Rat Prolactin Serum-1 were used for the first antibody.

REFERENCES

ALBE-FESSARD, D., STATINSKY, D. F. and LIBOUBAN, S. (1966): *Atlas Stéréotaxique du Diencéphale du Rat Blanc.* Centre National de la Recherche Scientifique, Paris.

ALTMAN, J. and DAS, G. D. (1965): Autoradiographic and histological evidence of postnatal hippocampal neurogenesis in rats. *J. comp. Neurol.* **124**, 319–335.

ANDY, O. J. and STEPHAN, H. (1964): *The Septum.* Thomas, Springfield.

ANDY, O. J. and KOSHINO, K. (1967): Duration and frequency patterns of the after-discharge from septum and amygdala. *Electroenceph. clin. Neurophysiol.* **22**, 167–173.

ANDY, O. J., WEBSTER, C. L., MUKAWA, J. and BONN, P. (1962): Electrophysiological comparisons of the dorsal and ventral hippocampus. In: *Physiologie de l'Hippocampe.* Ed. by Passouant. Centre National de la Recherche Scientifique, Paris. pp. 411–427.

BARRACLOUGH, C. A., YRARRAZAVAL, S. and HATTON, R. (1964): A possible hypothalamic site of action of progesterone in the facilitation of ovulation in the rat. *Endocrinology* **75**, 838–845.

BAR-SELA, M. E. and CRITCHLOW, V. (1966): Delayed puberty following electrical stimulation of amygdala in female rats. *Amer. J. Physiol.* **211**, 1103–1107.

BOGDANOVE, E. M. (1957): Selectivity of the effects of hypothalamic lesions on pituitary trophic hormone secretion in the rat. *Endocrinology* **60**, 689–697.

BUNN, J. P. and EVERETT, J. W. (1957): Ovulation in persistent-estrous rats after electrical stimulation of the brain. *Proc. Soc. exp. Biol.* (*N. Y.*) **96**, 369–371.

CAMPBELL, H. J., FEUER, G. and HARRIS, G. W. (1964): Effect of intrapituitary infusion of median eminence and other brain extract on anterior pituitary gonadotrophic secretion. *J. Physiol.* (*Lond.*) **170**, 474–486.

CLEMENS, J. A., SHAAR, C. J., KLEBER, J. W. and TANDY, W. A. (1971): Areas of the brain stimulatory to LH and FSH secretion. *Endocrinology* **88**, 180–184.

CRAMER, O. M. and BARRACLOUGH, C. A. (1971): Effect of electrical stimulation of the preoptic area on plasma LH concentration in proestrous rats. *Endocrinology* **88**, 1175–1183.

D'ANGELO, S. A. (1959): Thyroid hormone administration and ovarian and adrenal activity in rats bearing hypothalamic lesions. *Endocrinology* **64**, 685–702.

D'ANGELO, S. A. and KRAVATZ, A. S. (1960): Gonadotrophic hormone function in persistent estrous rats with hypothalamic lesions. *Proc. Soc. exp. Biol.* (*N. Y.*) **104**, 130–133.

DAVIDSON, J. M. (1969): Localization of inhibitory feedback by estrogen: Feedback control of gonadotropin secretion. In: *Frontiers in Neuroendocrinology.* Ed. by W. F. Ganong and L. Martini. Oxford University Press, Oxford. pp. 348–388.

DEY, F. L. (1941): Changes in ovaries and uteri in guinea-pigs with hypothalamic lesions. *Amer. J. Anat.* **69,** 61—87.
DEY, F. L. (1943): Evidence of hypothalamic control of hypophysial gonadotrophic function in the female guinea-pig. *Endocrinology* **33,** 75—82.
DONOVAN, B. T. and VAN DER WERFF TEN BOSCH, J. J. (1950): Precocious puberty in the rats with hypothalamic lesions. *Nature (Lond.)* **178,** 745.
DONOVAN, B. T. and VAN DER WERFF TEN BOSCH, J. J. (1959): The hypothalamus and sexual maturation in the rat. *J. Physiol. (Lond.)* **147,** 78—92.
DONOVAN, B. T. and VAN DER WERFF TEN BOSCH, J. J. (1965): *Physiology of Puberty*. Williams and Wilkins, Baltimore.
DORDOM, F. and TIMIRAS, P. S. (1952): Inhibitory action of stress on the release of luteinizing hormone by estrogen in the rat. *J. Pharmacol. exp. Ther.* **106,** 381—383.
ELWERS, M. and CRITCHLOW, V. (1960): Precocious ovarian stimulation following hypothalamic and amygdaloid lesions in rats. *Amer. J. Physiol.* **198,** 381—385.
ELWERS, M. and CRITCHLOW, V. (1961): Precocious ovarian stimulation following interruption of stria terminalis. *Amer. J. Physiol.* **201,** 281—284.
EVERETT, J. W. (1961): The preoptic region of the brain and its relation to ovulation. In: *Control of Ovulation*. Ed. by Villee. Pergamon Press, New York. pp. 101—112.
EVERETT, J. W. (1964): Preoptic stimulative lesions and ovulation in the rat: 'Thresholds' and LH-release time in late diestrus and proestrus. In: *Major Problems in Neuroendocrinology*. Ed. by E. Bajusz and G. Jasmin. Williams and Wilkins, Baltimore. pp. 346—366.
EVERETT, J. W. and RADFORD, H. M. (1961): Irritative deposits from stainless steel electrodes in the preoptic rat brain causing release of pituitary gonadotrophin. *Proc. Soc. exp. Biol. (N.Y.)* **108,** 604—609.
EVERETT, J. W. and QUINN, D. L. (1966): Differential hypothalamic mechanisms inciting ovulation and pseudopregnancy in the rat. *Endocrinology* **78,** 141—150.
EVERETT, J. W., RADFORD, H. M. and HOLSINGER, J. (1964): Electrolytic irritative lesions in the hypothalamus and other forebrain areas: Effects on luteinizing hormone release and the ovarian cycle. In: *Steroid, Biochemistry, Pharmacology and Therapeutics*. Ed. by L. Martini. Academic Press, New York. pp. 251—258.
FLERKÓ, B. (1953): Einfluss experimenteller Hypothalamus-Laesionen auf die Funktion des Sekretionsapparates im weiblichen Genitaltrakt. *Acta morph. Acad. Sci. hung.* **3,** 65—86.
FLERKÓ, B. (1954): Zur hypothalamischen Steuerung der gonadotrophen Funktion der Hypophyse. *Acta morph. Acad. Sci. hung.* **4,** 475—492.
FLERKÓ, B. (1956): Die Rolle hypothalamischer Strukturen bei der Hemmungswirkung des erhöhten Östrogenblutspiegels auf die Gonadotrophinsekretion. *Acta physiol. Acad. Sci. hung.* **9,** Suppl. 17—18.
FLERKÓ, B. (1957): Einfluss experimenteller Hypothalamusläsion auf die durch Follikelhormon indirekt hervorgerufene Hemmung der Luteinisation. *Endokrinologie* **34,** 202—208.
FLERKÓ, B. (1963): The central nervous system and the secretion and release of luteinizing hormone and follicle stimulating hormone. In: *Advances in Neuroendocrinology*. Ed. by S. Nalbandove. University of Illinois Press, Urbana. pp. 211—224.
FLERKÓ, B. and BÁRDOS, V. (1959): Zwei verschiedene Effekte experimenteller Läsion des Hypothalamus auf die Gonaden. *Acta neuroveg. (Wien)* **20,** 248—262.
FLERKÓ, B. and BÁRDOS, V. (1960): Pituitary hypertrophy after anterior hypothalamic lesion. *Acta endocr. (Kbh.)* **35,** 375—380.
FLERKÓ, B. and BÁRDOS, V. (1961): Absence of compensatory ovarian hypertrophy in rats with anterior hypothalamic lesions. *Acta endocr. (Kbh.)* **36,** 180—184.
GELLERT, R. J. and GANONG, W. F. (1960): Precocious puberty in rats with hypothalamic lesions. *Acta endocr. (Kbh.)* **33,** 569—576.
GLOOR, P. (1955a): Electrophysiological studies on the connections of the amygdaloid nucleus in the cat. Part I. The neuronal organization of the amygdaloid projection system. *Electroenceph. clin. Neurophysiol.* **7,** 223—242.
GLOOR, P. (1955b): Electrophysiological studies on the connection of the amygdaloid nucleus in the cat. Part II. The electrophysiological properties of the amygdaloid projection system. *Electroenceph. clin. Neurophysiol.* **7,** 243—264.

GOLDMAN, B. D. and MAHESH, V. B. (1968): Fluctuations in pituitary FSH during the ovulatory cycle in the rat and a possible role of FSH in the induction of ovulation. *Endocrinology* **83**, 97–106.

GORSKI, R. A. and BARRACLOUGH, C. A. (1963): Effect of low dosages of androgen on the differentiation of hypothalamic regulatory control of ovulation in the rat. *Endocrinology* **73**, 210–216.

GREEN, J. D. (1960): The Hippocampus. In: *Neurophysiology, Vol. II. Handbook of Physiology*. Ed. by J. Field, T. Magoun and M. Hall. American Physiological Society, Washington, D.C. pp. 1373–1390.

GREEN, J. D., CLEMENTE, C. D. and DE GROOT, J. (1957): Rhinencephalic lesions and behavior in cats: an analysis of the "Klüver-Bucy" syndrome with particular reference to normal and abnormal sexual behavior. *J. comp. Neurol.* **108**, 505–545.

GREER, M. A. (1953): The effect of progesterone on persistent estrus produced by hypothalamic lesion in the rat. *Endocrinology* **53**, 380–390.

HALÁSZ, B. and PUPP, L. (1965): Hormone secretion of the anterior pituitary gland after physical interruption of all nervous pathways to the hypophysiotrophic area. *Endocrinology* **77**, 553–562.

HALÁSZ, B. and GORSKI, R. A. (1967): Gonadotrophic hormone secretion in female rats after partial or total interruption of neural afferents to the medial basal hypothalamus. *Endocrinology* **80**, 608–622.

HALÁSZ, B., PUPP, L., UHLARIK, S. and TIMA, L. (1965): Further studies on the hormone secretion of the anterior pituitary transplanted into the hypophysiotrophic area of the rat hypothalamus. *Endocrinology* **77**, 343–355.

HILLARP, N. A. (1949): Studies on the localization of hypothalamic center controlling the gonadotropic function of the hypophysis. *Acta endocr. (Kbh.)* **2**, 11–23.

HOHLWEG, W. and JUNKMANN, K. (1932): Die hormonal-nervöse Regulierung der Funktion des Hypophysenvorderlappens. *Klin. Wschr.* **11**, 321–323.

JACOBSON, S. (1963): Sequence of myelinization in the brain of the albino rat. *J. comp. Neurol.* **121**, 5–29.

KALRA, S. P. and MCCANN, S. M. (1971): Changes in gonadotropin releasing factor content in the rat hypothalamus following electrochemical stimulation of the anterior hypothalamic area (AHA) and during estrous cycle. In: *Program of the 53rd Meeting of the Endocrine Society*. No. 58, San Francisco.

KALRA, S. P., AJIKA, K., KRULICH, L., FAWCETT, C. P., QUIJADA, M. and MCCANN, S. M. (1971): Effects of hypothalamic and preoptic electrochemical stimulation on gonadotropin and prolactin release in proestrus rats. *Endocrinology* **88**, 1150–1158.

KAWAKAMI, M. and TERASAWA, E. (1967): Differential control of sex hormone and oxytocin upon evoked potentials in the hypothalamus and midbrain reticular formation. *Jap. J. Physiol.* **17**, 65–93.

KAWAKAMI, M. and SAITO, H. (1967): Unit activity in the hypothalamus of the cat: Effect of genital stimuli, luteinizing hormone and oxytocin. *Jap. J. Physiol.* **17**, 466–486.

KAWAKAMI, M. and TERASAWA, E. (1970): Effect of electrical stimulation of the brain on ovulation during estrous cycle in the rats. *Endocr. jap.* **17**, 7–13.

KAWAKAMI, M. and KUBO, K. (1971): Neuro-correlate of limbic-hypothalamo-pituitary gonadal axis in the rat: Change in limbic-hypothalamic unit activity induced by vaginal and electrical stimulation. *Neuroendocrinology* **7**, 65–89.

KAWAKAMI, M., SETO, K. and YOSHIDA, K. (1966a): Influence of the limbic system on ovulation and on progesterone and estrogen formation in rabbit's ovary. *Jap. J. Physiol.* **16**, 254–273.

KAWAKAMI, M., TERASAWA, E., TSUCHIHASHI, S. and YAMANAKA, K. (1966b): Differential control by sex hormones of brain activity in the rabbit and its physiological significance. In: *Steroid Dynamics*. Ed. by G. Pincus, E. Nakao and I. A. Tait. Academic Press, New York and London. pp. 237–302.

KAWAKAMI, M., SETO, K., TERASAWA, E. and YOSHIDA, K. (1967): Mechanisms in the limbic system controlling reproductive functions of the ovary with special reference to the positive feedback of progestin to the hippocampus. *Progress in Brain Research*. Vol. 27. 69–102.

KAWAKAMI, M., KIMURA, F. and ISHIDA, S. (1968): Effect of the bilateral lesions of the fornix on the vaginal cycle in rats. *Folia endocr. Jap.* **43**, 154.

KAWAKAMI, M., TERASAWA, E. and IBUKI, T. (1970a): Changes in multiple unit activity of the brain during the estrous cycle. *Neuroendocrinology* **6**, 30—48.
KAWAKAMI, M., TERASAWA, E., IBUKI, T. and MANAKA, M. (1970b): Effects of sex hormones and ovulation-blocking steroids and drugs on electrical activity of the rat brain. In: *Santa Ynez Inn Steroid Conference*, Los Angeles 1970. (In press).
KAWAKAMI, M., SETO, K., KIMURA, F. and YANASE, M. (1971a): Brain mechanisms involved with adaptation to the immobilization stress. In: *Gunma Symposia on Endocrinology*, Vol. 8. (In press).
KAWAKAMI, M., SETO, K., KIMURA, F. and YANASE, M. (1971b): Difference in the buffer action between the limbic structures and the hypothalamus to the immobilization stress in rabbits. In: *Progress in Brain Research*. Ed. by D. H. Ford. Karger, Basel/New York. (In press.)
KAWAKAMI, M., TERASAWA, E., SETO, K. and WAKABAYASHI, K. (1971c): Effect of electrical stimulation of the medial preoptic area on hypothalamic multiple unit activity in relation to LH release. *Endocr. jap.* (In press.)
KIMURA, F. and KAWAKAMI, M. (1968): Effect of the hippocampal stimulation on the vaginal cycle in rats. *Folia endocr. jap.* **43**, 1059.
KLÜVER, H. and BUCY, P. C. (1937): Psychic blindness and other symptoms following bilateral temporal lobotomy on rhesus monkeys. *Amer. J. Physiol.* **119**, 352—353.
KOIKEGAMI, H. (1964): Amygdala and other related limbic structures: experimental studies on the anatomy and function. *Acta med. biol.* (*Niigato*) **12**, 73—266.
KOIKEGAMI, H., YAMADA, T. and USUI, K. (1954): Stimulation of the amygdaloid nuclei and periamygdaloid cortex with special reference to its effects on uterine movements and ovulation. *Folia psychiat. neurol. jap.* **8**, 7—31.
KOIKEGAMI, H., FUSE, S. and KAWAKAMI, K. (1960): Bilateral destruction experiments of hippocampus or amygdaloid nuclear region. *Neurol. Medico-Chirurg.* **2**, 49—55.
KÖVES, K. and HALÁSZ, B. (1970): Location of the neural structures triggering ovulation in the rat. *Neuroendocrinology* **6**, 180—193.
LAWTON, I. E. and SAWYER, C. H. (1970): Role of amygdala in regulating LH secretion in the adult female rat. *Amer. J. Physiol.* **218**, 622—626.
LEONARD, C. M. and SCOTT, J. W. (1971): Origin and distribution of the amygdalofugal pathways in the rat. An experimental neuroanatomical study. *J. comp. Neurol.* **141**, 313—330.
LISSÁK, K. and ENDRŐCZI, E. (1961): Neurohumoral factors in the control of animal behavior. In: *Brain Mechanisms and Learning*. Ed. by J. F. Delagresnaye. Blackwell Scientific Publications, Oxford. pp. 293—398.
LISSÁK, K. and ENDRŐCZI, E. (1962): Some aspects of the effect of hippocampal stimulation on the endocrine system. In: *Physiologie de l'Hippocampe*. Ed. by Passouant. Centre National de la Recherche Scientifique, Paris. pp. 463—471.
MACHIDA, T. (1970): Luteinization of ovarian transplants in gonadectomized male and female rats under stressful conditions and its relation to sexual differentiation of the hypothalamus. *Endocr. jap.* **17**, 189—193.
MACLEAN, P. D. (1957a): Chemical and electrical stimulation of hippocampus in unrestrained animals. Part I: Method and electroencephalographic findings. *Arch. Neurol. Psychiat.* (*Chic.*) **78**, 113—127.
MACLEAN, P. D. (1957b): Chemical and electrical stimulation of hippocampus in unrestrained animals. Part II: Behavioral findings. *Arch. Neurol. Psychiat.* (*Chic.*) **78**, 128—142.
MCCANN, S. M. (1962): Hypothalamic luteinizing hormone-releasing factor. *Amer. J. Physiol.* **202**, 395—400.
MCCANN, S. M., WATANABE, S., CRIGHTON, D. B., BEDDOW, D. and DHARIWAL, A. P. S. (1968): The physiology and biochemistry of luteinizing hormone-releasing factor and follicle stimulating hormone-releasing factor. In: *International Symposium on the Pharmacology of Hormonal Polypeptides*. Ed. by N. Back, L. Martini and R. Paoletti. Plenum Press, New York.
NEILL, J. D. (1970): Effect of "Stress" on serum prolactin and luteinizing hormone levels during the estrus cycle of the rat. *Endocrinology* **87**, 1192—1197.
NIKITOVITCH-WINER, M. B. (1962): Induction of ovulation in rats by direct intrapituitary infusion of median eminence extracts. *Endocrinology* **64**, 914—920.

Niswender, G. D., Midgley, A. R. Jr., Monroe, S. C. and Reichert, L. E. Jr. (1968): Radioimmunoassay for rat luteinizing hormone with antiovine LH serum and ovine LH-^{131}I. *Proc. Soc. exp. Biol.* (*N. Y.*) **128**, 807—811.

Ramaley, J. A. and Gorski, R. A. (1967): The effect of hypothalamic deafferentation upon puberty in the female rat. *Acta endocr.* (*Kbh.*) **56**, 661—674.

Ramirez, V. D. and Sawyer, C. H. (1965): Advancement of puberty in the female rat by estrogen. *Endocrinology* **76**, 1158—1168.

Redmond, W. C. (1968): Ovulatory response to brain stimulation or exogenous luteinizing hormone in progesterone-treated rat. *Endocrinology* **83**, 1013—1022.

Riss, W. (1958): Effect of limbic damage in infancy on subsequent endocrine development and running activity in rats. *Anat. Rec.* **130**, 364.

Riss, W., Burstein, S. D. and Johnson, R. W. (1963): Hippocampal or pyriform lobe damage in infancy and endocrine development of rats. *Amer. J. Physiol.* **204**, 861—866.

Rodrigues, J. A. (1959): Influence de l'écorce cérébrale sur le cycle sexuel du rat blanc. *C.R. Soc. Biol.* (*Paris*) **153**, 1271—1273.

Sawyer, C. H. (1970): Electrophysiological correlates of release of pituitary ovulating hormones. *Fed. Proc.* **29**, 1895—1899.

Schiavi, R. C. (1964): Effect of anterior and posterior hypothalamic lesions on precocious sexual maturation. *Amer. J. Physiol.* **206**, 805—810.

Schreiner, L. and Kling, A. (1953): Behavioral changes following rhinencephalic injury in cat. *J. Neurophysiol.* **16**, 643—659.

Sherwood, N. and Timiras, P. S. (1968): *Stereotaxic Atlas of the Developing Rat Brain.* University of California Press, Berkeley, Calif.

Stumpf, W. C. (1968): Estradiol-concentrating neurons: Topography in the hypothalamus by dry-mount autoradiography. *Science* **162**, 1001—1003.

Szentágothai, J., Flerkó, B., Mess, B. and Halász, B. (1968): *Hypothalamic Control of the Anterior Pituitary.* Akadémiai Kiadó, Budapest.

Takasugi, N. (1956): Untersuchungen über die hypophysäre gonadotrope Aktivität der dauroestrischen und normalen Ratten unter Stress-Situationen. *J. Fac. Sci. Univ. Tokyo.* Sec. IV, **7**, 605—623.

Talwalker, P. K., Ratner, A. and Meites, J. (1963): In vivo inhibition of pituitary prolactin synthesis and release by hypothalamic extract. *Amer. J. Physiol.* **205**, 213—218.

Tejasen, T. and Everett, J. W. (1967): Surgical analysis of the preoptic-tuberal pathway controlling ovulatory release of gonadotropins in the rat. *Endocrinology* **81**, 1387—1396.

Terasawa, E. and Timiras, P. S. (1968): Electrical activity during the estrous cycle of the rat: cyclic changes in limbic structures. *Endocrinology* **83**, 207—216.

Terasawa, E. and Sawyer, C. H. (1969a): Electrical and electrochemical stimulation of the hypothalamus—adenohypophyseal system with stainless steel electrode. *Endocrinology* **84**, 918—925.

Terasawa, E. and Sawyer, C. H. (1969b): Changes in electrical activity in the rat hypothalamus related to electrochemical stimulation of adenohypophyseal function. *Endocrinology* **85**, 143—149.

Terasawa, E. and Sawyer, C. H. (1970): Diurnal variation in the effects of progesterone on multiple unit activity in the rat hypothalamus. *Exp. Neurol.* **27**, 359—374.

Timiras, P. S., Vernadakis, A. and Sherwood, N. M. (1968): Development and plasticity of the nervous system. In: *Biology of Gestation.* Ed. by N. S. Assali. Academic Press, New York. pp. 261—319.

Velasco, M. E. and Taleisnik, S. (1969): Effect of hippocampal stimulation on the release of gonadotropin. *Endocrinology* **85**, 1154—1159.

Hormones and Brain Function, Budapest 1971, pp. 375–378 (1973)

STEROID SENSITIVITY OF THE NERVOUS SYSTEM

J. P. SCHADÉ and H. van WILGENBURG

Netherlands Central Institute for Brain Research
Amsterdam, the Netherlands

The nervous system of both vertebrates and invertebrates possesses groups of cells which release hormones. During the past decade, considerable attention has been paid to the output mechanisms of these so-called neuroendocrine cells. Much less is known about the input. In a previous paper (Schadé and van Wilgenburg 1970) we showed that neuroendocrine cells of a snail (*Helix pomatia*) responded to circulating steroids by either a decrease or an increase of the membrane potential and thus altered the firing rate.

It has become evident from investigations of neuroendocrine cells in mammals and snails, that these cells possess all properties of neurons as far as the excitatory and inhibitory synaptic potential shift is concerned. All cells are also shown to conduct action potentials. These cells may thus be defined as neuroendocrine transducers with the following properties: the output function is exerted by the release of a hormone or a monoamine; the receptive pole may be influenced by neurotransmitters or circulating hormones, and the transfer of information between the input and output parts of the cell is exerted by action potentials.

We have been interested in the translation properties of the receptive surface of the neuroendocrine transducer. In our investigation on snail neurons we found that these cells showed the same receptive properties for neurotransmitters. Iontophoretically applied neurotransmitters mimic the excitatory and inhibitory synaptic input. The sensor properties for circulating steroid of the neuronal membrane of the receptive pole of these cells have been subject of a detailed study. Since a review on the electrical properties of neuroendocrine transducers will be published (Schadé and van Wilgenburg 1971) we will limit ourselves to present here a few examples.

Figures 1 and 3 show the difference between dopamine and dexamethasone on the firing rate of snail neurons. After 20 to 30 seconds, a marked increase in firing rate is observed upon iontophoretic application of dopamine (Fig. 1). The effect may still be seen one to two minutes after cessation of the dopamine application, but five minutes after the onset of the experiment, a normal firing pattern is observed. In Fig. 2 a different response pattern is shown. Upon application of dexamethasone, initially a slight decrease in firing rate is observed. A considerable time after the initial application an effect upon the firing rate is noted. Apparently the substance has just to penetrate the neuronal membrane before an effect upon membrane polarization is accomplished. An additive effect is seen in Fig. 3, where the two substances have been applied simultaneously. The influence of dexamethasone apparently depends on the background level of synaptic inputs. In Fig. 4, the background level is considerably lower than in Fig. 3, resulting in a delayed increase in the firing rate. These and other experiments lend support to the postulation that steroids do not act like neurotransmitters as far as a specific receptor interaction is concerned, but probably influence ATP-ase activity, and thus may indirectly influence the polarization state of the membrane.

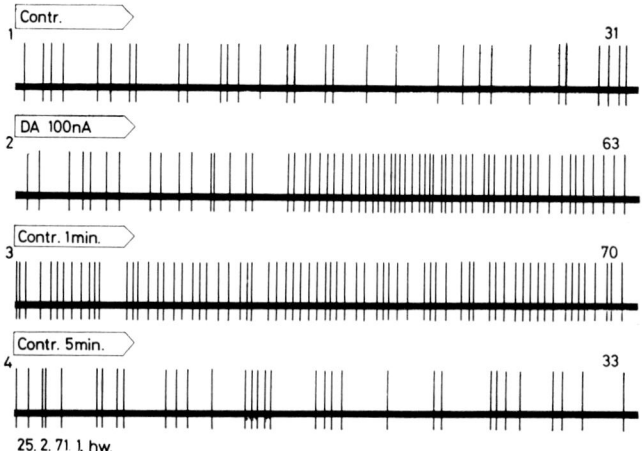

Fig. 1.

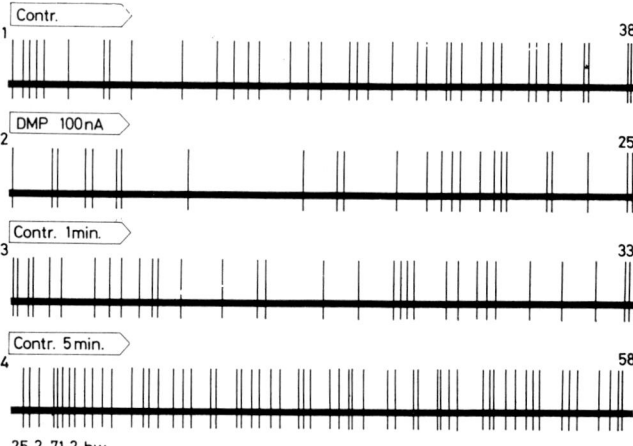

Fig. 2.

Perhaps the most characteristic difference between the transmission of signals by neurotransmitters and by hormones lies in the specific molecular properties of the mechanisms which regulate the membrane potential. The neurotransmitters alter the permeability for either sodium or potassium ions; the hormones alter the regulatory mechanism of the membrane pump, probably by increasing or decreasing the speed of one of the systems involved in the synthesis of cyclic AMP or ATP-ase. In this way a slow shift in the membrane potential is achieved. This shift in itself will not cause the generation of action potentials along the membrane, but if sufficient background synaptic activity is present, a considerable

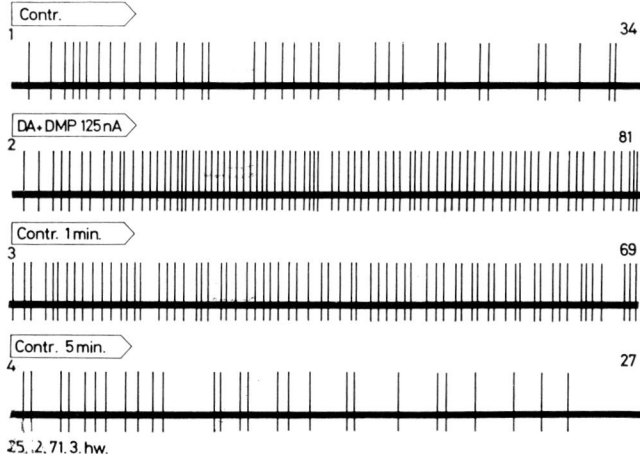

Fig. 3.

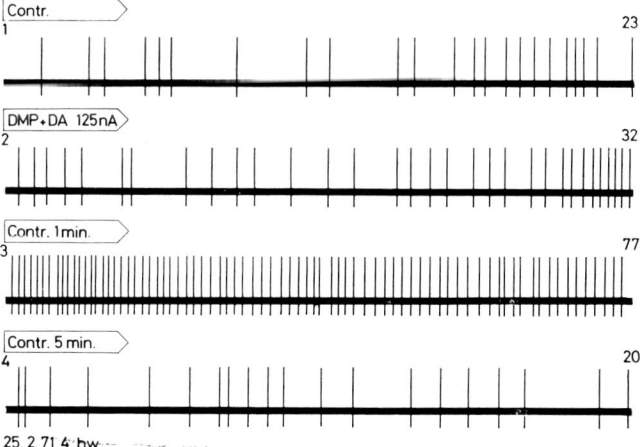

Fig. 4.

decrease or increase in the firing rate will occur. Neurotransmitters act via specific receptors of the receptive surface of the neuroendocrine transducers, but the circulating hormones act in a more dynamic way. Any major alteration of the concentration of a circulating hormone will, depending on the product released by the neuroendocrine transducer, activate or slow down the pump mechanism of the membrane. Thus, either a great many more impinging subthreshold stimuli will reach threshold value, or the resting value of the membrane is raised in such a way that considerably less action potentials are being generated. This mechanism thus acts as a modulator of the membrane activity. In the absence of background activity the effect of the membrane modulator is nil, but with sufficient background activity, provided by synaptic input, a major influence is exerted on the generation of action potentials, and thus on the output of the system.

REFERENCES

Schadé, J. P. and Wilgenburg, H. van (1970): The influence of hormones on the unit firing of neurons. In: *Influence of Hormones on the Nervous System*. First International Congress of Psychoneuroendocrinology. (In press).

Schadé, J. P. and Wilgenburg, H. van (1971): Electrophysiological aspects of neuroendocrine cells. *Progress in Brain Research*. (In press).

AN EVOLUTIONARY APPROACH TO THE INVESTIGATION OF PSYCHONEUROENDOCRINE FUNCTIONS

P. D. MacLEAN

Laboratory of Brain Evolution and Behavior
National Institute of Mental Health
Poolesville, Md., U.S.A.

INTRODUCTION

Evolutionary considerations are helpful in the approach to brain and behavior investigations, including those on neuroendocrine mechanisms. As diagrammed in Fig. 1, the primate forebrain evolves in hierarchic fashion along the lines of three basic patterns which, for purposes of discussion, I refer to as reptilian, paleomammalian, and neomammalian (MacLean 1962, 1964, 1967). Although markedly unlike in chemistry and structure, the three cerebrotypes establish extensive interconnections and function together as a *triune* brain (MacLean 1970a). Yet there is evidence that each is capable of operating somewhat independently.

The major counterpart of the reptilian *forebrain* in mammals includes the corpus striatum and globus pallidus which I will hereafter refer to as the *striatal*

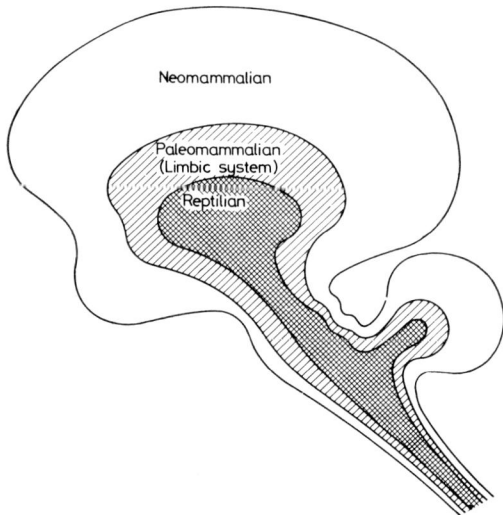

Fig. 1. In evolution the primate brain enlarges along the lines of three basic patterns that may be characterized in ascending order as reptilian, paleomammalian, and neomammalian (from MacLean 1967)

complex. Despite 150 years of investigation relatively little is known about the functions of the striatal complex. Comparative behavioral observations and some experimental findings (MacLean 1971) challenge the traditional clinical view that the *complex* is primarily a motor apparatus. At our new field Laboratory of Brain Evolution and Behavior we plan to test the hypothesis that the striatal complex of mammals is essential for such genetically constituted forms of behavior as selecting homesite, establishing and defending territory, hunting, homing, mating, rearing young, forming social hierarchies, and the like. We hope that this work will also give insight into brain mechanisms underlying compulsive, ritualistic, and imitative forms of behavior.

Paleoneurologists infer that in animals that were transitional between reptiles and mammals the rudimentary reptilian cortex increased in area and became further differentiated. In all existing mammals most of the phylogenetically old cortex is contained in a large convolution which Broca (1878) called the great limbic lobe because it encircles the brainstem. In 1952, I suggested the term "limbic system" as a designation for the limbic cortex and structures of the brainstem with which it has primary connections (MacLean 1952). By mid-century there had accumulated electroencephalographic and other clinical evidence that the limbic cortex is involved in emotional behavior. Epileptic discharges within or near the limbic cortex were known to be associated with a broad spectrum of emotional feelings. There were also indications that the limbic system is basic for affective feelings of reality of the self, and the environment, and that disruption of its functions may result in changes in mood, feelings of depersonalization, disorders of perception, hallucinations, and paranoid delusions characteristic of the endogenous and toxic psychoses (MacLean 1970b). Animal studies have provided additional evidence of the role of the limbic structures in emotional behavior and our own experiments have suggested that subdivisions of the limbic system are involved respectively in activities that promote self-preservation and the preservation of the species (MacLean 1958, 1962).

The human neocortex is the crowning development of the neomammalian brain. It has long been recognized that it is necessary for language functions. During the dark clinical days of prefrontal lobotomy it became evident that the prefrontal cortex is implicated in the anticipatory aspects of emotions that are best denoted by the word "anxiety". In those pitiful cases, for example, in which lobotomy was performed for the relief of pain there no longer appeared to be a dread or fear of impending death (White and Sweet 1969).

As regards psychoneuroendocrine functions the question arises as to how the three basic evolutionary formations of the forebrain exert an influence on hypothalamic–pituitary mechanisms. Figure 2 shows a section of the squirrel monkey's brain with the striatal complex selectively colored a deep brown by a stain for cholinesterase. The recent findings of Nauta and Mehler (1966) indicate that the so-called pallido-hypothalamic tract does not, in fact, project to the hypothalamus. They believe that the basal nucleus of Meynert may be the part of the striatal complex that establishes connections with the hypothalamus. The question of how the striatal complex anatomically and functionally plays upon the hypothalamus presents a challenging problem for future investigation.

As regards the limbic forebrain, there are large hypothalamic pathways, and I will return to this question when describing some new microelectrode and neuro-

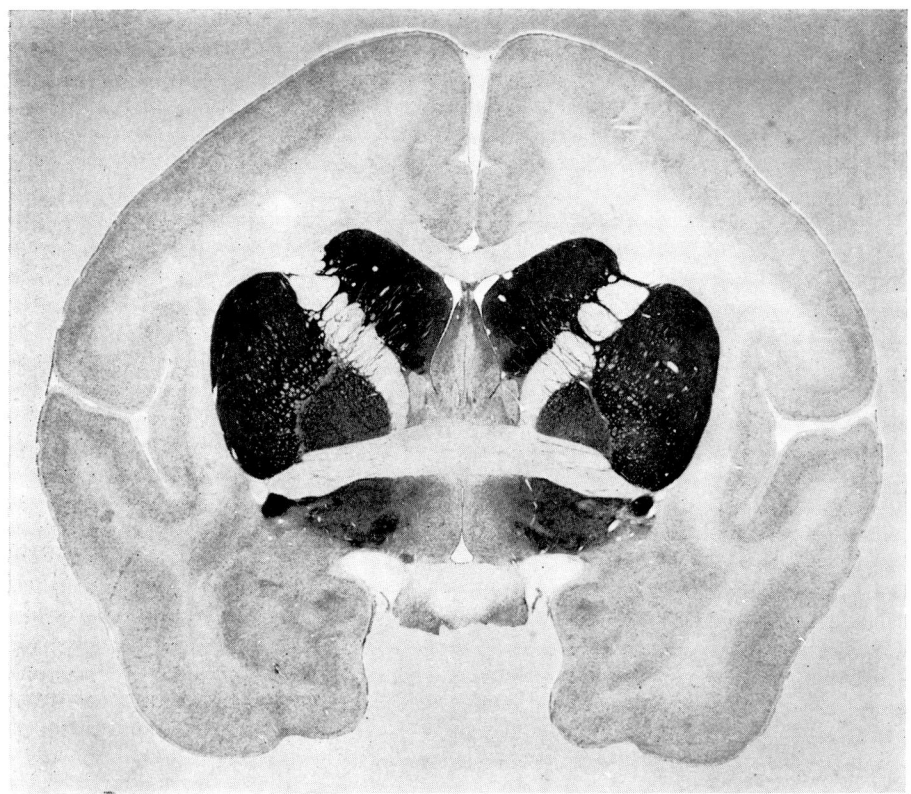

Fig. 2. The mammalian striatal complex (corpus striatum+globus pallidus) reflects the pattern of organization of a major part of the reptilian forebrain. This section from the brain of a squirrel monkey reveals how the corpus striatum (caudate+putamen+basal nucleus of Meynert), and to a lesser degree the globus pallidus, are selectively colored by a stain for cholinesterase. Note lack of staining of claustrum, a finding that conflicts with claims that it is part of the corpus striatum. Karnovsky's modification (1964) of the Koelle stain for cholinesterase; cresyl violet counterstain (from MacLean 1971)

anatomical findings. The neocortex, on the contrary, appears to have only sparse *direct* connections with the hypothalamus. There are, nevertheless, many possibilities by which it can influence the hypothalamus indirectly through the limbic system, the most notable being the prefrontal connections *via* the medial dorsal nucleus, cingulum, and uncinate fasciculus. The reticular system also provides indirect pathways for neocortical influences on the hypothalamus (Szentágothai et al. 1962).

Using different indices, Porter (1953), Mason (1958), and Endrőczi and Lissák (1959) uncovered evidence that stimulation of the hippocampus was followed by a suppression of the secretion of adrenocorticotrophic hormone (ACTH). Stimulation of the amygdala, on the contrary, resulted in a marked rise in ACTH. McHugh and Smith (1967) have since shown that unless amygdala stimulation induces a propagating afterdischarge a rise in ACTH does not occur. Such discharges propagate not only to the septum, medial thalamus, and hypothalamus, but also to the hippocampus (personal observations).

SOME NEW FINDINGS

In the remainder of this paper I will review some of our recent microelectrode and neuroanatomic findings that indicate a direct influence of the hippocampal archicortex on preoptic and tuberal structures involved in vegetative and endocrine function.

MICROELECTRODE FINDINGS

We performed experiments in awake, sitting squirrel monkeys in which we used a special stereotaxic device for exploring the brain with microelectrodes and testing the effects of hippocampal volleys on basal forebrain, preoptic, and hypothalamic neurons (Poletti et al. 1969, 1970, Kinnard et al. 1970). Coaxial bipolar stimulating electrodes were bilaterally implanted in the anterior and posterior hippocampus. Observations were made on 666 units. As shown in Table 1, hippocampal volleys regularly evoked unit responses in the basal forebrain and preoptic areas of more than 30 per cent of the units. Only 14 per cent of hypothalamic units, however, were responsive. As will be discussed, it was of special interest that more than 83 per cent of the responsive units in all regions were *initially* excited.

The effect of hippocampal afterdischarges, like hippocampal volleys, was also predominantly excitatory, with the ratio of excited and inhibited units being about 4 to 1. Units that were excited during afterdischarges showed a suppression of activity following afterdischarges for relatively long periods, ranging from 1 to 11 minutes. On the contrary, units inhibited during afterdischarges commonly showed an increase in their firing rate after cessation of the discharge.

Figure 3 shows the response of a unit in the medial preoptic area. Twenty-five (36 per cent) of 70 units recorded from the medial preoptic area were responsive

TABLE 1

Units responsive to hippocampal volleys

	Basal forebrain	Preoptic region	Hypothalamus
No. tested	177	99	390
No. and % responding	60 (34%)	30 (30%)	56 (14%)
% initially excited	87%	83%	86%
% initially inhibited	13%	17%	14%

to hippocampal volleys, with 25 showing initial excitation and two inhibition. Response latencies were as short as 11 msec. Other structures with units responding with comparably short latencies were the lateral preoptic area (10.0 msec), nucleus accumbens (12.5 msec), nucleus of the diagonal band (9.5 msec), lateral septum (10.0 msec), nucleus of the stria terminalis (11.0 msec), anterior hypothalamus (12.0 msec), the dorsal hypothalamus (10 msec), perifornical nucleus (10.0 msec), medial mamillary nucleus (11.0 msec), and posterolateral hypo-

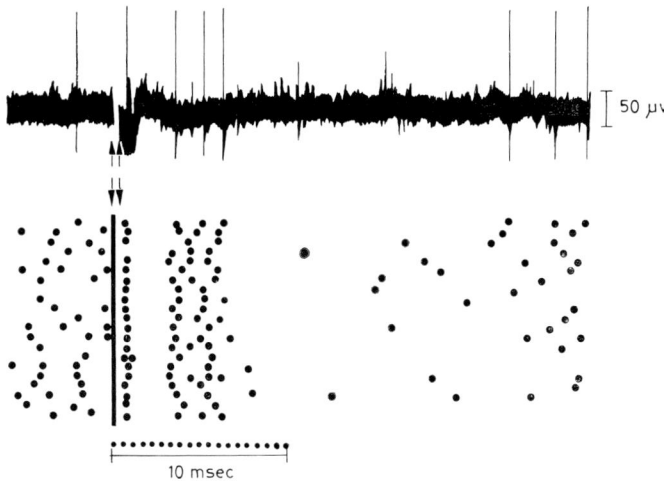

Fig. 3. Responses of a unit in medial preoptic area to paired shocks (arrows) applied to hippocampus. Dot display below oscilloscopic tracing illustrates reproducibility of the complex response characterized by excitation–inhibition–excitation–inhibition. Most medial preoptic units show only excitatory responses at regular latencies (from Poletti, Kinnard and MacLean, in preparation)

thalamus (12.5 msec). Units with these short latencies commonly showed a variability of less than 0.5 msec in the onset of the response to each stimulus, and tests of excitability cycles revealed an inability of such units to respond to a second stimulus within 25 msec. These findings suggested direct, orthodromic conduction.

Recordings were obtained from 26 units in the tuberal region, including three in the arcuate nucleus. Only one unit — located just lateral to the arcuate nucleus — was responsive (see anatomic findings below). Only a few units in the magnocellular, "neurosecretory" nuclei were tested: one of two units isolated in the paraventricular nucleus was excited, but neither of two units recorded in the supraoptic nucleus responded. It is also relevant to mention that two of six units in the suprachiasmatic nucleus were responsive, whereas only two of 20 in the anterior hypothalamus were affected.

ANATOMIC FINDINGS

The large percentage of responsive units in the medial preoptic region, as well as the evidence of direct orthodromic connection, was not expected in view of the lack of previous evidence of direct anatomical connections. Using Voneida and Trevarthen's (1969) modification of the Nauta stain, however, Poletti and Creswell in our laboratory found that section of the fornix in the squirrel monkey resulted in degenerated fibers and terminals in the medial preoptic area (in preparation). This stain, we find, is more effective than other recently reported silver methods for demonstrating very fine degenerating fibers in the squirrel monkey (MacLean and Creswell 1970). Dr. Poletti performed unilateral section of the fornix under direct vision. This procedure involved the use of a Horsley-Clarke instrument as a head holder and special "duck-bill" spreaders held in the carrier for gentle retraction of the hemispheres (MacLean, unpublished data). Control brains were prepared in which the entire operative procedure (including a midline incision of the corpus callosum) was performed except for unilateral section of the fornix. In histological section the degenerating fibers descending from the fornix into the medial preoptic area resembled falling rain (Fig. 4), contrasting with the corresponding clear area on the opposite side. Further findings of particular interest were degenerated fibers branching from the fornix into the perifornical nucleus and others that followed the course of the medial forebrain bundle before descending into the ventrolateral part of the tuber cinereum. None of the latter was seen entering the arcuate nucleus. The tuberal fibers follow an entirely different course from that of the "cornual band of the tuber cinereum" described by Cajal (see translation 1955) in macrosmatic forms and depicted as descending along the walls of the third ventricle. The "cornual band" is not seen in monkeys.

DISCUSSION

In prefacing the discussion of our results it deserves emphasis that the microelectrode experiments were carried out on awake, sitting, unmedicated monkeys. In a preceding study using quite similar preparations for the study of fornix and fifth nerve interaction, it was found that the hippocampus suppressed responses of thalamic intralaminar and midline units to fifth-nerve stimulation. These findings would be compatible with the conclusions of several investigators that the functions of the hippocampus are predominantly inhibitory (see e.g. Grastyán 1959). Consequently, it was surprising that the great majority of responding units in the basal forebrain, preoptic, and hypothalamic areas were initially excited by hippocampal volleys. These results would indicate that if the hippocampus had a predominantly inhibitory action on these structures, it would exert this effect through the agency of neurons that are initially excited. This statement requires qualification, however, because of a lack of information about the relative percentage of cells in which inhibitory postsynaptic potentials are induced by hippocampal volleys. Unlike a preceding study on the hippocampus (Yokota et al. 1970), we were unable in the present experiments to obtain satisfactory intracellular recordings in the awake, sitting monkey. Vascular pulsation appears to have been a major factor in contributing to this failure.

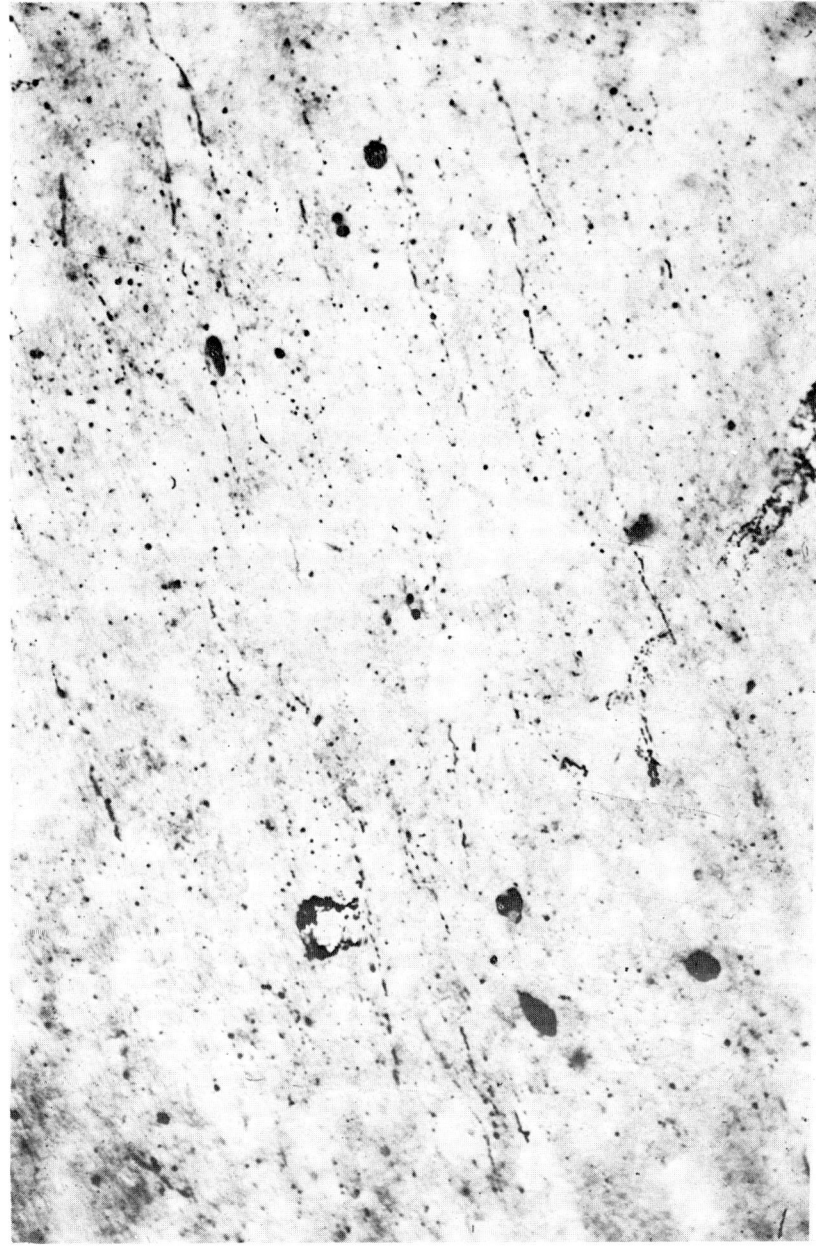

Fig. 4. Degeneration fibers and terminals in medial preoptic area following ipsilateral section of the fornix (see text; Voneida stain; from unpublished findings of Poletti and Creswell)

A large number of investigations has implicated the preoptic region in a variety of autonomic and endocrine functions. At the present meetings further consideration has been given to the role of the medial preoptic area in sexual differentiation (Gorski 1972, Dörner 1972, Flerkó 1971). Relevant to this matter, it is of great interest that radioautographic studies have shown that the medial preoptic area, as well as adjoining parts of the septum and anterior hypothalamus, have a special affinity for estradiol (Michael 1965, Pfaff 1968a, b, Stumpf 1968) and 1-testosterone (Pfaff 1968b). Michael (1965) inferred from his radioautograms in the cat that there is an "estrogen-sensitive neurological system involving the lateral septal area, preoptic region, and hypothalamus". According to one study (Lincoln and Cross 1967) estrogen enhances the responsiveness of medial preoptic neurons to stimulation of the cervix. In 1937 Haterius tentatively concluded on the basis of incomplete anatomical data that electrical stimulation of the preoptic area and adjoining parts of the septum induced ovulation in rabbits. The preoptic findings have been essentially confirmed by Everett (1965) (see also recent view by Sawyer 1969). Lisk (1962) has observed sexual receptivity in spayed rats following implantation of estrogen into the medial preoptic area. It has been both claimed (Larsson and Heimer 1964) and denied (Lott 1966) that medial preoptic lesions abolish mating behavior of male rats. Our own findings in squirrel monkeys have shown that electrical stimulation in the medial septopreoptic region is highly effective in eliciting penile erection (MacLean and Ploog 1962 and also see *Addendum*). The importance of the present studies lies in the demonstration by improved microelectrode and anatomical techniques of a direct hippocampal influence on preoptic neurons.

The observations I have described also indicate to a lesser degree a direct influence of the primate hippocampus on cells of the tuberal region, exclusive of the arcuate nucleus. These findings are of special interest in the light of the reports mentioned earlier of an inhibitory effect of hippocampal stimulation on the release of ACTH and the paper just presented by Kawakami on the influence of the hippocampus on the release of gonadotrophin. In view of neuroendocrine changes induced by light it is pertinent to mention that in a previous study we found units in the posterior hippocampal gyrus that gave sustained on-responses with ocular illumination (MacLean et al. 1968). The hippocampal gyrus is a major source of afferents to the hippocampus.

In regard to the regulation of the internal milieu perhaps the most striking evolutionary change one finds in passing from reptiles to mammals is the organism's ability to maintain a "constant" temperature. With respect to behavior the most striking change applies to care of the young. Of the four existing orders of reptiles only the crocodilia appear to have any disposition to look after their young. None of the living reptiles, to be sure, is considered representative of the forerunners of mammals. In mammals a major development of the limbic system is the subdivision comprising mamillary, thalamic, and cingulate structures. There is now evidence that this subdivision is involved in sexual functions (MacLean 1962) and maternal behavior (Stamm 1955, Slotnick 1967). The mamillo-thalamo-cingulate pathway articulates with the medial dorsal nucleus which projects to the prefrontal cortex. The progressive enlargement of these limbic and neocortical formations in higher primates and man appears to go hand in hand with an increasingly complicated social structure and a longer period of parent–offspring attachment. Is it possible that the neural mechanisms of the structures in question are unable to go fully into play until the hormonal changes of adolescence occur? If so, it would deny the claim of those who contend that the personality is fully formed by the age of 5 or 6, or at least before adolescence. Here, it seems, is a provocative psychoneuroendocrine question for future investigation.

SUMMARY

The primate forebrain evolves along the lines of three basic patterns that are here referred to as reptilian, paleomammalian, and neomammalian. Hence, it is basically a *triune* brain. The striatal complex (corpus striatum + globus pallidus) reflects the organization of a major part of the reptilian forebrain. The limbic system (limbic cortex + its primary nuclear connections) is largely a paleomammalian derivative. The human neocortex represents the culminating development of the neomammalian brain.

The question arises as to how each of the three basic formations of the forebrain influence neuroendocrine functions. The present paper focuses on one facet of limbic influences, describing the results of microelectrode and neuroanatomical studies on hippocampal (archicortical) efferent connections with basal forebrain, preoptic, and hypothalamic structures in the squirrel monkey (*Saimiri sciureus*).

The microelectrode experiments on awake, sitting, unmedicated monkeys reveal that hippocampal volleys have an initially excitatory effect on the great majority of *responsive* units in the three different regions. As discussed, it is of particular interest with respect to neuroendocrine mechanisms that the findings with improved microelectrode and neuroanatomic techniques indicate a direct hippocampal influence on neurons of the medial preoptic area and tuberal region.

Addendum. It is of interest to mention here some preliminary observations with M. A. Kinnard (unpublished) on the effects of depositing ACTH or MSH (melanin-stimulating hormone) in the septal and medial preoptic region of the squirrel monkey. These experiments were suggested by those of G. L. Gessa et al. (*Rev. Canad. Biol.*, 1967, **26**: 229), who reported that the intracisternal injection of ACTH in cats resulted in yawning, stretching, and penile erection). The hormones were deposited in solid form in amounts of 50–150 μg. The deposit of α-MSH in the region of the diagonal band and olfactory tubercle 1 mm from the midline and of β^{1-24} ACTH in the medial preoptic area close to the optic chiasm, resulted in episodes of stretching, yawning, scratching of the body, and full penile erection. The episodes developed within 1–1$^{1}/_{2}$ hrs and persisted for 5–5$^{1}/_{2}$ hrs. The peak activity occurred in about three hours, with episodes following immediately one after the other. The deposit of MSH in the ventromedial nucleus of the hypothalamus and of ACTH in the premamillary region had no apparent effect.

REFERENCES

Broca, P. (1878): Anatomie comparée des circonvolutions cérébrales. Le grand lobe limbique et la scissure limbique dans la série des mammifères. *Rev. Anthrop.* **1**, 385–498.

Dörner, G. (1972): Personal communication.

ENDRŐCZI, E. and LISSÁK, K. (1959): The role of the mesencephalon and archicortex in the activation and inhibition of the pituitary–adrenocortical system. *Acta physiol. Acad. Sci. hung.* **15**, 25.

EVERETT, J. W. (1965): Ovulation in rats from preoptic stimulation through platinum electrodes. Importance of duration and spread of stimulus. *Endocrinology* **76**, 1195–1201.

FLERKÓ, B. (1971): Personal communication.

GORSKI, R. A. (1972): Personal communication.

GRASTYÁN, E. (1959): The hippocampus and higher nervous activity. In: *Second Conference on the Central Nervous System and Behavior*. Transactions. New York, Josiah Macy, Jr. Foundation. pp. 119–205.

HATERIUS, H. O. (1937): Studies on a neuro-hypophyseal mechanism influencing gonadotropic activity. *Cold Spr. Harb. Symp. quant. Biol.* **5**, 280–288.

KARNOVSKY, M. J. (1964): A "direct-coloring" thiocholine method for cholinesterases. *J. Histochem. Cytochem.* **12**, 219.

KINNARD, M. A., POLETTI, C. E. and MACLEAN, P. D. (1970): Preoptic unit responses to hippocampal stimulation. *Fed. Proc.* **29**, 792.

LARSSON, K. and HEIMER, L. (1964): Mating behaviour of male rats after lesions in the preoptic area. *Nature (Lond.)* **202**, 413–414.

LINCOLN, D. W. and CROSS, B. A. (1967): Effect of oestrogen on responsiveness of neurones in the hypothalamus, septum and preoptic area of rats with light-induced persistent oestrus. *J. Endocr.* **37**, 191–203.

LISK, R. D. (1962): Diencephalic placement of estradiol and sexual receptivity in the female rat. *Amer. J. Physiol.* **203**, 493–496.

LOTT, D. F. (1966): Effect of preoptic lesions on the sexual behavior of male rats. *J. comp. physiol. Psychol.* **61**, 284–288.

MACLEAN, P. D. (1952): Some psychiatric implications of physiological studies on frontotemporal portion of limbic system (visceral brain). *Electroenceph. clin. Neurophysiol.* **4**, 407–418.

MACLEAN, P. D. (1958): Contrasting functions of limbic and neocortical systems of the brain and their relevance to psychophysiological aspects of medicine. *Amer. J. Med.* **25**, 611–626.

MACLEAN, P. D. (1962): New findings relevant to the evolution of psychosexual functions of the brain. *J. nerv. ment. Dis.* **135**, 289–301.

MACLEAN, P. D. (1964): Man and his animal brains. *Mod. Med.* **32**, 95–106.

MACLEAN, P. D. (1967): The brain in relation to empathy and medical education. *J. nerv. ment. Dis.* **144**, 374–382.

MACLEAN, P. D. (1970a): The triune brain, emotion, and scientific bias. In: *The Neurosciences Second Study Program*. Ed. by F. O. Schmitt. The Rockefeller University Press, New York. pp. 336–349.

MACLEAN, P. D. (1970b): The limbic brain in relation to the psychoses. In: *Physiological Correlates of Emotion*. Ed. by P. Black. Academic Press Inc., New York. pp. 129–146.

MACLEAN, P. D. (1971): Cerebral evolution and emotional processes. *Ann. N.Y. Acad. Sci.* (In press).

MACLEAN, P. D. and PLOOG, D. W. (1962): Cerebral representation of penile erection. *J. Neurophysiol.* **25**, 29–55.

MACLEAN, P. D. and CRESWELL, G. (1970): Anatomical connections of visual system with limbic cortex of monkey. *J. comp. Neurol.* **138**, 265–278.

MACLEAN, P. D., YOKOTA, T. and KINNARD, M. A. (1968): Photically sustained on-responses of units in posterior hippocampal gyrus of awake monkey. *J. Neurophysiol.* **31**, 870–883.

MASON, J. W. (1958): The central nervous system regulation of ACTH secretion. In: *Reticular Formation of the Brain*. Little and Brown, Boston. pp. 645–662.

MCHUGH, P. R. and SMITH, G. P. (1967): Plasma 17-OHCS response to amygdaloid stimulation with and without afterdischarges. *Amer. J. Physiol.* **212**, 619–622.

MICHAEL, R. P. (1965): Oestrogens in the central nervous system. *Brit. med. Bull.* **21**, 87–90.

NAUTA, W. J. H. and MEHLER, W. R. (1966): Projections of the lentiform nucleus in the monkey. *Brain Res.* **1**, 3–42.

Pfaff, D. W. (1968a): Uptake of ³H-estradiol by the female rat brain. An autoradiographic study. *Endocrinology* **82**, 1149—1155.

Pfaff, D. W. (1968b): Autoradiographic localization of radioactivity in rat brain after injection of tritiated sex hormones. *Science* **161**, 1355—1356.

Poletti, C. E., Kinnard, M. A. and MacLean, P. D. (1969): Effect of hippocampal stimulation on unit activity of hypothalamic, preoptic and basal forebrain areas. *Electroenceph. clin. Neurophysiol.* **24**, 686.

Poletti, C. E., Kinnard, M. A. and MacLean, P. D. (1970): Analysis of hippocampal influence on units of mamillary region in awake, sitting squirrel monkeys. *Electroenceph. clin. Neurophysiol.* **29**, 322.

Porter, R. W. (1953): The central nervous system and stress-induced eosinopenia. *Recent Progr. Hormone Res.* **10**, 1—27.

Ramon y Cajal, S. (1955): *Studies on the Cerebral Cortex (limbic structures)*. Translated from Spanish by L. M. Kraft. London, Lloyd-Luke Ltd. and Chicago, The Year Book Publishers, 1955. xii + 179 pp.

Sawyer, C. H. (1969): Regulatory mechanisms of secretion of gonadotrophic hormones. In: *The Hypothalamus.* Ed. by W. Haymaker, E. Anderson and W. J. H. Nauta. Charles C. Thomas, Springfield, Ill. pp. 389—430.

Slotnick, B. M. (1967): Disturbances of maternal behavior in the rat following lesions of the cingulate cortex. *Behaviour* **24**, 204—236.

Stamm, J. S. (1955): The function of the median cerebral cortex in maternal behavior of rats. *J. comp. physiol. Psychol.* **48**, 347—356.

Stumpf, W. E. (1968): Estradiol-concentrating neurons: topography in the hypothalamus by dry-mount autoradiography. *Science* **162**, 1001—1003.

Szentágothai, J., Flerkó, B., Mess, B. and Halász, B. (1962): *Hypothalamic Control of the Anterior Pituitary. An experimental-morphological study.* Akadémiai Kiadó, Budapest. p. 330.

Voneida, T. J. and Trevarthen, C. B. (1969): An experimental study of transcallosal connections between the proreus gyri of the cat. *Brain Res.* **12**, 384—395.

White, J. C. and Sweet, W. H. (1969): *Pain and the Neurosurgeon. A Forty-year Experience.* Charles C. Thomas, Springfield, Ill. p. 1000.

Yokota, T., Reeves, A. G. and MacLean, P. D. (1970): Differential effects of septal and olfactory volleys on intracellular responses of hippocampal neurons in awake, sitting monkeys. *J. Neurophysiol.* **33**, 96—107.

THE ROLE OF THE POSTERIOR PITUITARY AND ITS PEPTIDES ON THE MAINTENANCE OF CONDITIONED AVOIDANCE BEHAVIOUR

D. de WIED

Rudolf Magnus Institute for Pharmacology
Medical Faculty, University of Utrecht
Utrecht, the Netherlands

The pituitary–adrenal axis is the system "par excellence" of homeostasis and responsible for the relative freedom which higher organisms exhibit in a constantly changing environment. Every stressful situation therefore initiates a chain of events which results in the release of ACTH and the subsequent secretion of adrenocortical hormones.

Stress not only results in the discharge of ACTH from the anterior pituitary but also in the release of vasopressin from the posterior pituitary. The close association between the vasopressor and adrenocorticotropic response to stress led to the hypothesis that vasopressin may be responsible for the release of ACTH (Mirsky et al. 1954). In support of this assumption is the rapidity with which vasopressin as well as ACTH are released following stress (Mirsky et al. 1954, de Wied and Mirsky 1959), the efficacy with which vasopressin induces the release of ACTH, and the inhibition of ACTH release in animals with extensive lesions in the median eminence of the hypothalamus which at the same time cause diabetes insipidus as the result of destruction of the hypothalamic–neurohypophyseal connections (McCann 1957, de Wied et al. 1958).

Some ten years ago Smelik and I found that removal of the posterior lobe of the pituitary resulted in a disturbance in the release of ACTH in response to neurogenic or emotional stress while that to somatic or systemic stress remained unaltered (Smelik 1962, de Wied 1961). These findings were confirmed by Arimura et al. in 1965.

Posterior lobectomized rats subjected to emotional stress such as transfer to a strange environment, sound, or pain show less of an adrenocortical response to these stresses than sham-operated control animals. Posterior lobectomy, however, did not affect the release of ACTH in response to systemic stress like haemorrhage under ether anaesthesia, or the injection of histamine or nicotine.

This altered reaction of the anterior pituitary was thought to be the result of the absence of posterior lobe principles involved in the mechanism of ACTH release. In fact, treatment for 6 days with an extract of posterior pituitary tissue, pitressin in a long acting form, nearly completely restored the reaction of the pituitary–adrenal system in response to neurogenic stress.

These results suggested that the absence of posterior pituitary principles had caused the defect in the release mechanism of ACTH following neurogenic stress.

However, we felt that it might also be possible that the deficient pituitary–adrenal response to neurogenic stimulation resulted from a defective translation of environmental stimuli to the pituitary of posterior lobectomized rats. If this were true the origin of the reduced pituitary response to neurogenic stress might be located in higher central nervous structures. In other words, posterior lobectomy might result in alterations in behaviour.

For this reason it was decided to investigate the behaviour of posterior lobectomized rats. Since conditioned avoidance behaviour is thought to be motivated by fear, this type of behaviour was chosen for our studies (de Wied 1965).

Posterior lobectomized and sham-operated animals were trained to avoid an electric shock in a shuttle box. Ten trials a day were administered with intertrial intervals averaging from 60 sec in the beginning to 30 sec at the end of the training. Rats conditioned under a progressively diminishing intertrial interval procedure are more resistant to extinction than rats maintained on a fixed intertrial interval (Murphy and Miller 1956). After 14 days of acquisition, extinction was studied in all animals that had reached the conditioning criterion of 80 per cent avoidance responses during the last 3 days of conditioning. Posterior lobectomized rats exhibit a moderate diabetes insipidus. Acquisition in these animals is indistinguishable from that of sham-operated controls. However, posterior lobectomized rats are not resistant to extinction. Treatment of posterior lobectomized rats with pitressin tannate in oil (1 U subcutaneously) every 2 days during the extinction period restores the daily water intake toward normal levels and, in addition, results in normal extinction behaviour in these animals.

Pitressin is an extract of posterior and intermediate lobe tissue and contains various peptides. Among these are MSH, ACTH, vasopressin and oxytocin; peptides with marked biological activities. In fact, ACTH as well as α- and β-MSH are able to affect the rate of extinction of an avoidance response in posterior lobectomized rats in a fashion similar to that of pitressin. No effect of these peptides on daily water intake has been found, indicating that the disturbance in water metabolism is not a likely cause of the defective behaviour in the posterior lobectomized rat.

It is well known that vasopressin is capable of stimulating the release of ACTH (de Wied et al. 1968). Therefore, it might be that the effect of pitressin on extinction is caused by chronic stimulation of pituitary ACTH release. However, pitressin also affects the rate of extinction of an avoidance response in rats in which the anterior pituitary has been removed (de Wied 1965).

Accordingly, two different classes of peptides seem to be able to substitute for the posterior pituitary with respect to the behavioural deficiency of the posterior lobectomized rat. This rather puzzling phenomenon was studied further and it was found that the treatment of posterior lobectomized rats with pitressin tannate during the acquisition period only has the same effect on extinction as when this treatment is given only during extinction (de Wied 1969). The effect manifests itself at the time that daily water intake has reached the level of that of placebo-treated posterior lobectomized rats. In contrast, a similar treatment with long-acting ACTH during the acquisition period hardly affects the rate of extinction of the avoidance response of the posterior lobectomized rat.

From these experiments it was inferred that pitressin preserves a conditioned avoidance response irrespective of the time of treatment, while ACTH and related peptides affect extinction only during the period of treatment. Accordingly, the mechanism by which pitressin and ACTH analogues or posterior, intermediate, and anterior pituitary principles affect avoidance behaviour is basically different.

Bohus and I subsequently studied the effect of pitressin as compared to α-MSH on extinction of a shuttle-box avoidance response in intact rats (de Wied and Bohus 1966). In this case rats were conditioned under a procedure slightly different from that used in the posterior lobectomized rat. The reason for this was that the animals had to extinguish the avoidance response in a relatively short period of time in order to allow the demonstration of an inhibitory effect of pitressin and of α-MSH on the rate of extinction of the avoidance response. Animals were trained in the shuttle box under a fixed intertrial interval procedure averaging 60 sec till they made 80 per cent or more avoidances for 3 consecutive days. As soon as they had reached this criterion, extinction trials were run. Under this procedure animals extinguish within 2 weeks. Treatment with 1 U pitressin tannate in oil and 10 μg of α-MSH as a long-acting zinc phosphate preparation per 2 days has an identical effect in delaying extinction of the avoidance response of intact rats when the treatment is given during the extinction period. However, when a similar treatment is given during acquisition and discontinued during extinction pitressin does, but α-MSH does not exhibit its inhibitory effect on the rate of extinction of the avoidance response. When animals were subjected to a second extinction session 3 weeks after the first one, the effect of pitressin was still present. Pitressin, then, exhibits a long-term effect on the maintenance of an avoidance response whereas the influence of ACTH and its analogues manifests itself only for a relatively short period of time.

The principle present in the posterior pituitary responsible for this long-term effect could be vasopressin but a definitive proof, using synthetic preparations, is difficult to provide because the preparation of long-acting synthetic vasopressin or oxytocin is not easily accomplished. To circumvent this difficulty we examined the influence of various peptides which were not prepared for long-lasting activity. Animals were conditioned to jump onto a pole in order to avoid electric shocks (de Wied 1966, van Wimersma Greidanus and de Wied 1969). Ten conditioning trials were given each day for 3 days with a fixed intertrial interval averaging 60 sec. Rats which made 10 or more avoidances during the 3 acquisition sessions were used for extinction studies which started on the 4th day. Only rats that made 8 or more avoidances in the first extinction session were used for subsequent extinction sessions which were run 2, 4, 24, 48 or 72 hours later. Injections were given subcutaneously immediately after the first extinction session.

As mentioned above, the inhibitory effect of ACTH on extinction could be obtained with either α- or β-MSH. These peptides have the sequence ACTH 4–10 in common. In fact, this heptapeptide has the same effect on extinction as ACTH (Greven and de Wied 1967) and was used in the subsequent study. A dose of 100 μg of ACTH 4–10 inhibits extinction significantly at 2 and 4 hours after injection as compared to placebo treatment but there was no observable effect 24 hours after administration of this heptapeptide. In contrast, lysine vasopressin in a dose of 1 μg (60 mU) not only inhibits extinction at 2 and at 4 hours, but also at 24 and 72 hours after injection (de Wied 1971).

Other structurally and physiologically related peptides like oxytocin, angiotensin II, insulin or growth hormone in a dose of 1 μg do not affect the rate of extinction of the pole jumping avoidance response.

Thus the peptide in the pitressin preparation responsible for the long-term effect on extinction is lysine vasopressin. The effect is rather specific since structurally and physiologically related peptides in similar amounts are without effect.

A subsequent experiment was performed to determine if there was a critical period for the effect of lysine vasopressin on the maintenance of the avoidance response. For this purpose rats were injected immediately or 1 or 6 hours after the first extinction session. Administration of lysine vasopressin immediately after the first extinction session again results in inhibition of extinction (Fig. 1). Injection of this peptide 1 hour later also delays extinction, although the effect does not appear to be as complete as that produced by the immediate injection. When administration is delayed for 6 hours, the effect on extinction is not observed. Accordingly, there appears to be a critical period for the influence of vasopressin on the maintenance of the avoidance response; to be completely effective, vasopressin must be administered within 1 hour after an extinction session.

To determine the duration of action of vasopressin a similar experiment was performed but now the peptide was administered 6, 3 or 1 hour prior to the first extinction session. The results clearly show that vasopressin must be injected within 1 hour of the first extinction session to be completely effective. It is of interest to note that the half-life of vasopressin has been estimated to be between 1 and 5 min (Ginsburg 1968). The half-life for the behavioural effect, however, seems to be more than an hour since the administration of vasopressin 1 hr before the first extinction session has approximately the same effect on extinction as an injection immediately after this session. One possibility is that some breakdown product exerts identical behavioural effects as vasopressin. For example, trypsinated vasopressin which almost completely lacks the biological activities exhibits

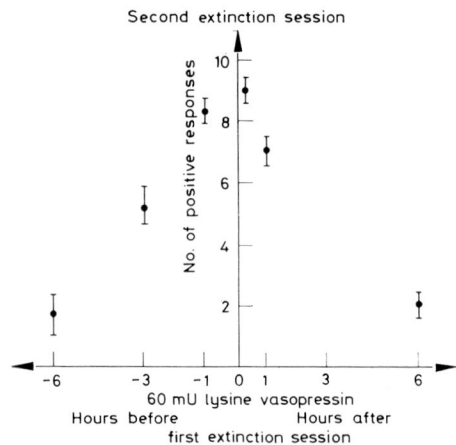

Fig. 1. The inhibitory effect of lysine vasopressin on extinction of a pole jumping avoidance response (as related to the time of injection before and after the first extinction session). Right: the administration of 60 mU of lysine vasopressin, immediately and 1 and 6 hrs after the first extinction session. To be effective vasopressin had to be administered within 1 hr following the session. Left: the administration of 60 mU of lysine vasopressin, 6, 3 and 1 hr before the first extinction session. To obtain an optimal effect, vasopressin had to be injected at least 1 hr prior to the session

an effect similar to that of vasopressin on the maintenance of a pole jumping avoidance response (de Wied et al. 1971, in preparation).

Vasopressin not only affects the maintenance of conditioned avoidance behaviour, it also affects acquisition of the pole jumping avoidance response. Injection of lysine vasopressin or a related peptide, ornithine vasopressin one hour before training is begun significantly improves avoidance learning (Fig. 2). Interestingly, a single injection of the peptide influences the rate of extinction in the same way as when it is injected after acquisition has been completed.

Accordingly, vasopressin or related peptides from the posterior pituitary affect acquisition as well as extinction of a conditioned avoidance response and it seems as if these peptides are involved in the long-term retention of behaviour. This is not the case with ACTH and its analogues. These peptides exhibit a short-term effect which lasts only as long as the peptide is present.

The foregoing reveals that the posterior pituitary and vasopressin can determine the rate of extinction of conditioned avoidance behaviour. The removal of the posterior lobe of the pituitary interferes with the maintenance of the avoidance response while the administration of vasopressin has a consolidating effect. Consolidation of learned responses requires time and appears to be susceptible to a variety of influences for several hours after training (McCaugh 1966). Temporary (those occurring within seconds and minutes) and permanent (lasting several hours) changes occur in the CNS, and these have been designated as short-term and long-term memory processes. ACTH analogues seem to facilitate those processes involved in short-term memory processes because they inhibit extinction only when they are present. Vasopressin induces long-term effects since a single injection of this peptide is capable of influencing retention for a long period of time.

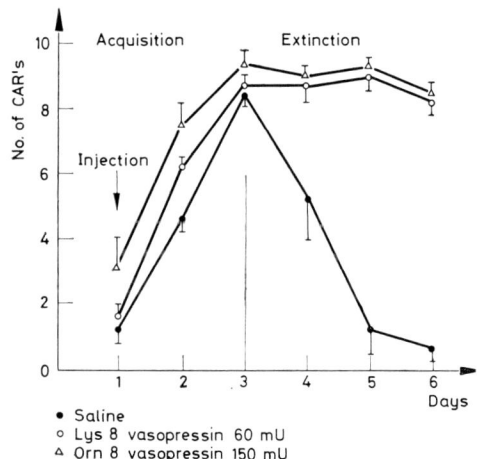

Fig. 2. Effect of vasopressin on acquisition and extinction of a pole jumping avoidance response. Peptides and placebo were administered once at, 1 hr prior to the first training session. A single injection of these peptides induces a significant increase in the rate of acquisition of the avoidance response at day 1 for the ornithine and at day 2 for both the ornithine and the lysine vasopressin. Extinction is delayed by this treatment in the same way as when peptide treatment is started immediately following completion of avoidance training

The way in which these peptides act is unknown. Consolidation of learned responses has been reported for a number of drugs which are known to alter synaptic transmission (Glassman 1969). The sensitive period for these drugs, however, seems shorter than that for lysine vasopressin. In addition, repeated injections of these drugs are necessary to affect performance. This is also true for the ACTH analogues. Moreover, the difference between centrally acting drugs and neuropeptides is that the former exhibit rather general effects in the CNS in contrast to that of neuropeptides. These peptides, e.g., do not affect the general level of activity or other gross behavioural patterns (Bohus and de Wied 1966).

The effect of lysine vasopressin resembles the long-term influences of RNA precursors on extinction of a shuttle box avoidance response (Matthies et al. 1971). Also, the effect is the reverse of the influence of antibiotics which inhibit protein synthesis in the brain and at the same time interfere with the consolidation of learned responses if the antibiotic is administered within a critical period of time following learning. For example, puromycin interferes with retention of a learned response in goldfish only if it is given within an hour after the training session (Agranoff et al. 1965, Davis and Agranoff 1966). Although the effect of puromycin on protein synthesis in relation to its effect on behaviour is still under debate (Glassman 1969), it has been suggested that puromycin interferes with retention by producing peptidyl-puromycin (Flexner and Flexner 1967, 1968). Such abnormal peptides are thought to prevent consolidation by displacement of normal peptides from nerve cell membranes. The present findings support this view and indicate that acquisition and extinction of new behavioural patterns are, to some extent at least, under the control of the pituitary through the influence of pituitary neuropeptides.

REFERENCES

Agranoff, B. W., Davis, R. E. and Brink, J. J. (1965): Memory fixation in the Goldfish. *Proc. nat. Acad. Sci. (Wash.)* **54**, 788.

Arimura, A., Yanaguchi, T., Yoshimura, K., Imazeki, T. and Itoh, S. (1965): Role of the neurohypophysis in the release of adrenocorticotrophic hormone in the rat. *Jap. J. Physiol.* **15**, 278–295.

Bohus, B. and Wied, D. de (1966): Inhibitory and facilitatory effect of two related peptides on extinction of avoidance behavior. *Science* **153**, 318–320.

Davis, R. E. and Agranoff, B. W. (1966): Stages of memory formation in goldfish: evidence for an environmental trigger. *Proc. nat. Acad. Sci. (Wash.)* **55**, 555.

Flexner, J. B. and Flexner, L. B. (1967): Restoration of expression of memory lost after treatment with puromycin. *Proc. nat. Acad. Sci. (Wash.)* **57**, 1651.

Flexner, L. B. and Flexner, J. B. (1968): Intracerebral saline: effect on memory of trained mice treated with puromycin. *Science* **159**, 330.

Ginsburg, M. (1968): Production, release, transportation and elimination of the neurohypophyseal hormones. In: *Handbook of Experimental Pharmacology*. Vol. 23. Ed. by B. Berde. Springer, New York. pp. 286–352.

Glassman, E. (1969): The biochemistry of learning: an evaluation of the role of RNA and protein. *Ann. Rev. Biochem.* **38**, 606.

Greven, H. M. and Wied, D. de (1967): The active sequence in the ACTH molecule responsible for inhibition of the extinction of conditioned avoidance behavior in rats. *Europ. J. Pharmacol.* **2**, 14–16.

Matthies, H., Fähse, C. and Liets, W. (1971): Die Wirkung von RNS-Präcursoren auf die Erhaltung des Langzeitgedächtnisses. *Psychopharmacologia (Berl.)* **20**, 10–15.

McCann, S. M. (1957): ACTH-releasing activity of extract of the posterior lobe of the pituitary in vivo. *Endocrinology* **60**, 664.

McCaugh, J. L. (1966): Time-dependent processes in memory storage. *Science* **153**, 1351.

Mirsky, I. A., Stein, M. and Paulish, G. (1954): The secretion of an antidiuretic substance into the circulation of rats exposed to noxious stimuli. *Endocrinology* **54**, 491.

Murphy, J. V. and Miller, R. E. (1956): Spaced and massed practice with a methodological consideration of avoidance conditioning. *J. exp. Psychol.* **52**, 77–81.

Smelik, P. G., Gaarenstroom, J. H., Konojnendijk, W. and Wied, D. de (1962): Evaluation of the role of the posterior lobe of the hypophysis in the reflex secretion of corticotrophin. *Acta physiol. pharmacol. neerl.* **11**, 20–33.

Wied, D. de (1961): The significance of the antidiuretic hormone in the release mechanism of corticotrophin. *Endocrinology* **68**, 956–970.

Wied, D. de (1965): The influence of the posterior and intermediate lobe of the pituitary and pituitary peptides on the maintenance of a conditioned avoidance response in rats. *Int. J. Neuropharmacol.* **4**, 157–167.

Wied, D. de (1966): Inhibitory effects of ACTH and related peptides on extinction of conditioned avoidance behavior in rats. *Proc. Soc. exp. Biol. (N. Y.)* **122**, 28–32.

Wied, D. de (1969): Effects of peptide hormones on behavior. In: *Frontiers in Neuroendocrinology.* Ed. by W. F. Ganong and L. Martini. Oxford University Press, New York. pp. 97–140.

Wied, D. de (1971): Long-term effect of vasopressin on the maintenance of a conditioned avoidance response in rats. *Nature (Lond.)* (In press).

Wied, D. de and Mirsky, I. A. (1959): The action of hydrocortisone on the antidiuretic and adrenocorticotrophic responses to noxious stimuli. *Endocrinology* **64**, 955.

Wied, D. de and Bohus, B. (1966): Long-term and short-term effects on retention of a conditioned avoidance response in rats by treatment with long-acting Pitressin and α-MSH. *Nature (Lond.)* **212**, 1484–1486.

Wied, D. de, Bouman, P. R. and Smelik, P. G. (1958): The effect of a lipid extract from the posterior hypothalamus and of pitressin on the release of ACTH from the pituitary gland. *Endocrinology* **62**, 605.

Wied, D. de, Bohus, B., Ernst, A. M., Jong, W. de, Nieuwenhuizen, W., Pieper, E. E. M. and Yasumura, S. (1967): Several aspects of the influence of vasopressin on pituitary–adrenal activity. In: *Proceedings of the Royal Society of Medicine, September 1967.* Vol. 60. No. 9. 907.

CORRELATIONS BETWEEN THE PITUITARY–ADRENAL FUNCTION AND THE EXPLORATORY ACTIVITY, LEARNING BEHAVIOUR AND LIMBIC FUNCTIONS

E. ENDRŐCZI and T. FEKETE

Central Research Division
Postgraduate Medical School
Budapest, Hungary
and
Department of Neurology and Psychiatry
University Medical School
Pécs, Hungary

Exploratory activity, learning and memory functions are related phenomena of brain activities. Humoral factors exert a modifying influence on these behavioural processes and neuroendocrine interrelationships may be regarded as a functional bond between internal and external environment. There are data indicating that hormones produce changes in the excitability state of the nervous system and lead to alteration of the sensory input and of the ongoing motor activity.

This paper gives a short survey of the recent findings concerning the correlations between the pituitary–adrenal function and exploratory activity, passive avoidance learning and limbic functions in the rat.

EXPLORATORY ACTIVITY

The exploratory activity of adult male rats was tested in a 12-cell maze for 10 minutes and blood samples for determination of plasma corticosterone response levels were obtained in the 20th minute after the beginning of the behavioural session. The rats with high plasma corticosterone response values showed a lesser degree of the exploratory activity, although there were animals with extremely high exploration and high plasma corticosterone concentration which indicated a U-shape correlation between the two parameters (Fig. 1). Nevertheless, the main tendency of the relationship between the exploratory activity and pituitary–adrenal response levels is an inverse correlation at a low or moderate degree of exploration.

Both the exploratory activity and the pituitary–adrenal function go through a circadian variation but show maximal values in the opposite phases under a synchronizing influence of light and dark periods (light: from 6.00 till 18.00 hours). High exploratory activity had been observed in night hours (tested in red light) when the plasma corticosterone resting level is extremely low. On the other hand, the exploratory activity was very low in the afternoon when the plasma corticosterone concentration reaches a peak during the daily variation (Fig. 2). These observations demonstrated an inverse correlation of the daily rhythm of pituitary–

adrenal function to the exploratory activity, although did not indicate a causative relation between the two parameters.

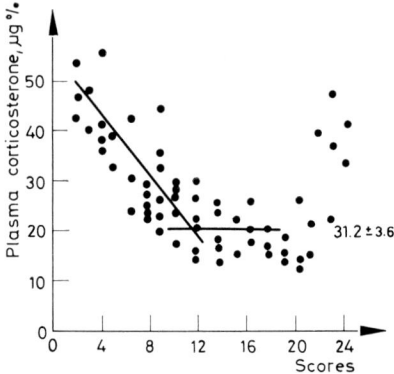

Fig. 1. Relation between exploratory activity and plasma corticosterone response level in the adult male rats

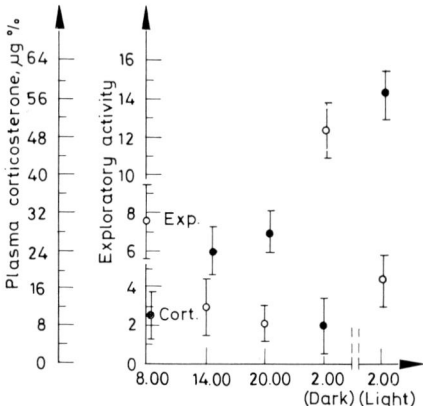

Fig. 2. Circadian variations of plasma corticosterone concentration and the exploratory activity in the rat. The illumination of the animals for 1 hour during night hours (light: 2.00) led to an increased plasma corticosterone concentration and a decrease in the exploratory activity

In further experiments, for studying the causative relationship between the exploratory activity and the pituitary–adrenal function adrenalectomized rats were tested for exploratory activity after the intravenous injection of different amounts of corticosterone and dexamethasone as well as physiological saline solution. A significant suppression of the exploratory activity was observed following corticosterone administration and a similar action of the dexamethasone treatment lasted at least for 2 days (Figs 3 and 4). These observations clearly indicated that corticosteroids exert a suppressive influence on the exploratory behaviour and this effect may explain the inverse correlation of the pituitary–adrenal function to the exploratory behaviour under physiological conditions.

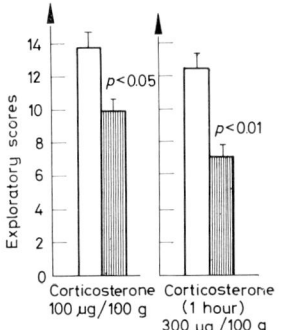

Fig. 3. Suppressive effect of corticosterone administration on the exploratory activity of adrenalectomized rats

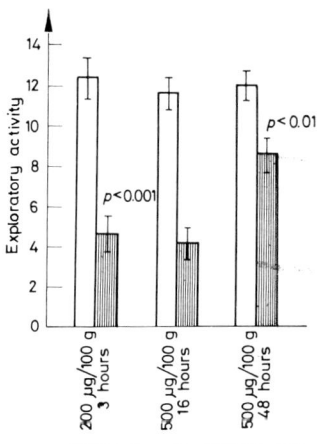

Fig. 4. Suppressive effect of dexamethasone administration on the exploratory activity of adrenalectomized rats

EXPLORATORY ACTIVITY AND PASSIVE AVOIDANCE LEARNING

Passive avoidance learning was studied in a conflict situation of thirst versus fear. The rats were kept on a fixed schedule of 23-hour water deprivation and were provided with water only in the experimental box for 5 days to achieve habituation to the experimental conditions. On the 6th day, in the early morning hours, each drinking attempt was associated with the administration of electric shock through an electrified grid for 20 minutes. It was found that the rats with different exploratory scores tested in a 12-cell maze before the passive avoidance training, showed marked differences in the rate of passive avoidance learning. Rats with a low exploratory activity displayed a faster learning rate than rats with moderate or high exploratory scores (Fig. 5). The difference is shown by a steeper slope and less trials.

The intravenous administration of 0.3 mg/100 g corticosterone or 0.1 mg/100 g dexamethasone 1 hour prior to the passive avoidance procedure led to a significant modification of the rate of passive avoidance learning in adrenalectomized rats. The experiments were performed according to the same procedure as indicated in the study mentioned in the foregoing. Corticosteroid treatment resulted in a

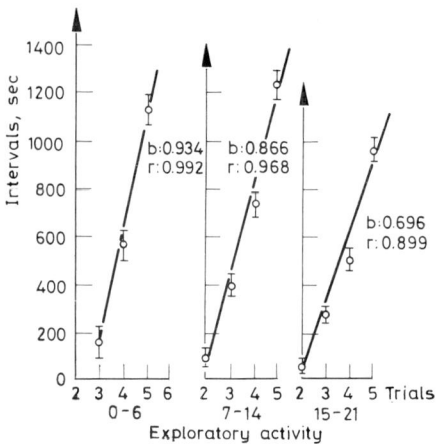

Fig. 5. Differences between the rates of passive avoidance learning by the rats showing low, moderate or high exploratory activity

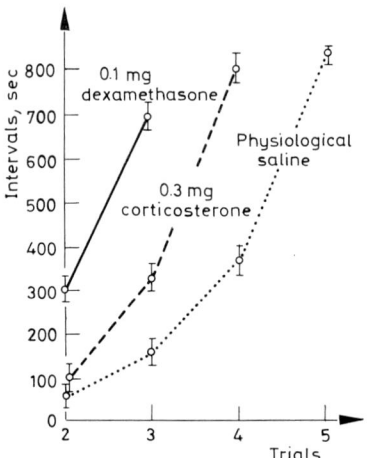

Fig. 6. Effect of the corticosterone and dexamethasone administration on passive avoidance learning of adrenalectomized rats

marked facilitation of the acquisition of passive avoidance response (Fig. 6). If we consider that an inverse correlation exists between the exploratory activity and pituitary–adrenal function, on the one hand, and an inverse correlation between the exploratory activity and the passive avoidance behaviour, on the other, we may presume a causative relationship between the pituitary–adrenal activity and the behavioural phenomena.

EFFECT OF SEPTAL LESION ON EXPLORATORY ACTIVITY, PASSIVE AVOIDANCE LEARNING AND PITUITARY–ADRENAL FUNCTION

Bilateral electrolytic lesions which destroyed the dorsal septal area and the descending fornices were performed with a stereotaxic apparatus 3 weeks prior to observations. The "exploratory activity" of septal-lesioned rats tested in a 12-cell maze cannot be identified with the exploration of the sham-operated or intact animals since there was a great number of perseverative movements (moving through the same gate more frequently than the controls) which virtually increased the number of the exploratory scores, but this activity might be considered better than an increased general motor behaviour. The rats with septal lesion showed a great number of exploratory scores although plasma corticosterone response level was higher than in the control animals (Fig. 7). An intravenous injection of 0.4 mg/100 g corticosterone 3 hours prior to the exploration test did not produce a change in exploratory behaviour. In contrast to these observations, the administration of 0.5 mg/100 g dexamethasone led to a significant decrease in the exploratory activity of septal-lesioned animals (Fig. 8). These findings revealed a resistance of the septal-lesioned rats against the suppressive effect of corticosterone administration, however, dexamethasone as a more potent steroid remained still effective. Testing the rats with septal lesion for passive avoidance learning in the same conflict situation as mentioned already, it

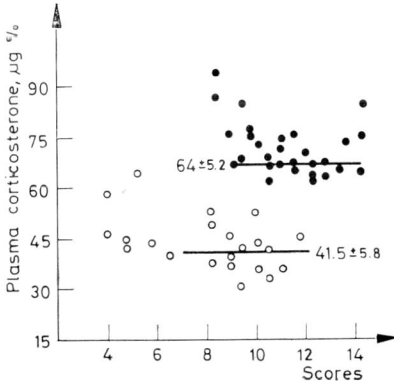

Fig. 7. Relation between the plasma corticosterone response level and the exploratory activity of sham-operated (○) and septal-lesioned (●) rats

was found that these animals show a deficit in this learning situation which confirmed the earlier data of the relevant literature (Douglas 1967, Kimble 1970). Such a change in passive avoidance behaviour following destruction of the septo-hippocampal connections may be attributed to increased perseverative responding and a weakening to withhold an approaching response in a conflict situation. Also, this interpretation of the septal-lesioned animals' behaviour is in accordance with the concept that the exploratory activity or an increased initiation of goal-directed motor pattern is in an inverse correlation to the performance of a passive avoiding animal (Dupont et al. 1970). Figure 9 shows the difference between the rates of passive avoidance learning of sham-operated and septal-lesioned rats.

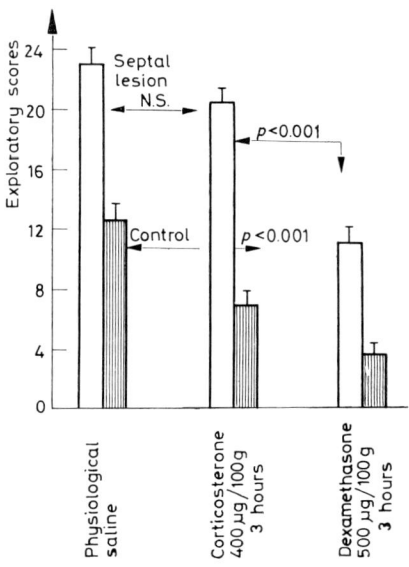

Fig. 8. Effect of corticosterone and dexamethasone administration on the exploratory activity of sham-operated (empty bars) and septal-lesioned (shaded bars) rats

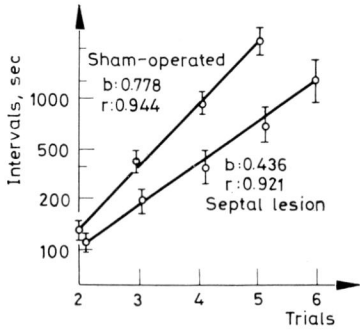

Fig. 9. Rate of passive avoidance learning of the sham-operated and the septal-lesioned rats

CORRELATIONS BETWEEN HIPPOCAMPAL THETA ACTIVITY AND PASSIVE AVOIDANCE LEARNING IN ADRENALECTOMIZED AND CORTICOSTERONE-TREATED RATS

Appearance of the hippocampal theta rhythm during exploration and goal-directed motor response is known from earlier studies (Grastyán et al. 1959, Adey et al. 1960, etc.). In the present investigations the rate of passive avoidance learning was correlated to the appearance of theta rhythm in adrenalectomized rats without and after treatment with corticosterone. The adrenals were removed 2 to 3 weeks prior to the implantation of bipolar electrodes into the dorsal hippocampus. The establishment of a passive avoidance response was performed according to the procedure which has already been described in this paper. To carry out the study on adrenalectomized rats our aim was to avoid the influence of the endogenous corticosteroid production on the behavioural and electrophysiological parameters.

The rat displays two different frequency ranges of theta rhythm (Gray 1970): (i) with a frequency range from 8 to 9.6 cps which occurs during the integration and the approaching of a known reward, and (ii) with a lower frequency range (from 6 to 8 cps) which appears during the exploratory activity in a novel situation. In passive avoidance conditioning the theta rhythm with a high frequency could be observed during the first intertrial interval and only for a short period in the consecutive intervals when the animal showed a preparatory phase to approach the water. Total duration of theta activity was progressively decreasing in the consecutive intertrial intervals which means a decreasing interest in the environment during the development of passive avoidance conditioned response. This interpretation of the relationship between passive avoidance behaviour and hippocampal theta activity corroborates well with our previous concept, nevertheless, it still requires approval that theta rhythm would express certain expectation by the animal to satisfy its needs. Appearance of theta rhythm is unrelated to the type of motivation and cannot be simplified as an electrical correlate of the movement (Endrőczi and Nyakas 1971). A progressive decline in the appearance of theta rhythm during the consecutive intertrial intervals is shown in Fig. 10.

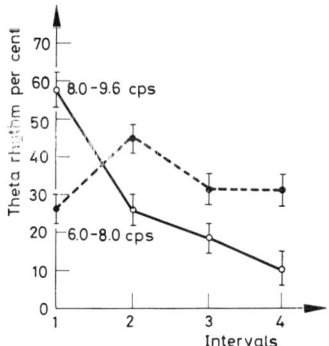

Fig. 10. Changes in theta rhythm both in the frequency range and the total duration of their appearances in the intertrial intervals during the course of the development of a passive avoidance response

The intravenous injection of 0.5 mg/100 g corticosterone produced a dissociation between the development of passive avoidance behaviour and the appearance of theta rhythm. Thus, corticosterone facilitated learning and led to the suppression of the genesis of hippocampal theta activity. The proportions of the time of the intertrial interval and the duration of theta activity in the interval are shown on the sequence of the consecutive intertrial intervals in Fig. 11.

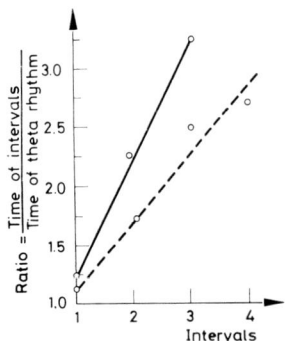

Fig. 11. Changes in the ratios of time of intervals and the time of theta rhythm in the interval following 0.5 mg/100 g corticosterone administration (solid line) in adrenalectomized rats. The broken line corresponds to the values obtained by the rats with physiological saline injection

GENERAL CONCLUSIONS

The role of the rhinencephalic structures in the control of motivated behaviour and neuroendocrine processes has been suggested by a great number of observations (Douglas 1967, Endrőczi 1968, 1970, Lissák and Endrőczi 1960, 1965, Sawyer 1967, etc.). Studying the influence of pituitary–adrenocortical hormones on the conditioned reflex behaviour on different mammals we have concluded that corticosteroids exert a facilitatory action on the internal inhibition and such action manifests itself by an enhanced extinction of both the alimentary and defensive conditioned response (Lissák et al. 1957, Endrőczi and Lissák 1962), a decreased intertrial activity (Endrőczi and Lissák 1962) and may interfere with the acquisition of a two-way active avoidance response (Endrőczi 1970). Moreover, an inverse correlation of the pituitary–adrenal function to the rate of a passive avoidance learning has been observed in both the recent and the earlier studies (Endrőczi et al. 1959, Dupont et al. 1970).

The participation of rhinencephalic structures in the mediation of corticosterone-adjusted behaviour seems to be strongly supported by the facts that the elimination of hippocampal–brainstem connections has led to the resistance of the suppressive effect of corticosterone in a passive avoidance situation or in term of the exploratory activity. The hippocampus which exhibits a control on the sensory input and probably other activities of the brainstem and diencephalon may be considered a chemoreceptive area for corticosterone. This assumption is supported by the observations of McEwen et al. (1969) and Dupont et al. (1970)

who found that the hippocampal cells can accumulate corticosterone in a much greater amount than other parts of the brain and the corticosterone-binding property of these cells is highly specific for 11-beta-hydroxy- but not 17,11-dihydroxy-steroids. In other words, neither cortisol nor dexamethasone can compete for the hippocampal binding sites under conditions far above the physiological concentration of plasma corticosterone level. The assumption of a corticosterone-specific receptor system at the septo-hippocampal level does not exclude the possibility of the existence of many quasi-specific corticosteroid-sensitive cells distributed over the brainstem and the diencephalon. Iontophoretic application of dexamethasone revealed a large population of these cells sensitive to this substance (Steiner 1970).

A correlation between the exploratory activity and the appearance of theta rhythm in the hippocampus, on the one hand, and an inverse relationship between these parameters and the rate of passive avoidance learning, on the other, suggested that the influence of adrenocortical hormones on the behavioural reactions manifests itself by changing the initiation of the exploratory activity or of the goal-directed motor response. This concept is in accordance with the view that theta rhythm is an electrical correlate of the expectation to do something and unrelated to the specificity of the need of the organism, on the one hand, and that the corticosteroids exert a suppressive influence on the initiation of the integration of motor pattern, on the other hand.

REFERENCES

Adey, W. R., Dunlop, C. W. and Hendrix, C. E. (1960): Hippocampal slow waves *Arch. Neurol. (Chic.)* **3**, 74–90.

Douglas, J. R. (1967): The hippocampus and behavior. *Psychol. Bull.* **67**, 416–442.

Dupont, A., Endrőczi, E. and Fortier, C. (1970): Relationship of pituitary–thyroid and pituitary–adrenocortical activities to conditioned behaviour in the rat. In: *The Influence of Hormones on the Central Nervous System*. Ed. by D. H. Ford. Karger, Basel–New York.

Endrőczi, E. (1968): Effect of hormones on the brainstem and limbic structures. In: *Symposium on Hormones and Behavior*. Ed. by G. C. Gual. Mexico City, Intern. Congr. Endocrinology.

Endrőczi, E. (1970): Pituitary–adrenocortical function, exploration and passive avoidance behaviour in the rat. In: UCLA Workshop Conference. Ed. by C. H. Sawyer and R. Gorski. Univ. Calif. Press.

Endrőczi, E. and Lissák, K. (1962): Spontaneous goal-directed motor activity related to the alimentary conditioned reflex behaviour and its regulation by neural and humoral factors. *Acta physiol. Acad. Sci. hung.* **21**, 265–283.

Endrőczi, E. and Nyakas, Cs. (1971): Effect of septal lesion on exploratory activity, passive avoidance learning and pituitary–adrenal function in the rat. *Acta physiol. Acad. Sci. hung.* **39**, 351–360.

Endrőczi, E., Telegdy, Gy. and Lissák, K. (1957): Analysis of the individual variation of adaptation in the rat on the basis of conditioned reflex and endocrine studies. *Acta physiol. Acad. Sci. hung.* **11**, 393–398.

Grastyán, E., Lissák, K., Madarász, I. and Donhoffer, H. (1959): Hippocampal electrical activity during the development of conditioned reflexes. *Electroenceph. clin. Neurophysiol.* **11**, 409–430.

Gray, A. J. (1970): Sodium amobarbital, the hippocampal theta rhythm and the partial reinforcement extinction effect. *Psychol. Rev.* **77**, 465–480.

Kimble, D. P. (1970): Possible inhibitory functions of the hippocampus. *Neuropsychologia* **7**, 235–244.

Lissák, K. and Endrőczi, E. (1960): *Die neuroendokrine Steuerung der Adaptationstätigkeit.* Akadémiai Kiadó, Budapest.

Lissák, K. and Endrőczi, E. (1965): *The Neuroendocrine Control of Adaptation.* Pergamon Press, Oxford.

Lissák, K., Endrőczi, E. and Medgyesi, P. (1957): Somatisches Verhalten und Nebennierenrindentätigkeit. *Pflügers Arch. ges. Physiol.* **265**, 117—124.

McEwen, B. S. and Weiss, J. M. (1970): The uptake and action of corticosterone: Regional and subcellular studies on rat brain. In: *Pituitary, Adrenal and the Brain.* Ed. by D. de Wied and J. A. W. M. Weijnen. Elsevier, Amsterdam. pp. 200—213.

McEwen, B. S., Weiss, J. M. and Schwartz, L. S. (1969): Uptake of corticosterone by rat brain and its concentration by certain limbic structures. *Brain Res.* **16**, 227—241.

Routtenberg, A. (1968): The two arousal hypothesis: reticular formation and limbic system. *Psychol. Rev.* **75**, 51—80.

Sawyer, C. H. (1967): Some endocrine aspects of forebrain inhibition. *Brain Res.* **6**, 48—59.

Steiner, F. A. (1970): Effects of ACTH and corticosteroids on single neurons in the hypothalamus. In: *Pituitary, Adrenal and the Brain.* Ed. by D. de Wied and J. A. W. M. Weijnen. Elsevier, Amsterdam. pp. 102—107.

BRAIN–ENDOCRINE INTERACTION: ARE SOME EFFECTS OF ACTH AND ADRENOCORTICAL HORMONES ON NEUROENDOCRINE REGULATION AND BEHAVIOUR MEDIATED VIA CENTRAL CATECHOLAMINE NEURONS?

K. FUXE, T. HÖKFELT, G. JONSSON and P. LIDBRINK

Department of Histology
Karolinska Institutet
Stockholm, Sweden

INTRODUCTION

During the last decade it has become increasingly clear that hormonal steroids and pituitary hormones exert important actions on the brain influencing particularly neuroendocrine and behavioural functions (Martini and Ganong 1966, Ganong and Martini 1967, 1969, Martini et al. 1970, Martini and Meites 1970, De Wied and Weijnen 1970). Many physiological, pharmacological and biochemical studies suggest that the central catecholamine (CA) neurons could be involved in the control of the secretions of the various releasing and inhibitory factors regulating the secretion of the hormones from the anterior pituitary (Sawyer et al. 1949, Stefano et al. 1965, Donoso and Stefano 1967, Fuxe et al. 1967, Stefano and Donoso 1967, Fuxe and Hökfelt 1967, 1969, Schneider and McCann 1969, Kamberi et al. 1969) and various behavioural functions (Seiden and Carlsson 1964, Carlsson 1966, Hansson 1967, Stein 1968, Randrup and Munkvad 1968, Reis and Fuxe 1968, Arbuthnott et al. 1971). Of great interest is a small tubero-infundibular DA system (Jonsson et al. 1971a, b, c) which probably is involved in the control of gonadotrophin secretion (Fuxe et al. 1967). Our studies on turnover in these dopamine (DA) neurons suggest that the system via an axo-axonic influence could act to inhibit luteinizing hormone releasing factor (LHRF) and follicle stimulating hormone releasing factor (FSHRF) secretion and stimulate prolactin inhibitory factor (PIF) secretion from peptidergic nerve terminals in the median eminence (Fuxe et al. 1969a, b, 1971a, b, Ahrén et al. 1971, Hökfelt and Fuxe 1971a). Since several review articles recently have been written on this system (Fuxe and Hökfelt 1969, 1970a, b, Hökfelt and Fuxe 1971b) the present article will mainly deal with our turnover studies on the ascending noradrenaline (NA) and DA neurons in relation to changes in the activity of the pituitary–adrenal axis and associated unconditioned and conditioned behavioural responses. Some of these findings have been briefly reported in previous review articles (Fuxe and Hökfelt 1969a, b, Fuxe et al. 1970a). It may be emphasized that this article is based on preliminary results. In spite of this we would like to take the opportunity to advance a hypothetical discussion on a possible correlation between changes in amine turnover and various behavioural parameters in neuroendocrine states.

METHODOLOGY

Information as to the functional role of the central CA neurons can be obtained by investigating the nervous activity of the neurons during various physiological and experimental states. An indication of the activity can be reached by studying the amine turnover which is highly dependent on ongoing nervous activity. There are several ways of measuring amine turnover and the various methods have been thoroughly discussed in several papers (see Andén et al. 1969, Iversen and Simmonds 1969, Costa 1970, Costa and Neff 1970, Fuxe et al. 1970b, Persson and Waldeck 1970). The approach used in this study has been to analyse the rate of decline of CA stores following amine synthesis inhibition with either tyrosine or DA-β-hydroxylase inhibitors (Corrodi and Hansson 1966, Andén et al. 1966a, Corrodi et al. 1970, Florvall and Corrodi 1970, Svensson and Waldeck 1969). The inhibitors used were H44/68 (α-methyl-p-tyrosine methylester, tyrosine hydroxylase inhibitor) and PLA63 [(bis-(4-methyl-1-homopiperazinyl-thiocarbonyl) disulphide, DA-β-hydroxylase inhibitor]. Supramaximal doses of the inhibitors have always been used. CA analysis has been performed both biochemically (Bertler et al. 1958, Carlsson and Lindqvist 1962) and histochemically (Falck et al. 1962, Corrodi and Jonsson 1967). The histochemical approach enables one to evaluate changes in the various CA nerve terminal systems of the brain. Although the histochemical techniques for CA analysis cannot be regarded as exact quantitatively like a chemical-analytical procedure, several investigations have clearly shown that careful semiquantitative estimation of fluorescence intensity will allow determination of changes in CA levels (Olson et al. 1968, Jonsson 1969, 1971, Lidbrink and Jonsson 1971). The biochemical analyses have so far been made on whole brain, since the changes in NA turnover have usually been found to be wide-spread as revealed histochemically and whole brain DA mainly reflects changes in the large nigro-neostriatal DA system (Fuxe et al. 1970).

RESULTS

CHANGES IN CENTRAL CA TURNOVER IN VARIOUS ENDOCRINE STATES

Adrenalectomy. Using both histochemical and biochemical amine analyses it was found that there was an increase in MA disappearance in most parts of the brain, e.g., in the hypothalamus and cerebral cortex after tyrosine or DA-β-hydroxylase inhibition in both male and female rats. These results suggest that there is a general increase in NA turnover in the brain both of ascending coerulocortical NA neurons and the medullo-ponto-subcortical NA systems (Fuxe et al. 1970d, Ungerstedt 1971a, Olson and Fuxe 1971). Clearcut increases in NA turnover were observed only after about 6 to 8 days and persisted for at least 1 to 2 months (Jonsson et al. 1971c). The DA turnover in the neostriatum seemed to be relatively unaffected by adrenalectomy, since the rate of disappearance of DA was more or less unchanged after H44/68 treatment.

Hypophysectomy. Histochemically and biochemically it was found that there was a decrease in the disappearance of NA after tyrosine and DA-β-hydroxylase inhibition in most parts of the brain of both male and female rats. These results suggested a general decrease in amine turnover in the central NA neurons after hypophysectomy. The effects were clearcut only after about a week and persisted for several months (Jonsson et al. 1971). The rate of H44/68 induced disappearance of DA fluorescence from the neostriatum, while it was not changed following hypophysectomy.

Castration. In male rats it has been found that castration did not change the rate of NA depletion following tyrosine and DA-β-hydroxylase inhibition. After many months a slight deceleration was observed (Jonsson et al. 1971b).

CHANGES IN CENTRAL CA TURNOVER AFTER HORMONAL TREATMENTS

Effect of glucocorticoids and mineralocorticoids

NA turnover. In normal rats single or multiple doses of corticosterone (in doses up to 50 mg/kg), hydrocortisone (up to 25 mg/kg) and dexamethasone (1 mg/kg) not at all or only slightly decreased NA disappearance after H44/68 in the cerebral cortex and the hypothalamus as observed histochemically. These results suggest no clearcut changes in NA turnover after treatment with glucocorticoids in normal rats. Also, the stress-induced acceleration of NA turnover (Corrodi et al. 1968) was only slightly or not at all counteracted by corticosterone and dexamethasone given several times before the stress.

In adrenalectomized animals corticosterone, hydrocortisone, dexamethasone and desoxycorticosterone in multiple doses were capable of completely counteracting the increase in NA turnover found after adrenalectomy in a dose-dependent manner.

DA turnover. Corticosterone (5–50 mg/kg) and dexamethasone (0.5–10 mg/rat) given in multiple doses were capable of causing a slight increase in the disappearance of DA fluorescence from the neostriatum and the limbic forebrain of adrenalectomized rats (Figs 1 and 2). These results suggest that these steroids can increase DA turnover in the nigro-neostriatal and the mesolimbic DA neurons. Similar effects on DA turnover have been observed in hypophysectomized rats but not in normal rats following treatment with corticosterone or dexamethasone (Fuxe et al. 1970a, Jonsson et al. 1971a, b).

Effect of pituitary hormones

In normal male rats purified ACTH and the synthetic β1-24 corticotrophine (Synacten®) have been found to slightly increase NA turnover in most NA terminal systems of the brain when given intravenously or subcutaneously (long-acting ACTH) in multiple doses of 10–60 I.U. as revealed with H44/68 and PLA63 (Figs 3 and 4). FSH (300 γ/rat), LH (300 γ/rat) and prolactin (5 mg) have proved ineffective in this respect (Hökfelt and Fuxe 1971a). The decrease in NA turnover already found in hypophysectomized rats, however, was not counteracted.

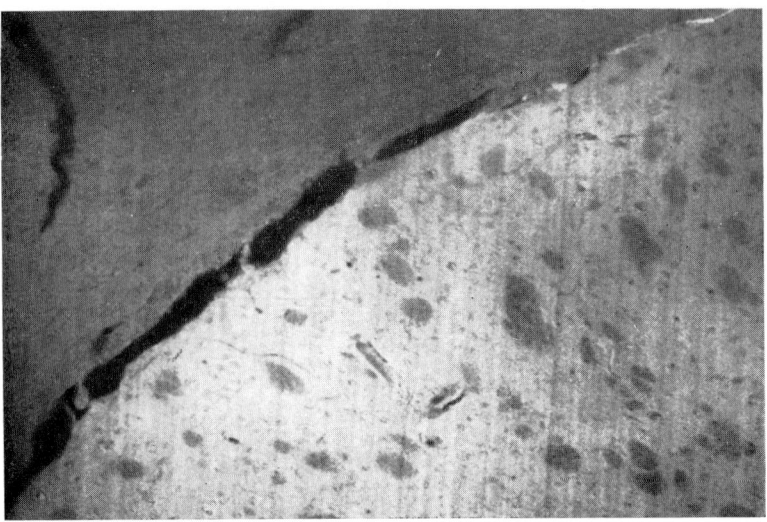

Fig. 1. Neostriatum of adrenalectomized male rats 2 hrs after treatment with a tyrosine-hydroxylase inhibitor (H 44/68, 250 mg/kg). A green DA fluorescence of moderate intensity is observed in the neostriatum. ×160

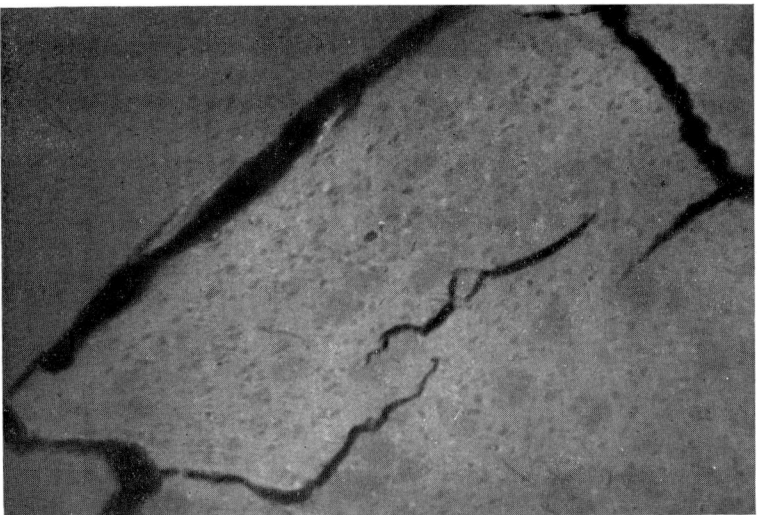

Fig. 2. Same area and treatment as in text to Fig. 1 except that dexamethasone had been given i.m. 24 and 2 hours before the inhibitor in a dose of 10 mg/kg. After this treatment only a weak DA fluorescence remains in the neostriatum. ×160

In hypophysectomized rats intravenous injections of ACTH, Synacten or subcutaneous injections of long-acting ACTH (30–60 I.U.) have been found to slightly decrease DA turnover in the neostriatum and limbic forebrain.

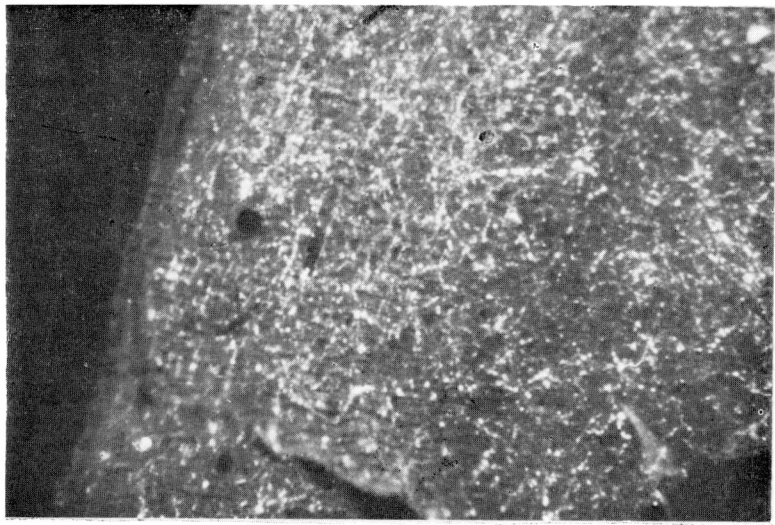

Fig. 3. Dorsomedial nucleus of hypothalamus of a normal male rat 4 hrs after treatment with a tyrosine-hydroxylase inhibitor (H 44/68, 250 mg/kg). A large number of strongly fluorescent NA nerve terminals are still observed. ×160

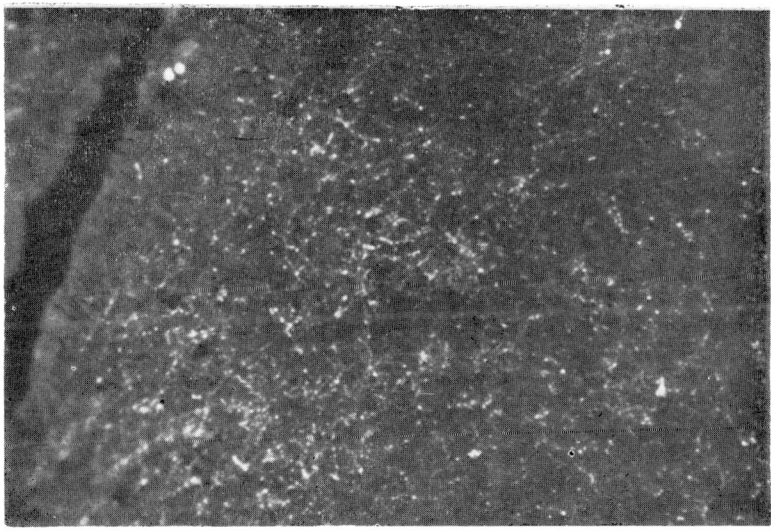

Fig. 4. The same area and treatment as in text to Fig. 3 except that ACTH, in a slowly releasable form and in a dose of 30 I.U., had been given subcutaneously 24, 12 and 2 hrs before the injection of the inhibitor. An additional dose of 15 I.U. was given 2 hrs after the injection of the inhibitor. As can be seen only weakly to moderately fluorescent nerve terminals are observed. ×160

DISCUSSION

The present results demonstrate that the tubero-infundibular DA neurons are not the only monoamine neurons which are responsive to changes in the endocrine state. The ascending NA neurons both to cortical and subcortical areas have been shown to exhibit changes in turnover in response to treatment with both hormonal steroids and pituitary hormones and with the variations of endocrine states. Certain changes in amine turnover in the ascending DA neurons have also been observed. It seems reasonable to conclude from this hormone–CA interaction that the pituitary–adrenal axis plays a role in the regulation of turnover in the ascending CA neurons. However, the influence of gonadal steroids on the ascending CA neurons should not be underestimated in view of the high turnover increase found after daily oestradiol treatment with or without progesterone in castrated female rats, suggesting that the ascending CA neurons are not exclusively concerned with the regulation of only one hormonal axis (unpublished data from this laboratory).

The mechanisms for the changes in CA turnover found after treatment with exogenous hormones or after experimentally induced changes in hormone levels are unknown.

We think that the following two principal possibilities are the most likely ones: (i) The hormones act directly on the central CA neuron systems via a direct effect on the CA cell bodies and/or nerve terminals facilitating or counteracting the nervous impulse induced release of catecholamines in the brain. (ii) The hormones could act indirectly via other neuron systems, which in turn could change the nervous impulse flow in the central CA neurons. It may be pointed out that in this case the hormones may act either directly on central neurons or via peripheral afferent pathways. Direct effects of hydrocortisone on NA nerve terminals have in fact been demonstrated in studies on NA uptake in vitro in which it was demonstrated that hydrocortisone stimulated NA uptake (Maas and Mednieks 1971). Similar findings have been obtained in this laboratory with corticosterone, the natural adrenocortical steroid in rats.

On the effects of pituitary–adrenal activity on central NA neurons

It is now of interest to evaluate whether the effects on CA turnover by adrenocortical steroids and ACTH can be related to other well-known effects of these hormones such as changes in electrolyte balance, changes in sensory detection (Henkin 1970), changes in brain excitability (Woodbury 1954, Woodbury and Vernadakis 1966) and/or changes in behaviour (e.g., De Wied 1969). To elucidate this question it is important to note that glucocorticoids such as hydrocortisone and mineralocorticoids such as desoxycorticosterone (DOCA) have similar actions on the central NA neurons, i.e. they counteract the NA turnover increases found after adrenalectomy.

These results make it unlikely that the effects are secondary to changes in abnormal electrolyte balance found e.g. in adrenalectomized rats, since carbohydrate-active steroids are as effective as DOCA in normalizing activity in the NA neurons. Nor can changes in sensory detection be responsible for the turnover changes, since DOCA does not change the increased sensory detection following adrenalectomy as do glucocorticoids. Furthermore, it does not seem probable that the effects of the gluco-mineralosteroids on the control NA neurons are mediating the increase in brain excitability (Woodbury and Vernadakis 1966) found after e.g., hydrocortisone treatment, since a similar increase in brain excitability is found after adrenalectomy (Woodbury 1954) in which state the NA turnover is increased and not decreased.

Instead, it is our view that the NA turnover changes may at present best be related to behavioural changes induced by these hormones. Thus, the retardation of NA turnover found all over the brain in adrenalectomized rats after treatment with corticosterone, dexamethasone, hydrocortisone and DOCA could partly mediate the facilitation of extinction of conditioned avoidance responses found after treatment with these steroids especially after treatment with glucocorticoids (De Wied 1967, Bohus and Lissák 1968, De Wied et al. 1968, Weiss et al. 1970). Thus, many pharmacological and physiological studies on the central NA neurons suggest that they could be involved in psychomotor stimulation and in the mediation of tonic cortical arousal (Carlsson et al. 1966, Jones 1969, Jones et al. 1969, Bobon et al. 1970, Fuxe et al. 1970d, Corrodi et al. 1970, 1971, Fuxe and Lidbrink 1971). Morphologically, they could be regarded as belonging to the ascending reticular activating system. Furthermore, it should be pointed out that probably DA and particularly NA neurons are activated in the performance of negatively reinforced conditioned avoidance behaviour (Fuxe and Hansson 1967), and pharmacological studies with apomorphine and amphetamine also underline the important role of both DA and NA neurons in this type of behaviour (Butcher and Andén 1969). Also the NA neurons probably play an important role in reinforcement mechanisms, since the central NA neurons are activated in self-stimulation behaviour (Arbuthnott et al. 1971) and extensive pharmacological analysis points out the importance of NA in this behaviour (Stein and Wise 1969, Wise and Stein 1969). Therefore, a decrease in NA turnover as seen after the steroids mentioned above probably results in a decrease in wakefulness and psychomotor drive which could be one of the mechanisms for the facilitation of the extinction of conditioned avoidance response(s) (CAR) observed. This hypothesis is further strengthened by the fact that the testosterone and β-oestradiol which do not facilitate extinction of CAR do not decrease NA turnover, whereas progesterone which facilitates extinction (Van Wimersma Greidanus 1970) also decreases NA turnover in adrenalectomized rats as found recently (Jonsson et al. 1971c). Thus, the features of steroids decreasing NA turnover and facilitating extinction of CAR are parallel phenomena. They are C_{21} steroids with a double bond and with keto groups at C_3 and at C_{20}. It is interesting to note that these steroids have small if any effect on DA turnover in the median eminence, whereas testosterone and β-oestradiol cause a marked increase in amine turnover in the tubero-infundibular DA neurons (Fuxe et al. 1969a, 1971a) demonstrating a relative specificity and in this case the importance of the OH groups at C_3 and C_{17} for the effects.

ACTH treatment, on the other hand, slightly increased amine turnover in NA nerve terminals all over the brain, particularly when given subcutaneously in a slowly releasable form. It may be that the ACTH induced increase in amine turnover in the central NA neurons, though small, could partly mediate the retardation of extinction of CAR induced by ACTH (Miller and Ogawa 1962, De Wied 1966a, b, 1967, Bohus and De Wied 1966, Weiss et al. 1970).

It is also known that ACTH treatment can somewhat improve the rate of avoidance acquisition in hypophysectomized rats (Applezweig and Baudry 1955, De Wied 1964); an effect which does not seem to be mediated via the adrenal cortex, since ACTH analogues lacking corticotrophic activity exert similar effects on the rate of acquisition (De Wied 1969, De Wied et al. 1970). In hypophysectomized rats there is a severe impairment in the ability to acquire a CAR. These effects on acquisition ability by ACTH could possibly be mediated via activation of the reticular NA neurons which could result in improvement of reinforcement and in increased arousal facilitating learning, but no evidence for an effect by ACTH on NA neurons in hypophysectomized rats has been obtained in the present study. In agreement with this view, however, the activity of the NA neurons is low in hypophysectomized rats which show difficulties to learn a CAR.

Since the NA neurons should be regarded as a part of the ascending reticular activating system (ARAS) the mechanism by which ACTH exerts its behavioural effects could partly be by activation of parts of the ARAS. It is not known, however, whether the effects of ACTH and pituitary–adrenal steroids are primarily on the ARAS or on the descending inhibitory pathways from the basal forebrain which probably are concerned with internal inhibition and are involved in motivated behavioural processes and could control activity in ascending NA neurons. A number of findings suggest, e.g., that adrenocortical hormones could enhance internal inhibition under conditioned reflex circumstances (Lissák et al. 1957, Lissák and Endrőczi 1964, Endrőczi and Lissák 1962, Bohus and Endrőczi 1965, De Wied 1967, Korányi and Endrőczi 1967, 1970, Bohus and Lissák 1968, Levine 1968). It is possible that ACTH in turn could directly or indirectly counteract activity in these inhibitory pathways.

None of the other pituitary hormones tested so far have been found in our models to increase NA turnover in normal male rats. The hormones tested are FSH (300 γ/100 g), LH (300 γ/100 g) and prolactin (mg doses). It is most probable that the ACTH induced (both the natural peptide and the synthetic β 1–24 adrenocorticotrophin have been tested) increase in NA turnover is not mediated via release of adrenocortical hormones, since these hormones reduce NA turnover. Therefore, the ACTH effect must be due to an extra-adrenal action. However, the action may not necessarily be a neural extra-adrenal effect, since ACTH induced e.g., lipid mobilization, ketosis, hypoglycaemia and hypotension which could influence CNS activity and, in this way, behaviour. Insulin treatment in high doses, however, will not result in the same degree of activation of the NA neurons as will ACTH treatment (unpublished data). Also the ACTH induced retardation of extinction of CAR is independent of stimulation of the adrenals since the action is present also in adrenalectomized rats and since ACTH analogues, which lack the adrenocortical effects of ACTH have the same behavioural effects as ACTH (Miller and Ogawa 1962, De Wied 1967, Greven and De Wied 1967, De Wied 1969).

It could be argued that the action of the adrenocortical steroids on NA turnover is due to a reduction of ACTH secretion, since rapid and dramatic rises of corticosteroid levels in blood are known to inhibit ACTH secretion with a latency of about 2 hours (Smelik 1963). Such an action could very well contribute to the reduction of NA turnover observed but cannot be the only effect of the corticosteroids in view of the relatively weak effects obtained with exogenous ACTH on NA turnover even in high doses. Similarly, the effects of the glucocorticoids on extinction of CAR are present also in hypophysectomized rats (De Wied 1967). Furthermore, Bohus (1968) has shown that cortical implants in the rostral reticular formation caused a faster extinction of CAR than implants in the median eminence which, however, caused a higher degree of suppression of ACTH secretion. These results again suggest an action of the corticoids independent of effects on ACTH secretion probably directly on the reticular formation. The results of Bohus (1968) with effective implants of cortisol also in several limbic–diencephalic regions clearly suggest that enhancement of descending inhibitory pathways to the reticular core in the brainstem could play an important role in causing the inactivation of the ascending reticular NA neurons observed and also in the behavioural effects of cortisol.

Also, the NA turnover changes found after adrenalectomy and hypophysectomy are in good agreement with the view mentioned above that reticular NA neurons are partly mediating the behavioural effects of the pituitary–adrenal axis on the brain. Thus, in adrenalectomized rats the NA turnover is increased and in hypophysectomized rats it is decreased. These changes are correlated with a retardation and enhancement of the extinction of CAR (De Wied 1967, Bohus and Lissák 1968, Weiss et al. 1970, De Wied 1969). It seems likely that in adrenalectomized rats the increase in NA turnover is partly mediated via the increase in ACTH secretion and partly via the loss of circulatory levels of glucocorticoids. In agreement with this view the latency (several days) for onset of increase in NA turnover in adrenalectomized rats (Javoy et al. 1968, Fuxe et al. 1971) is similar to that for onset of ACTH hypersecretion (Brodish and Long 1956). It seems logical to think that the decrease in NA turnover found after hypophysectomy should partly be due to removal of ACTH secretion. However, so far the results are negative.

In view of the above it seems possible that behavioural effects found in relation to extinction of CAR after changes of pituitary–adrenal activity are partly mediated via changes in activity of reticular NA neurons. Weiss et al. (1970) have suggested that the pituitary–adrenal axis mainly moderates fear-motivated responses, ACTH increases fear and glucocorticoids decrease fear in this way increasing and decreasing fear-motivated responses, respectively. Our results are in good agreement with this view, since fear could probably be of a higher intensity and better retained with increased arousal, which probably is present in states with high activity of the NA neuron systems (adrenalectomy, ACTH treatment) from the reticular formation. The reverse is true with low activity of the NA neuron systems (hypophysectomy, glucocorticoid treatment). It should be added that performance of CAR is to be regarded as a relatively stressful situation, and it is known that the central NA neurons are activated in stressful conditions in general (Gordon et al. 1966, Bliss et al. 1968, Corrodi et al. 1968, Thierry et al. 1968). These results suggest that glucocorticoids could act to reduce stress and anxiety and to normalize overstimulated behaviour (Woodbury 1958) by reducing activity in the NA neurons.

It should be mentioned that many antidepressant drugs of the imipramine type, such as protriptyline and desipramine, seem to have potent blocking effects on the NA membrane pump (Carlsson et al. 1966) thereby facilitating transmission in the central NA neurons. It is believed by many workers (Carlsson et al. 1966, Glowinski and Baldessarini 1966, Schildkraut et al. 1967) that this action on the NA neurons could mediate a part of the antidepressant effects of these drugs, especially recovery of psychomotor drive. In this context it might be of interest to mention that a small increase in adrenocortical activity has been observed in depressive illness but not in mania (Coppen 1970). It has also been reported that adrenalectomized patients on fixed doses of adrenocortical steroids can develop depression (Crisp and Roberts 1963, Lindqvist and Lindqvist 1964, Bunney and Davis 1965, Schildkraut 1965). These results are consistent with the view that decrease in activity in the central NA neurons is induced by these steroids. The euphoria found on ACTH treatment of patients could in turn be speculated to be partly related to the induction by this hormone of increased activity in the NA neurons.

Role of the central NA neurons in control of ACTH secretion

There exists evidence that the ascending NA neurons could be involved in the inhibition of ACTH secretion by reducing activity in the corticotrophin releasing factor (CRF) containing neurons. The evidence is mainly based on pharmacological experiments demonstrating that CA depletors and receptor blocking agents such as reserpine and chlorpromazine and tyrosine-hydroxylase inhibitors increase ACTH secretion, whereas CA releasing agents such as amphetamine or CA precursors such as Dopa inhibit stress-induced hypersecretion of corticosterone secretion (Van Loon et al. 1969, Van Loon and Ganong 1969, Bhattacharya and Marks 1969a, b, Ganong 1970, Marks et al. 1970, Scapagnini et al. 1970). The inhibitory systems seem to be noradrenergic and not dopaminergic, since dopamine β-hydroxylase inhibitors block Dopa-induced inhibition of ACTH secretion (Ganong 1971) and in view of the increase of tonic hypersecretion of corticosterone after selective 6-hydroxy-DA (6-OH-DA) induced lesions of the ascending NA pathway or after intraventricular injections of 6-OH-DA (Lidbrink et al., unpublished data).

In view of the above the NA turnover changes found in hypothalamus and the limbic system in relation to changes in the pituitary–adrenal axis activity should be interpreted along the lines that the noradrenergic system is inhibitory with regard to release of CRF and subsequently of ACTH.

The inhibitory feedback action of circulating corticosteroids on ACTH secretion can therefore not be mediated via the NA neurons, since the corticosteroids decrease NA neuronal activity (Fuxe et al. 1970a). Such an action would aim at increasing ACT H secretion and could possibly explain the low capacity and slow action of this feedback mechanism (Smelik 1963), since obviously corticoids also inhibit inhibitory and not only excitatory systems in relation to ACTH secretion.

However, there is also evidence for a "short" feedback mechanism for the control of ACTH secretion (Halász and Szentágothai 1960, Motta et al. 1965, Dallman and Yates 1968). Since ACTH increases the activity of the inhibitory NA system it may be that the short-negative feedback of ACTH is partly mediated via the ventral NA pathway from the reticular formation innervating the hypothalamus and subcortical limbic areas and the dorsal NA pathway innervating e.g., the hippocampal formation (Fuxe et al. 1970d, Ungerstedt 1971a). If this is true the NA neurons are involved in mediating both the neuroendocrine and behavioural effects of ACTH on the brain.

On the effects of pituitary–adrenal activity on ascending DA neurons

In contrast to the case with the central NA neurons glucocorticoids induced a small increase in the amine turnover in the ascending DA neurons of adrenalectomized rats, whereas natural or synthetic ACTH caused a small decrease in the activity in these neurons of hypophysectomized rats.

It is well known that the nigro-neostriatal DA neurons constitute an important locomotor system probably mediating unconditioned behavioural responses (Carlsson 1959, Poirier and Sourkes 1965, Andén et al. 1966b, Hornykiewicz 1966, Randrup and Munkvad 1968, Corrodi et al. 1970, Fuxe and Ungerstedt 1970, Andén 1970, Ungerstedt 1971b). It is possible that the decreased DA turnover found after ACTH treatment could partly mediate the facilitation of conditioned avoidance *performance* found after ACTH treatment (Bohus and Endrőczi 1964, Bohus et al. 1968, Levine and Brush 1967, Wertheim et al. 1969) by decreasing locomotion and favouring conditioned behaviour. Such an effect could also partly mediate the ACTH induced increase in rate of acquisition of a CAR and retardation of its extinction. The effect of ACTH is probably not caused by release of glucocorticoids since these increase DA turnover.

The increased DA turnover, found after treatment with glucocorticoids, is also of great interest, since running activity in male rats is increased by dexamethasone (Kendall 1970). Also this increase in DA turnover could be of importance for the enhancement of extinction of CAR induced by glucocorticoids, since the action on the DA neurons will favour the performance of unconditioned behaviour such as locomotion, sniffing, etc. This action of the glucocorticoids could partly be due to inhibition of ACTH secretion by their negative feedback action. However, the glucocorticoids must have in addition an action of their own, since they were capable of increasing DA turnover in hypophysectomized rats.

It should be pointed out that glucocorticoids and ACTH induced similar changes in DA turnover in the limbic forebrain in the tuberculum olfactorium and nucleus accumbens as in the neostriatum. It may be speculated that since tuberculum olfactorium is a relay in the central olfactory pathways the glucocorticoid induced increase in DA turnover in this area could partly mediate the decrease in smell detection observed after treatment with glucocorticoids (Henkin 1970).

SUMMARY

Although it is premature to make any definite conclusions, on the basis of the present data, we would like to point out the following possibilities as a neurochemical basis for the changes in behaviour and neuroendocrine regulation found in relation to changes in activity of the pituitary–adrenal axis.

1. The enhancement of the rate of acquisition of CARs and the retardation of the rate of extinction of CARs induced by ACTH may partly be mediated via a general increase in the activity of the reticular NA neurons by ACTH, resulting in increased arousal. A decrease in activity in the nigro-neostriatal DA neurons, an important locomotor system, could also contribute to these behavioural changes by reducing unconditioned behaviour. This could also be the mechanism for the ACTH induced enhancement of avoidance performance.

2. The reverse effects induced by glucocorticoids on these conditioned processes may partly be mediated via a decreased activity in the reticular NA neurons decreasing arousal and an increased activity in the nigro-neostriatal DA neurons facilitating the appearance of unconditioned behaviour.

3. The "short" negative feedback action by ACTH on CRF release may partly be mediated via increased activity in the NA pathway to the hypothalamus and the limbic system.

ACKNOWLEDGEMENTS

This work has been supported by grants (B72-14C-715-07, B72-14X-2887-03B, B72-14X-2295-05A, B72-14P-3262-02B) from the Swedish Medical Research Council and grants from M. Bergwalls Stiftelse and C. and E. Ericssons Stiftelse.

REFERENCES

AHRÉN, K., FUXE, K., HAMBERGER, L. and HÖKFELT, T. (1971): Turnover changes in the tubero-infundibular dopamine neurons during the ovarian cycle of the rat. *Endocrinology* **88**, 1415—1424.

ANDÉN, N.-E. (1970): Effects of amphetamine and some other drugs on central catecholamine neurons. In: *Amphetamines and Related Compounds*. Raven Press, New York.

ANDÉN, N.-E., CORRODI, H., DAHLSTRÖM, A., FUXE, K. and HÖKFELT, T. (1966a): Effects of tyrosine hydroxylase inhibition on the amine levels of central monoamine neurons. *Life Sci.* **5**, 561—568.

ANDÉN, N.-E., DAHLSTRÖM, A., FUXE, K. and LARSSON, K. (1966b): Functional role of the nigro-neostriatal dopamine neurons. *Acta pharmacol. (Kbh.)* **24**, 263—274.

ANDÉN, N.-E., CORRODI, H. and FUXE, K. (1969): Turnover studies using synthesis inhibition. In: *Metabolism of Amines in the Brain*. MacMillan, London.

APPLEZWEIG, M. H. and BAUDRY, F. D. (1955): The pituitary–adrenocortical system in avoidance learning. *Psychol. Rep.* **1**, 417—420.

ARBUTHNOTT, C., FUXE, K. and UNGERSTEDT, U. (1971): Central catecholamine turnover and self-stimulation behaviour. *Brain Res.* **27**, 406—413.

BERTLER, A., CARLSSON, A. and ROSENGREN, E. (1958): A method for the fluorimetric determination of adrenaline and noradrenaline in tissues. *Acta physiol. scand.* **44**, 273—292.

BHATACHARYA, A. N. and MARKS, B. H. (1969a): Reserpine and chlorpromazine-induced changes in hypothalamo–hypophyseal–adrenal system in rats in the presence and absence of hypothermia. *J. Pharmacol. exp. Ther.* **165**, 108—116.

BHATTACHARYA, A. N. and MARKS, B. H. (1969b): Effects of pargyline and amphetamine upon acute stress responses in rats. *Proc. Soc. exp. Biol. (N.Y.)* **130**, 1194—1198.

BLISS, E. L., AILION, J. and ZWANZIGER, J. (1968): Metabolism of norepinephrine, serotonin and dopamine in rat brain with stress. *J. Pharmacol. exp. Ther.* **164**, 122—134.

BOBON, D. P., JANSSEN, P. A. J. and BOBON, J. (Eds) (1970): *Modern Problems in Pharmacopsychiatry, Vol. 5. The Neuroleptics*. Karger, Basel, München, Paris, New York.

BOHUS, B. (1968): Pituitary ACTH release and avoidance behaviour of rats with cortisol implants in mesencephalic reticular formation and median eminence. *Neuroendocrinology* **3**, 355—365.

BOHUS, B. and ENDRŐCZI, E. (1965): The influence of pituitary–adrenocortical functions on the avoiding conditioned reflex activity. *Acta physiol. Acad. Sci. hung.* **26**, 183—189.

BOHUS, B. and WIED, D. DE (1966): Inhibitory and facilitatory effect of two related peptides on extinction of avoidance behavior. *Science* **153**, 318—320.

BOHUS, B. and LISSÁK, K. (1968): Adrenocortical hormones and avoidance behaviour of rats. *Int. J. Neuropharmacol.* **7**, 301—306.

Bohus, B., Nyakas, Cs. and Endrőczi, E. (1968): Effects of adrenocorticotropic hormone on avoidance behavior of intact and adrenalectomized rats. *Int. J. Neuropharmacol.* **7**, 307—314.
Brodish, A. and Long, C. N. H. (1956): Changes in blood ACTH under various experimental conditions studied by means of a cross-circulation technique. *Endocrinology* **59**, 666—676.
Bunney, W. E. Jr. and Davies, J. M. (1965): *Arch. gen. Psychiat.* **13**, 483.
Butcher, L. L. and Andén, N.-E. (1969): Effects of apomorphine and amphetamine on schedule-controlled behaviour: reversal of tetrabenazine suppression and dopaminergic correlates. *Europ. J. Pharmacol.* **6**, 255.
Carlsson, A. (1959): The occurrence, distribution and physiological role of catecholamines in the nervous system. *Pharmacol. Rev.* **11**, 490—493.
Carlsson, A. (1966): Drugs, which block the storage of 5-hydroxytryptamine and related amines. In: *Handbuch der experimentellen Pharmakologie.* Springer, Berlin, Heidelberg, New York.
Carlsson, A. and Lindqvist, M. (1962): In vivo decarboxylation of α-methyl Dopa and α-methyl metatyrosine. *Acta physiol. scand.* **54**, 87—94.
Carlsson, A., Fuxe, K., Hamberger, B. and Lindqvist, M. (1966): Biochemical and histochemical studies on the effects of imipramine-like drugs and (+)-amphetamine on central and peripheral catecholamine neurons. *Acta physiol. scand.* **67**, 481—497.
Coppen, A. (1970): Pituitary-adrenal activity during psychosis and depression. In: *Pituitary, Adrenal and the Brain.* Ed. by D. DeWied and J. A. W. M. Weijnen. *Progr. Brain Res.* **32**. Elsevier, Amsterdam. pp. 336—342.
Corrodi, H. and Hansson, L. (1966): Central effects of an inhibition of tyrosine hydroxylation. *Psychopharmacologia (Berl.)* **10**, 116—125.
Corrodi, H. and Jonsson, G. (1967): The formaldehyde fluorescence method for the histochemical demonstration of biogenic monoamines. A review on the methodology. *J. Histochem. Cytochem.* **15**, 65—78.
Corrodi, H., Fuxe, K. and Hökfelt, T. (1968): The effect of immobilization stress on the activity of central monoamine neurons. *Life Sci.* **7**, 107—112.
Corrodi, H., Fuxe, K., Hamberger, B. and Ljungdahl, Å. (1970): Studies on central and peripheral noradrenaline neurons using a new dopamine-β-hydroxylase inhibitor. *Europ. J. Pharmacol.* **12**, 145—155.
Corrodi, H., Fuxe, K., Lidbrink, P. and Olson, L. (1971): Minor tranquillizers, stress and central catecholamine neurons. *Brain Res.* **29**, 1—16.
Costa, E. (1970): Simple neuronal models to estimate turnover rate of noradrenergic transmitters in vivo. In: *Biochemistry of Simple Neuronal Model. Advance in Biochemical Psychopharmacology.* Raven Press, New York.
Costa, E. and Neff, N. H. (1970): Estimation of turnover rates to study the metabolic regulation of the steady-state level of neuronal monoamines. In: *Handbook of Neurochemistry* Plenum Press, New York, London.
Crisp, A. H. and Roberts, F. J. (1963): The response of an adrenalectomised patient to ECT. *Amer. J. Psychiat.* **119**, 784—785.
Dallman, M. F. and Yates, F. E. (1968): Anatomical and functional mapping of central neural input and feedback pathways of the adrenocortical system. *Mem. Soc. Endocr.* **17**, 39—72.
Donoso, A. O. and Stefano, F. J. E. (1967): Sex hormones and concentration of noradrenaline and dopamine in the anterior hypothalamus of castrated rats. *Experientia (Basel)* **23**, 665—666.
Endrőczi, E. and Lissák, K. (1962): Spontaneous goal-directed motor activity related to the alimentary conditioned reflex behaviour and its regulation by neural and humoral factors. *Acta physiol. Acad. Sci. hung.* **21**, 265—283.
Falck, B., Hillarp, N.-Å., Thieme, G. and Torp, A. (1962): Fluorescence of catecholamines and related compounds condensed with formaldehyde. *J. Histochem. Cytochem.* **10**, 348—354.
Florvall, L. and Corrodi, H. (1970): Dopamine β-hydroxylase inhibitors. The preparation and the dopamine β-hydroxylase inhibitory activity of some compounds related to dithiocarbamic acid and thiuramdisulfide. *Acta pharmacol. suec.* **7**, 7—22.

FUXE, K. and HANSSON, L. C. F. (1967): Central catecholamine neurons and conditioned avoidance behaviour. *Psychopharmacologia. (Berl.)* **11**, 439–447.
FUXE, K. and HÖKFELT, T. (1967): The influence of central catecholamine neurons on the hormone secretion from the anterior and posterior pituitary. In: *Neurosecretion.* Springer Verlag, New York.
FUXE, K. and HÖKFELT, T. (1969): Catecholamines in the hypothalamus and the pituitary gland. In: *Frontiers in Neuroendocrinology.* Ed. by W. F. Ganong and L. Martini. Oxford University Press, New York, London, Toronto.
FUXE, K. and HÖKFELT, T. (1970a): Participation of central monoamine neurons in the regulation of anterior pituitary function with special regard to the neuroendocrine function of tubero-infundibular dopamine neurons. In: *Aspects of Neuroendocrinology.* Springer Verlag, Berlin, Heidelberg, Göttingen, New York.
FUXE, K. and HÖKFELT, T. (1970b): Central monoaminergic systems and hypothalamic function. In: *The Hypothalamus.* Ed. by L. Martini, M. Motta and F. Fraschini. Academic Press, New York, London.
FUXE, K. and UNGERSTEDT, U. (1970): Histochemical, biochemical and functional studies on central monoamine neurons after acute and chronic amphetamine administration. In: *Amphetamine and Related Compounds.* Raven Press, New York.
FUXE, K. and LIDBRINK, P. (1971): On the function of central catecholamine neurons – their role in cardiovascular and arousal mechanisms. In: *Pharmacology and Physiology of Monoamines in the Central Nervous System.* (In press).
FUXE, K., HÖKFELT, T. and NILSSON, O. (1967): Activity changes in the tubero-infundibular DA neurons of the rat during various states of the reproductive cycle. *Life Sci.* **6**, 2057–2061.
FUXE, K., HÖKFELT, T. and NILSSON, O. (1969a): Castration, sex hormones and tubero-infundibular dopamine neurons. *Neuroendocrinology* **5**, 107–120.
FUXE, K., HÖKFELT, T. and NILSSON, O. (1969b): Factors involved in the control of the activity of the tubero-infundibular dopamine neurons during pregnancy and lactation. *Neuroendocrinology* **5**, 257–270.
FUXE, K., CORRODI, H., HÖKFELT, T. and JONSSON, G. (1970a): Central monoamine neurons and pituitary–adrenal activity. *Progr. Brain Res.* **32**, 42–56.
FUXE, K., HÖKFELT, T. and JONSSON, G. (1970b): Participation of central monoaminergic neurons in the regulation of anterior pituitary secretion. In: *Neurochemical Aspects of Hypothalamic Function.* Ed. by L. Martini and J. Heites. Academic Press, New York, London.
FUXE, K., HÖKFELT, T., JONSSON, G. and UNGERSTEDT, U. (1970c): Fluorescence microscopy in neuroanatomy. In: *Contemporary Research in Neuroanatomy.* Springer, New York.
FUXE, K., HÖKFELT, T. and UNGERSTEDT, U. (1970d): Morphological and functional aspects of central monoamine neurons. *Int. Rev. Neurobiol.* **13**, 93–126.
FUXE, K., HÖKFELT, T. and JONSSON, G. (1971a): The effect of gonadal steroids on the tubero-infundibular dopamine neurons. In: *Excerpta Medica International Congress Series.* (In press).
FUXE, K., HÖKFELT, T. and NILSSON, O. (1971b): Effect of constant light and androgen-sterilization of the amine turnover of the tubero-infundibular dopamine neurons: blockade of cyclic activity and induction of a persistent high dopamine turnover in the median eminence. *Acta endocr. (Kbh.)* (In press).
GANONG, W. F. (1970): Control of adrenocorticotropin and melanocyte-stimulating hormone secretion. In: *The Hypothalamus.* Ed. by L. Martini, M. Motta and F. Fraschini. Academic Press, New York, London.
GANONG, W. F. (1971): Evidence that adrenergic systems in the brainstem inhibit ACTH secretion. In: *Median Eminence.* Karger, Basel, München, Paris, New York.
GANONG, W. F. and MARTINI, L. (Eds) (1967): *Neuroendocrinology.* Vol. II. Academic Press, New York, London.
GANONG, W. F. and MARTINI, L. (Eds) (1969): *Frontiers in Neuroendocrinology.* Oxford University Press, New York, London, Toronto.
GLOWINSKI, J. and BALDESSARINI, R. J. (1966): Metabolism of norepinephrine in the central nervous system. *Pharmacol. Rev.* **18**, 1201–1238.
GORDON, R., SPECTOR, S., SJOERDSMA, A. and UDENFRIEND, S. (1966): Increased

synthesis of norepinephrine and epinephrine in the intact rat during exercise and exposure to cold. *J. Pharmacol. exp. Ther.* **153**, 440—447.

GREVEN, H. M. and WIED, D. DE (1967): The active sequence in the ACTH molecule responsible for inhibition of the extinction of conditioned avoidance behaviour in rats. *Europ. J. Pharmacol.* **2**, 14—16.

HALÁSZ, B. and SZENTÁGOTHAI, J. (1960): Control of adrenocorticotrophin function by direct influence of pituitary substance on the hypothalamus. *Acta morph. Acad. Sci. hung.* **9**, 251—261.

HANSSON, L. C. F. (1967): Evidence that the central action of (+)-amphetamine is mediated via catecholamines. *Psychopharmacologia (Berl.)* **10**, 289—297.

HENKIN, R. J. (1970): The effects of corticosteroids and ACTH on sensory systems. *Progr. Brain Res.* **32**, 270—293.

HÖKFELT, T. and FUXE, K. (1971a): Effects of prolactin and ergot alkaloids on the tubero-infundibular dopamine (DA) neurons. *Neuroendocrinology.* (In press).

HÖKFELT, T. and FUXE, K. (1971b): On the morphology and neuroendocrine role of the hypothalamic catecholamine neurons. In: *Median Eminence.* Karger, Basel, München, Paris, New York.

HORNYKIEWICZ, O. (1966): Dopamine (3-hydroxytyramine) and brain function. *Pharmacol. Rev.* **18**, 925—964.

IVERSEN, L. L. and SIMMONDS, M. A. (1969): Studies of catecholamine turnover in rat brain using ^{3}H-noradrenaline. In: *Metabolism of Amines in the Brain.* MacMillan, London.

JAVOY, F., GLOWINSKI, J. and KORDON, C. (1968): Effects of adrenalectomy on the turnover of norepinephrine in the rat brain. *Europ. J. Pharmacol.* **4**, 103—104.

JONES, B. E. (1969): Catecholamine containing neurons in the brainstem of the cat and their role in waking. Thesis. University of Delaware. Tixier et Fils, Lyon.

JONES, B. E., BOBILLIER, P. and JOUVET, M. (1969): Effets de la destruction des neurones contenant des catécholamines du mésencéphale sur le cycle veilles-sommeils du chat. *C.R. Soc. Biol. (Paris)* **163**, 176—180.

JONSSON, G. (1969): Microfluorometric studies on the formaldehyde-induced fluorescence of noradrenaline in adrenergic nerves of rat iris. *J. Histochem. Cytochem.* **17**, 714—723.

JONSSON, G. (1971): Quantitation of fluorescence of biogenic monoamines demonstrated with the formaldehyde fluorescence method. *Progr. Histochem. Cytochem.* (In press).

JONSSON, G., FUXE, K. and HÖKFELT, T. (1971a): On the catecholamine innervation of the hypothalamus, with special reference to the median eminence. *Brain Res.* (In press).

JONSSON, G., FUXE, K. and HÖKFELT, T. (1971b): Effect of castration and hypophyseal hormones on central catecholamine neurons. (In preparation).

JONSSON, G., FUXE, K., HÖKFELT, T. and LIDBRINK, P. (1971c): Pituitary-adrenal activity and central catecholamine neurons. (In preparation).

KAMBERI, I. A., MICAL, R. S. and PORTER, J. C. (1969): Luteinizing hormone-releasing activity in hypophyseal stalk blood and elevation by dopamine. *Science* **166**, 388—390.

KENDALL, J. W. (1970): Dexamethasone stimulation of running activity in the male rat. *Hormones and Behavior* **1**, 327—336.

KORÁNYI, L. and ENDRŐCZI, E. (1967): The effect of ACTH on nervous processes. *Neuroendocrinology* **2**, 65—75.

KORÁNYI, L. and ENDRŐCZI, E. (1970): Influence of pituitary-adrenocortical hormones on thalamo-cortical and brainstem limbic circuits. *Progr. Brain Res.* **32**, 120—130.

LEVINE, S. (1968): Hormones and conditioning. In: *Nebraska Symposium on Motivation.* Ed. by J. M. R. Jones. Univ. Nebraska Press.

LEVINE, S. and BRUSH, F. (1967): Adrenocortical activity and avoidance learning as a function of time after avoidance training. *Physiology and Behavior* **2**, 385—388.

LIDBRINK, P. and JONSSON, G. (1971): Semiquantitative estimation of noradrenaline induced fluorescence in central noradrenaline nerve terminals. *J. Histochem. Cytochem.* (In press).

LINDQVIST, B. E. R. and LINDQVIST, G. (1964): The antidepressant effect of amitriptyline in an adrenalectomised patient. *Amer. J. Psychiat.* **120**, 912—913.

LISSÁK, K. and ENDRŐCZI, E. (1964): Neuroendocrine interrelationships and behavioural processes. In: *Major Problems in Neuroendocrinology.* Karger, Basel.

LISSÁK, K., ENDRŐCZI, E. and MEDGYESI, P. (1957): Somatisches Verhalten und Nebennierenrindentätigkeit. *Arch. ges. Physiol.* **117**, 265—273.

MAAS, J. W. and MEDNIEKS, M. (1971): Hydrocortisone-mediated increase in norepinephrine uptake by brain slices. *Science* **171**, 178—179.

MARKS, B. H., HALL, M. M. and BHATTACHARYA, A. N. (1970): Psychopharmacological effects and pituitary–adrenal activity. *Progr. Brain Res.* **32**, 58—70.

MARTINI, L. and GANONG, W. F. (Eds) (1966): *Neuroendocrinology.* Vol. I. Academic Press, New York, London.

MARTINI, L. and MEITES, J. (Eds) (1970): *Neurochemical Aspects of Hypothalamic Function.* Academic Press, New York, London.

MARTINI, L., MOTTA, M. and FRASCHINI, F. (Eds) (1970): *The Hypothalamus.* Academic Press, New York, London.

MILLER, R. E. and OGAWA, N. (1962): The effect of adrenocorticotrophic hormone (ACTH) on avoidance conditioning in the adrenalectomized rat. *J. comp. physiol. Psychol.* **55**, 211—213.

MOTTA, M., MANGILI, G. and MARTINI, L. (1965): A "short" feedback loop in the control of ACTH secretion. *Endocrinology* **77**, 392—395.

OLSON, L. and FUXE, K. (1971): On the projections from the locus coeruleus noradrenaline neurons: The cerebellar innervation. *Brain Res.* **28**, 165—171.

OLSON, L., HAMBERGER, B., JONSSON, G. and MALMFORS, T. (1968): Combined fluorescence histochemistry and ^{3}H-noradrenaline measurements of adrenergic nerves. *Histochemie* **15**, 38—45.

PERSSON, T. and WALDECK, B. (1970): Some problems encountered in attempting to estimate catecholamine turnover using labelled tyrosine. *J. Pharm. Pharmacol.* **22**, 473—478.

POIRIER, L. J. and SOURKES, T. L. (1965): Influence of the substantia nigra on the catecholamine content of the striatum. *Brain* **88**, 181—192.

RANDRUP, A. and MUNKVAD, I. (1968): Behavioural stereotypes induced by pharmacological agents. *Pharmakopsychiat. Neuro-Psychopharmacol.* (Stuttgart) **1**, 18—26.

REIS, D. J. and FUXE, K. (1968): Depletion of noradrenaline in brain stem neurons during sham rage behaviour produced by acute brainstem transection in cat. *Brain Res.* **7**, 448—451.

SAWYER, C. H., MARKEE, J. E. and TOWNSEND, B. F. (1949): Cholinergic and adrenergic components in the neurohumoral control of the release of LH in the rabbit. *Endocrinology* **44**, 18—37.

SCAPAGNINI, U., VAN LOON, G. R., MOBERG, G. P. and GANONG, W. F. (1970): Effect of α-methyl-p-tyrosine on the circadian variation of plasma corticosterone in rats. *Europ. J. Pharmacol.* **11**, 266—268.

SCHILDKRAUT, J. J. (1965): *Amer. J. Psychiat.* **122**, 509.

SCHILDKRAUT, J. J., SHANBERG, S. M., BREESE, G. R. and KOPIN, J. (1967): Norepinephrine metabolism and drugs used in the affective disorders: A possible mechanism of action. *Amer. J. Psychiat.* **124**, 600—608.

SCHNEIDER, H. P. G. and MCCANN, S. M. (1969): Possible role of dopamine as transmitter to promote discharge of LH-releasing factor. *Endocrinology* **85**, 121—132.

SEIDEN, L. S. and CARLSSON, A. (1964): Brain and heart catecholamine levels after L-Dopa administration in reserpine treated mice: correlations with conditioned avoidance response. *Psychopharmacologia* (Berl.) **5**, 178—181.

SMELIK, P. G. (1963): Failure to inhibit corticotrophin secretion by experimentally induced increases in corticoid levels. *Acta endocr.* (Kbh.) **44**, 36—46.

STEFANO, F. J. E. and DONOSO, A. O. (1967): Norepinephrine levels in rat hypothalamus during estrous cycle. *Endocrinology* **81**, 1405—1406.

STEFANO, F. J. E., DONOSO, A. O. and CUKIER, J. (1965): Hypothalamic noradrenaline changes in ovariectomized rats. *Acta physiol. lat.-amer.* **15**, 425—427.

STEIN, L. (1968): Chemistry of reward and punishment. In: *Psychopharmacology. A Review of Progress 1957—1967.* U.S. Publ. Health Service Publn. No. 1836, Washington, D.C.

STEIN, L. and WISE, C. D. (1969): Release of norepinephrine from hypothalamus and amygdala by rewarding medial forebrain bundle stimulation and amphetamine. *J. comp. physiol. Psychol.* **67**, 189—198.

SVENSSON, T. H. and WALDECK, B. (1969): On the significance of central noradrenaline for motor activity: experiments with a new dopamine-β-hydroxylase inhibitor. *Europ. J. Pharmacol.* **7**, 278–282.

THIERRY, A. M., JAVOY, F., GLOWINSKI, J. and KETY, S. S. (1968): Effects of stress on the metabolism of norepinephrine, dopamine and serotonin in the central nervous system of the rat. *J. Pharmacol. exp. Ther.* **163**, 163–171.

UNGERSTEDT, U. (1971a): Stereotaxic mapping of the monoamine pathways in the rat brain. *Acta physiol. scand.* Suppl. **367**, 1–48.

UNGERSTEDT, U. (1971b): On the anatomy, pharmacology and function of the nigro-neostriatal dopamine system. Thesis. Karolinska Institutet, Stockholm.

VAN LOON, C. R. and GANONG, W. F. (1969): Effect of drugs which alter catecholamine metabolism on the inhibition of stress-induced ACTH secretion produced by L-dopa. *Physiologist* **12**, 381.

VAN LOON, C. R., HILGER, L., COHEN, R. and GANONG, W. F. (1969): Evidence for a hypothalamic adrenergic system that inhibits ACTH secretion in the dog. *Fed. Proc.* **28**, 438.

VAN WIMERSMA GREIDANUS, TJ. B. (1970): Effects of steroids on extinction of an avoidance response in rats. A structure–activity relationship study. In: *Pituitary, Adrenal and the Brain.* Ed. by D. De Wied and J. A. W. M. Weijnen. *Progr. Brain Res.* **32**. Elsevier, Amsterdam. pp. 185–191.

WEISS, J. M., MCEWEN, B. S., SILVA, M. T. and KALKUT, M. (1970): Pituitary–adrenal alterations and fear responding. *Amer. J. Physiol.* **218**, 864–868.

WERTHEIM, G., CONNER, R. and LEVINE, S. (1969): Avoidance conditioning and adrenocortical function in the rat. *Physiology and Behavior* **4**, 41–44.

WIED, D. DE (1964): Influence of anterior pituitary on avoidance learning and escape behavior. *Amer. J. Physiol.* **207**, 255–259.

WIED, D. DE (1966a): Inhibitory effect of ACTH and related peptides on extinction of conditioned avoidance behavior in rats. *Proc. Soc. exp. Biol. (N. Y.)* **122**, 28–32.

WIED, D. DE (1966b): Antagonistic effect of ACTH and glucocorticoids on avoidance behaviour of rats. In: *2nd International Congress on Hormonal Steroids.* Excerpta Medica International Congress Series **111**, Amsterdam. p. 89.

WIED, D. DE (1967): Opposite effect of ACTH and glucocorticosteroids on extinction of conditioned avoidance behavior. In: *Proceedings of Second International Congress on Hormonal Steroids*, Milan, May 1966. Excerpta Medica International Congress Series **132**, Amsterdam. pp. 945–951.

WIED, D. DE (1969): Effects of peptide hormones on behavior. In: *Frontiers in Neuroendocrinology.* Oxford University Press, New York.

WIED, D. DE and WEIJNEN, J. A. W. M. (Eds) (1970): *Pituitary, Adrenal and the Brain. Progr. Brain Res.* **32**. Elsevier, Amsterdam.

WIED, D. DE, BOHUS, B. and GREVEN, H. M. (1968): Influence of pituitary and adrenocortical hormones on conditioned avoidance behaviour in rats. In: *Endocrinology and Human Behaviour.* Oxford University Press, London.

WIED, D. DE, WITTER, A. and LANDE, S. (1970): Anterior pituitary peptides and avoidance acquisition of hypophysectomized rats. In: *Pituitary, Adrenal and the Brain.* Ed. by D. De Wied and J. A. W. M. Weijnen. *Progr. Brain Res.* **32**. Elsevier, Amsterdam. pp. 213–218.

WISE, C. D. and STEIN, L. (1969): Facilitation of brain self-stimulation by central administration of norepinephrine. *Science* **163**, 299–301.

WOODBURY, D. M. (1954): Effect of hormones on brain excitability and electrolytes. *Recent Progr. Hormone Res.* **10**, 65–107.

WOODBURY, D. M. (1958): Relation between the adrenal cortex and the central nervous system. *Pharmacol. Rev.* **10**, 275–357.

WOODBURY, D. M. and VERNADAKIS, A. (1966): Effects of steroids on the central nervous system. *Methods Hormone Res.* **5**, 1–57.

PITUITARY–ADRENOCORTICAL HORMONE INFLUENCES ON MULTIPLE UNITS IN THE BRAINSTEM AND FOREBRAIN STRUCTURES[1]

L. KORÁNYI[2] and C. GUZMÁN-FLORES

Institute of Physiology
University Medical School
Pécs, Hungary
and
Departamento de Investigaciónes Cientifica, IMSS,
Universidad Nacional Autonóma de México
Mexico City, Mexico

There is growing evidence in the literature that the unit firing frequency changes in diverse subcortical structures during various stages of vigilance and sleep–wakefulness cycle. According to these observations the unit activity is high during attentive behaviour, it declines to a low level during slow-wave sleep and in paradoxical sleep it increases to higher levels than those observed during attention (Evarts et al. 1962, Goodman and Mann 1967, Guzmán-Flores and Alcaraz 1970, Huttenlocker 1961, Korányi et al. 1971a, Mori et al. 1968, Podvoll and Goodman 1967, Winters et al. 1967). It is also well proven that the changes of multiple unit activity at the midbrain reticular formation reflect the states of excitation or inhibition of the central nervous system (Mori et al. 1968, Winters et al. 1967). Recently a high correlation was shown between the variability of multiple unit activity and different emotional stages, rage reaction, aggressive behaviour, orienting reflex and diverse phases of attentive behaviour (Guzmán-Flores and Alcaraz 1970, Guzmán-Flores and Garcia-Castells 1970, Garcia-Castells and Guzmán-Flores 1970).

The present experiments were devoted to study the multiple unit activity in the brainstem and forebrain structures of cats in the course of habituation to a novel environment and the influencing effect of ACTH and adrenocortical hormones on this process. The experiments were carried out on chronically implanted freely moving animals. The habituation sessions were started 10 to 60 days after the operation. Each session lasting for 3 hours was performed on consecutive days following the strictest schedule. EEG and multiple unit activity were simultaneously recorded with Guzmán-Flores and Alcaraz's technique (1970). This technique records the discharge frequency of a small neuronal pool and registers the actual activity level of diverse subcortical structures. The voltage gate was adjusted at the start of the experiments and an identical electronic window detector was used throughout the sessions for the same animal. In this way the activity level can be evaluated numerically. The changes of multiple unit activity in different

---

[1] This work was partially supported by a grant from the Ford Foundation
[2] IBRO/UNESCO Fellow in 1970/71 at the Instituto de Investigaciónes Biomédicas, UNAM de México, México.

behavioural stages were calculated as per cent values of the average activity recorded during the animal's quiet attention in the course of the first session.

We found that the multiple unit activity of the mesencephalic reticular formation, the preoptic area, the medial forebrain bundle, the midline thalamic

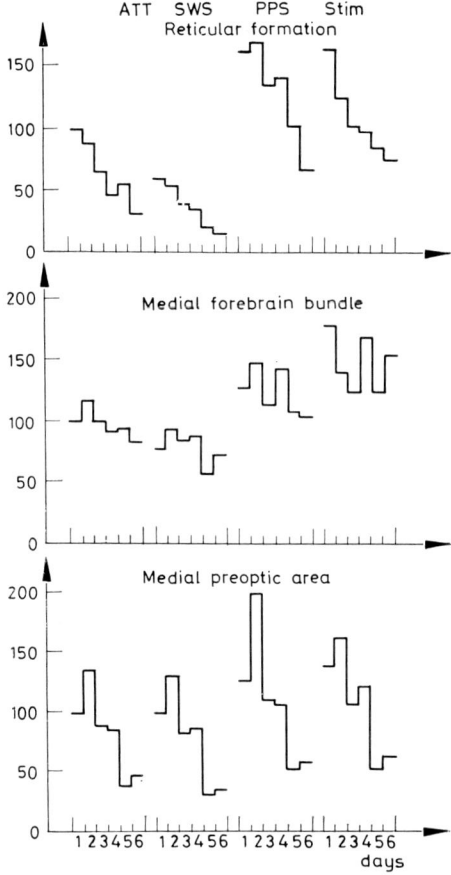

Fig. 1. Changes in multiple unit activity level in different subcortical structures in the course of habituation. ATT: attentive behaviour; SWS: slow-wave sleep; PPS: paradoxical sleep; Stim: somatic stimulation

nuclei and the nucleus fornicis showed a gradual and marked decrease in the course of the consecutive sessions (Figs 1 and 2). However, the multiple unit activity levels were very variable in the different phases of attentive behaviour, during transition from quiet attention to slow-wave sleep and paradoxical phase of sleep. We have already described (Korányi et al. 1971b) that the base level in terms of activity recorded during slow-wave sleep did not change significantly during one session. The animals were considered habituated to the environment when the multiple unit activity levels were stationary at a constant low value.

Hormone injections (ACTH, hydrocortisone, cortisone, corticosterone) were given to non-habituated and habituated animals. All these hormones resulted in a marked, general decrease in multiple unit activity levels in all structures (Figs 3, 4 and 5).

Furthermore, we have studied the effect of electric stimulation of the mesencephalic reticular formation on the changes of multiple unit activity in normal and adrenalectomized cats, and the influence of ACTH and hydrocortisone on the

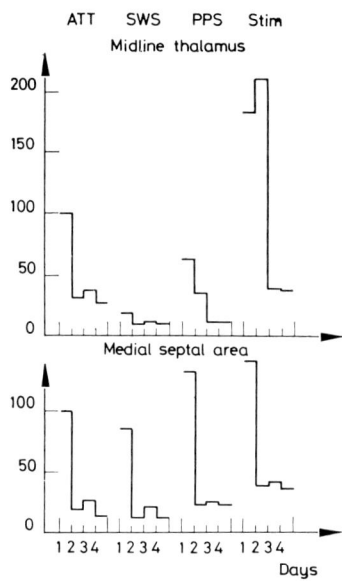

Fig. 2. For abbreviations *see* Fig. 1

responsiveness of neuronal pools in the brainstem and extrahypothalamic structures of habituated animals. Five to 15 habituation sessions were given prior to hormone injections. Moreover, 90 min control recordings were made on each animal before hormone injections. Stimulation parameters were: 100 cps frequency, 0.2 msec duration. The impulse train lasted for 10 sec. Stimulation intensities were different in each individual cat, but identical stimulation intensity was used throughout the session for the same animal. The activity recorded during stimulation was left out of consideration.

In freely moving cats the multiple unit activity showed a slight increase when the stimulation was administered during attentive behaviour, a large and consistent increase during slow-wave sleep and a significant decrease during paradoxical sleep. Due to the variability of reactivity of the neuronal pools during the different states of the CNS, the stimulations were performed exclusively when the multiple unit activity showed a stable low level, i.e., under slow-wave sleep.

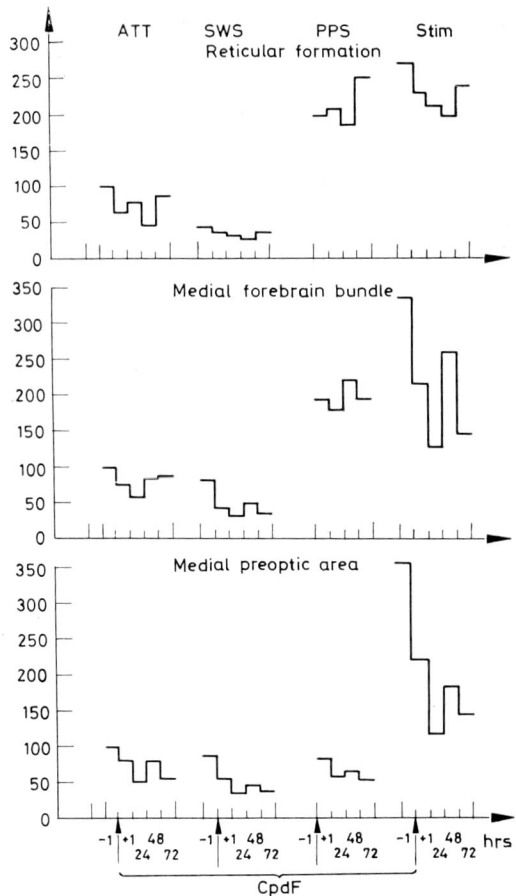

Fig. 3. Effect of a single injection of hydrocortisone (CpdF) on multiple unit activity level in non-habituated cat. For abbreviations see Fig. 1

We have found that the responsiveness of the subcortical structures to electrical stimulation was significantly lower in adrenalectomized animals than in normal cats. In Fig. 6 the cell firing rate is expressed in per cent of the average activity recorded during the 30 sec prior to the stimulation (Fig. 6a and b).

Hydrocortisone injection resulted in a decrease of responsiveness of the mesencephalic reticular formation, medial forebrain bundle, preoptic area and the midline thalamic nuclei (Fig. 7). The trend of the changes was similar in ACTH-treated intact cats, except for the nucleus fornicis where the ACTH resulted in an increase (Fig. 8). In adrenalectomized animals the responsiveness increased in the medial forebrain bundle both after hydrocortisone and ACTH treatment (Fig. 9). In these cases the multiple unit activity recorded 30 sec prior to and 30 sec following stimulation was expressed in per cent of the corresponding activity reg-

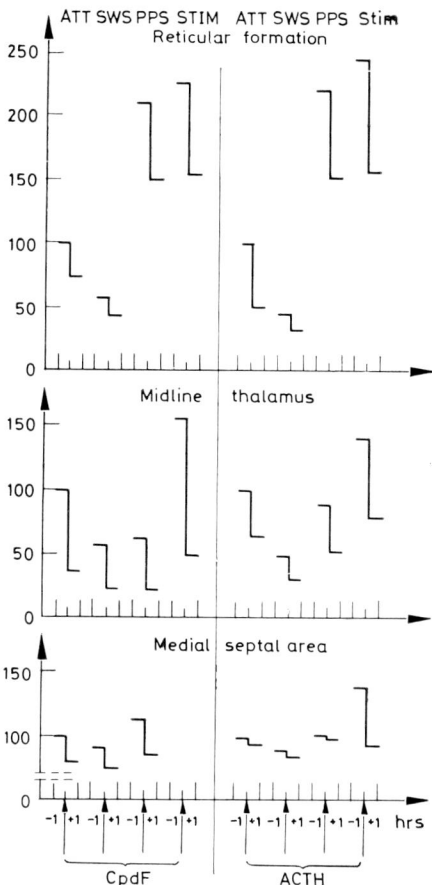

Fig. 4. Effect of a single injection of hydrocortisone (CpdF) and ACTH on multiple unit activity level in non-habituated cats. For abbreviations *see* Fig. 1

istered before hormone injection. In this way the general decreasing effect of the hormones could also be demonstrated.

It would be far-fetched to draw conclusions from the earlier and the present experiments as to the mechanisms of different mental and psychic disturbances described in humans suffering from hyperadrenocorticism or Addisonian disease, or as to the mechanisms by which the pituitary–adrenocortical hormones influence behavioural events, conditioned reflex performance or learning processes.

We have demonstrated a significant decrease in the multiple unit activity level during habituation to the environment in the cat. The process of habituation is based first of all on neural mechanisms and the hormonal effects manifesting themselves in lowering the activity level may influence, modify or support the process of habituation. A difference was shown in the electric stimulation induced

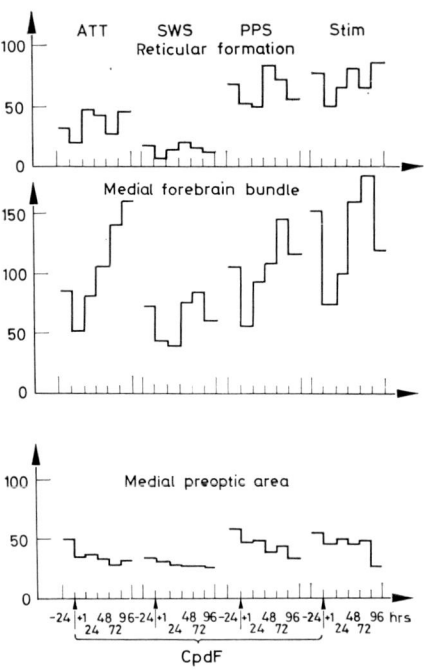

Fig. 5. Effect of a single injection of hydrocortisone on multiple unit activity level in habituated cat. For abbreviations *see* Fig. 1

firing rate of the neuronal pools in the nucleus fornicis and the medial forebrain bundle of habituated cats. This finding may reflect those neural mechanisms which integrate or influence the function of the pituitary–adrenal axis. As long as there is an overlap between the function of these structures participating in the intrinsic endocrine regulatory mechanisms and in the integration of behaviour, the hormones secondarily may play a role in the modification of behavioural processes by influencing the neuronal excitability state.

The neuronal and/or CNS excitability level should be considered when evaluating the behavioural experiments and conditioned reflex studies. It is known that the relation which exists between the level of performance of conditioned reflex activity or behavioural efficiency and the excitability of the central nervous system is described by an inverted U-shape function (Broadhurst 1957, Brush 1957, Finch 1957, Malmo 1959, Lát 1965, 1966, Yerkes and Dodson 1908). It is obvious that in the acquisition or extinction of a conditioned reflex both an increase or a decrease of the CNS' excitability level may lead to a lower level of performance; or vice versa, a better conditioned reflex performance or long-lasting extinction can be the result of both increasing or decreasing brain excitability. This implies that diverse treatments may result in the same behavioural manifestation, although they can activate two different central nervous mechanisms (Fig. 10).

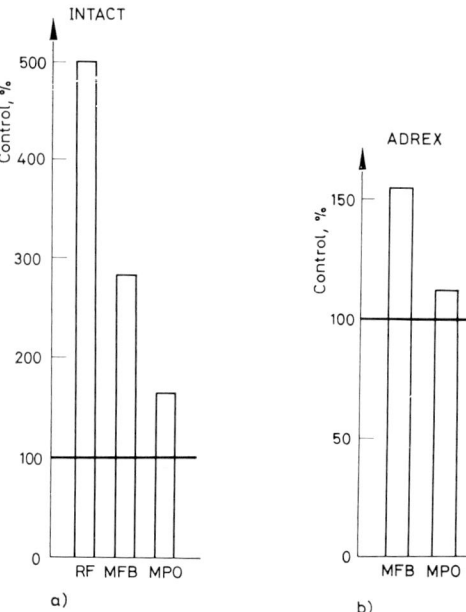

Fig. 6a and b. Stimulation-induced firing rate of multiple units in different subcortical structures of intact and adrenalectomized cats. Stimulation was performed during slow-wave sleep. 100 per cent represents the average activity recorded prior to stimulation. RF: reticular formation; MFB: medial forebrain bundle; MPO: preoptic area

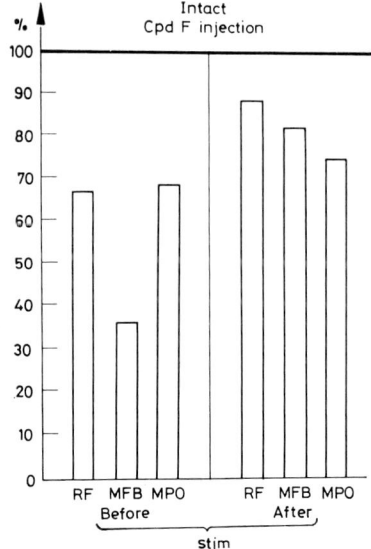

Fig. 7. Firing rate of multiple units in response to electric stimulation in different subcortical structures of hydrocortisone injected habituated cat. Multiple unit activity level recorded 30 sec prior to and 30 sec following the stimulation is expressed in per cent of the corresponding activity registered before hormone injection. For abbreviations see Fig. 6a and b

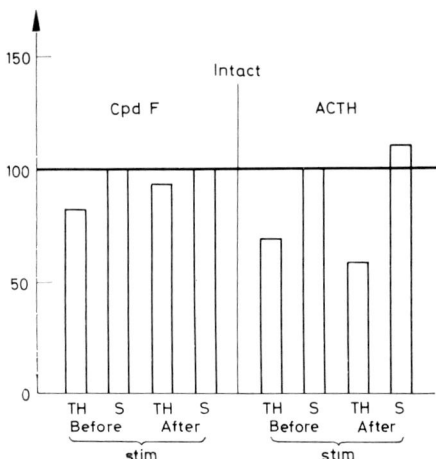

Fig. 8. Stimulation induced changes in the multiple unit activity in intact habituated cats following hydrocortisone and ACTH injection. TH: n. centromedianus; S: nucleus fornicis

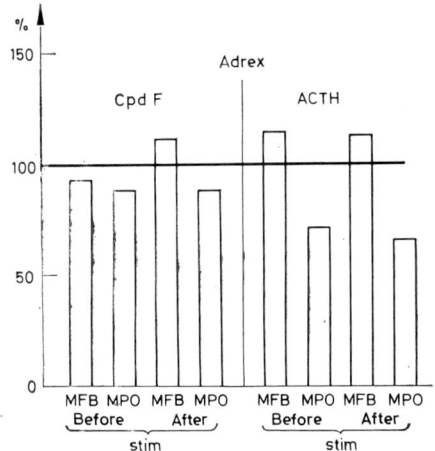

Fig. 9. Stimulation-induced changes of multiple unit activity in adrenalectomized and habituated cats following hydrocortisone and ACTH injection. MFB: medial forebrain bundle; MPO: preoptic area

The study of spontaneous and electric stimulation induced changes of the multiple unit activity levels with Guzmán-Flores and Alcaraz' method gives an excellent reflection of the CNS excitation and inhibition. The present findings fit in well with our earlier experiments in which we have concluded that the hormones of the pituitary–adrenal axis may exert an inhibitory influence on the function of

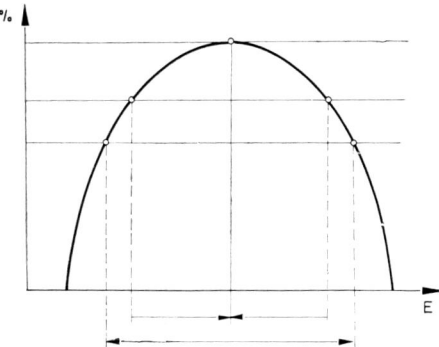

Fig. 10. Inverted U shape relation between the level of behavioural efficiency (%) and the excitability of the central nervous system (E). Opposite changes in E may lead to the same level of behavioural performance

the central nervous system, and the results may serve as a neurophysiological basis for the previously described behavioural phenomena (Endrőczi and Lissák 1962, Korányi et al. 1965/66, 1969, Korányi and Endrőczi 1967, 1970, Levine 1968, Lissák et al. 1957, Lissák and Endrőczi 1961, 1964).

REFERENCES

BROADHURST, P. L. (1957): Emotionality and the Yerkes–Dodson law. *J. exp. Psychol.* **54**, 345—352.
BRUSH, F. R. (1957): The effect of shock intensity on the acquisition and extinction of an avoidance response in dogs. *J. comp. physiol. Psychol.* **50**, 547—552.
ENDRŐCZI, E. and LISSÁK, K. (1962): Spontaneous goal-directed motor activity related to the alimentary conditioned reflex behaviour and its regulation by neural and humoral factors. *Acta physiol. Acad. Sci. hung.* **21**, 265—283.
EVARTS, E. V., BENTAL, E., BIHARI, B. and HUTTENLOCKER, P. R. (1962): Spontaneous discharge of single neurons during sleep and waking. *Science* **135**, 726—728.
FINCH, G. (1938): Hunger as a determinant of conditional and unconditional salivary response magnitude. *Amer. J. Physiol.* **123**, 379—382.
GARCIA-CASTELLS, E. and GUZMÁN-FLORES, C. (1970): Efectos de la clormadinona soble la conducta emocional de la gata. In: *XIII. Congreso Nacional de Ciencias Fisiologicas*. 27—31 de Agosto de 1970. Morelia, Mich. México.
GOODMAN, S. J. and MANN, P. E. G. (1967): Reticular and thalamic multiple unit activity during wakefulness, sleep and anesthesia. *Exp. Neurol.* **19**, 11—24.
GUZMÁN-FLORES, C. and ALCARAZ, M. (1970): A technique for recording and integrating unit activity. *Bol. Inst. Estud. méd. biol. (Méx.)* 1970.
GUZMÁN-FLORES, C. and GARCIA-CASTELLS, E. (1970): Análisis de la actividad eléctrica de los nucleos amigdalinos y la conducta emocional. In: *XIII. Congreso Nacional de Ciencias Fisiologicas*, 27—31 de Agosto de 1970. Morelia, Mich. México.
HUTTENLOCKER, P. R. (1961): Evoked and spontaneous activity in single units of the medial brainstem during natural sleep and waking. *J. Neurophysiol.* **24**, 451—468.
KORÁNYI, L. and ENDRŐCZI, E. (1967): The effect of ACTH on nervous processes. *Neuroendocrinology* **2**, 65—75.
KORÁNYI, L. and ENDRŐCZI, E. (1970): Influence of pituitary-adrenocortical hormones on thalamo-cortical and brainstem-limbic circuits. In: *Pituitary, Adrenal and the Brain*. Ed. by D. de Wied and J. A. W. M. Weijnen. Progress in Brain Research. Vol. 32. Elsevier, Amsterdam. pp. 120—130.

Korányi, L., Endrőczi, E. and Tárnok, F. (1965/1966): Sexual behavior in the course of avoidance conditioning in male rabbits. *Neuroendocrinology* **1,** 144—157.

Korányi, L., Endrőczi, E. and Tamásy, V. (1969): Influence of pituitary–adrenocortical hormones on the central nervous system. Electrophysiological and behavioural studies on rats and chicks. *Acta physiol. Acad. Sci. hung.* **36,** 73—82.

Korányi, L., Beyer, C. and Guzmán-Flores, C. (1971a): Multiple unit activity during habituation, sleep–wakefulness cycle and the effect of ACTH and corticosteroid treatment. *Physiol. Behav.* **7,** 321—329.

Korányi, L., Beyer, C. and Guzmán-Flores, C. (1971b): Effect of ACTH and hydrocortisone on multiple unit activity in the forebrain and thalamus in response to reticular stimulation. *Physiol. Behav.* **7,** 331—335.

Lát, J. (1965): The spontaneous exploratory reactions as a tool for psychopharmacological studies. A contribution towards a theory of contradictory results in psychopharmacology. In: *Pharmacology of Conditioning, Learning and Retention.* Ed. by M. Ya. Mikhelson and V. G. Longo. Pergamon Press, Oxford. pp. 47—66.

Lát, J. (1966): The phenomena of extinction (habituation, adaptation) and spontaneous recovery. A confrontation with the Lorenzian RSE hypothesis. In: *Symposium on Ecology and Etiology in Behavioral Studies.* XVIII. International Congress of Psychology, Moscow. pp. 41—54.

Levine, S. (1968): Hormones and conditioning. In: *Nebraska Symposium on Motivation.* Ed. by J. M. R. Jones. Vol. XIV. Univ. of Nebraska Press, Lincoln. pp. 85—102.

Lissák, K. and Endrőczi, E. (1961): Neurohumoral factors in the control of animal behavior. In: *Brain Mechanisms and Learning.* Ed. by G. J. F. Delafresnaye. Blackwell, Oxford. pp. 293—308.

Lissák, K. and Endrőczi, E. (1964): Neuroendocrine interrelationships and behavioral processes. In: *Major Problems in Neuroendocrinology.* Ed. by E. Bajusz and G. Jasmin. S. Karger, Basel. pp. 1—14.

Lissák, K., Endrőczi, E. and Medgyesi, P. (1957): Somatisches Verhalten und Nebennierenrindentätigkeit. *Pflügers Arch. ges. Physiol.* **117,** 265—273.

Malmo, R. B. (1959): Activation: a neurophysiological dimension. *Psychol. Rev.* **66,** 367—386.

Mori, K., Winters, W. D. and Spooner, C. W. (1968): Comparison of reticular and cochlear multiple unit activity with evoked response during various stages induced by anesthetic agents, II. *Electroenceph. clin. Neurophysiol.* **24,** 242—248.

Podvoll, E. M. and Goodman, S. J. (1967): Averaged neural electrical activity and arousal. *Science* **155,** 223—225.

Winters, W. D., Mori, E., Spooner, C. E. and Kado, R. T. (1967): Correlation of reticular and cochlear multiple unit activity with auditory evoked responses during wakefulness and sleep, I. *Electroenceph. clin. Neurophysiol.* **23,** 539—545.

Yerkes, R. M. and Dodson, J. D. (1908): The relation of strength of stimulus to rapidity of habit formation. *J. comp. Neurol. Psychol.* **18,** 459—465.

EFFECT OF SEPTAL LESIONS ON ADRENAL CORTICAL AND MEDULLARY ACTIVITY DURING STRESS

K. MURGAŠ and R. KVETŇANSKÝ

Institute of Experimental Endocrinology
Slovak Academy of Sciences
Bratislava, Czechoslovakia

Acute stress in animal organism may induce changes not only in the "classical stress-dependent organs" (Selye 1936), but also in the functions of other structures, which fact renders it difficult to understand processes underlying mutual neuroendocrine relationships (Charvát 1964, Murgaš and Jonec 1967).

As regards chronic stress situations or chronically repeated acute stress and the ensuing changes, literary data on the function of the adrenal cortex and medulla are far more abundant than those on other organs (Mikulaj and Sciba 1963, Mikulaj and Kvetňanský 1966). These data seem to imply, that a characteristic feature of the function of the adrenal cortex following repetition of stress stimuli is a decline in its responsiveness, but the intensity of each stimulus during repetition remains unchanged (Mikulaj and Sciba 1963, Mikulaj and Kvetňanský 1966). This, however, does not hold true for the adrenal medullary function (Kvetňanský and Mikulaj 1970).

Another question coming to the foreground is that of centrally regulated humoral reactions in the organism under stressful conditions (e.g., Lissák and Endrőczi 1965, Jonec et al. 1966). Furthermore, data are available on the role of higher nervous activity on humoral reactions of the organism and on efforts at correlate neuroendocrine events with behavioural parameters (Ader 1969, Brain and Nowell 1970, Paré and Cullen 1965).

In the present study an attempt has been made to follow some of the indicators of adrenal cortex and medulla of rats in a stress situation after electrocoagulation of the septal area.

MATERIAL AND METHODS

Male Wistar rats SPF, weighing approximately 180 to 200 g and having free access to food and water, were used in these experiments.

Septal lesions were made by means of bilateral electrocoagulation (2 mA/15 sec, DC) according to stereotaxic coordinates (Maršala and Fifková 1960). Animals were taken into the experiments 10 to 12 days after the operation. The lesioned area was kept under control.

As stress stimulus we chose:

1. Carrying the experimental animals into another room of the animal house and transferring them into a different cage.
2. Daily immobilization. The animals were attached by the legs with adhesive tape to metal clamps fixed to a board for 150 min daily (Kvetňanský and Mikulaj 1970). This immobilization was repeated on 7 consecutive days.

After application of the stress stimuli, the animals were decapitated, blood was collected into test tubes containing heparin, and the adrenals were extirpated.

We followed plasma corticosterone levels (Van den Vies et al. 1960), total catecholamine content in adrenal homogenate (Euler and Lishajko 1961) and catecholamine synthetizing enzymes (CSE) tyrosine hydroxylase (Nagatsu et al. 1964) and dopamine-β-hydroxylase (Viviros et al. 1969) in adrenal. When the activity of these enzymes was to be followed, the animals were decapitated 6 hrs after the last immobilization.

RESULTS

The septal lesions alone, without additional application of stress stimulus, failed to induce any notable change in the majority of the parameters except for some behavioural changes.

Similarly, no changes were observed in parameters of the adrenal function of lesioned rats as against the controls when the animals had been transferred to another environment, although plasma corticosterone levels following transfer increased in the sense of our previous findings (Jonec et al. 1966).

Plasma corticosterone levels rose significantly in the controls and the sham-operated animals ($p < 0.01$) following repeated immobilization. Even though the septal lesion in non-stressed rats did not by itself alter the plasma corticosterone

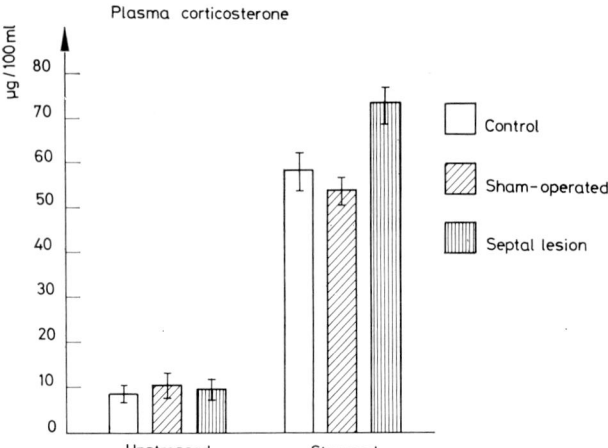

Fig. 1. Effect of septal lesion on plasma corticosterone in rats after repeated immobilization. Rats were immobilized for 2.5 hrs for 7 consecutive days and killed immediately after the last immobilization. Each group contains 7 to 8 animals and the results are expressed as mean values ($\pm$ SEM)

values, repeated immobilization in lesioned animals caused them to rise significantly ($p < 0.01$) in comparison with both the control and sham-operated groups (Fig. 1).

The level of total catecholamines in adrenal tissues decreased significantly ($p < 0.05$) following repeated immobilization and in the group with septal lesions the decrease was even more pronounced ($p < 0.01$) in comparison with that of the controls (Fig. 2).

Thyrosine hydroxylase, an enzyme with a rate limiting function, shows an increased activity following repeated immobilization ($p < 0.001$). The septal lesion alone without immobilization, does not bring about any significant change in the activity of these enzymes, but immobilization of animals with septal lesions enhances further its activity, which differs significantly ($p < 0.05$) also from that of immobilized controls (Fig. 3).

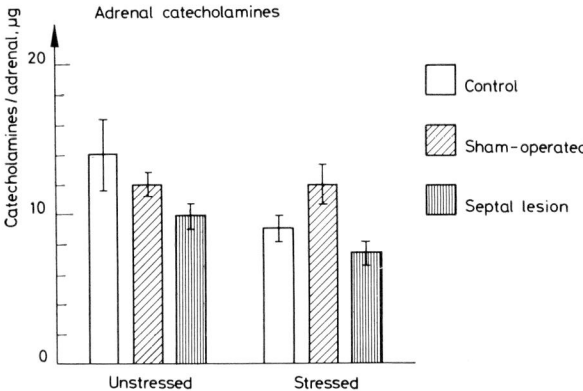

Fig. 2. Effect of septal lesions on total adrenal catecholamines after a daily 2.5 hrs' immobilization for 7 consecutive days. Animals were killed 6 hrs after the last immobilization. Each group contained 8 to 14 animals (mean values ± SEM)

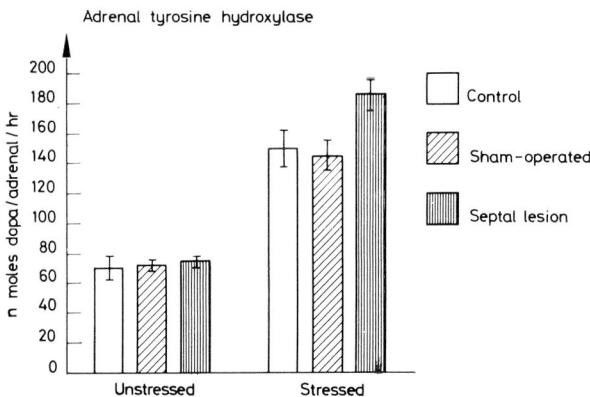

Fig. 3. Effect of septal lesions on thyroxine hydroxylase after a daily 2.5 hrs' immobilization for 7 consecutive days. Animals were killed 6 hrs after the last immobilization. Each group contained 8 to 14 animals (mean values ± SEM)

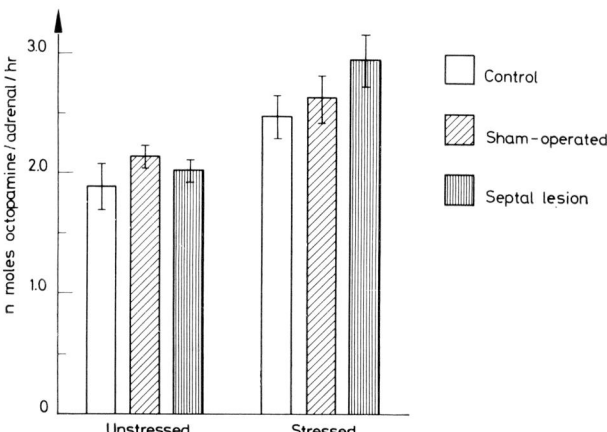

Fig. 4. Effect of septal lesions on dopamine-β-hydroxylase after a daily 2.5 hrs' immobilization for 7 consecutive days. Animals were killed 6 hrs after the last immobilization. Each group contained 8 to 14 animals (mean values $\pm$ SEM)

Dopamine-β-hydroxylase activity does not change following septal lesions in non-stressed animals, but in lesioned animals, repeatedly immobilized, it rises significantly in comparison with immobilized controls ($p < 0.02$).

DISCUSSION AND CONCLUSIONS

Judged by emotionality rating scales, rats with septal lesions show characteristic behavioural changes like hypersensitivity and agressivity (Horovitz 1965, Igič et al. 1970). However, it has not been confirmed, whether rats or mice of a different emotionality level would differ in the activation of their adrenal cortex (Ader 1969, Brain and Nowell 1970). It is known that the activation of catecholamine synthesis in the adrenal medulla occurs following stimulation to the hypothalamus, if the electrical stimulation is accompanied by behavioural manifestation such as aggressivity (Reis et al. 1970). Repeated immobilized stress which alters the catecholamine content in adrenal tissues (Kvetňanský and Mikulaj 1970) induces always a simultaneous activation of enzymes involved in the catecholamine synthesis (Kvetňanský et al. 1970, 1971). This effect, however, may be suppressed by a lesion to the splanchnic nerve immediately above the adrenal (Kvetňanský et al. 1970, 1971).

Animals with septal lesions in our experiments manifested marked behavioural changes, especially in the first days following the intervention, in terms of hyperirritability and aggressivity (Stark and Henderson 1966).

At the same time we found that the lesion alone, without any stress stimulus, as also only a weak stress stimulus, fails to induce any difference in the adrenal reaction between rats with septal lesions and the controls. However, following a stronger stress stimulus (repeated immobilization), the adrenal activity was more intense in lesioned rats than in immobilized controls.

At present we cannot interpret the results obtained or the mechanism responsible for the changes in the adrenal cortex and medulla that occur during stress induced by electrocoagulation of the septal area. However, in terms of the findings by Horovitz (1965), Igič et al. (1970) and some other authors, it may be postulated that the function of the septal and amygdaloid area resides in an excitatory or inhibitory effect on numerous autonomic and behavioural functions and this probably by way of projection into brainstem reticular formation and hypothalamic structures.

The mechanism of action by which septal lesions lead to a further increase of adrenal activation following stress is interpreted in the same way.

SUMMARY

The effect of septal lesions was followed on adrenal cortex and medulla following immobilization.

Plasma corticosterone levels and catecholamine synthetizing enzyme activity were found to increase while adrenal catecholamine levels to decrease in animals with septal lesions as against immobilized controls.

REFERENCES

ADER, R. (1969): *Ann. N.Y. Acad. Sci.* **159**, 791.
BRAIN, F. P. and NOWELL, W. N. (1970): *Physiol. Behav.* **5**, 259.
CHARVÁT, J. (1964): *Čas. Lék. čes.* **103**, 761.
EULER, U. S. VON and LISHAJKO, F. (1961): *Acta physiol. scand.* **51**, 348.
HOROVITZ, Z. P. (1965): *Psychosomatics* **6**, 281.
IGIČ, R., STERN, P. and BAJAGIČ, E. (1970): *Neuropharmacology* **9**, 73.
JONEC, V., MURGAŠ, K. and KVETŇANSKÝ, R. (1966): *Fed. Proc.* **25**, 1200.
KVETŇANSKÝ, R. and MIKULAJ, L. (1970): *Endocrinology* **87**, 783.
KVETŇANSKÝ, R., WEISE, V. K. and KOPIN, I. J. (1970): *Endocrinology* **87**, 744.
KVETŇANSKÝ, R., GEWIRTZ, G. P., WEISE, V. K. and KOPIN, I. J. (1971): *Mol. Pharmacol.* **7**, 81.
LISSÁK, K. and ENDRŐCZI, E. (1965): *The Neuroendocrine Control of Adaptation.* Akadémiai Kiadó, Budapest.
MARŠALA, J. and FIFKOVÁ, E. (1960): *Stereotaxic Atlases for the Cat, Rabbit and Rat Brain.* SZN, Praha.
MIKULAJ, L. and SCIBA, J. (1963): *Čs. Fysiol.* **12**, 330.
MIKULAJ, L. and KVETŇANSKÝ, R. (1966): *Physiol. bohemoslov.* **15**, 439.
MURGAŠ, K. and JONEC, V. (1967): *Čs. Fysiol.* **16**, 246.
NAGATSU, T., LEVITT, M. and UDENFRIEND, S. (1964): *Analyt. Biochem.* **9**, 122.
PARÉ, W. P. and CULLEN, J. W., JR. (1965): *Psychol. Rep.* **16**, 283.
REIS, D. J., MOORHEAD, D. T., RIFIKIN, M., JOH, T. and GOLDSTEIN, M. (1970): *Fed. Proc.* **28**, 277.
SELYE, H. (1936): *Brit. J. exp. Path.* **17**, 234.
STARK, P. and HENDERSON, J. K. (1966): *Int. J. Neuropharm.* **5**, 379.
VIES, J. VAN DEN, BAKKER, R. F. M. and WIED, D. DE (1960): *Acta endocr. (Kbh.)* **34**, 513.
VIVIROS, O. H., ARQUEROS, L., CONNOT, R. J. and KIRSHNER, N. (1969): *Mol. Pharmacol.* **5**, 60.

SEXUAL MOTIVATION IN THE NEONATALLY ANDROGEN-TREATED FEMALE RAT

B. J. MEYERSON and L. LINDSTRÖM

Department of Pharmacology
University of Uppsala
Uppsala, Sweden

In most mammalian species used as laboratory animals it is now well established that the psychosexual differentiation is possible to be influenced by exogenous hormone treatment during a critical pre- or postnatal period (Harris and Levine 1962, Barraclough and Gorski 1962, Young et al. 1964). As to sexual behaviour in the female, most investigations have been concerned with the effect of an early hormone treatment on the adult display of the sex-typical mating behaviour. Less is known about the effect on the urge of the adult subject to seek heterosexual contact, i.e. sexual motivation.

In a recent investigation three different methods were employed to study sexual motivation and it was demonstrated that oestradiol treatment (25–100 µg/kg s.c.) of the ovariectomized rat induced an urge to seek contact with a vigorous male. In analogous experiments, an oestrous female or castrated male was not the same incentive as a vigorous male (Meyerson and Lindström 1970). The present investigation was conducted to study the effect of neonatal testosterone propionate treatment on the sexual motivation in the female rat.

Female Sprague-Dawley rats were given testosterone propionate (TP) 1 mg/animal s.c. at 5 days of age (Neo-TP), or oil blank solution 0.05 ml (Neo-oil). The size of each litter was reduced to six members. At least one male was bred in each litter, and separated shortly after weaning (about day 22). The animals were ovariectomized when about 90 days old. Vaginal smears were taken for at least two weeks before ovariectomy. All Neo-TP animals were found to have persistent cornified vaginal smears. Two weeks after surgery a standard test for mating behaviour was performed which revealed that oestradiol benzoate (EB, 10 µg/kg s.c. followed 48 hours later by progesterone (0.4 mg/animal s.c.) did not activate lordosis response on mounting by a vigorous male in the early androgen-treated females. The Neo-oil subjects displayed a clearcut lordosis response after this treatment.

The animals were used in the motivational experiments when about 120 days of age (250 g). From weaning the animals were kept in laboratories with reversed day–night rhythm (light from 9 p.m. to 9 a.m.).

To test the sexual motivation three methods were employed. They differ in respect to the operant behaviour the subject has to perform to reach sexual contact. The sexual contact was in the present investigation restricted, i.e. contact with the stimulus animal was allowed but the animals were separated by a wire mesh. The animals were used only in one method but were taken from the same breeding colony. A detailed description of care of animals, training procedure, statistical evaluation and the different techniques used will be published elsewhere (Meyerson and Lindström 1972). The essentials of the methods and the effect of oestradiol benzoate in androgenized females are as follows:

In the *open field method* (Fig. 1) the animals are observed in an observation arena with the incentive animal (vigorous male) placed in a mesh cage in the centre of the field. A wall runs straight across the field to separate the experimental animal, which was placed in one of the semicircular areas and the control subject which was placed in the other one. In the circumference of each semicircular area a mesh cage is located which holds another stimulus animal (spayed female). The location of the subject was recorded by a film-camera located in the cage ceiling, and triggered every minute. The subjects were observed for one hour per day during nine consecutive days. The percentage of records with the animal found to stay in the vicinity of the male is shown in Fig. 2. (Vicinity of the male means area a in Fig. 1.) Oestradiol benzoate, 100 μg/kg s.c., was given on day 0. In the

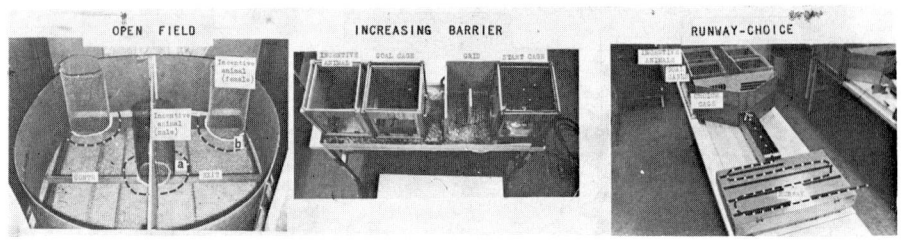

Method	Open field	Increasing barrier	Runway-choice
Recorded	No. of records with subject located in the vicinity of the male (a) or female (b)	No. of grid crossings	The specific choice
Program	Camera located in the cage ceiling. Triggered every minute	Grid current increases every second time subject crosses the grid. 15 sec allowed in goal cage	15 sec allowed in goal cage
		Inter-trial time = 0 If subject hesitates >5 min run is ended	Intertrial time = 0 20 trials per run
Trial	One hour recording = 60 records	From start until subject is in goal cage	From start until subject is in goal cage
Run		No. of trials subject is willing to perform	20 trials

Fig. 1. Test schedule of the experimental animals

non-androgenized female (Neo-oil controls) there is an obvious increase in the number of records with the female staying with the male after the oestradiol treatment as compared to oil blank controls. (Fig. 2). The Neo-TP oil blank controls have a greater day-to-day variability than was seen in the Neo-oil experiment. No significant effect was found in the Neo-TP group by the oestradiol treatment.

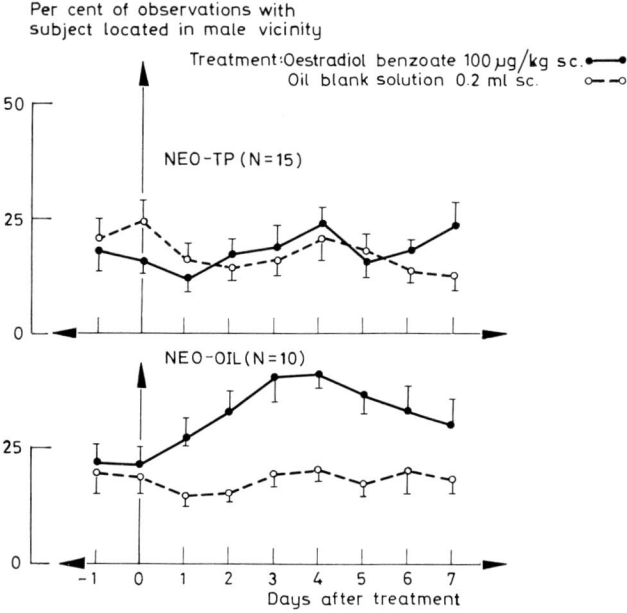

Fig. 2. The effect of oestradiol benzoate on the urge of neonatally testosterone propionate (1 mg) or oil (0.05 ml) treated female rats to stay in the vicinity of a vigorous male (animal located in area a, as in Fig. 1). The subjects were spayed as adults. Vertical bars $1 \times$ S.E.M.

In the *increasing barrier method* (Fig. 1) we make use of an electric grid to tell how much of a negative stimulus the subject is willing to bear to reach sexual contact. The animals have to pass from one cage via an electric grid to a second cage which holds the incentive object. The intensity of the grid current is stepwise increased every second time the animal passes.

EB, 100 μg/kg, was given on day 0. The animals were tested one run per day and animal, except for the day after the treatment had been given (day 1). In agreement with our previous study in the neonatally non-treated female the oestrogen treatment significantly increased the number of passages over the grid the Neo-oil subject was willing to pay to reach contact with a sexually active male (Fig. 3). In the Neo-TP animal no such oestrogen effect was obtained. The rewarding situation was changed but the experiment otherwise analogously performed. As incentive animal served a spayed female brought into oestrus by oestradiol (100 μg/kg) followed 48 hours later by progesterone (1 mg/animal). This object did

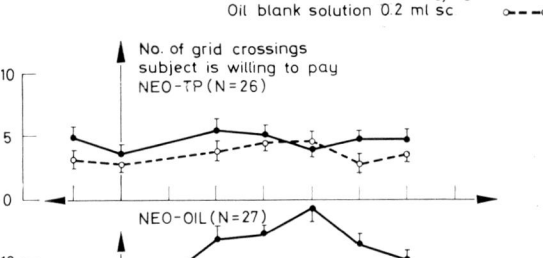

Fig. 3. The effect of oestradiol benzoate on the amount of electric grid shock neonatally testosterone propionate (1 mg) or oil (0.05 ml) treated female rats are willing to pay to reach contact with a vigorous male. The subjects were spayed as adults. Vertical bars 1 × S.E.M.

not attract the Neo-oil female to the same extent as did the vigorous male (Fig. 4). The difference between oestrogen and oil treated Neo-oil subjects is not significant. However, there is a slight increase in grid-crossings considering the whole period. Also in this experiment there was no increased urge to seek contact with the oestrous female after oestrogen treatment of the Neo-TP animals.

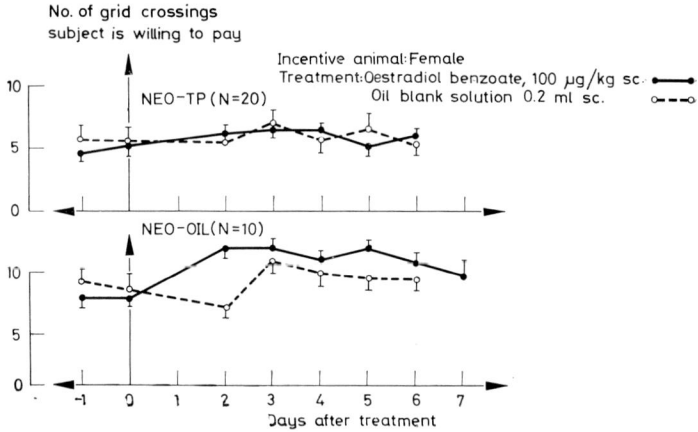

Fig. 4. The effect of oestradiol benzoate on the amount of electric grid shock neonatally testosterone treated (1 mg) or oil (0.05 ml) treated female rats are willing to pay to reach contact with an oestrous female. The subjects were spayed as adults. Vertical bars 1 × S.E.M.

The third technique employed for the study of sexual motivation is a *runway-choice* method. The experimental animal runs through a runway which brings it to a chamber the opposite wall of which has two doors. In the present experiments one door leads into a cage with a vigorous male the other door to a female brought into oestrus by oestradiol + progesterone (see above). The subjects were run 20 consecutive trials (trial = each time the animal is started) once a day except days 1 and 8 after the EB treatment. The effect of EB, 100 µg/kg s.c. on the choice of male versus female is shown in Fig. 5. In this experiment data are given for comparison of three different groups of animals, namely neonatally androgen treated (Neo-TP), neonatally oil blank treated (Neo-oil) and controls which were purchased and ovariectomized as adults (250 g). The latter group was from the same breeding colony as the parents of the two former categories.

Preference is calculated as the excess choice of male over that expected from random. In the controls (Fig. 5) the not oestrogen treated animals had throughout

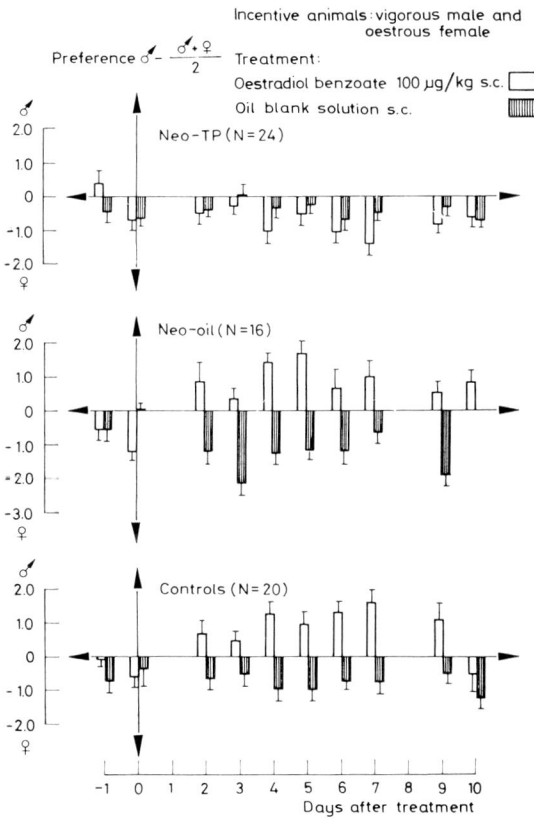

Fig. 5. The effect of oestradiol benzoate on the preference for a vigorous male over an oestrous female in neonatally testosterone propionate (1 mg), oil (0.05 ml) or neonatally not treated female rats. The subjects were spayed as adults. Vertical bars $1 \times$ S.E.M.

the test period a slight preference to seek contact with the oestrous female. After EB treatment this preference obviously changed. From day 2 to 9 there was a preference for the male. The day-to-day variability of the Neo-oil group is greater than that in the controls but the change of preference is analogous; the preference for the female stimulus animal is changed by the oestrogen treatment to a preference for the male. In the Neo-TP animals there is a slight preference for the female after the adult oil blank treatment. However, in contrast to controls and the Neo-oil group no preference for the male was seen after the EB treatment but rather an augmented preference for the female.

CONCLUSIONS

In the female rat ovariectomized as adult, EB induced an urge to seek contact with a vigorous male. This was a consistent finding in the three methods used. The neonatally androgen-treated female did not respond to EB in this way. No heterosexual motivation was seen. The possibility of a homosexual preference needs further experiments to be elucidated.

REFERENCES

HARRIS, G. W. and LEVINE, S. (1962): *J. Physiol.* **163**, 42.
BARRACLOUGH, C. A. and GORSKI, R. A. (1962): *J. Endocr.* **25**, 175.
MEYERSON, B. J. and LINDSTRÖM, L. (1970): *Proceedings of the Congress on Steroid Hormones*. Hamburg, 1970.
MEYERSON, B. J. and LINDSTRÖM, L. (1972): *Acta physiol. scand.* (In preparation).
YOUNG, W. C., GOY, R. W. and PHOENIX, C. H. (1964): *Science* **143**, 212.

AFFERENT BRAINSTEM PATHWAYS TO HYPOTHALAMUS AND TO LIMBIC SYSTEM IN THE RAT

L. ZÁBORSZKY, CS. LÉRÁNTH, J. MARTON and M. PALKOVITS

1st Department of Anatomy
Semmelweis Medical University
Budapest, Hungary

Institute of Experimental Medicine
Hungarian Academy of Sciences
Budapest, Hungary

It has been shown in physiological experiments that certain peripheral stimuli affecting the hypothalamo–pituitary system reach the hypothalamus through neural pathways. Among others the neural stress pathways are of significance (Ganong 1970), the interruption of which, at the border between the mesencephalon and diencephalon (Halász and Gorski 1967, Makara et. al 1972) prevents ACTH release in response to certain stresses. Numerous authors have described fibre systems ascending from the brainstem (see the text) their hypothalamic ermination, however, has not been convincingly elucidated (Raisman 1970).

MATERIAL AND METHODS

In searching for the possible anatomical substrate of these effects bi- and unilateral transections were made in the upper brainstem of rats at the level of the posterior hypothalamus–mamillary body (Fig. 1 a). The operations were performed in rats of both sexes, weighing about 200 to 250 g of a local breed of the Wistar strain.

The animals were killed 2 days after the operation for electron microscopic purposes. Their brains were fixed by perfusion with Karnowsky's solution and the different hypothalamic areas and parts of the amygdaloid complex were dissected and embedded after postosmification into Durcupan. The removed areas were controlled on semithin sections (staining with methylene blue). Tesla II S 413 EM-device was used for electron microscopy.

Another group of the animals was killed 4 days after the operation by perfusion under 10 per cent formaline solution anaesthesia. After fixation 20 μ thick frontal and sagittal sections were made and the distribution of degenerated fibres and endings was examined on sections impregnated according to Fink–Heimer's method (1967).

Direct pathways could be traced from the site of the lesion to most parts of the hypothalamus, in particular to the medial basal hypothalamus (MBH), the arcuate and ventromedial nuclei (NA, NVM), furthermore, to the dorsomedial nucleus (NDM), dorsal premamillary nucleus (NPMD), and posterior hypothalamic area (PHA). Degeneration could be traced even to the neurosecretory supraoptic and the paraventricular nuclei (NSO, NPV).

Direct connections from the brainstem ascend also to certain parts of the limbic system (septum, hippocampus, amygdala, habenula).

The exact origin of several ascendig fibre bundles cannot be defined in our study, but it appears that the ventral and dorsal tegmental nucleus of Gudden (Nauta and Kuypers 1958, Morest 1961), the ventral tegmental area, the tegmental reticular nucleus (Cowan et al. 1964) are among the chief sources of ascending systems to the hypothalamus and related limbic structures.

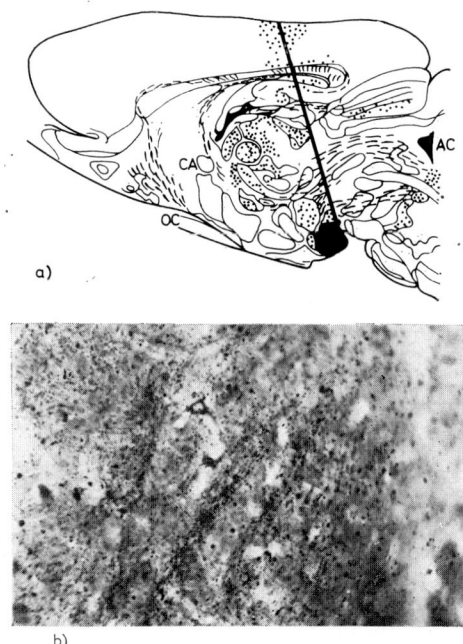

Fig. 1. (a) Solid black line indicates the channel of penetration (about 0.7 mm wide), the lower black area shows the cutting area. Broken black lines and dots represent the location of degenerated fragments projected into the median sagittal plane. (Note the absence of degeneration in the NVM, NDM at this level.) Diagram after König and Klippel (1963). CA = anterior commissure, OC = optic chiasma, AC = cerebral aqueduct. (b) Degenerated fibres in the FLD of the same preparation as demonstrated in Fig. 1a

The following afferent tracts might be involved in the transmission of impulses to the hypothalamus.

Periventricular fibre system (dorsal longitudinal fasciculus—Fig. 1b). There is now ample evidence that the pathway, originally described as an efferent system (Krieg 1932), forms a reciprocal association system between the hypothalamus and the central grey substance of the midbrain (Nauta 1958). Krieg (1932) subdivided the fibre system forming itself in the area of the cerebral aqueducts into an anterior and a posterior component. The ascending fibres of this system are proceeding in periventricular position and are fanning out to the medial hypothalamus and to various parts of the medial thalamus. Szentágothai et al. (1968)

report similar observations, showing that the pathways directed to the hypothalamus become detached along the 3rd ventricle from the main bundles and reach the medial hypothalamus.

Our examinations showed that the afferent fibre system is not closely related to the wall of the 3rd ventricle but deviates in lateral direction at the level of NDM, to which nucleus the tract issues preterminal fibres. The fibres directed toward the MBH cannot be traced with the light microscope. Conversely, those running forward in the direction of the paraventricular nucleus can be recognized

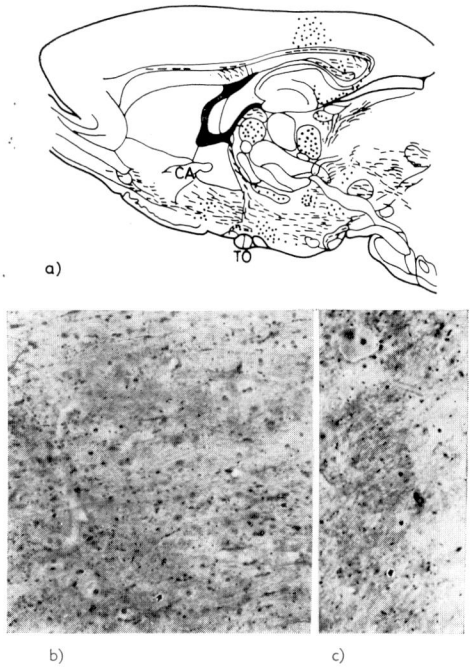

Fig. 2. (a) Distribution of degenerated fibres of the MFB, charted from a single paramedian section, more lateral than in Fig. 1a. TO = optic tract. (b) Fibre degeneration in the sagittal section and (c) in the frontal section of the MFB. Fink–Heimer's method

both with the light and the electron microscope. The pathway is lost from sight in the oral and ventral region to the paraventricular nucleus.

Medial forebrain bundle (MFB). This bundle is first recognizable caudally in the ventral tegmental area of Tsai (Cowan et al. 1964). In our material the fibres run through the whole lateral hypothalamic area (Fig. 2), while giving off side branches to the cells situated here as well as in medial direction to the MBH and to the NSO. They proceed forward in the lateral part of the preoptic region and reach the diagonal band nucleus, the medial septal nucleus, and the rostral part of the olfactory tubercle (Fig. 2). Similar data were published by Nauta and Kuypers (1958), Guillery (1957), Ban (1964), Cowan et al. (1964) and Raisman (1966) following rostral midbrain lesion.

Some fibres reach the dorsal fornix over the septum where the fibres may be traced as far as the subiculum. A few fibres terminate in the stratum lacunosum of the area CA_1 of the hippocampus (CA fields of Lorente de No). These observations accord with the findings of Guillery (1957), while Raisman et al. (1965) did not succeed in demonstrating degeneration in the hippocampus proper after lesions to the MFB.

From the fibres of the MFB a few become laterally detached and terminate in the medial nucleus of the amygdaloid complex as it is revealed by axonal degeneration method.

From the MFB a considerable number of fibres can be traced through the inferior thalamic peduncle to the stria medullaris and eventually to the lateral nucleus of the habenula. Similar data were published by Ban (1964); conversely, Cragg (1961), Massopoust and Thompson (1962) describe the following pathway: ventromedial tegmental area of the midbrain—fasciculus retroflexus—stria medullaris—lateral preoptic region. We could not find such a pathway in the present study. Nauta and Kuypers (1958) traced a few fibres to the lateral habenular nucleus through the fasciculus retroflexus.

Mamillary peduncle (PM). The majority of the ascending fibres terminate in the mamillary nuclei, however, some join the MFB. In this study it was not possible to isolate the mamillary component from the MFB proper, but according to Guillery (1957), Morest (1961), Nauta and Kuypers (1958), Cowan et al. (1964) the fibres terminate in the posterior hypothalamic area, in the dorsal premamillary nucleus and in the lateral part of the tuberal region (Kuypers 1956) and may be traced as far as the septum.

TERMINAL DEGENERATION IN THE VARIOUS HYPOTHALAMIC NUCLEI

Supraoptic nucleus. Only few literary data can be found on the fibre connections of NSO (Leontowich 1970). The afferent fibres directed towards the nucleus are very thin and near the nucleus they lose their myelin sheath. With the Fink–Heimer method only few fibres could be traced through the MFB to this nucleus. With the light microscope, terminal degeneration was only occasionally observed in the nucleus, while a considerable number of them was revealed electron microscopically. In intact animals axo-dendritic, axo-somatic, with neurosecretory axons axo-axonic synapses are found in abundance in the electron microscopic picture. After posterior deafferentation the axo-axonic synapses remain intact without exception. Axo-somatic and axo-dendritic synapses were found often to degenerate after positive lesions at the border between the posterior hypothalamus and the midbrain (Fig. 3).

Paraventricular nucleus. Degeneration of ascending fibres may be demonstrated in both the parvo- and magnocellular parts of the nucleus. The fibres reach the nucleus through the dorsal longitudinal fasciculus, from cranial and dorsal direction. Apart from these, the nucleus receives degenerated fibres also from the lateral side. These fibres come most probably from the subthalamic region and from the zona incerta—though they can be well seen—their origin is so far not elucidated. In electron microscopic studies the degeneration of synapses is similar to that in the NSO.

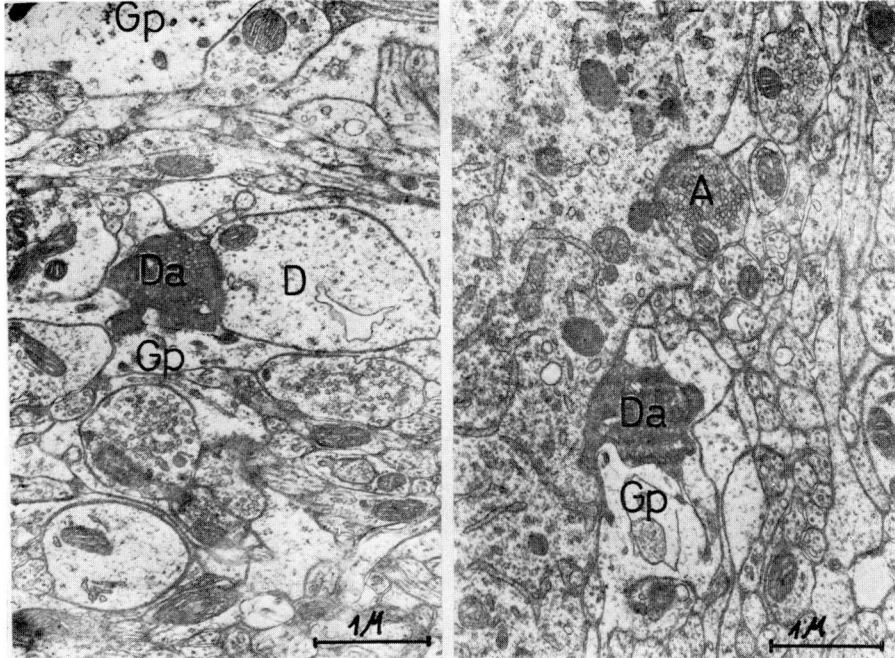

Fig. 3. Terminal degeneration in the NSO. The degenerated axon (Da) is surrounded by glial processes (Gp). Left, axo-dendritic synapse. D = dendrite. Right, axo-somatic synapse. On the right of the picture the intact axon (A) is in synaptic contact with the soma

Dorsomedial nucleus. The majority of ascending fibres reaches the nucleus from behind through the periventricular system, however, the degeneration is concentrated only in the lateral part of the nucleus. Another fibre group reaches the nucleus laterally, from the direction of the zona incerta, from beneath the fasciculus mamillothalamicus and from above the fornix and the MFB.

A small number of degenerated fibres was observed originating from the MFB. If the MFB is separated from the lateral hypothalamus by a parasagittal cut, degenerated fibres may be traced as far as the medial hypothalamic nuclei. Following lateral lesions of the hypothalamus Guillery (1957) and Chi (1970) also traced fibres to the NDM.

Ventromedial nucleus. A great part of the fibres reach the nucleus from cranial and lateral direction as may be well seen both in sagittal and frontal sections. The fibres reach the nucleus partly through the periventricular system (Ban 1964, Szentágothai et al. 1968) and partly from the side, from the component of the PM, proceeding in the MFB (Kuypers 1956, Ban 1964). Lesion of the MFB causes the degeneration of a small number of fibres in the lateral part of the nucleus.

A few fibres come from above the MFB, from the zona incerta, ventrally or dorsally from the fornix and may be traced to the lateral part of the NVM. In

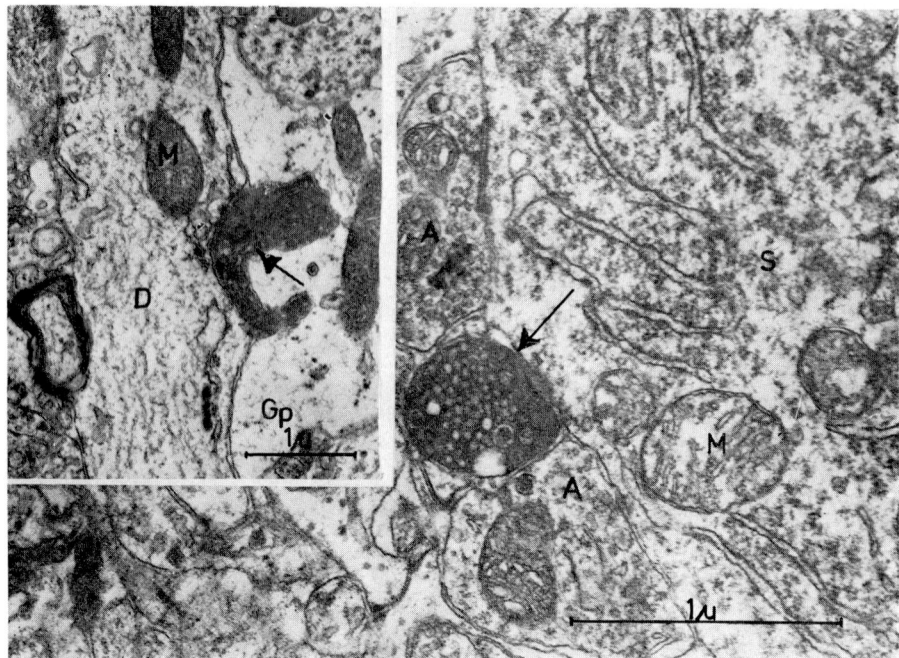

Fig. 4. Terminal degeneration in the NVM. Inset, axo-dendritic synapse. Axo-somatic synapse. Degenerated axon (A) marked by arrow. Gp = glial process, D = dendrite, M = mitochondrion

our material the subthalamic area of Forel was damaged. Le Gros Clark (1938) traced fibres from this region to the NVM and Bard and Rioch (1937) from the palladium. A part of these fibres might belong to the Ganser's commissure. The field of Forel gets fibres also from the reticular formation of the brainstem (Nauta and Kuypers 1958). Szentágothai et al. (1968) relying upon Golgi and degeneration studies consider these fibres as emerging from the MFB. Electron microscopically degenerated axons were found in the nucleus. These axons terminate either on the soma or on the dendrites (Fig. 4).

Arcuate nucleus. In the parvocellular neurosecretory nucleus only axo-dendritic and axo-somatic synapses may be found under the electron microscope. After transection of the ascending systems degeneration is discernible on both types of synapses. With Fink–Heimer's method we did not succeed in tracing fibres directly into the nucleus. Regarding the origin of these fibres we refer to the examinations of Krieg (1932) who from the most medial group of the MFB traced a few fibres as far as the NA (Fig. 5).

Suprachiasmatic nucleus. Szentágothai et al. (1968), traced fibres to the nucleus following lesions of the anterior midbrain central grey matter and this group corresponds exactly to the posterior component of the periventricular system of Krieg (1932). In our examinations, we could not detect these fibres with Fink–

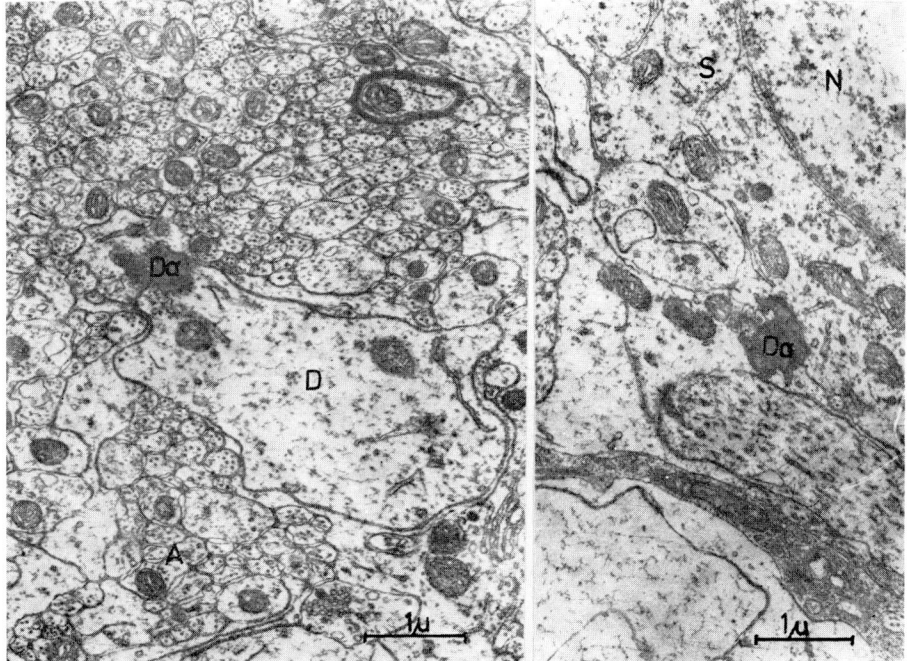

Fig. 5. Terminal degeneration in the NA. Left, axo-dendritic synapse. The picture shows furthermore transections of many intact axons. D=dendrite. Right, axo-somatic synapse. A = axon, Da = degenerated axon, N = nucleus, S = soma

Heimer's method (1967) under the electron microscope, however, the degenerated axo-somatic and axo-dendritic synapses can be well demonstrated.

Posterior hypothalamic area, premamillary nuclei. In accordance with the data of many authors (Nauta and Kuypers 1956, Szentágothai et al. 1968) ascending fibres reach the posterior hypothalamic area by the way of the periventricular system and through the PM, respectively. In our material a massive degeneration was found only in the dorsal part of the premamillary nuclei (NPMD) which, in agreement with Krieg (1932), can be considered to be mainly of MFB and periventricular origin.

SUMMARY

Ascending inputs from and through the lower brainstem may reach hypothalamic and related limbic structures through the following pathways:

1. The ascending portion of the dorsal longitudinal fasciculus, the fibres of which reach mainly the medial hypothalamus (ventromedial, dorsomedial, paraventricular, dorsal premamillary nuclei, posterior hypothalamic area).

2. In the medial forebrain bundle the majority of the fibres are ascending and

they give branches mainly to the lateral hypothalamus itself, further in medial direction to the medial basal hypothalamus and to the supraoptic nucleus. Some fibres ascending through the dorsal fornix terminate in the hippocampus and those laterally detached from the medial forebrain bundle in the amygdaloid complex. The lateral nucleus of the habenula is also in connection with the brainstem by the medial forebrain bundle—inferior thalamic peduncle—stria medullaris.

3. Mamillary peduncle. A large portion of the fibres terminate in the mamillary nuclei, but a few fibres join the medial forebrain bundle and terminate in the dorsal premamillary, dorsomedial nuclei and in the posterior hypothalamic area.

4. The subthalamic region of Forel might be the relay station of many transit-systems (pallido-hypothalamic, incerto-hypothalamic fibres, the fibres of Ganser's commissure, and the fibres originating in the reticular formation of the midbrain), which might reach the ventromedial and dorsomedial nuclei.

REFERENCES

BAN, T. (1964): The hypothalamus, especially on its fiber connections, and the septo-preoptico-hypothalamic system. *Med. J. Osaka University* **15**, 1.
BARD, P. and RIOCH, D. MCK. (1937): A study of four cats deprived of neocortex and additional portions of the forebrain. *Johns Hopk. Hosp. Bull.* **60**, 73.
CHI, C. C. (1970): Afferent connections to the ventromedial nucleus of the hypothalamus in the rat. *Brain Res.* **17**, 439.
COWAN, W. M., GUILLERY, R. W. and POWELL, T. P. S. (1964): The origin of the mamillary peduncle and other hypothalamic connections from the midbrain. *J. Anat. (Lond.)* **98**, 345.
CRAGG, B. G. (1961): The connections of the habenula in the rabbit. *Exp. Neurol.* **3**, 388.
FINK, R. P. and HEIMER, L. (1967): Two methods for selective silver impregnation of degenerating axons and their synaptic endings in the central nervous system. *Brain Res.* **4**, 369.
GANONG, W. F. (1970): Control of adrenocorticotropin and melanocyte-stimulating hormone secretion. In: *The Hypothalamus.* Ed. by L. Martini, M. Motta and F. Fraschini. Academic Press, New York, London. p. 313.
GUILLERY, R. W. (1957): Degeneration in the hypothalamic connections of the albino rat. *J. Anat. (Lond.)* **91**, 91–115.
HALÁSZ, B. and PUPP, L. (1965): Hormone secretion of the anterior pituitary gland after physical interruption of all nervous pathways to the hypophysiotropic area. *Endocrinology* **77**, 553.
HALÁSZ, B. and GORSKI, R. A. (1967): Gonadotrophic hormone secretion in female rats after partial or total interruption of neural afferents to the medial basal hypothalamus. *Endocrinology* **80**, 608.
KÖNIG, J. F. R. and KLIPPEL, R. A. (1963): *The Rat Brain.* Williams and Wilkins, Baltimore.
KRIEG, W. J. S. (1932): The hypothalamus of the albino rat. *J. comp. Neurol.* **55**, 19.
KUYPERS, H. A. I. M. (1956): Certain fiber connections of the mesencephalic central gray matter. In: *Progress in Neurobiology.* Ed. by J. Ariens Kappers. Elsevier, Amsterdam. p. 246.
LE GROS CLARK, W. E. (1938): Morphological aspects of the hypothalamus. In: *The Hypothalamus.* Ed. by E. E. Le Gross Clark. Oliver and Boyd, Edinburgh. p. 1.
LEONTOWICH, T. A. (1970): The neurons of the magnocellular neurosecretory nuclei of the dog's hypothalamus. *J. Hirnforsch.* **11**, 499.
MAKARA, G. B. Stark, E., Marton, J. and Mészáros, T. (1972): Corticotrophin release induced by surgical trauma after transection of various afferents to the hypothalamus. *J. Endocr.* **53**, 389.

Massopoust, L. G. and Thompson, R. (1962): A new interpedunculo-diencephalic pathway in rats and cats. *J. comp. Neurol.* **118,** 97.

Morest, D. K. (1961): Connections of the dorsal tegmental nucleus in rat and rabbit. *J. Anat. (Lond.)* **95,** 229.

Nauta, W. J. H. (1958): Hippocampal projections and related neural pathways to the midbrain in the cat. *Brain* **81,** 319.

Nauta, W. J. H. and Kuypers, H. G. J. M. (1958): Some ascending pathways in the brain stem reticular formation. In: *Reticular Formation of the Brain.* Ed. by H. Jasper et al. Little and Brown, Boston. p. 3.

Raisman, G. (1966): The connections of the septum. *Brain* **89,** 317.

Raisman, G. (1970): Some aspects of the neural connections of the hypothalamus. In: *The Hypothalamus.* Ed. by L. Martini, M. Motta and F. Fraschini. Academic Press, New York and London.

Raisman, G., Cowan, W. M. and Powell, T. P. S. (1965): The extrinsic afferent, commissural and association fibers of the hippocampus. *Brain* **88,** 963.

Szentágothai, J., Flerkó, B., Mess, B. and Halász, B. (1968): *Hypothalamic Control of the Anterior Pituitary.* An Experimental-Morphological Study. 3rd ed. Akadémiai Kiadó, Budapest.

Hormones and Brain Function, Budapest 1971, pp. 459–474 (1973)

SOME PHYSIOLOGICAL ASPECTS OF EMOTIONAL STRESS

G. PETERFY and E. J. PINTER

Allan Memorial Institute of Psychiatry and
Department of Psychiatry, Reddy Memorial Hospital
and
Clinical Investigation Unit, Queen Mary Veterans Hospital and
Department of Medicine, Reddy Memorial Hospital and
Allan Memorial Institute of Psychiatry
Montreal, Canada

This paper reports on studies of the correlations of measures of affect, plasma corticoids (PC) and free fatty acids (FFA) in hypnotic state, while specific hypnotic instructions were given, and during anticipation of repetition of the experimental procedure. Under these experimental conditions the following specific interactions could be examined:

1. The relative magnitude and temporal sequence of PC and FFA changes.
2. The relationship of PC to the lipid mobilization of emotional stress (Cleghorn et al. 1972, Pinter et al. 1967a) as compared with the established role of catecholamines and the beta adrenergic receptors (Cleghorn et al. 1969, Pinter and Pattee 1967, Pinter et al. 1967b).
3. The relationship of measures of verbal anxiety and hostility to PC and FFA changes.

METHODS AND PROCEDURES

The subjects were 14 women aged 22–42 (average 26), and 4 men with average age 37. All were free of organic diseases, and all had a trial experience with two of the experimental conditions: hypnosis and talking unprompted into a tape recorder to give a 5-minute verbal sample. This rehearsal was an attempt to minimize novelty effect (Mason 1968).

The studies were begun at 9 a.m. after a 12–14-hour overnight fast. Subjects rested in bed in a darkened room after initial venipuncture with an indwelling needle inserted into the antecubital vein. The needle was kept patent with a steady rate intravenous infusion of normal saline (60 ml/hr). The subjects were unaware of blood sampling.

The following design was adopted for each experimental trial: after the venipuncture subjects rested quietly in a darkened room for 40 minutes. Hypnosis was induced to a medium depth of trance according to the Davis–Husband scale (Davis and Husband 1931). Twenty minutes later three different hypnotic instructions were given to each subject for 10 minutes, on 3 different trials: SI (Active)— "You face a difficult problem and are struggling hard to solve it"; SII (Passive)— indicated that the subject could do nothing but hold tight and wait for help with a difficult problem; and SIII (No suggestion)—consisted of hypnotic relaxation suggestions. A two-way block design was employed with the order of presentation of these 3 hypnotic instructions balanced within each of 5 blocks or 3 subjects (45 experiments).

Immediately after the suggestions, subjects were asked to speak into a tape recorder for 5 minutes about anything on their minds. This produced a transcript ready to be scored for measures of affect, by coders unaware of the aims of the study. Following verbal sampling the hypnotic state was maintained for 20 minutes, then terminated.

The above procedure was repeated in 6 subjects (18 experiments) following the intravenous administration of a beta adrenergic blocking agent (Propranolol, 0.3 mg/kg/15 min) 30 minutes prior to commencement of hypnosis.

In all studies blood specimens were obtained for PC and FFA determinations on two occasions during the pre-experimental control period and at regular intervals during the hypnotic state (3 measurements for PC and 8 for FFA).

After these studies were completed the experimental procedure was begun again for 13 subjects. On these occasions, however, the hypnotist simply entered the room on schedule, said "good morning" and then left. Thus, the effect of anticipation on PC was examined.

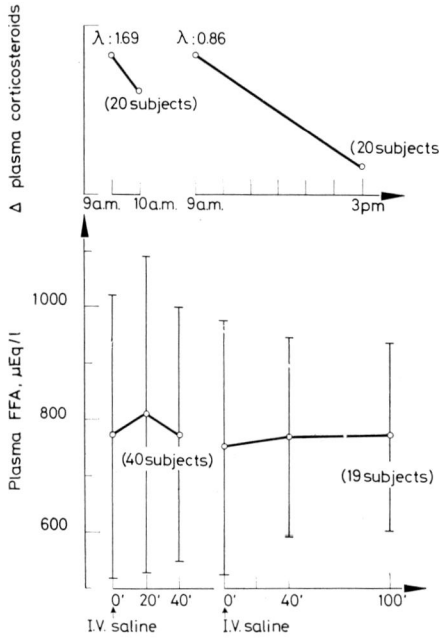

Fig. 1. Mean slopes of PC levels between 9–10 a.m. and 9 a.m.–3 p.m., respectively, in groups of 20 normal subjects in order to illustrate the diurnal variation of these hormone levels. The spontaneous variation of plasma FFA (with i.v. saline infusion started at 0 min) is also shown up to 40 minutes in 40 subjects. Saline infusion experiments in an additional 19 subjects indicated virtually stable FFA levels during a 40-min control and a 60-min simulated experimental period

PC were measured by competitive protein binding using the microassay previously described employing ³H-corticosterone and Florisil (Murphy 1967). Plasma FFA were determined by Dole's method (Dole 1956).

Anxiety and hostility levels were estimated by the methods of Gottschalk and Gleser (Gleser et al. 1961, Gottschalk and Gleser 1969, Gottschalk et al. 1966), applied to 5-minute samples of unprompted speech recorded on audiotape.

RESULTS

Careful attention was paid to establish a reliable baseline for both PC and FFA in order to obtain valid reference points for the evaluation of changes (Fig. 1).

The assessment of PC changes was based on comparisons with the diurnal decline of PC. We will explain how PC changes were categorized as positive or negative. Figure 1 illustrates the slope of decline from 9–10 a.m. as well as between 9 a.m. and 3 p.m. in a large group of subjects. Experimental trials in which PC failed to rise (40 per cent of subjects), the mean slope of decline did not differ significantly from the mean slope during the 40-minute pre-experimental rest period, nor from the mean 9 a.m.–3 p.m. slopes of the larger groups. Each of 3 PC determinations on every trial in which the slope continued to decline remained below the

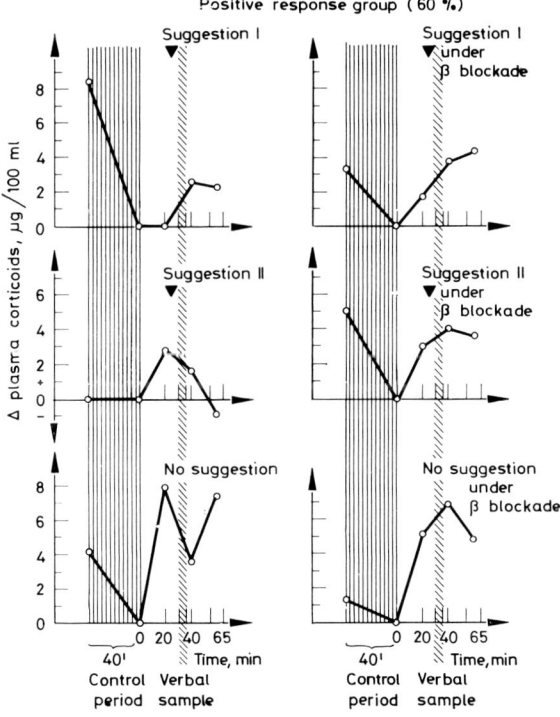

Fig. 2. Temporal sequence of mean plasma corticoid changes during the pre-experimental control period and during hypnotic state with and without suggestions in those subjects who showed an increment of circulating corticoids

baseline value at the induction of hypnosis. The difference between mean maximal increases and decreases was significantly different to a high degree, therefore, it was thought reasonable to categorize PC responses as positive or negative, the latter being a failure to deviate from the mean diurnal change. While this approach to the data may be cogent physiologically, a median split is more cogent statistically. Hence some of the data are presented both ways (Figs 2 and 3, Table 1).

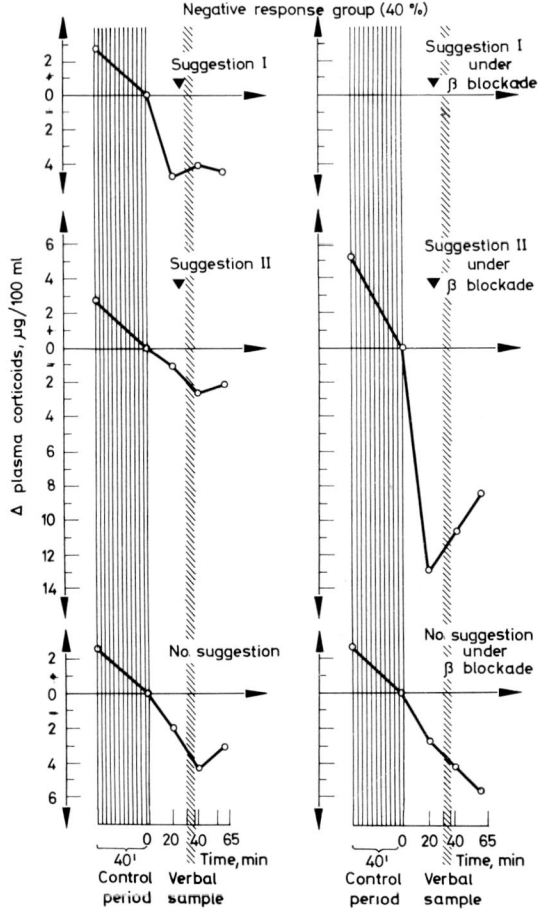

Fig. 3. Mean plasma corticoid changes in the negative reactors (no data are shown for "Suggestion I, under beta blockade", as in all subjects PC increased in this study)

CHANGES IN PC AND THEIR RELATIONSHIP TO AFFECT SCORES, PLASMA FFA AND BETA ADRENERGIC BLOCKADE

When trials are categorized into positive and negative PC responses (Table 2) we see that high levels of anxiety and hostility-out tend to be associated with positive PC response.

TABLE 1

Peak Δ PC, μg/100 ml ($\pm$SD)

	SI	SII	SO	SI	SII	SO	Anticipating stress
				with β blockade			
Positive PC response groups	+5.05 ± 3.40	+3.54 ± 2.50	+8.84 ± 7.50	+4.78 ± 4.16	+5.17 ± 4.00	+7.23 ± 3.69	+8.89 ± 5.18
Mean and difference vs negative PC response groups		+6.19 ± 3.17 S ($p < 0.001$)			+5.62 ± 4.08 S ($p < 0.001$)		S ($p < 0.01$)
			+5.96 ± 3.44				
Negative PC response groups	−6.34 ± 4.33	−2.85 ± 0.82	−4.98 ± 2.51	*	−12.73 ± 7.87	−6.05 ± 1.48	−6.80 ± 4.61
Mean		−4.85 ± 3.20			−10.50 ± 7.03		
			−6.63 ± 5.28				

* No data; all subjects showed positive response.

TABLE 2

Relationship between affect scores and direction of PC chance

Suggestion	Mean anxiety scores			D.F.*	t*	p*
	N	PC positive	PC negative			
1. Active (SI)	4	2.45	1.92	6	3.666	0.011
2. Passive (SII)	3	3.33	2.70	4	2.497	0.067
3. Relax (SIII)	4	2.20	2.32	6	0.554	0.600

Suggestion	Mean hostility-out			D.F.*	t*	p*
	N	PC positive	PC negative			
1. Active (SI)	4	2.07	1.50	6	3.560	0.012
2. Passive (SII)	3	1.66	0.60	4	4.764	0.009
3. Relax (SIII)	4	2.20	1.57	6	4.486	0.004

* Symbols of Student's t test.

Table 3 shows PC levels divided at the medium. Those trials with a rise in PC above the median PC change are compared with those below the median. In general when PC levels rose above the median they again had higher anxiety,

TABLE 3

T tests on affect scores for subjects above and below median change on plasma corticoids

Suggestion	Variables	X for subjects above median	X for subjects below median	D.F.*	t*	p*
I Active	Anxiety	2.57	1.95	7	1.123	0.299
	Hostility-Out	2.19	1.35	7	2.939	0.022
	Hostility-In	1.11	1.63	7	8.209	0.001
	Hostility-Environ.	1.89	1.10	7	4.799	0.002
II Passive	Anxiety	3.12	2.68	6	3.519	0.013
	Hostility-Out	1.31	0.97	6	2.078	0.083
	Hostility-In	1.83	1.67	6	1.063	0.329
	Hostility-Environ.	1.67	1.32	6	4.908	0.003
III Relax	Anxiety	3.06	1.98	9	5.435	0.001
	Hostility-Out	1.76	1.70	9	2.407	0.039
	Hostility-In	2.01	1.74	9	0.704	0.499
	Hostility-Environ.	1.57	0.86	9	6.652	0.001

* Symbols of Student's t test.

outward hostility and environmental hostility* scores. Correlations (Table 4) were in the same direction but the associations are not powerful enough to attain significance. The inward hostility scale, unlike the other scales, appears to be

TABLE 4

Correlations between PC change (μg/100 ml) and affect scores

Variables	Suggestion I	Suggestion II	Suggestion III N = 9
Anxiety	0.33	+0.48	0.14
Hostility-Out	0.49	−0.03	0.44
Hostility-In	−0.40	0.08	0.07
Hostility-Environ.	0.48	0.66	0.25

With D.F. = 7, r = 0.666 at 5% level.

unrelated to elevated PC. For Suggestion I it appears to be inversely related but here, inward and outward hostility correlate (r = −0.93.) Correlations amongst the different affect scales are seen in Table 5.

TABLE 5

Correlations between affect scores

Suggestion	Variables	Anxiety	Hostility-Out	Hostility-In N = 12
I	Anxiety	—	—	—
	Hostility-Out	0.09	—	—
	Hostility-In	0.08	−0.93	—
	Hostility-Environ.	0.47	0.07	0.14
II	Anxiety	—	—	—
	Hostility-Out	0.13	—	—
	Hostility-In	0.28	−0.54	—
	Hostility-Environ.	−0.44	0.07	−0.07
III	Anxiety	—	—	—
	Hostility-Out	−0.30	—	—
	Hostility-In	0.46	−0.22	—
	Hostility-Environ.	0.01	0.26	−0.01

With D.F. = 10, r = 0.576 at 5% level.

* The term environmental hostility refers to hostility perceived by the subject as being located in the environment. Gottschalk and Gleser (1969) categorize this type of hostility as ambivalently directed. This is their scale and the term "environmental" is ours.

Direction of PC change was not related to magnitude of mean FFA level during the experiment (Table 6, Fig. 4). When peak FFA levels are compared (Table 7) differences are magnified but are in opposite directions with different suggestions. Therefore, changes in PC cannot be said to contribute to lipid mobilization.

TABLE 6

Relationship of mean FFA level and direction of PC change

Sug-gestion	Mean FFA level		D.F.*	t^*	p^*
	PC positive	PC negative			
I	1,072	720	6	1.69	N.S.
II	777	771	6	0.06	N.S.
III	563	820	6	1.40	N.S.

* Symbols of Student's t test.

TABLE 7

Relationship between mean peak FFA levels and direction of PC change

Sug-gestion	No.	Mean FFA µEq/L		D.F.*	t^*	p^*
		PC positive	PC negative			
I	4	1,112.5	724.3	6	9.365	0.001
II	3	950.0	838.7	4	1.417	0.229
III	4	625.8	844.5	6	4.367	0.005

* Symbols of Student's t test.

When propranolol is given, the magnitude of PC change is not influenced (Table 8, Figs 2 and 4) in a meaningful manner.

TABLE 8

Effect of beta adrenergic blockade on changes in plasma corticoid levels

Hypnotic sug-gestion	No.	$\bar{X}$ Δ PC µg/100 ml		D.F.*	t^*	p^*
		Saline	Propranolol			
I	5	0	+4.55	4	1.20	N.S.
II	5	+2.8	−10.4	4	2.38	< 0.10 0.05
III	4	−1.7	+7.2	3	3.06	< 0.10 0.05

* Symbols of Student's t test.

Peak PC changes occurred at variable times following the induction of hypnosis, sometimes immediately but most frequently 5–10 minutes after peak FFA developed.

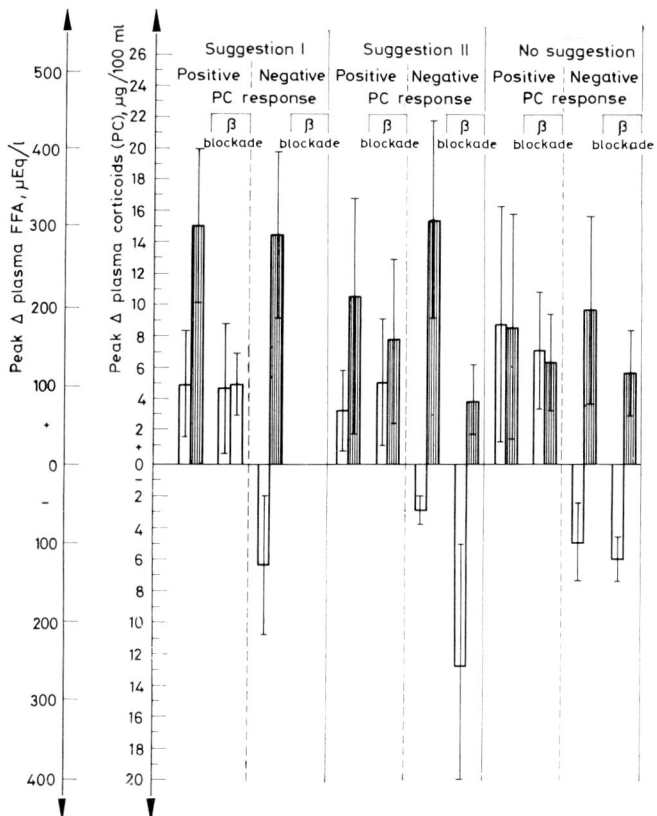

Fig. 4. A comparative representation of mean plasma corticoid (white bars) and FFA (shaded bars) changes ($\Delta \pm SD$). Grouped according to suggestions I, II and no suggestion (with and without beta adrenergic blockade), the positive and negative reactors are contrasted. FFA increased in all trials (but least when there was no suggestion given). FFA rise was markedly diminished by beta adrenergic blockade. Plasma corticoid changes showed no correlation with the variations of FFA and remained uninfluenced by beta blockade. (No PC data are shown under Suggestion I. Negative PC response, beta blockade, as all subjects reacted with a rise in PC)

Latin square analysis showed no effects on PC attributable to the content of suggestions nor to the order of experimental days (Table 9). This indicates that there was no 'novelty' effect (the first experimental day was a rehearsal).

Anticipation of repetition of the experiment in 13 subjects elicited a positive PC response in 8 subjects, negative in 5 (Fig. 5). The difference in mean peak PC was significant ($p < 0.01$) vs the baseline.

Of seven individuals studied over a number of experimental days, only one had consistently positive PC and only one consistently negative PC response.

TABLE 9

Latin square analysis of variance on plasma corticoid peak values by order and hypnotic instruction

Variables	Ss*	DF*	MS*	F*	p*
Between subjects	1,020.92	5			
Groups	541.87	2	270.93	1.70	0.321
Error	479.05	3	159.68		
Within subjects	519.95	12			
Treatments	14.82	2	7.41	0.16	0.856
Order	25.82	2	12.91	0.27	0.767
Treatments × order	127.06	2	63.53	1.35	0.290
Error	658.00	14	47.00		
Total	1,540.86	17			

* Symbols of latin square analysis.

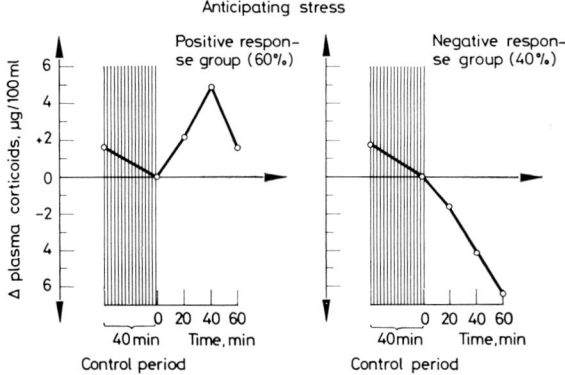

Fig. 5. The temporal sequence of plasma corticoid changes in 13 subjects, only anticipating stress.' A clear separation into positive and negative reactors was possible

CHANGES IN PLASMA FFA, THEIR RELATIONSHIP TO BETA RECEPTORS AND TO MEASURES OF AFFECT

Plasma FFA increased significantly reaching a peak at 40 minutes. In 2/3 of the trials the FFA peak was reached between 35 and 45 minutes while 3/4 PC peaks occurred at 40 to 55 minutes.

Beta adrenergic blockade markedly diminished lipid mobilization in these studies (55 and 60 per cent blockade in SI and SII groups, respectively). Decrease in mean FFA for each suggestion is shown in Table 10. These observations have been corroborated by kinetic studies of FFA production and pool sizes (Figs 6 and 7). No significant difference in anxiety or hostility scores was noted in trials with propranolol, a finding which is being documented in detail elsewhere (Cleghorn et al., in press).

TABLE 10

Analysis of variance showing effect of beta adrenergic blockade on plasma FFA levels in different experimental conditions

Source	Ss*	DF*	MS*	F*	p*
Subjects	6,164.535	191			
Suggestions (S)	29.092	2	11,546.000	2.281	N.S.
Blocker (B)	2,874.589	1	2,874,589.000	272.587	< 0.001
FFA (F)	416.269	3	138,756.333	337.442	< 0.001
S × B	53.627	2	26,813.500	6.834	< 0.01
S × F	14.422	6	2,403.667	9.470	< 0.005
B × F	121.554	3	40,518.000	70.999	< 0.001
S × B × F	23.100	6	3,850.000	19.073	< 0.001
Error Total	6,531.099	4,393			
Error$_S$	1,933.365	382	5,061.164		
Error$_B$	2,014.206	191	10,545.581		
Error$_F$	235.618	573	411.200		
Error$_{S \times B}$	1,498.715	382	3,923.337		
Error$_{S \times F}$	290.876	1,146	253.818		
Error$_{B \times F}$	326.998	573	570.677		
Error$_{S \times B \times F}$	231.321	1,146	201.850		
Total	16,222.287	4,607			

* Symbols of analysis of variance.

Comparison of peak FFA levels and direction of PC change revealed no consistent relationship (Table 7). For Suggestion I (SI), mean peak FFA was significantly higher when PC rose. In Suggestion III (SIII) the opposite was true. For Suggestion II (SII), no significant association was noted. This method of analysis exaggerates extremes and hence more emphasis is to be attached to the direction of association than to the degree of significance.

Finally, correlations between affect scores and (i) FFA levels and (ii) FFA changes were computed for each of the ten times FFA measured. Thus, there are 20 correlations for each condition (i.e. each hypnotic suggestion).

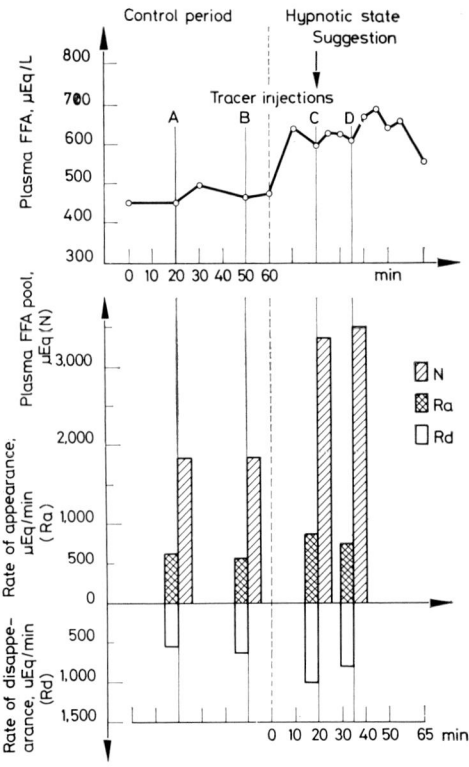

Fig. 6. A representative illustration of the influence of emotional stress on plasma FFA production, utilization and pool in one subject given anxiety-provoking suggestion in hypnotic state

Anxiety and FFA levels are positively and significantly ($p < 0.05$) correlated for SI nine out of ten times. Environmental hostility and FFA levels covary significantly ten out of ten times ($p < 0.05$). Maximum correlations are as follows: $r = +0.64$ and $r = +0.81$, respectively.

Increase in FFA hostility-out tended to be inversely related. Correlations reach significance at $p < 0.05$ ($r = 0.57$) three out of ten times for SI, none for SII and two out of ten times for SIII.

In general, PC change is weakly associated with anxiety, FFA levels on the other hand, are quite strongly associated with anxiety. PC is weakly but positively associated with outward hostility, while FFA is negatively and rather weakly associated. FFA and environmental hostility are strongly associated with SI while PC is weakly associated with this variable for all hypnotic suggestions. Relationships between affects and FFA vary with hypnotic conditions to a greater extent than do relationships between affects and PC.

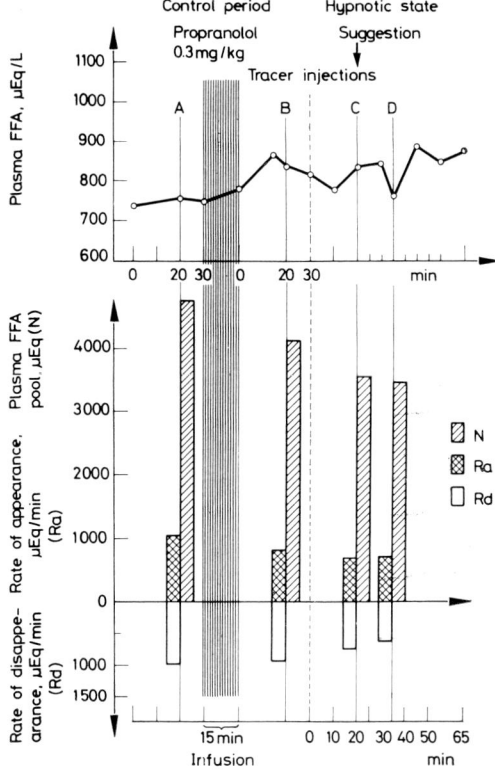

Fig. 7. Absence of the adipokinetic effect of emotional stress, as illustrated by the plasma FFA level, FFA production, utilization and pool determinations in one subject (same as Fig. 6) with propranolol administration prior to the stressful hypnotic session

DISCUSSION

The experimental conditions appear to stimulate the pituitary–adrenocortical system in 60 per cent of trials. Inasmuch as fat mobilization is substantially mediated by an adrenergic mechanism (Pinter and Pattee 1967, Pinter et al. 1967a, b) the sympathetic nervous system, on the other hand, can be said to respond in almost all trials.

Beta adrenergic blockade inhibits lipid mobilization of emotional stress to a significant degree and it is unrelated to PC levels. In the absence of beta blockade the direction of PC change is inconsistently related to the magnitude of FFA response. The two were dissociated in some experiments, negatively associated in others and positively associated in still others. These observations, coupled with the fact that FFA changes tend to precede PC changes, suggest that PC have no relationship with the lipid mobilization of emotional arousal.

The finding that the two variables (FFA and PC) are differently associated under different experimental conditions adds to existing evidence that mechanisms of regulation must discriminate between the two systems involved (Mason 1968).

We suggest that behavioural observations may, in time, reveal some indications about these regulatory processes. Our work in the past (Cleghorn et al., in press), along with that of Gottschalk et al. (1965) and Stone et al. (1968), have revealed a positive significant correlation between plasma FFA and verbal anxiety levels (but not hostility) in several different samples of subjects under more simple experimental conditions.

Plasma corticoid increases, in contrast, appear to be positively associated with measures of verbal hostility-out as previously reported by Sholiton et al. (1963) and to a significant degree with anxiety under most conditions. Inconsistency in the direction of PC changes for individuals is also related to their hostility-out levels during experiments on different days. Perksy (1962) and many others (Wolff et al. 1964a, b, Tecce et al. 1965, Florica and Huehl 1962, Sholiton et al. 1963) were found associations between anxiety and 17-OHCS, and measurements of corticoids have related also with a number of other behavioural variables, thus elevation is now taken to be an index of nonspecific emotional arousal. The relationship of FFA to affective states appears to be more specific (Cleghorn et al., in press). Therefore, we postulate that different central mechanisms of activation may be triggered by processes which underlie the different behavioural variables.

The trance relationship as well as affects also appear to be important. Sachar et al. (1965, 1966) have noted rapid changes in 17-OHCS levels in response to the induction of trance. This was also observed immediately after induction of trance in the present study in which positive PC changes were observed in 11 trials, negative in 7. But such prompt responses were seen in only 25 per cent of trials. Few very low PC levels were observed in our subjects and no systematic attempt was made to assess the quality of the hypnotic relationship in those cases as Sachar has done.

It seems that simultaneous precise analysis of affects, together with measurements of relationship phenomena and other factors such as effectiveness of defense, merit continued study. While such investigations admittedly add more complexity to an already complicated phenomenon, they may ultimately contribute to a behavioural description of processes relevant to central regulation of some endocrine and metabolic processes.

SUMMARY

1. Emotional stress constitutes both pituitary–adrenal and adipokinetic stimuli.
2. While fat mobilization occurs in all subjects, PC increases only in 60 per cent of those given suggestions and also in a similar proportion of those anticipating stress (mean Δ PC $+ 5.9 + 3.4$ $\mu g/100$ ml; $p < 0.001$). The remaining 40 per cent of subjects showed the usual diurnal decline of PC.
3. Outward hostility was positively associated with PC increases and negatively with FFA increases.
4. Anxiety scores were positively related with both PC and FFA increases.
5. Beta adrenergic blockade had no significant effect on PC changes, but significantly inhibited FFA mobilization.

6. Thus, the frequency and magnitude of PC and FFA changes are dissociated yet are differentially associated with concurrent measures of affective behaviour.

7. Peripheral mediation of FFA response relies primarily on catecholamines and beta receptors; pituitary–adrenal activity definitely does not contribute to the adipokinetic mechanism.

8. It is suggested that the two systems are activated by different modes of transmission at the higher neural level.

9. It is undecided from these acute studies whether PC and FFA changes may contribute to somatic morbidity. A sustained state of stimulation, however, can lead to protein catabolism, superfluous glucose mobilization, potentiation of adipokinesis, impaired carbohydrate tolerance, increased thrombogenicity of the blood and hyper-β-lipoproteinaemia.

ACKNOWLEDGEMENTS

The authors wish to express their gratitude to Dr. B.E.P. Murphy, Queen Mary Veterans Hospital, Montreal, for all corticosteroid determinations, and for her helpful discussion of corticosteroid metabolism and the experimental design in connection with corticosteroids; to Dr. J. M. Cleghorn, McMaster University, Hamilton, for his substantial contribution to the experimental design, and for his great help in evaluating all affect scores and in carrying out all statistical analysis; to Dr. G. Hetenyi, University of Toronto, for his help in the kinetic studies of FFA; to Dr. T. Zsoter, University of Toronto, for his discussion of autonomic physiology and adrenergic receptors; and to Miss H. Wetzel, Queen Mary Veterans Hospital, Montreal, for her expert technical assistance.

REFERENCES

CLEGHORN, J. M., PETERFY, G. and PINTER, E. J. (1969): Experimenter effects on lipid mobilization in human subjects. (In preparation).
CLEGHORN, J. M., PETERFY, G. and PINTER, E. J. (1972): *Psychophysiology of Lipid Mobilization. Dysnutrition in the Seven Ages of Man.* Univ. of Calif. Press, Los Angeles. (In press).
CLEGHORN, J. M., PETERFY, G., PINTER, E. J. and PATTEE, C. J.: Verbal anxiety and the beta adrenergic receptors. *J. nerv. ment. Dis.* (In press).
DAVIS, L. W. and HUSBAND, R. W. (1931): Study of hypnotic susceptibility in relation to personality traits. *J. abnorm. soc. Psychol.* **26**, 175.
DOLE, V. P. (1956): Relations between non-esterified fatty acids in plasma and metabolism of glucose. *J. clin. Invest.* **35**, 150.
FLORICA, V. and HUEHL, S. (1962): Relationship between plasma levels of 17-OHCS and a psychological measure of manifest anxiety. *Psychosom. Med.* **24**, 6.
GLESER, G. C., GOTTSCHALK, L. A. and SPRINGER, K. J. (1961): An anxiety scale applicable to verbal samples. *Arch. gen. Psychiat.* **5**, 593.
GOTTSCHALK, L. A. and GLESER, G. C. (1969): *The Measurement of Psychological States through the Content Analysis of Verbal Behaviour.* Univ. of Calif. Press, Los Angeles.
GOTTSCHALK, L. A., GLESER, G. C. and SPRINGER, K. J. (1963): Three hostility scales applicable to verbal samples. *Arch. gen. Psychiat.* **9**, 254.
GOTTSCHALK, L. A., CLEGHORN, J. M., GLESER, G. C. and IACONO, J. M. (1965): Studies of relationships of emotions to plasma lipids. *Psychosom. Med.* **27**, 2.
GOTTSCHALK, L. A., STONE, W. N., GLESER, G. C. and IACONO, J. M. (1966): Anxiety levels in dreams: Relation to changes in plasma free fatty acids. *Science* **153**, 654.

Mason, J. W. (1968): A review of psychoendocrine research on the pituitary–adrenal cortical system. *Psychosom. Med.* **30**, 2.

Murphy, B. E. P. (1967): Some studies of the protein-binding of steroids and their application to the routine micro- and ultramicro-measurement of various steroids in body fluids by competitive protein-binding radioassay. *J. clin. Endocr.* **27**, 973.

Persky, H. (1962): Adrenocortical function during anxiety. In: *Physiological Correlates of Psychological Disorder*. Ed. by N. S. Greenfield. Univ. of Wisconsin Press.

Pinter, E. J. and Pattee, C. J. (1967): Effect of beta adrenergic blockade on resting and stimulated fat mobilization. *J. clin. Endocr.* **27**, 1441.

Pinter, E. J., Peterfy, G., Cleghorn, J. M. and Pattee, C. J. (1967a): Observations on the adrenergic mechanism of hyperadipokinesis in emotional stress. *Amer. J. med. Sci.* **254**, 5.

Pinter, E. J., Pattee, C. J., Peterfy, G. and Cleghorn, J. M. (1967b): Metabolic effects of autonomic blockade. *Lancet* **ii**, 101.

Sachar, E. J., Fishman, J. B. and Mason, J. W. (1965): Influence of hypnotic trance on plasma 17-OHCS concentration. *Psychosom. Med.* **27**, 230.

Sachar, E. J., Cobb, J. C. and Shor, R. E. (1966): Plasma cortisol changes during hypnotic trance relation to depth of hypnosis. *Arch. gen. Psychiat.* **14**, 482.

Sholiton, L. J., Wohl, T. H. and Week, E. E. Jr. (1963): The correlation of two psychological variables, anxiety and hostility, with adrenocortical function in patients with lung cancer. *Cancer* **16**, 2.

Stone, W. M., Gleser, G. C., Gottschalk, L. A. and Iacono, J. M. (1968): Variations in plasma FFA following verbal samples or venipuncture and relationship to anxiety. Psychosom. Med. Presented to the American Psychosomatic Society Annual Meeting, New Orleans, 1968.

Tecce, J. J., Friedman, S. B. and Mason, J. W. (1965): Anxiety, defensiveness and 17-OHCS excretion. *J. nerv. ment. Dis.* **141**, 549.

Wolff, C. T., Hofer, M. A. and Mason, J. W. (1964a): Relationship between psychological defenses and mean urinary 17-hydroxycorticosteroid excretion rates. II. Methodologic and theoretical considerations. *Psychosom. Med.* **26**, 5.

Wolff, C. T., Friedman, S. B., Hofer, M. A. and Mason, J. W. (1964b): Relationship between psychological defenses and mean urinary 17-hydroxycorticosteroid excretion rates. I. A predictive study of parents of fatally ill children. *Psychosom. Med.* **26**, 5.

SECTION V
RECENT DEVELOPMENTS IN CLINICAL NEUROENDOCRINOLOGY

Chairman: N. HATOTANI

ENDOCRINOLOGICAL STUDIES ON PERIODIC PSYCHOSES

N. HATOTANI

Department of Psychiatry
Mie Prefectural University Medical School
Tsu, Japan

Under the concept of periodic psychoses various clinical conditions can be included according to the degree and mode of the mental breakdown. It is characteristic of typical manic-depressive psychosis, which is the prototype of periodic psychoses, that the lowering of personality level remains relatively slight. If the dissolution of mental function goes further, disturbed states of consciousness such as acute hallucinatory-delusional states and oneiroid or confusional states make their appearance, and sometimes a catatonic syndrome becomes predominant. As a rule, the more acute and serious the breakdown of mental function, the more intense the disturbance of consciousness.

The clinical features common to the periodic psychoses may be summarized as follows:

1. The onset of illness is usually acute and prognosis for each psychotic episode is generally favourable. However, there is a tendency toward periodic recurrence.

2. The basic character of the mental symptom is disturbance of consciousness in a broad sense, manifested by emotional disturbance, distorted perception, confusional thinking and psychomotor disturbances, etc.

3. The emotional and psychomotor disturbances tend to alternate in opposite direction such as manic-depressive and hyperkinetic-akinetic. Such bipolar manifestations can be seen not only in mental symptoms, but also in such somatic phenomena as insomnia–hypersomnia, anorexia–polyphagia, oliguria–polyuria, etc.

These three characteristics, periodic recurrence, pathology of consciousness and bipolar manifestation of the symptom seem to indicate the underlying biological basis of this group of psychoses. For this reason, we have examined a group of periodic psychoses with extremely frequent relapses and followed their clinical course from the endocrinological point of view.

The incidence of psychoses in this group, especially that of the monthly relapsing type, was found to be overwhelmingly high in females. Also, the time of onset seemed to be in close relationship with the menstrual cycle.

RELATIONSHIP BETWEEN THE ONSET OF PSYCHOSES AND THE MENSTRUAL CYCLE

Forty-seven cases displaying more than three psychotic periods were examined in order to elucidate the relationship between the onset of the psychotic episodes and the menstrual cycle. As is shown in Table 1, about half of the cases showed repeated psychotic states during the middle through the latter half of the menstrual cycle. There was no case showing regular periodicity restricted exclusively to the first half of the cycle. There were only 3 cases where the onset never failed to appear during menstruation. Even in cases that reveal apparent simultaneousness of the psychotic period and menstruation, when studied carefully, the majority proved to have had the onset already during the premenstrual period. In other cases relationship between the psychotic onset and menstrual cycle was not always constant.

TABLE 1

Relationship between onset of the psychotic period and the phase of the menstrual cycle

Time of onset of psychosis	No. of cases	%
First half of the menstrual cycle	0	0
Middle or latter half of the menstrual cycle	23	49.1
During menstruation	3	6.3
Irregular	21	44.6
Total	47	100.0

These results indicate that the periodic psychoses in the female are apt to relapse during the premenstrual period. This synchronization of psychotic recurrence and menstrual cycle suggests that the functional vulnerability of the hypothalamo–pituitary–gonadal system may be of great importance in some cases of this group of psychoses.

CASE HISTORY

Only one representative case shall be discussed in this report.

H. A. 32-year-old female patient (Fig. 1). She is the fourth of six children of consanguinous parents. Her father, two brothers and one sister suffered from periodic psychoses. Her previous history includes 14 psychoses, 1 epileptic seizure and 5 suicidal attempts. Menarche occurred at the age of 16 followed by a series of irregular periods. Since March, 1959, the patient, without apparent reason, became depressed, avoided company, and had once made an unsuccessful suicidal attempt. From the following June, somewhat regular stupor spells, of about 10 days' duration, accompanied by perspiration, fever, mydriasis and tachycardia were

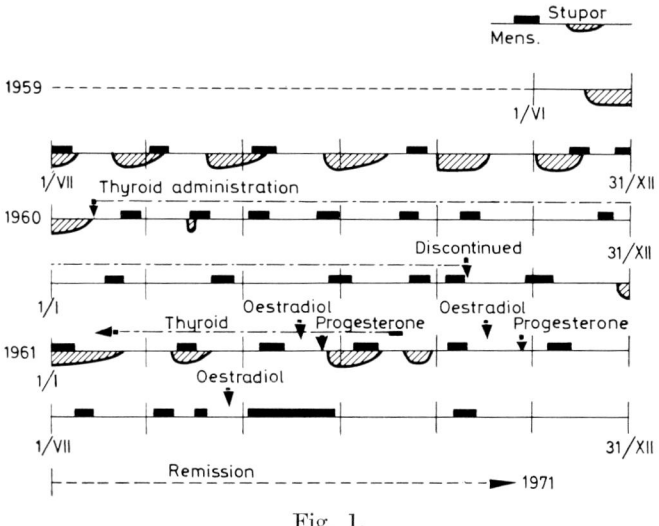

Fig. 1.

noted every month. Rapid recovery would be followed by a hypomanic state of a few days' duration. Her physical development is poor; infantilism was displayed by poor secondary sexual characteristics and a small sella turcica.

LABORATORY FINDINGS

Urinary oestrogens in the normal individuals are characterized by the presence of biphasic peaks corresponding to the ovulation and the premenstrual period, respectively (Fig. 2). This case showed a lack of such biphasic peaks. Pregnanediol was undetectable and periodic elevation in basal temperature was also absent.

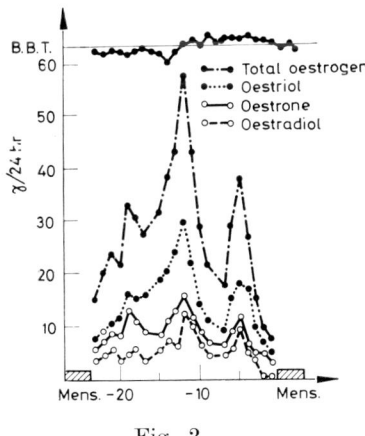

Fig. 2.

479

Thus, anovulatory menstruation was suggested. The oestrogen fraction pattern was abnormal during psychoses, in which oestrone fraction exceeded oestriol fraction (Fig. 3).

During lucidity, the 17-KS fraction pattern was normal in that the androsterone fraction (IV) was greater than the etiocholanolone fraction (V). But during psychosis, this ratio was reversed (Fig. 4).

Serum cholesterol increased during psychosis and returned to normal during lucidity.

Serum NPN (non-protein nitrogen) decreased during the normal interval and then tended to increase during the psychotic phase.

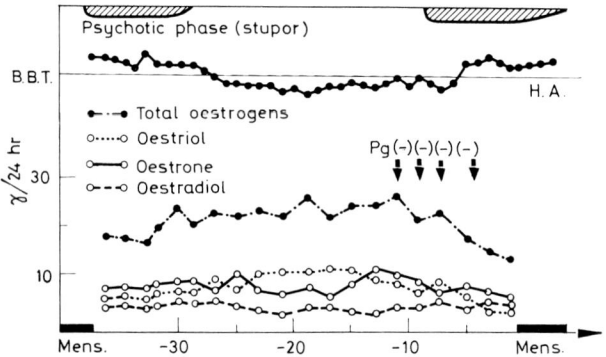

Fig. 3. Oestrogen excretion curve

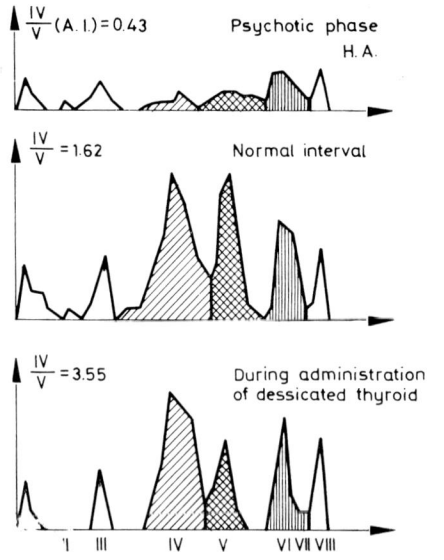

Fig. 4. Fraction pattern of 17-KS

Changes in urine volume and body temperature closely parallelled the clinical course, but 17-KS, and 17-OHCS, and PBI correlations with the clinical course were difficult to establish despite the great changes in these variables (Fig. 5).

The insulin tolerance test and ultra-short wave irradiation aimed at the diencephalon were performed during remission. Both yielded abnormal patterns of blood sugar responses which will be discussed later (Fig. 6).

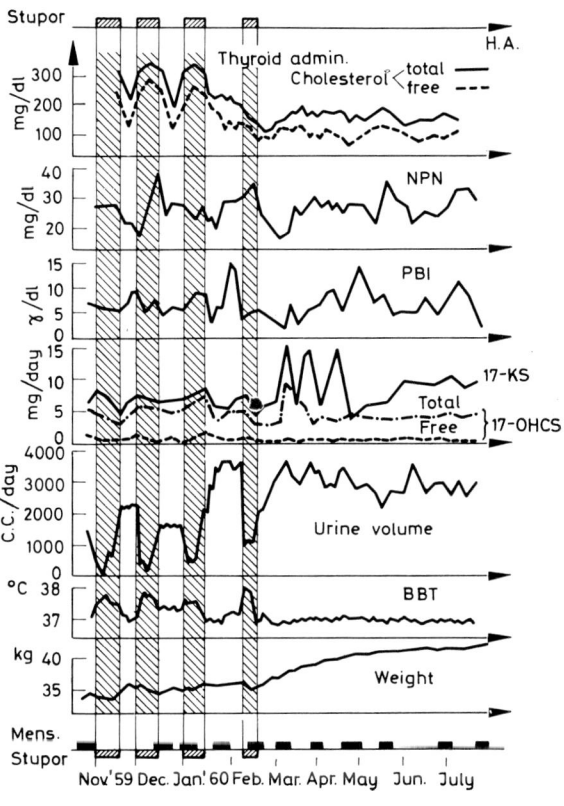

Fig. 5.

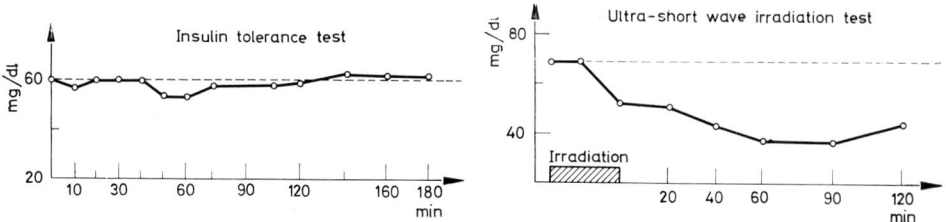

Fig. 6. Result of insulin tolerance test and effect on the blood sugar level of ultrashort wave irradiation in case H. A. following remission

TREATMENT

Desiccated thyroid administration curbed psychotic onset for about one year (Fig. 1).

At the same time, the ratio of androsterone over etiocholanolone increased (Fig. 4).

Moreover, serum cholesterol and NPN levels became stabilized within the normal ranges; however, total amounts of 17-KS, 17-OHCS and PBI continued to show great variations (Fig. 5).

Discontinuation of thyroid medication led to relapse. Resumption of medication, however, yielded insufficient response and even produced side-effects.

Because of data suggesting anovulatory menstruation, oestrogen and progesterone were injected during the latter halves of three successive menstrual cycles. The result of this treatment has been complete recovery and good health up to the present time.

DISCUSSION

As this case has demonstrated, some variables accord with fluctuations in the clinical picture; others do not, despite great variation. Having examined the results obtained from numerous cases, we found the same traits and learned that endocrinological variations in psychotic periods may be, in general, merely homeostatic reactions of non-specific nature, but, at the same time, these findings can be most useful therapeutic indicators.

Of these, the most frequent and consistent findings obtainable during the psychotic phase are those of abnormal fraction patterns in the androgen and oestrogen, which are indicators of abnormal steroid metabolism.

It should be also pointed out that anovulatory menstruation can be observed in the great majority of these cases.

Therefore, a few problems regarding sex steroid metabolism and hypothalamic function in periodic psychoses will be discussed here.

In 17-KS chromatography, with the method applied by the author, androsterone fraction (IV) is greater than etiocholanolone fraction (V) in normal individuals (Fig. 7).

If the ratio between androsterone and etiocholanolone is designated tentatively as the androgen index (A.I.), as is shown in Fig. 8, the A.I. in normal individuals is over 1.5. In periodic psychotic patients, during the psychotic phase, it scores below 1.5 or even lower than 1.0. This is due to the relative decrease of androsterone, so that the quantitative relationship between androsterone and etiocholanolone is reversed. On remission this ratio returns to the normal range.

It should be mentioned here that A.I. also reaches a very low value in most hepatic diseases (Fig. 8).

Biochemically, both androsterone and etiocholanolone are isomers having testosterone of 4-androstene-3,-17-dione as precursors (Fig. 9).

One possible explanation for the above findings may be that androgens, such as testosterone and androstenedione, are predominantly metabolized to androsterone during normalcy, but that abnormal conditions disturb this tendency so that they are metabolized to etiocholanolone in excess during abnormalcy. The

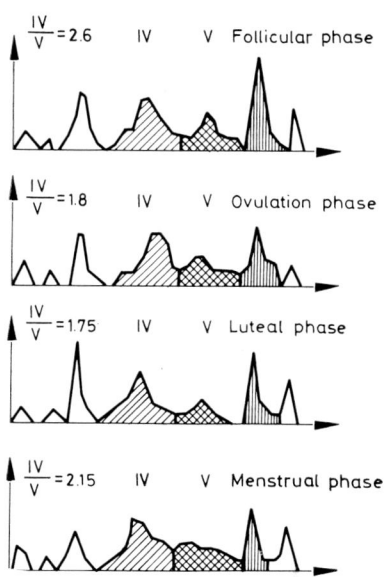

Fig. 7. Fraction patterns of 17-KS in normal female

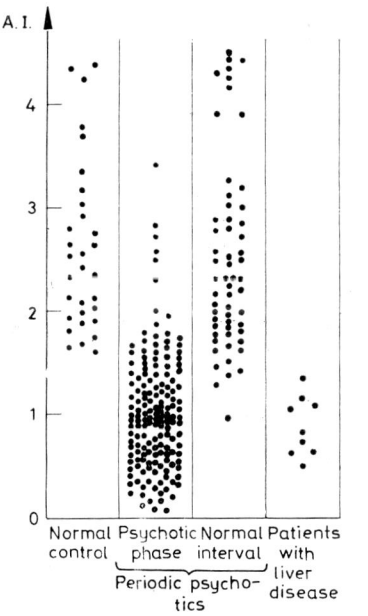

Fig. 8. Androgen index (A.I.) demonstrated under various clinical conditions.
$$\text{A.I.} = \frac{\text{Androsterone}}{\text{Etiocholanolone}}$$

liver being the main site of steroid metabolism explains the A.I. similarity found in hepatic diseases.

As to oestrogen fraction pattern, the ratio between oestradiol, oestrone and oestriol is approximately 1.0 : 2.0 : 3.0, respectively, as has been known. During the psychotic phase, the oestrone value far exceeds oestriol value in 25 of the 28 observed cases (Fig. 10). The same abnormality was found in all 4 cases of hepatic disorder under our observation.

It is thus reasonable to suppose that metabolic abnormalities in androgen and oestrogen indicate metabolic disturbance in the liver.

In this connection, various liver tests were performed in periodic psychotics. Quick's hippuric acid synthetic test, e.g., revealed obvious abnormality in 70 per cent of the cases; as with the A.I., normalcy was spontaneously restored upon remission (Fig. 11).

This spontaneous recovery of steroid metabolism and detoxication functioning in parallel with the recovery of lucidity suggests some cerebro-hepatic interrelationship.

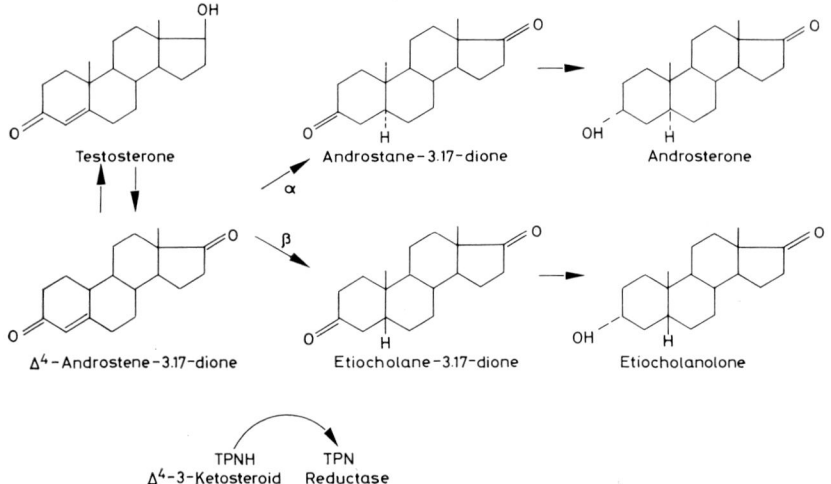

Fig. 9. Metabolism of testosterone

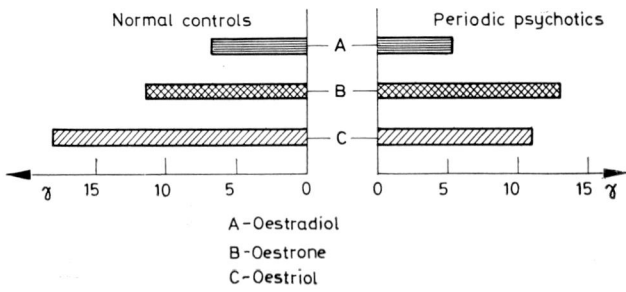

A—Oestradiol
B—Oestrone
C—Oestriol

Fig. 10. Fraction patterns of urinary oestrogens

This parallelism was pursued by investigating the 17-KS fraction patterns in LSD-induced psychoses (Fig. 12).

After the administration of 100 to 150 μg of LSD-25, 10 out of 14 cases presented a remarkably low A.I. within 12 to 24 hours; normal values were restored within 48 to 72 hours. It is of interest to note that the 4 cases showing little or no change in A.I. displayed hardly any mental symptoms. These findings become highly significant because of the closely resembling diencephalic characters of the two psychoses.

Thereupon, when 17-KS fraction patterns were examined in the hypothalamo–pituitary disorders, a lowered A.I. was found in most cases (Table 2). This finding

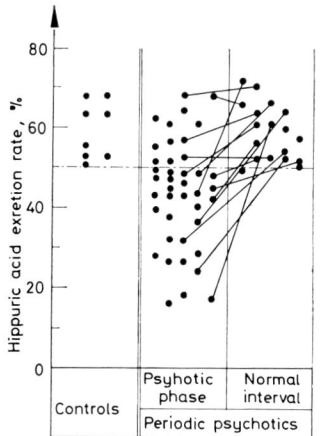

Fig. 11. Results of Quick's hippuric acid synthetic test

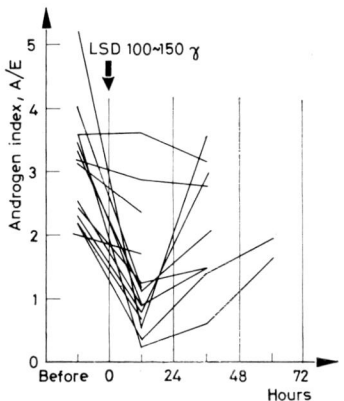

Fig. 12. Change in metabolic pattern of androgen during LSD experimental psychosis

TABLE 2

Androgen index in hypothalamo–pituitary disorders

Hypothalamo–pituitary disorder	A.I.
Simmond's disease	0.61
Simmond's disease	0.18
Pituitary dwarfism	1.00
Infantilism	0.63
"Diencephalose"	0.48
"Diencephalose"	0.47
"Diencephalose"	0.81
Marfan's syndrome	1.45
"Periodische Schlafsucht"	0.77

suggests a functional interdependence between the hypothalamo–pituitary system and the liver.

Findings concerning the hypothalamic control of metabolism in the liver have been reported (Shimazu and Fukuda 1962, Shimazu 1964, Shimazu et al. 1966).

The foregoing clinical observations make it reasonable to assume that in periodic psychoses hepatic dysfunction in steroid metabolism and detoxication capacity may not be primary, but should be considered as an aspect in the breakdown of the cerebro-hepatic homeostasis.

In order to verify this hypothesis, we carried out the following experiment: 50 μg of LSD-25 were injected intraperitoneally into adult male rats of Wistar strain. The rats were sacrificed 12 hours after the injection and the livers excised and homogenized. Δ4-androstenedione (the precursor of androstene and etiocholanolone) was added to the homogenate which was then incubated at 37°C for 3 hours. Then, their ratio of androsterone to etiocholanolone (A/E) was compared with that of controls by gas chromatography.

In the test group, this ratio decreased to about 1/5 to 2/5 of that of the controls (Fig. 13).

This result points to a decline in 5α-reductase activity in the liver.

The experimental result strongly supports our clinically based hypothesis that disturbance in cerebro(hypothalamo)hepatic homeostasis plays a significant role in the pathogenesis of such acute psychoses as the periodic and LSD-induced psychoses.

However, the distinguishing traits of the periodic psychoses are their strong recurring tendency with definite periodicity, disturbance of consciousness, and bipolar manifestation of symptoms. These are the criteria whereby diencephalic dysfunction is indicated.

To examine diencephalic function, both the insulin tolerance test and ultra-short wave irradiation of the diencephalon were applied to determine blood sugar levels during remission.

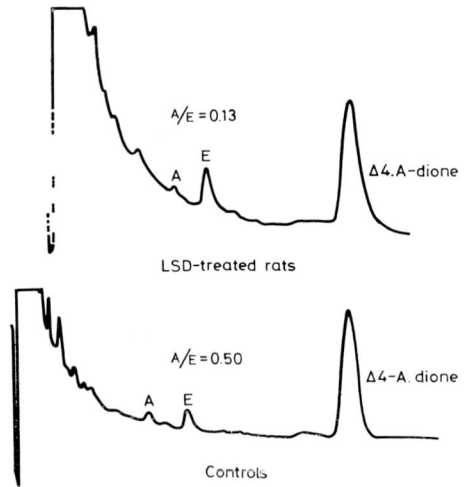

Fig. 13. Gas chromatogram of androgen metabolism in the liver of control and LSD-treated rats

The periodic psychotics presented highly abnormal responses to the insulin tolerance resistance (Type II) and hypoglycaemia unresponsiveness (Type III) (Fig. 14).

Normal blood sugar response to ultra-short wave irradiation is that of the upward (hyperglycaemic) pattern (Type I), but periodic psychotics tended to present the abnormal downward (hypoglycaemic) pattern (Type III); this was especially true for the cases with frequent recurrence (Fig. 15).

To some extent, these findings may be taken as evidence of a predisposition in many periodic psychotics towards functional vulnerability of the diencephalo-pituitary system.

As to therapy, we have had many cases which responded well to thyroid medication. Since few such cases, however, give unequivocal indications of hypothyroidism, this treatment was not primarily a replacement, because:

1. It is well known that the thyroid hormone increases the amount of androsterone by activating Δ4-3-ketosteroid reductase (5α) in the liver (McGuire and Tomkins 1959).

2. It is also well known that the thyroid hormone participates in Co-A biosynthesis and in the activation of various oxidative enzymes (Danziger et al. 1954, Tissières 1946, McShau et al. 1947, Tipton 1950, Minz and Cohen 1949, Cohen and Minz 1950).

3. It has recently been reported that thyroxine promotes the synthesis of adenyl cyclase and thereby increases the response to catecholamine which stimulates the formation of cyclic 3,5-AMP (Krishna et al. 1968, Leak 1970).

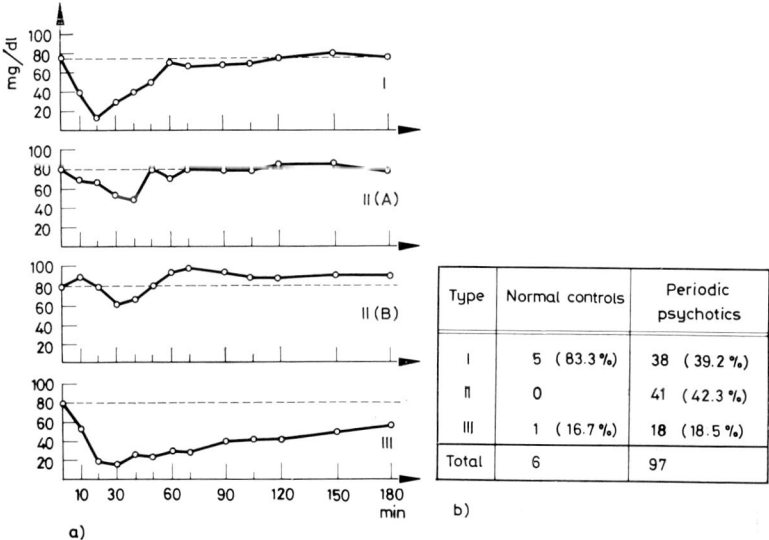

Fig. 14. (a) Patterns of response to insulin tolerance test, (b) pattern distribution of the response to insulin tolerance test in normal controls and periodic psychotics

Thus, the influence of thyroid hormone on these enzymes can be assumed to be one of the mechanisms involved in metabolic correction. In addition, the feedback mechanisms of the thyroid hormone to the hypothalamo–pituitary system should also be considered.

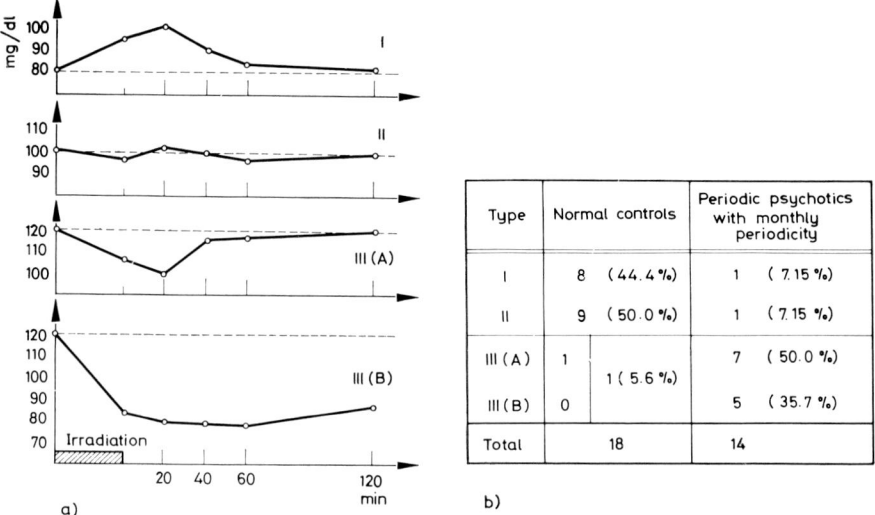

Fig. 15. (a) Response patterns of blood sugar level to ultra-short wave irradiation, (b) pattern distribution of the response to ultra-short wave irradiation test in normal controls and periodic psychotics

There have been cases, however, where thyroid medication produced side-effects and aggravated mental symptoms.

In such cases, ovarian hormone medication, given according to the findings of anovulatory menstruation, have resulted in complete remission. In these cases, the pathogenesis may be said to involve functional disturbance somewhere in the hypothalamo–pituitary–ovarian system.

SUMMARY

In summary, it may be concluded that:

1. One of the underlying constitutional factors in this group of periodic psychoses is a functional vulnerability of the diencephalo–pituitary system.

2. This predisposition makes patients psycho-biologically unstable and thereby exposes them to various physical reactions.

3. While these physical reactions themselves may be nonspecific in nature, they are important as guides to therapy. Especially those findings which indicate some disturbance in the hypothalamo–hepatic and/or hypothalamo–pituitary–gonadal function are of great significance.

REFERENCES

COHEN, G. N. and MINZ, B. (1950): *Arch. Sci. physiol.* **4,** 145.
DANZIGER, L. et al. (1954): *Dis. nerv. Syst.* **15,** 35.
KRISHNA, G., HYNIN, S. and BRODIE, B. B. (1968): *Proc. nat. Acad. Sci. (Wash.)* **59,** 884.
LEAK, D. (1970): *The Thyroid and the Autonomic Nervous System.* Heinemann, London.
MCGUIRE, J. S. and TOMKINS, G. M. (1959): *J. biol. Chem.* **234,** 791.
MCSHAU, W. H. et al. (1947): *Arch. Biochem.* **15,** 99.
MINZ, B. and COHEN, G. N. (1949): *C.R. Soc. Biol. (Paris)* **143,** 803.
SHIMAZU, T. (1964): *J. Biochem.* **55,** 163.
SHIMAZU, T. and FUKUDA, A. (1962): *Biochim. biophys. Acta (Amst.)* **65,** 373.
SHIMAZU, T., FUKUDA, A. and BAN, T. (1966): *Nature (Lond.)* **210,** 1178.
TIPTON, S. R. (1950): *Amer. J. Physiol.* **161,** 29.
TISSIÈRES. A. (1946): *Arch. Int. Physiol.* **54,** 305.

ENDOCRINOLOGICAL TREATMENT OF PSYCHOSES

T. WAKOH and N. HATOTANI

Department of Neuropsychiatry
Mie Prefectural University School of Medicine
Tsu, Japan

While disturbances in endocrine balance often occurring during psychosis may be considered non-specific biological reactions, it is probable that in some cases these findings might have a great significance on the pathogenesis and the course of some psychopathological conditions, although the aetiological factors remain unclear. At least, these findings have been found therapeutically useful giving important indices for treatment, so that they could be a clue to clarifying the pathophysiology of some types of psychoses (Hatotani et al. 1962).

Hoping for pathogenetic clarification, we re-examined 227 patients who had received endocrinological therapy during the past 15 years and attempted to find the relationship between clinical picture, endocrinological findings, and the endocrinological therapeutic measures taken.

These 227 cases comprised 124 periodic psychotics, 23 postpartum psychotics, and 63 typical schizophrenics. The great majority were female patients who had not well responded to other types of treatment.

Endocrinological treatments aimed at modifying the disturbed endocrine equilibrium were administered according to the particular endocrinological findings.

RESULTS

Table 1 shows that the cases which responded well to this type of treatment were to be found among the periodic and postpartum psychotics, but not among schizophrenics. Four types of individual hormone therapy were given:

1. Anterior-lobe hormone administration

Prehormone, a crude product of animal anterior pituitary gland, in a dose of 100 to 500 units was administered daily for two to four weeks. The most prominent characteristics of the cases which had shown a marked improvement through this therapy were as follows:

(i) The majority belonged to the group of periodic or postpartum psychotics.
(ii) Some had had prolonged pathological phases which failed to respond to other types of treatment.

TABLE I

Effects of endocrinological

Type of treatment	Periodic psychosis				Postpartum psychosis			
	a	b	c	d	a	b	c	d
Anterior-lobe hormones	8	15	15	13	1	5		2
Thyroid hormones	11	9	9	9	6	1	4	3
Corticoids	1			2	1			
Ovarian hormones	11	4	8	5				1
Testoids		1	2	1				
	31	29	34	30	8	6	4	6
	60		64		14		10	

a Dramatically improved; *b* improved; *c* partially or temporarily improved;

(*iii*) Laboratory findings in most cases had revealed gonadal, thyroidal, and adrenocortical hypofunction.

(*iv*) Electroshock therapy (EST) which proved to be ineffective during the prolonged state of postpartum psychosis, became effective after anterior-lobe hormone administration.

2. Thyroid hormone administration

Cases where thyroid hormone had proved effective fell into three types according to clinical and endocrinological characteristics:

Type I included patients who had shown long-lasting periodic courses and had failed to respond to all other treatments: hepatic metabolic disturbances such as androgen and oestrogen metabolic abnormalities, or where abnormal results in the hippuric acid synthetic test had been found. While the thyroid functions of such patients are well within normal limits, thyroid administration often not only normalizes endocrinological disturbances but also exerts a dramatic effect on the psychotic course.

Type II comprised the postpartum cases, whose response to EST was only temporary improvement followed by stupor or perplexity. Laboratory findings are frequently similar to those found in Type I.

Type III was characterized by depressive states. Lowered basal metabolic rate (BMR) and disturbed androgen metabolism are frequent although protein-bound iodine (PBI) level remains within normal range. Sometimes, serum BEI is low against PBI, a finding suggesting a possible abnormality in thyroid hormone metabolism.

3. Oestrogen and progesterone administration

Cases with anovulatory menstrual cycles displaying a deterioration in the mental condition in the premenstrual period respond fairly well to combined oestrogen and progesterone administration given in the premenstrual phase for three to five months.

treatments on psychoses

Schizophrenia				Other psychoses				Total
a	b	c	d	a	b	c	d	
	1	5	35	1	1	1	9	112
		7	11					70
								4
			4			1	2	36
				1				5
1		12	50	2	2	1	11	
1		62		4		12		227

d not improved.

4. Corticoid administration

Despite general contraindication of corticoids in psychosis, cortisone or cortisol has been found effective in acute pernicious catatonia in producing rapid recovery from febrile delirium.

To illustrate the course of these therapies, a few case reports are presented.

Case 1. A 21-year-old periodic psychotic female patient with a continuous stuporous state, which could not be alleviated by EST or neuroleptics, and became almost fixed for months after periodically depressed, anxious states. Incidentally, she had amenorrhoea from the beginning of this condition. Laboratory findings revealed continuously low oestrogen and 17-KS levels, serum PBI level was also relatively low. These findings suggested hypofunction of the anterior pituitary system. Prehormone, 500 U, was administered daily for 20 days. The EST given immediately after treatment had a marked effect in bringing about recovery from the stuporous state.

In this case, the hypothalamo–pituitary system could be regulated by replacement therapy in bringing about a condition responsive to EST.

Case 2. An 18-year-old periodic psychotic female patient. Since menarche, mental disturbances had accompanied the premenstrual periods. Delusions of reference and persecution as well as depressed, aggressive, or agonized states were added to the various premenstrual tension symptoms. Normally, these states disappeared rapidly following menstruation (Fig. 1). Laboratory findings revealed low urinary oestrogen and an abnormal oestrogen fraction ratio, the amount of oestrone exceeding that of oestriol (Fig. 2). The ratio of androsterone to etiocholanolone in the 17-KS fractions was also abnormally low. Desiccated thyroid administration proved effective. The psychotic phases and premenstrual tensions ceased and the 17-KS fraction pattern became normal. Temporary withdrawal of thyroid led to a temporary relapse; otherwise, continuous remission has been maintained for more than 10 years (Fig. 3). This case is illustrative of Type I.

Case 3. A 29-year-old female patient with postpartum psychosis. The onset of disturbances was in the second month after delivery. Periodic recurrence of anxiety and psychomotor restlessness followed by stupor had continued for more than 12 months.

Chlorpromazine and other neuroleptics yielded no substantial therapeutic effect and the effect of EST was only temporary. An abnormally low androgen index (androsterone over etiocholanolone) in the 17-KS fractions, an abnormal result in testosterone metabolic test, and lowered values in the hippuric acid synthetic test were found in the laboratory examination suggesting hepatic metabolic dys-

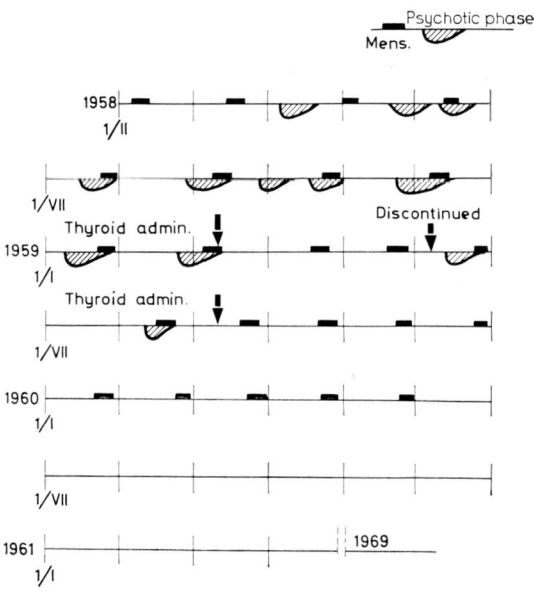

Fig. 1. *Case 2.* Thyroid hormone. Type I. 18 yrs, female, periodic psychosis

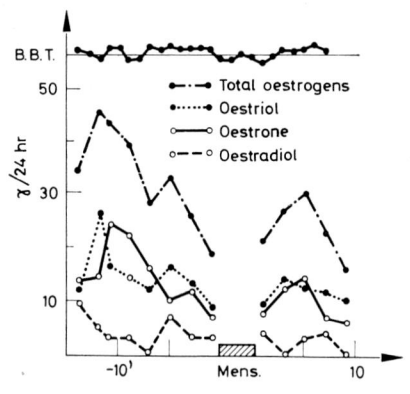

Fig. 2. *Case 2.*

function. Desiccated thyroid administration resulted in a continuous remission (Fig. 4). This case belongs to Type II.

The abnormal sex steroid metabolism found in these two cases obviously reflects disturbed hepatic metabolic function. The authors are of the opinion that functional disturbance is a partial manifestation of homeostatic disturbance in the cerebro–hepatic axis. However, the effective mechanism in thyroid therapy yet remains unclear. Several possibilities arise: the thyroid hormone might act directly upon the hypothalamo–pituitary system. Or it might do so indirectly through the adrenocortical system, or the gonadal system, or through influence upon hepatic metabolic function. That this hormone activates 5α-reductase in the liver is well known (McGuire and Tomkins 1959, Leak 1970). There is strong

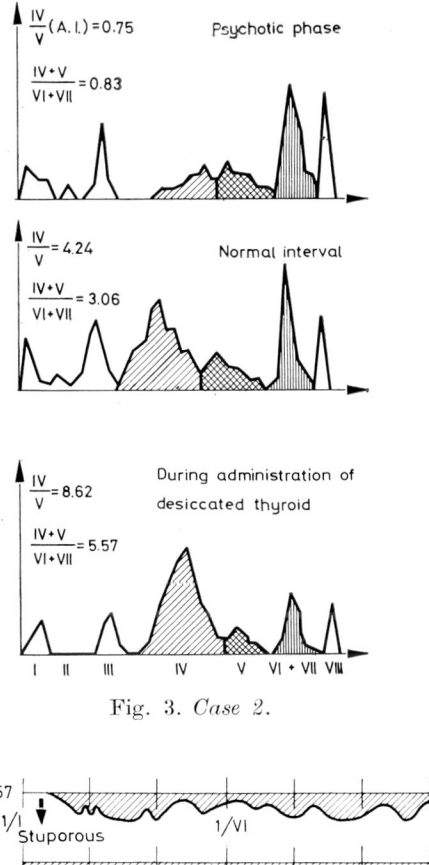

Fig. 3. *Case 2.*

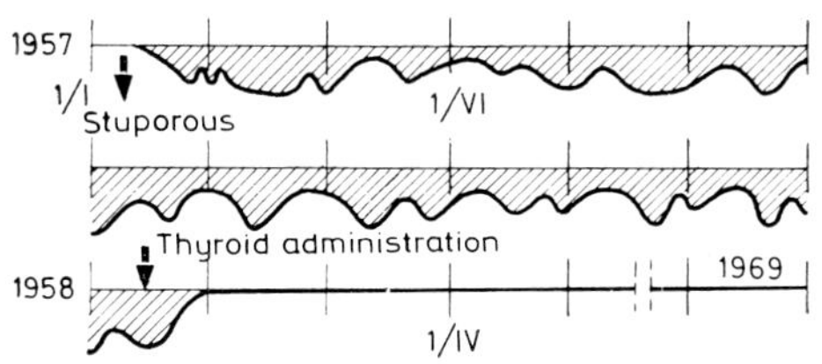

Fig. 4. *Case 3.* Thyroid hormone. Type II. 29 yrs, female, postpartum psychosis

evidence that this hormone not only normalizes disturbed androgen metabolism but also regulates various other hepatic metabolisms. Its function in the brain is still unclear. However, it has recently been reported that thyroxine promotes the synthesis of adenyl cyclase and thereby increases the response to catecholamine which stimulates the formation of cyclic 3,5 AMP (Krishna et al. 1968).

Case 4. A 22-year-old male patient with periodic psychosis. Onset took place while preparing for college board tests. He suffered from severe anxiety accompanied by ideas of persecution and his depressive state continued for many months. Laboratory tests revealed a continuously low BMR showing a -20% level for three months. Desiccated thyroid therapy corrected the BMR level to $+20\%$ and the patient rapidly recovered from the depressive state (Fig. 5). This case of depression accompanied by hypometabolism is representative of Type III.

Case 5. A 15-year-old female patient with periodic psychosis. Periodic episodes accompanied the menstrual periods (Fig. 6). Hormonal metabolic disturbance was not doubted as the oestrogen and 17-KS fraction patterns were found normal (Fig. 7). Anovulatory menstruation was discovered through the nonphasic oestrogen excretion and basal temperature curves and the immeasurably low pregnanedione excretion. Thyroid administration resulted in a state similar to hyper-

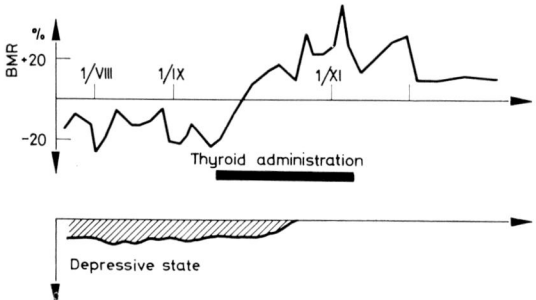

Fig. 5. *Case 4.* Thyroid hormone. Type III. 22 yrs, male, hypometabolic depressive state

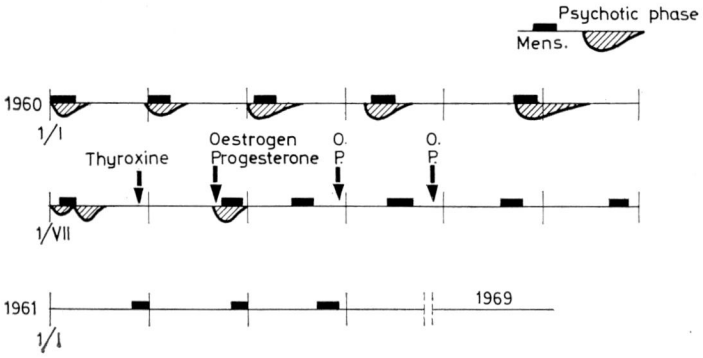

Fig. 6. *Case 5.* Ovarian hormone. 15 yrs, female, periodic psychosis

thyroidism and aggravation of the mental condition. Our findings indicated that combined follicular and luteal hormone administration, given for three months at the stages corresponding to the luteal phase, produced complete remission (Fig. 8). The pathogenesis of this illness may lie in disturbances in the diencephalo–pituitary–gonadal system which could recover on the administration of female sex hormones.

Case 6. A 23-year-old female patient with acute pernicious catatonia. Acute delirium accompanied by a 40°C fever led to a comatose state. The laboratory

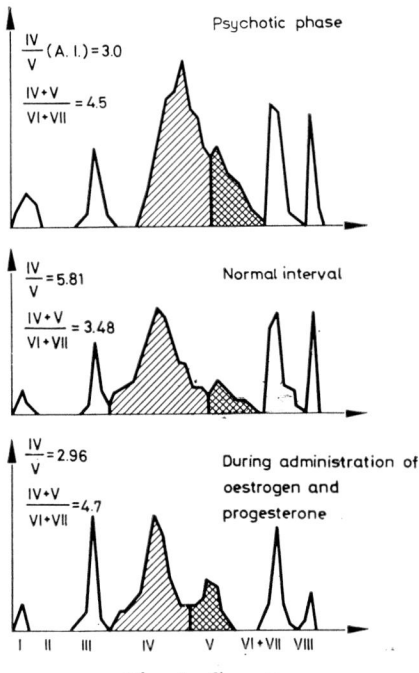

Fig. 7. *Case 5.*

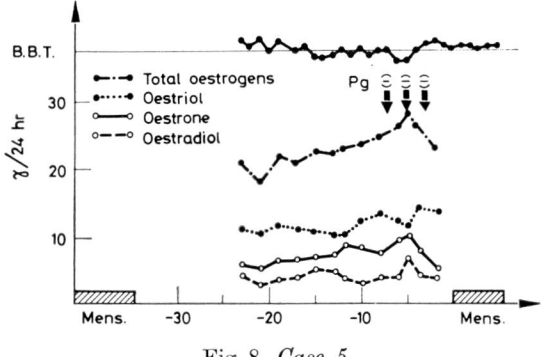

Fig 8. *Case 5.*

tests did not reveal any infection. Lowered 17-KS fractions suggested adrenocortical exhaustion. Cortisone administration produced rapid recovery of consciousness and the fever subsided (Fig. 9).

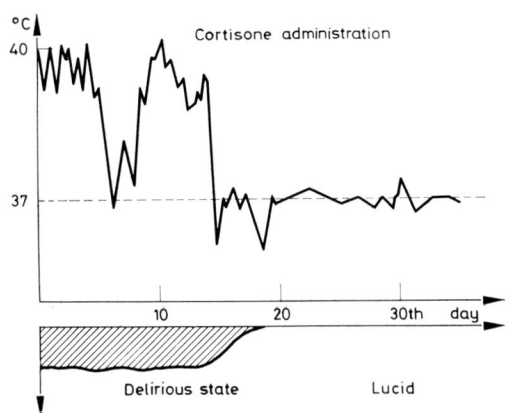

Fig. 9. *Case 6*. Corticoid hormone. 23 yrs, female, acute pernicious catatonia

CONCLUSIONS

Results of endocrinological treatment of 227 cases of various psychoses have revealed that adequate hormone therapy aimed at the correction of homeostatic imbalance can exert marked effects on some types of psychoses.

Thyroid hormones, anterior pituitary hormones, ovarian hormones and corticoids have proved to be effective, particularly in cases of periodic and postpartum psychoses, if properly administered. The therapeutic principles are considered to be applications of hormone in terms of replacement, feed-back, and the regulation of metabolic functions.

These therapies might some day yield solid clues to the pathogenesis of a number of the psychoses.

REFERENCES

HATOTANI, N., ISHIDA, C., YURA, R., MAEDA, M., KATO, Y., NOMURA, Y., WAKAO, T., TAKEKOSHI, A., YOSHIMOTO, S., YOSHIMOTO, K. and HIRAMOTO, K. (1962): Psychophysiological studies of atypical psychosis — endocrinological aspect of periodic psychoses. *Folia psychiat. neurol. jap.* **16**, 248.

KRISHNA, G., HYNIN, S. and BRODIE, B. B. (1968): Effects of thyroid hormones on adenyl cyclase in adipose tissue and on free fatty acid mobilization. *Proc. nat. Acad. Sci. (Wash.)* **59**, 884.

LEAK, D. (1970): *The Thyroid and the Autonomic Nervous System*. Heinemann, London.

MCGUIRE, J. S. and TOMKINS, G. M. (1959): The effects of thyroxine administration on the enzymic reduction of Δ^4-3-ketosteroids. *J. biol. Chem.* **234**, 791.

LONGITUDINAL STUDY OF CATECHOLAMINE METABOLISM IN PERIODIC CATATONIA

S. TAKAHASHI and L. R. GJESSING

Central Laboratory
Dikemark Hospital
Solberg, Norway

Biochemical changes accompanying the clinical cycle in periodic catatonia have been studied in this laboratory since 1927. Gjessing first suggested that cyclic variation in thyroid function might be involved in the clinical symptomatology of the illness. Clinical observations of a stuporous patient revealed many signs of adrenal activation. The symptoms during the switch from interval to psychotic phase were similar to those seen after an epinephrine injection. Further extensive studies of phenolic amines and phenolic acids have confirmed the overactivity of the sympathetic nervous system present during the catatonic phase in these cases.

The catecholamines themselves were, however, not investigated in urine specimens collected during previous studies. It is therefore quite appropriate to complete the metabolic study by measuring norepinephrine, epinephrine and dopamine and then to reconsider the biochemical aspects of catecholamine metabolism in periodic catatonia with our previous data on phenolic amines and phenolic acids.

In this study, a typical case of periodic catatonia was studied longitudinally for a period of 4 years including over 22 psychotic episodes. One of the problems, of course, is the contamination of such a clinical study by the therapeutic manipulations of the patient, and the limited allowances for experimental trials for research activities. Definitive interpretation of the data is limited since most urinary norepinephrine and its metabolites may be assumed to derive from the peripheral sympathetic nervous system rather than the brain.

CASE HISTORY

The patient (E. L.) was born in 1912 and admitted to this hospital in 1935. The diagnosis was established by clinical observation of mental symptoms and measurements of physical concomitants over many years according to our criteria of periodic catatonia. Schizophrenia-like symptoms with exacerbations were first observed and treated with insulin coma therapy and sulphur fever therapy with no effect. Gradually, periodic catatonic symptoms developed with quiet intervals in between. The patient has had very regular periods of catatonic stupor since 1952. The stuporous states and the intervals each last 3 to 4 weeks. The onset of the stupor is very sudden with a remarkable increase in pulse rate, basal metabolic rate and a decrease in sleeping time. The stupor is most profound in the first week of the catatonic phase, then it gradually disappears over a period of 2 to 3 weeks. No catatonic symptoms remain in the interval.

This patient has not received treatment such as ECT or leucotomy, nor has he previously been treated with psychotropic drugs.

The clinical course of the patient during this study was calculated on the basis of a 57.7 ± 13.9 day observation period (mean $\pm$ S.D.) in the years 1963 to 1966.

METHODS

CLINICAL ASSESSMENT

Daily psychiatric evaluation was subjectively carried out by the authors, based on the observation of psychiatric and neurological symptomatology. They were graded 1 to 5, where 1 represents the status in the interval and 5 deep stupor as seen at the peak of an exacerbation. Descriptive notes of the patient's behaviour by the nursing staff were also evaluated.

Daily notes of several physical measurements were also evaluated as an objective assessment of the clinical course. Pulse rate, body temperature and sleeping time were measured daily, as well as body weight and BMR 3 times a week by a Krogh spirometer.

DRUGS

Inhibitors of enzymes involved in catecholamine synthesis were first examined in this study. Three well-known commercially available enzyme inhibitor drugs, the monoamine oxidase inhibitor (Nardil), α-methyl dopa (Aldomet) and disulfiram (Antabus) were examined.

Thyroid hormones were repeatedly administered, because these drugs have been most effective in many cases of this disorder.

Among the psychotropic drugs, reserpine and lithium salt were chosen. They were administered as a maintenance therapy for 3 months each, because of their suppressive effect on catecholamine metabolism and prophylactic effect against recurring tendency.

Drugs were given 3 to 7 days after the onset of the active phase, in order to examine the immediate effect on the catatonic symptoms of the patient.

BIOCHEMICAL DETERMINATIONS

Urine was collected in 24-hour pools each day during the periods of investigation. Urine creatinine was determined using Jaffe's method. The daily excretion of creatinine was variable, mainly because of differences in collection time. It ranged 1.12 ± 0.35 g (mean $\pm$ S.D.).

The patient received the same constant fluid diet excluding vegetables and fruits, called H diet in this laboratory. In between the periods of investigations, the patient was partly on the ordinary hospital diet.

Free catecholamines, norepinephrine (NE), epinephrine (E) and dopamine (DA), were determined fluorometrically with a modification of the ethylenediamine condensation method combined with thin-layer chromatography.

Total (free + conjugated) normetanephrine (NMN) and metanephrine (MN) were determined by the method of Kakimoto and Armstrong (1962). To determine 3-methoxy-4-hydroxy-mandelic acid (VMA) and 3-methoxy-4-hydroxy-phenylacetic acid (HVA) the method of Armstrong et al. (1956) was employed.

About two-thirds of the determinations on NMN, MN, VMA and HVA in this study have been performed in this laboratory (Takahashi and Gjessing 1972, and in press).

ANALYSIS OF DATA

The onset of the active phase was easily identified by an abrupt increase in pulse rate, body temperature and BMR accompanied by psychic changes. The transition from the active psychotic phase to interval was less sharp, but the catatonic symptoms disappeared, the pulse rate settled below the baseline of 80 and the BMR curve crossed down the 0 per cent line.

Biochemical data were dealt with statistically after they were divided into the 4 parts of a period according to the clinical course mentioned above. Namely, the phase called A1 is the first half of the active phase in calender days, A2, second half of the active phase, R1 is the first half of the remission phase, and R2 is the second half.

Baseline levels of catecholamines and their metabolites from the periods without drug administration were calculated, summing up individual figures together in the sense of clinical state defined above.

RESULTS AND DISCUSSION

BASELINE EXCRETION LEVELS OF URINARY CATECHOLAMINES AND THEIR METABOLITES

Urinary excretion of all catecholamines and their metabolites showed a remarkable increase at the beginning of the catatonic symptoms.

Pulse rate increased sharply when the patient suddenly fell into stupor, and remained elevated during the entire stuporous phase. The BMR was also elevated to +30 to +40 per cent. Other parameters, such as body temperature, body weight and sleeping time followed these two main indices concomitantly. Creatinine excretion was constant during the entire period of observation.

E and MN reached the maximum value immediately after the onset of stupor, whereas NE and NMN were delayed and reached their peak 1 to 2 weeks after the onset and sustained the higher levels longer. VMA followed the NE values. Along with the waning of catatonic symptoms, urinary excretion of catecholamines and their metabolites gradually decreased. In the remission phase, both NE and E, as well as NMN and MN returned to the lowest levels of excretion.

The baseline levels of urinary catecholamines and their metabolites are shown in Table 1. It is clear that NE and its 3-methoxy metabolite NMN show no significant fall from the 1st half of active phase (A1) to the second half of the active

TABLE 1

Baseline levels of BMR and urinary excretion of catecholamines
and metabolites without drug administration
(Urinary excretion of catecholamines and metabolites in 10 normal subjects:
NE 26.2 ± 8.8 (46), E 5.5 ± 1.7, DA 91 ± 24, NMN 44 ± 14, MN 36 ± 12,
VMA 1490 ± 490 and HVA 1610 ± 480)

	Clinical state			
	First half of active phase (A1)	Second half of active phase (A2)	First half of remission phase (R1)	Second half of remission phase (R2)
BMR (%)	20.0^b ± 11.4 (79)*	12.7 ± 10.8 (53)*	−7.4 ± 10.2 (61)	−12.0 ± 8.4 (58)
NE^a	63.5 ± 28.6 (110)	59.5 ± 24.5 (91)*	35.8 ± 15.9 (66)*	27.7 ± 13.2 (55)
E	25.9 ± 11.9*	18.8 ± 7.8	16.2 ± 6.2	13.4 ± 5.7
DA	152 ± 41	143 ± 50	131 ± 31*	110 ± 29
NMN	222 ± 49 (65)	199 ± 60 (53)*	79 ± 37 (40)*	48 ± 18 (35)
MN	73 ± 26*	45 ± 16	36 ± 15	39 ± 15
VMA	3,090 ± 790 (75)	2,950 ± 790 (63)*	1,950 ± 720 (42)*	1,480 ± 310 (40)
HVA	2,160 ± 370	2,100 ± 570	1,850 ± 610*	1,400 ± 180

[a] Values for biochemical measurements are given in μg/g creatinine.
[b] Figures are given as mean ± standard deviation with number of determinations in parenthesis.
* $p < 0.01$, significantly higher than the value in the following clinical state.

phase (A2), while E and MN decreased significantly. On the other hand, NE and NMN as well as VMA decreased significantly from A2 to the first half of the remission phase (R1). All the figures show the lowest values in the second half of the remission phase (R2). They are very close to the values gained from 10 normal male subjects. DA and HVA also showed a waxing and waning excretion pattern but with less consistency. High levels of urinary NE and E were widely reported in the acute exacerbation of schizophrenia, and in patients with emotional outbursts.

NE, the neurotransmitter at the terminals of the peripheral sympathetic nervous system, has also been found in neurons of the central nervous system where it is also presumed to function as a neurotransmitter. NE, released from neurons in a physiologically active form, is thought to be inactivated mainly by re-uptake into the presynaptic neuron and by catechol-o-methyl transferase to form NMN. E is formed mainly in the adrenal medulla. It is also o-methylated to form MN. Both NMN and MN then undergo the secondary deamination to form VMA and vanylglycol (VG or HMPG). Thus, the levels or urinary NE and NMN may reflect the levels of activity of the noradrenergic nervous system whereas E and MN levels reflect adrenal medullary activity. The discrepancy between NE and E suggests a profile of pathology in periodic catatonia. Initially, at the onset of stupor, some unknown events in the central nervous system may intensely stimulate both the adrenals and the sympathetic nervous system. After intense activity for a week, the sympathetic response gradually wanes. The patient's acute psychic symptoms may in part be due to the high levels of E, which increased corresponding to the quantitative fluctuation of stuporous symptoms.

In this case of periodic catatonia, the increase in NE and E may be a result of the adrenergic overactivity rather than of the influence of elevated motor activity. Differing from patients in the manic state, this catatonic patient apparently had less motor activity because of the stupor.

The free catecholamines increased while the patient was active and decreased while he was quiet, whereas the conjugated amines were rather constant under both conditions. This finding suggests that the measurements of free catecholamines reflect the activity of the sympathetic nervous system. On the other hand, once they were o-methylated, a major part of NMN and MN were conjugated and excreted in the urine.

EFFECTS OF ENZYME INHIBITORS INVOLVED IN CATECHOLAMINE METABOLISM

During loading with a monoamine oxidase inhibitor (Nardil) for 4 weeks, the active phase occurred without a definite alteration of the cycle. The psychic state during the remission phase appeared to be somewhat unsettled, and BMR levels in the remission phase were also somewhat elevated by the drug.

NE and DA increased slightly due to the drug. Of the biochemical results, increased levels of NMN were the most pronounced (5–10-fold of baseline levels). Decrease in VMA and HVA was statistically consistent.

The administered α-methyl-dopa was metabolized to α-methyl-normethanephrine and exchanged itself nearly quantitatively with the natural NMN. In addition, it markedly suppressed VMA but not completely. It had no prophylactic effect on the catatonic attacks, but catatonic stupor was itself markedly improved.

Moderate dosage of Disulfiram for 5 days in the active phase significantly suppressed BMR from levels of 36.3 per cent to -2.3 per cent. The stupor became less pronounced, pulse rate decreased and sleep was better. After the withdrawal of the drug, BMR returned to the higher levels and there was exacerbation of the catatonic symptoms. This transient effect of Disulfiram was accompanied by the decreased excretion of NE, E, NMN and VMA.

These results of administration of enzyme inhibitors allow to glimpse at the metabolic spectrum in this case of periodic catatonia. Intense inhibition of MAO results in a decreased excretion of the acid and products of the metabolism of many amines. On the other hand, there is an increase in urinary excretion of those amines which lack alternate efficient means of metabolism, reflecting their accumulation in body tissue. In this patient with a higher production of catecholamines than in depressive patients or normal subjects, accumulation of o-methylated metabolites might cause the overflow of unmethylated catecholamines when monoamine oxidase inhibitor is administered and subsequently cause slightly increased excretion of NE and DA. The more than 10-fold increase in NMN and MN in the urine indicates the ample activity of catechol-o-methyl transferase, the principal enzyme in the inactivation of NE and E. The reaction of these enzyme inhibitors did not differ when the patient was in stupor or in remission.

THYROID HORMONES

A 6-month study of psychic symptoms, BMR, pulse rate, creatinine excretion as well as urinary excretion of catecholamines and metabolites was made during the administration of thyroxine. BMR showed higher levels with fluctuations of greater amplitude throughout the period of the administration. Urinary excretion of three catecholamines was markedly elevated.

As compared to the baseline levels, increase in these values of NE, E and DA was statistically significant in parallel with the BMR. The increase in other catecholamine metabolites was not significant.

PSYCHOTROPIC DRUGS

The administration of 3 mg of reserpine was started in the active phase and continued in the same dosage for 84 days. The drug gradually stabilized the pulse at 60 to 70 beats per minutes and the BMR below -10 per cent.

Urinary excretion of NE, E, NMN, MN and VMA also gradually decreased in the first week of administration, corresponding to the improvement in catatonic symptoms. NE values amounted to less than 20 $\mu g/g$ creatinine and E to less than 7 $\mu g/g$ creatinine, which are about half of the baseline level.

During the whole period of reserpine administration, the relapse of catatonia was completely suppressed, but the patient reacted with a recurrence of catatonic symptoms about a week after withdrawal of the drug. Physical measurements as well as urinary excretion of catecholamines and metabolites promptly returned to the levels seen in the active phase. DA and HVA were not significantly changed by reserpine.

When reserpine, which is said to be a potent agent of NE depletion in the brain, was administered to the patient, it abolished the relapse of the catatonic attack. Urinary excretion of NE was significantly suppressed as well. Our results showed, in addition, corresponding changes in the 3-methoxy-4-hydroxy metabolites. Decrease in the values of E and NE during long-term reserpine treatment was reported by some authors. This action of reserpine suggests that NE in the brain could have some association with the development of the catatonic symptoms. The action of Disulfiram, which effectively suppressed the psychotic phase mentally as well as somatically, supports this line of thought as Disulfiram is said to act as an inhibitor of hydroxylase, converting dopamine to norepinephrine, in addition to being an aldehyde-dehydrogenase inhibitor.

There were beneficial clinical effects of lithium citrate on this patient with periodic catatonia. Lithium citrate prolonged the remission phase, and alleviated the psychic symptoms. Maintenance therapy with 35 mEq lithium, which kept the serum lithium concentration within the range of 0.5 to 1.5 mEq/l, proved to have no prophylactic effect on the catatonic attack in this case.

During lithium administration, BMR and E were moderately reduced in accord with the milder psychic symptoms. Suppression of DA excretion was the most consistent finding of the many biochemical measurements throughout the whole period of lithium administration, while NE did not show any significant decrease. The 3-methoxy amine metabolites were also moderately decreased. Phenolic acids were hardly affected by lithium administration. It has recently been reported that the excretion of NMN and MN decreased significantly when lithium carbonate was administered to manic-depressive patients. The excretion of catecholamines, VMA and MHPG, however, appeared to be more consistently related to changes in the clinical state than to the administration of lithium itself. From the limited information obtained here, decrease in urinary excretion of DA may imply suppressed DA production in the kidney due to mild lithium intoxication.

Recently, Bunney et al. (1970) reported an increase in urinary NE excretion just before the manic period and presented a hypothesis that the switch process into mania is associated with an increase in functional biogenic amines in the brain. He also showed a marked elevation of urinary adenosine 3',5'-monophosphate on the day of rapid switch from the depressed to the manic state, proposing that this increase might serve as a trigger mechanism for the process by which catecholamines are elevated during the manic phase of the illness. Switch process in periodic catatonia is also of great interest. Elevation of urinary catecholamine excretion, as well as clinical signs, suggest a periodic intense stimulation of the sympathetic nervous system during the catatonic attacks. However, the abrupt rise of NE and E and their metabolites was observed concomitantly with the sudden manifestation of catatonic symptoms, and no preceding signs of increase in urinary catecholamine levels or clinical symptoms were recognized. The biochemical data obtained here cannot explain the periodicity of this disease.

REFERENCES

Armstrong, M. D., Shaw, K. N. F. and Wall, P. E. (1956): The phenolic acids in human urine. *J. biol. Chem.* **218**, 293–303.

Bunney, W. E. Jr., Murphy, D. L., Goodwin, F. K. and Borge, G. (1970): The switch process from depression to mania: relationship to drugs which alter brain amines. *Lancet* **1**, 1022–1027.

Carlsson, A., Rasmussen, E. B. and Kristjansen, P. (1959): The urinary excretion of adrenaline and noradrenaline by schizophrenic patients during reserpine treatment. *J. Neurochem.* **4**, 318–320.

Gjessing, L. R. (1932): Beiträge zur Kenntnis der Pathophysiologie des katatonen Stupors: I. Mitteilung. Über periodisch rezidivierenden katatonen Stupor, mit kritischem Beginn und Abschluss. *Arch. Psychiat. Nervenkr.* **96**, 319–392.

Gjessing, L. R. (1935): Beiträge zur Kenntnis der Pathophysiologie der katatonen Erregung: III. Mitteilung. Über periodisch rezidivierende katatone Erregung, mit kritischem Beginn und Abschluss. *Arch. Psychiat. Nervenkr.* **104**, 355–416.

Gjessing, L. R. (1953): Beiträge zur Somatologie der periodischen Katatonie: VIII. Mitteilung. Wertung der Befunde II. *Arch. Psychiat. Nervenkr.* **191**, 297–326.

Gjessing, L. R. (1964a): Studies of periodic catatonia: I. Blood levels of protein-bound iodine and urinary excretion of vanillylmandelic acid in relation to clinical course. *J. psychiat. Res.* **2**, 123–134.

Gjessing, L. R. (1964b): Studies of periodic catatonia: II. The urinary excretion of phenolic amines and acids with and without loads of different drugs. *J. psychiat. Res.* **2**, 149–162.

Gjessing, L. R. (1965): Studies on urinary phenolic compounds in man. II. Phenolic acids and amines during a load of α-methyldopa and Disulfiram in periodic catatonia. *Scand. J. clin. Lab. Invest.* **17**, 549–557.

Gjessing, L. R. (1967a): Lithium citrate loading of a patient with periodic catatonia. *Acta psychiat. scand.* **43**, 372–375.

Gjessing, L. R. (1967b): Effect of thyroxine, pyridoxine, orphenadrine-HCl, reserpine and Disulfiram in periodic catatonia. *Acta psychiat. scand.* **43**, 376–384.

Greenspan, K., Schildkraut, J. J., Gorden, E. K., Baer, L., Aronoff, M. S. and

Durell, J. (1970): Catecholamine metabolism in affective disorders — III. MHPG and other catecholamine metabolites in patients treated with lithium carbonate. *J. psychiat. Res.* **7**, 171—183.

Hatotani, N., Ishida, C., Yura, R., Maeda, M., Kato, Y., Nomura, Y., Wakao, T., Takekoshi, A., Yoshimoto, S., Yoshimoto, K. and Hiramoto, K. (1962): Psychophysiological studies of atypical psychosis — endocrinological aspect of periodic psychoses. *Folia psychiat. neurol. jap.* **16**, 248—292.

Kakimoto, Y. and Armstrong, M. D. (1962): The phenolic amines of human urine. *J. biol. Chem.* **237**, 208—214.

Paul, M. I., Cramer, H. and Bunney, W. E., Jr. (1971): Urinary adenosine 3',5'-monophosphate in the switch process from depression to mania. *Science* **171**, 300—303.

Pllin, W. and Goldin, S. (1961): The physiological and psychological effects of intravenously administered epinephrine and its metabolism in normal and schizophrenic men — II. Psychiatric observations. *J. psychiat. Res.* **1**, 50—67.

Pscheidt, G. R., Berlet, H. H., Bull, C., Spaide, J. and Himwich, H. E. (1964): Excretion of catecholamines and exacerbation of symptoms in schizophrenic patients. *J. psychiat. Res.* **2**, 163—168.

Schildkraut, J. J., Klerman, G. L., Hammond, R. and Friend, D. G. (1964): Excretion of 3-methoxy-4-hydroxy-mandelic acid (VMA) in depressed patients treated with antidepressant drugs. *J. psychiat. Res.* **2**, 257—266.

Takahashi, S. and Gjessing, L. R. (1972): Fluorometric method combined with thin-layer chromatography for the determination of epinephrine, norepinephrine and dopamine in human urine. (In preparation).

Takahashi, S. and Gjessing, L. R.: Studies of periodic catatonia—IV. Longitudinal study of catecholamine metabolism, with and without drugs. *J. psychiat. Res.* (In press).

METABOLISM OF ANDROGENIC STEROIDS IN HUMAN SKIN

M. JULESZ

1st Department of Medicine
University Medical School
Szeged, Hungary

In our view, the endocrine system is a system of five centres (Fig. 1). In the "heroic age" of endocrinology, the endocrine system was presumed to consist of endocrine glands directed by the anterior pituitary as a "mastergland". Cawadias (1947) deserves credit for having referred to the importance of the hypothalamus in controlling endocrine functions. He was blaming the foregoing conception for having beheaded the endocrine system between hypothalamus and anterior pituitary. He has made, essentially, the same mistake for which the previous conception had been blamed, only he denoted the endocrine system one level higher, above the hypothalamus. It is quite unnecessary just at this Congress to emphasize that the endocrine system is controlled through the suprahypothalamic pathways including neocortical association areas. Moreover, the regulation does not terminate at the level of the peripheral endocrine glands but includes actions at the cellular level of the target organs. I call the latter the periphery in a strict sense of the endocrine system.

It is easy to understand that the emphasis in the endocrine hierarchy is laid by the psychoneuroendocrinologist on the psyche and the hypothalamo–pituitary system. Until recently, the endocrine periphery was a neglected part of endocrinology. It is rewarding, therefore, if the attention of some endocrinologists is drawn to the enzyme systems of the periphery as factors determining the final endocrine events.

For more than ten years, our attention has been attracted by hirsutism. In my working hypothesis, I have started from the fact that hirsutism is decided in the enzyme systems of the skin and its appendages. Every female becomes hairy in whose skin, respectively more exactly around the follicles, the androgen : oestrogen ratio is shifted in the direction of androgens. In a part of hirsutisms we know well the cause. In more than 40 per cent of our hirsute patients, however, the cause of hirsutism is still unknown. In these cases we speak about essential, respectively, idiopathic hirsutism. According to our working hypothesis, in at least one part of the idiopathic hirsutisms it is possible that 17-ketosteroids of androgenic effect develop in the skin itself.

For approaching the problem, we had first of all to prove that there are androgenic steroids in the skin. My chemist co-workers, I. Faredin and I. Tóth, have undertaken the task of elaborating suitable methods for studying the steroid economy of the skin (Julesz et al. 1966a, b, Faredin et al. 1966, Tóth et al. 1966, Faredin et al. 1967a, b, Julesz 1968, Julesz et al. 1971).

The first step was to investigate the Zimmermann chromogens of human skin and hair and the more specific ketonic fraction of extracts separated by means

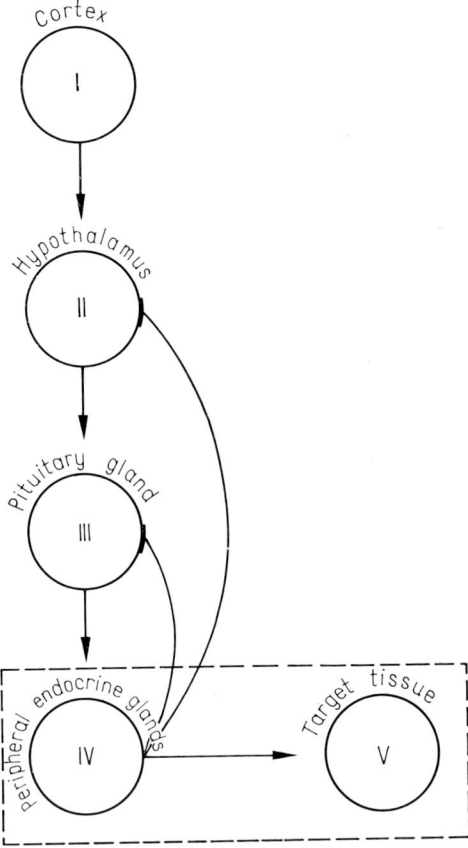

Fig. 1. Schematic drawing of the correlation existing between the endocrine system and target tissues

of the Girard's reagent. Zimmermann chromogens obtained by the enzymatic and hydrochloric acid hydrolysis of skin have been investigated on silica-gel-G thin layer plate with phosphoric acid colour reaction, in U.V. light. With that method the intensely fluorescent spots of cholesterol and authentic dehydroepiandrosterone and those of androsterone were excellently visible (Fig. 2). On the strips of extracts obtained by enzymatic and hydrochloric acid hydrolysis there are several smaller fluorescent spots observable, besides the spots already mentioned.

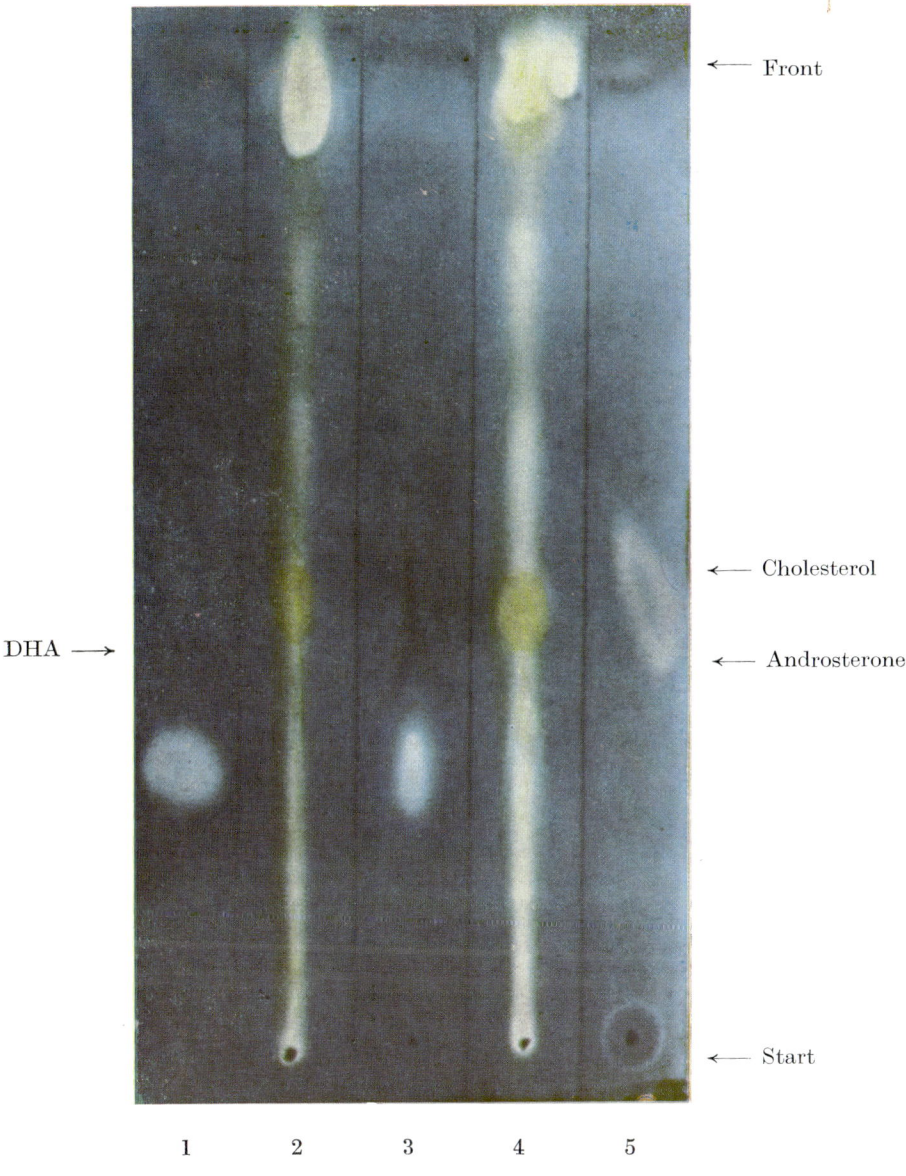

Fig. 2. Thin layer chromatogram of the total Zimmermann chromogens obtained from skin by enzymatic (strip 2) and hydrochloric acid (strip 4) hydrolysis. TLC: silica-gel-G; solvent system: ethanol (4)-benzene (96), (v/v); development: with 50 per cent phosphoric acid in U.V. light

We have been encouraged by the promising results of our investigations, to commence to investigate in details the androgenically active steroids in human skin and appendages by applying finer methods.

At first, we attempted to identify the steroids demonstrated in the course of thin layer chromatographic experiments only with approximative methods. Some informative data were given by the identical R_f values and by the so-called specific colour reactions, rendering the presence of dehydroepiandrosterone in human skin highly probable.

In 1965, we (Julesz and Horváth) demonstrated first by histochemical reaction that in the epidermal cells (stratum spinosum) round the hair follicles and in the sweat glands an expressed Δ^5-3β-hydroxysteroid dehydrogenase activity could be observed. The fact that in the skin we have found dehydroepiandrosterone and demonstrated Δ^5-3β-hydroxysteroid dehydrogenase activity with a histochemical method, made highly probable the occurrence of androst-4-ene-3,17-dione among the so far unknown 17-ketosteroids. In fact, the presence of this compound could be made later probable by thin layer chromatography and then identified.

In the following we are showing the chromatograms of 17-ketosteroids demonstrated on a silica-gel-G thin layer of the extracts of axillary hairs obtained from healthy females (Fig. 3). We see on strip 1 the extracts of thin layer chromatograms acidified with hydrochloric acid, on strip 2 those acidified with sulphuric acid. On strip 3 we have run authentic steroids. The development of colours was achieved with ferric chloride-sulphuric acid reagent — Zlatkis' colour reaction (Zlatkis et al. 1953). In this Figure, I should like to call attention to the following: dehydroepiandrosterone manifests itself in the shape of a very large spot both in the extracts obtained with hydrochloric acid and in those obtained with sulphuric acid hydrolysis. There runs a spot of considerable size at the height of authentic cholesterol as well. On strip 1 we see a large spot at the height of 3β-chlorodehydroepiandrosterone.

In Fig. 4 hair extracts obtained from males are shown. On strip 1 the extract of pubic hair can be seen chromatographed on an Al_2O_3-G thin layer and detected by Zimmermann reaction, on strip 3 that of axillary hair, and on strip 5 that of hair extracts from the scalp. On strip 2, the following authentic steroids can be observed, from above downwards: 3β-chlorodehydroepiandrosterone, dehydroepiandrosterone, and 11β-hydroxyandrosterone. On strip 4, the following authentic steroids are run: 3β-chlorodehydroepiandrosterone, androsterone, etiocholanolone and 11-ketoandrosterone. We can ascertain at first sight that the most 17-ketosteroids are contained in the axillary hair. We have obtained nearly exactly the same picture also when studying female hair. The most intensive spots have been obtained at the height of 3β-chlorodehydroepiandrosterone and dehydroepiandrosterone.

The 3β-chlorodehydroepiandrosterone was regarded as a product formed artificially. Our experiments could only be really evaluated as we succeeded in elaborating a method that enabled us to extract the ketosteroids without a harsh chemical treatment of hairs.

It was ascertained in a set of experiments that even boiling with 2.5 per cent NaOH solution for 3 minutes was sufficient for exploring the human hair and under such conditions the 17-ketosteroid esters were not damaged appreciably. It appeared that in the extract of female axillary hair we found prevailingly

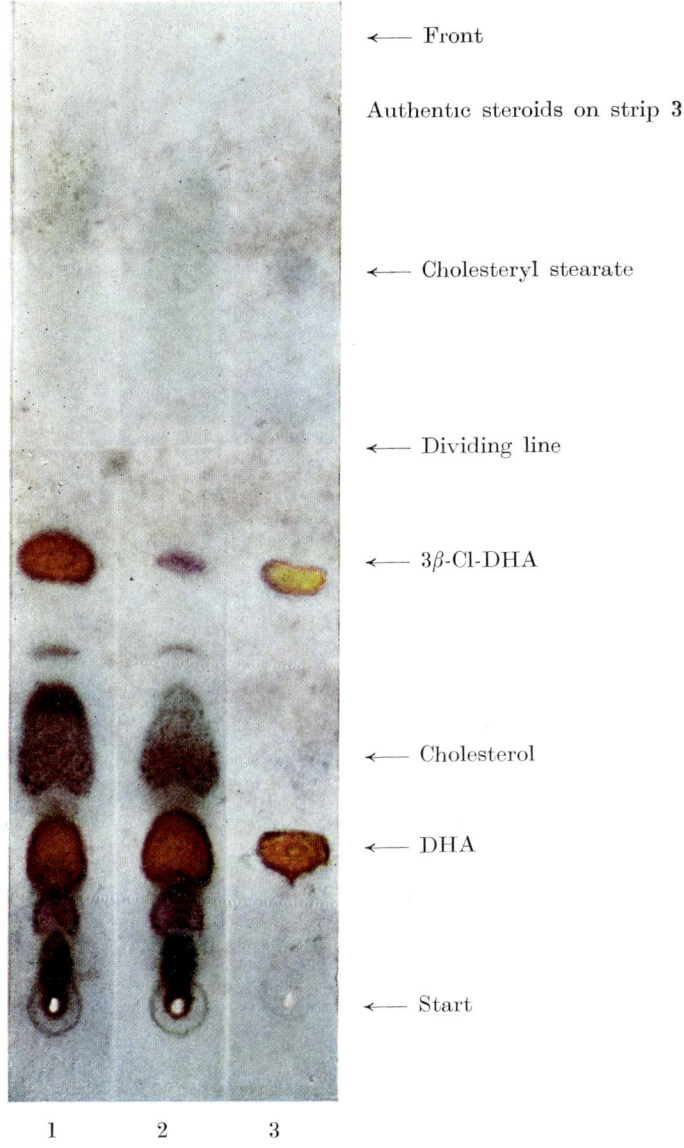

Fig. 3. Thin layer chromatogram of the extracts of axillary hair obtained from healthy females. Strip 1: extract after 11 N hydrochloric acid hydrolysis; strip 2: extract after 10 N sulphuric acid hydrolysis; TLC: silica-gel-G; solvent system: first running in benzene; second running in ethanol (6)-benzene (94) (v/v); detection: with Zlatkis colour reaction

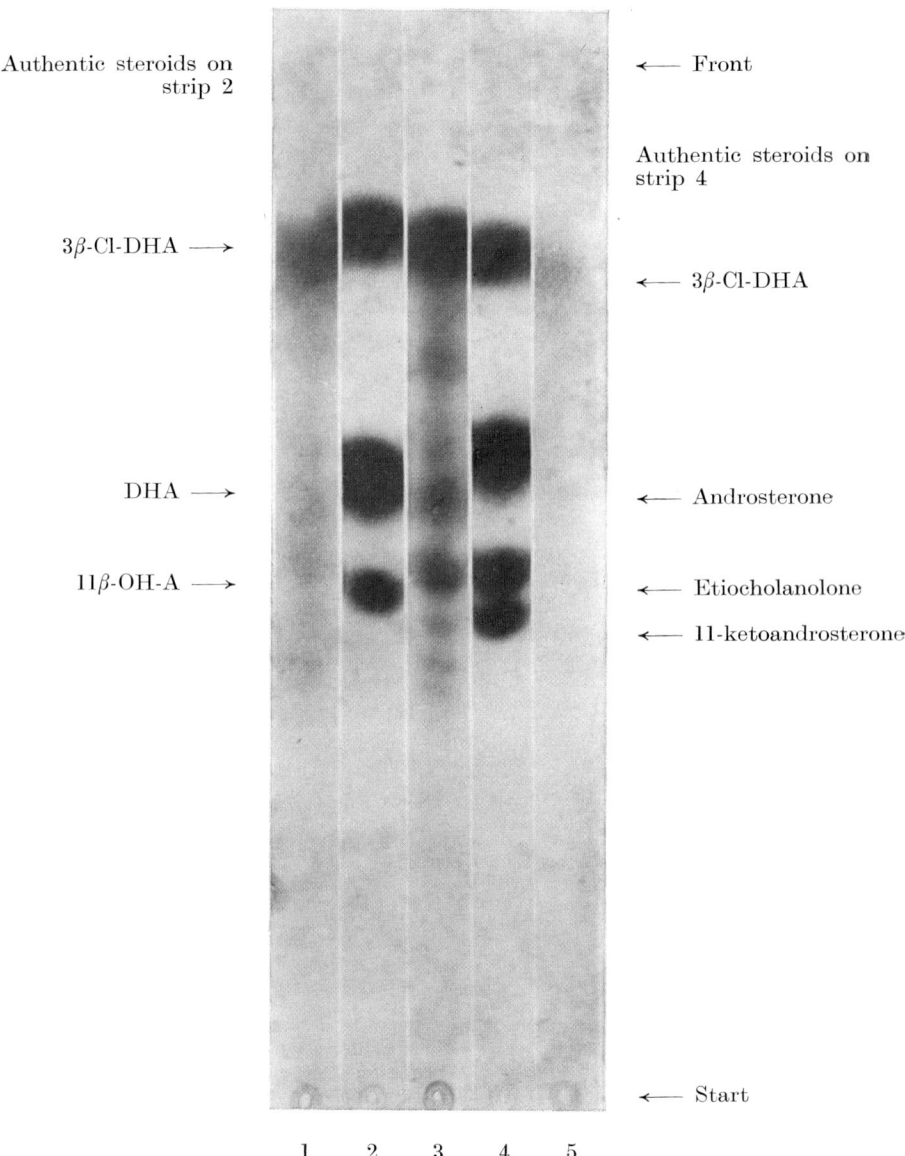

Fig. 4. Thin layer chromatogram of hair extracts obtained from healthy males. Strip 1: extract of pubic hair; strip 3: extract of axillary hair; strip 5: extract of hair from the scalp; TLC: Al_2O_3-G, 10×35 cm; solvent system: System "G"; detection: with Zimmermann colour reaction

dehydroepiandrosterone sulphate. After solvolysis, the latter proved to be dehydroepiandrosterone and androsterone.

Later on, we used [4-^{14}C] steroids for identification. The extracts were transferred on an Al_2O_3 column of 3 g and the radioactivity of the elutions obtained from the column was determined with Packard TriCarb's Liquid Scintillation Spectrometer (Model 3375) and the identifications were carried out with separated [4-^{14}C] dehydroepiandrosterone and [4-^{14}C] androsterone. In this way we have proved that the two steroids isolated from the female and male axillary hairs are: dehydroepiandrosterone and androsterone and these steroids occur in the human axillary hair originally in sulphate ester conjugation.

There arose early the problem, how the 17-ketosteroids get into the hairs. A large amount of axillary hair collected from healthy females was soaked in various solvents.

The best "eluent" proved to be 2 N NH_4OH. If we applied that solvent combined with ether for 8 to 10 days, the 17-ketosteroid content of hairs could be extracted nearly in 100 per cent. In this way we had a possibility for separating the free and ester 17-ketosteroids from each other. With this method we identified in the axillary hair a small amount of free 17-ketosteroids, apart from the water-soluble sulphate ester 17-ketosteroids.

Dehydroepiandrosterone sulphate and androsterone sulphate are water-soluble and we have thought probable that these water-soluble androgens may have reached by perspiration the surface of hairs and from there imbibed into the hairs. It seemed to be logical, therefore, to extend our research also over the investigation of the 17-ketosteroid content of sweat.

For our investigations some *sweat* collected from the surface of armpit was used. Our examinations were carried out on healthy females and males in the age of sexual maturity, as well as on hirsute females. The extracts purified appropriately were chromatographed on an alumina thin layer and then the thin layer was sprayed with Zimmermann reagent. We show as an example Fig. 5, which demonstrates the thin layer chromatogram of the 17-ketosteroid ester extract of female axillary sweat; the detection was carried out with Zimmermann reaction. On the right the authentic steroids are developed, and on the left the axillary sweat extract. It is apparent that the latter contains mostly dehydroepiandrosterone sulphate. After solvolysis it turned out that the sweat extract was containing dehydroepiandrosterone and androsterone.

In the course of our investigations we have ascertained that the sweat collected from the axillary area has in every case contained a determinable amount of 17-ketosteroid sulphate. At the same time, in the sweat collected from the abdominal area we have not found in any case a measurable amount of 17-ketosteroid sulphates.

We have investigated in incubation experiments in vitro, what happens with the steroids in the skin, whether they are only stored or they are metabolized in skin.

On the basis of our previous experiments it seemed practicable to continue our incubation experiments with dehydroepiandrosterone.

The possibility of accomplishing a successful in vitro study of the enzyme activity of human skin was supported by the experiments of János Julesz (1969) which proved that slices of skin excised under general anaesthesia utilized sugar and oxygen in the incubation medium for at least six hours.

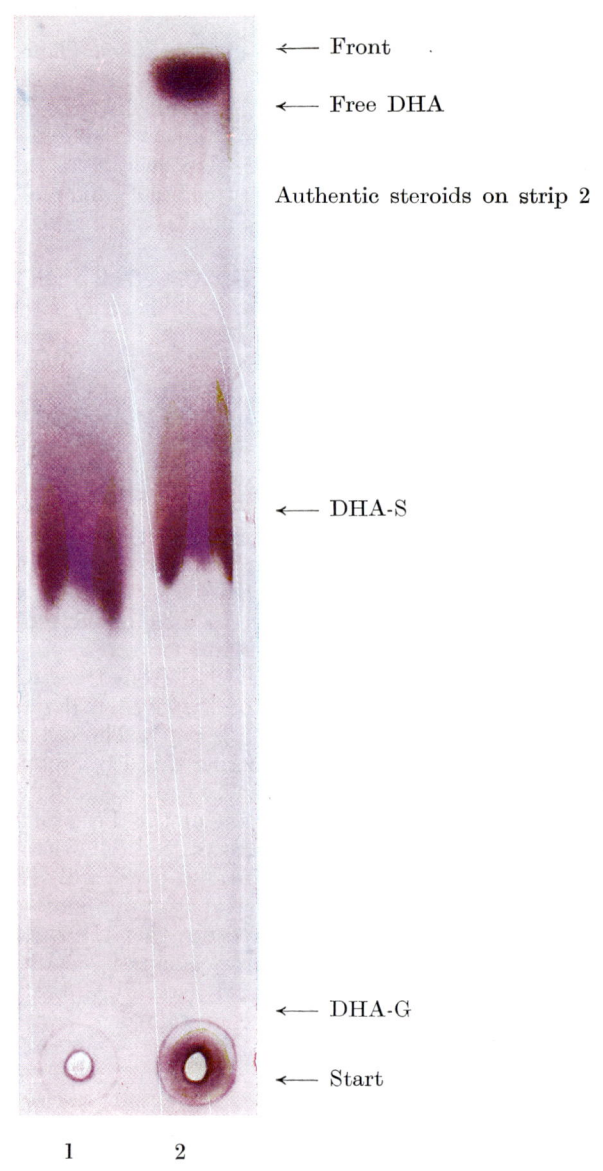

Fig. 5. Thin layer chromatogram of 17-ketosteroid sulphates (17-Ks-S) isolated from healthy female axillary hair. TLC: Al_2O_3-G, 5×20 cm; solvent system: System "I" (Sarfaty and Lipsett 1966); detection: with Zimmerman colour reaction

The essence of our method is as follows. First we incubated slices of skin, excised from the pubic (hair-bearing) and abdominal (hairless) regions of endocrinologically healthy females and males, with [4-^{14}C] dehydroepiandrosterone. The medium contained NAD, ATP, and NADP, in a 10^{-3} M concentration. The incubation was carried out in air atmosphere, between pH = 7.2–7.4, at 37°C, for five hours. The incubation medium and skin slices were extracted by organic solvents and the radioactive extract obtained in this way (organic phase) was chromatographed on an alumina column. In the chromatogram obtained in this way we have collected the steroids dissolved corresponding to their polarity in peaks from I to VIII (Fig. 6).

The Figure shows the distribution of radioactivity in the eluates obtained from the column. Curve A contains the column chromatograms of the incubated female skin slices, curve B those of the male ones. Curve C represents a chromatogram of an extract of skin slices, inactivated by boiling before incubation and that of [4-^{14}C] dehydroepiandrosterone, while curve D illustrates only the chromatogram of an extract obtained after a five-hour incubation period of the substrate [4-^{14}C] dehydroepiandrosterone, without any skin present. It is evident from curves C and D that there are no metabolites formed in significant quantities in either case in the course of incubation. Curve E shows the order and areas of elution of authentic steroids from the alumina column.

Then we investigated in detail the radioactive metabolites eluted from the single peaks.

Making no mention of details, I shall discuss only some of the final results. The radioactive eluate identified from peak I is 5α-androsterone-3,17-dione. From peak II there were isolated and identified androst-4-ene-3,17-dione and [4-^{14}C] dehydroandrosterone applied as a substrate. The female and male chromatograms differ from each other mainly in peak III. Although a significant amount of radioactivity was found in peaks III of both chromatograms, for want of proper authentic steroids we could not elucidate any of the metabolites of this peak. Peak IV is the most important from the point of view of our experiments as the two steroids of the strongest androgenic activity, androsterone and testosterone, are eluted together in that peak. We have identified, indeed, both testosterone and androsterone in peak IV. From peak V there could be demonstrated, in addition to the identified 7-keto-dehydroepiandrosterone and androst-5-ene-3β,17β-diol, also 16α-hydroxydehydroepiandrosterone. In peak VI in both sexes 7β-hydroxydehydroepiandrosterone was formed, while in peak VII 7α-hydroxydehydroepiandrosterone. In peak VIII we have obtained a practically insignificant radioactivity, without attaching major importance to it.

In the course of control, we found in the aqueous phase, remaining after extraction of the incubate with organic solvents, a not negligible amount of radioactivity. At that time there appeared a short publication by Gallegos and Berliner (1967) in which they described the formation of water-soluble dehydroepiandrosterone sulphate (DHA-S) when [4-^{14}C] dehydroepiandrosterone was incubated with male abdominal skin slices. This made us suspect that perhaps the radioactivity detected in the aqueous phase might be due to the formation of water-soluble sulphate esters of steroids. We have succeeded, indeed, in proving that in the course of the incubation of *female* and *male* skin slices steroid sulphate esters are formed from which we have identified the main metabolite, dehydroepiandrosterone sulphate.

In Fig. 7 we have indicated the possible ways of the in vitro metabolism of dehydroepiandrosterone with healthy female and male abdominal skin slices. Nine metabolites are produced.

The main direction of metabolism is 7α- and 7β-hydroxylation, respectively, oxidation of atom C_7. By the appearance of these steroids the presence of 7α- and 7β-hydroxylase is proved, as well as that of 7-hydroxysteroid dehydrogenase in the skin. The second main direction shows, through the intermediary androst-

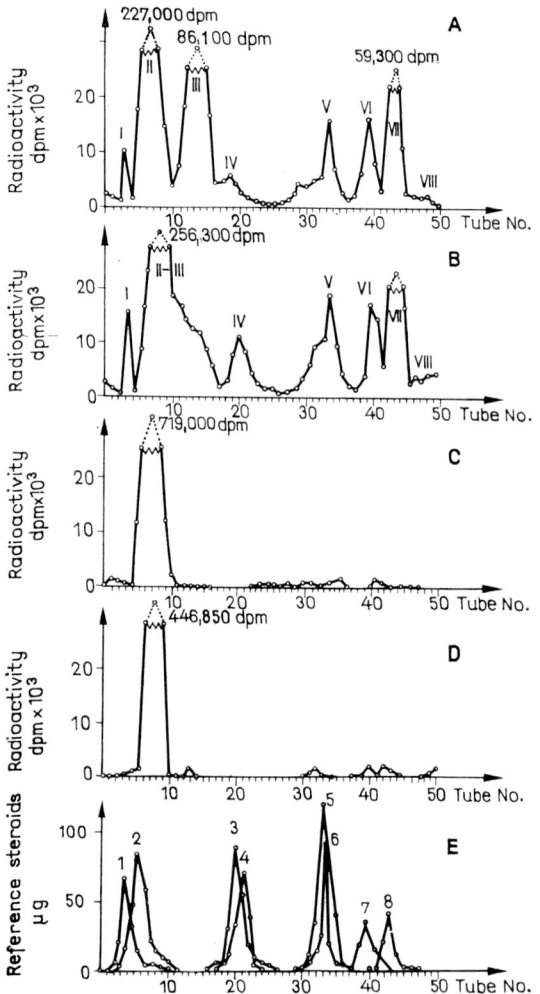

Fig. 6. Distribution of radioactivity in the eluates of the alumina column. Nos I–VIII represent peaks of radioactive steroids in order of increasing polarity. Curve A: normal female skin; curve B: normal male skin; curve C: boiled skin; curve D: [4–^{14}C] DHA substrate; curve E: reference steroids: 1. 5α-androstane-3,17-dione, 2. androst-4-ene-3,17-dione, 3. androsterone, 4. testosterone, 5. androst-5-ene-3,17-diol, 6. 7-keto-DHA, 7. 7β-OH-DHA, 8. 7α-OH-DHA

4-ene-3,17-dione, the formation of the two main androgenically active steroids, testosterone and androsterone. A third direction of metabolism is towards the formation of water-soluble dehydroepiandrosterone sulphate. It is proved by these metabolites that in the skin Δ^5-3β-hydroxysteroid dehydrogenase, 17β-hydroxysteroid dehydrogenase, Δ^4-5α-reductase and Δ^5-3β-hydroxysteroid sulphokinase enzyme systems are present. In this way, there is a possibility for the formation of a steroid of high androgenic activity, the testosterone, from the dehydroepiandrosterone of low androgenic activity at the periphery, in the skin.

We have extended our investigations also over the skin slices of an agonadal male and of a female with hirsutism of ovarian origin. As to the agonadal male, we made sure surgically and with various biochemical methods that he had neither testes nor ovary. Karyotyping: XY (male-type karyogram), Bar's sex-chromatin: negative (male type). The distribution of radioactivity in the eluates of the alumina column in shown in Fig. 8, reminding us very much of the female curve seen in Fig. 6. As in the female curve, too, column 4 containing the main androgens gave a small peak, the same can be seen in case of the agonadal male. This male, lacking sexual hair, has in his skin testosterone and androsterone of measurable radioactivity.

Later on, we used [4-^{14}C]androst-4-ene-3,17-dione as substrate. In Fig. 9 on the top, we can see the distribution of radioactivity in the eluates of the alumina column of a normal female (A), and below it that of a female with hirsutism of adrenocortical origin (B). In curve C the substrate itself was incubated without skin. It is evident from these experiments that [4-^{14}C]androst-4-ene-3,17-dione is intensively metabolized by the abdominal skin slices both of the normal female and of that with hirsutism of adrenocortical origin under in vitro

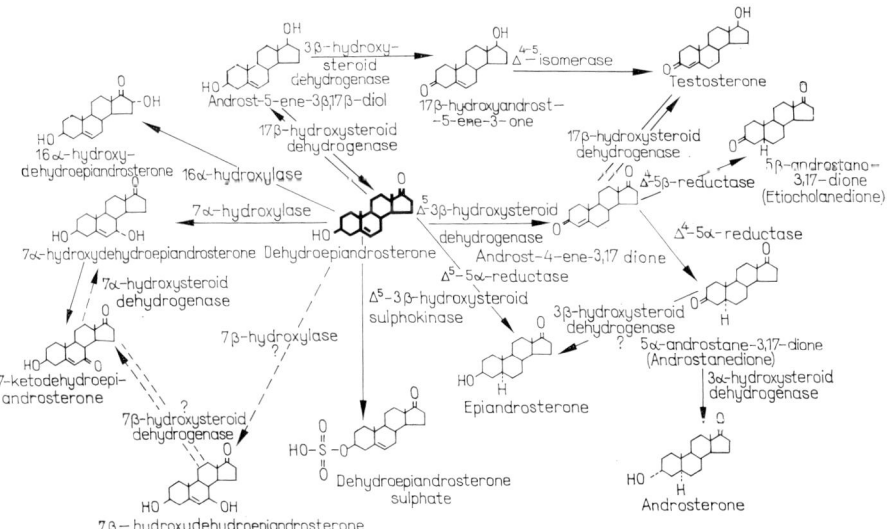

Fig. 7. Possible routes of metabolism of [4–^{14}C] dehydroepiandrosterone by abdominal skin slices of healthy females and males

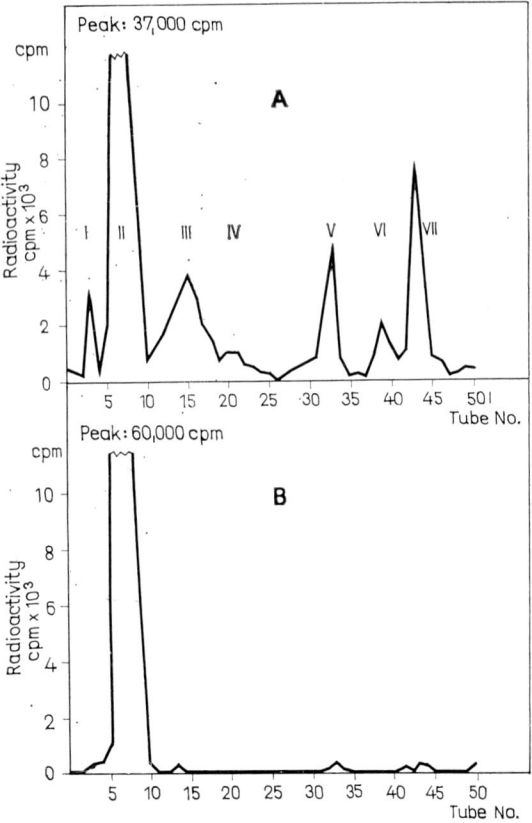

Fig. 8. Distribution of radioactivity in the eluates of the alumina column. Nos I–VII represent peaks of radioactive steroids with increasing polarity. Curve A: agonadal male pubic skin; curve B: [4–^{14}C]DHA substrate

conditions, and, from among the metabolites formed, we have identified 5α-androstane-3,17-dione, androsterone and testosterone. This, too, is an evidence for the androst-4-ene-3,17-dione being an important precursor of testosterone and androsterone formed in the skin.

It is proved by our investigations that in the skin water-soluble and free androgenically active steroids are present, as well. We could demonstrate in the skin an intensive steroid metabolism and have proved that dehydroepiandrosterone and androsterone-dione are important precursors of testosterone and androsterone with high androgenic activity, formed locally in the skin.

On the basis of our experiments we think the presumption well-founded that some of the idiopathic hirsutisms are a result of the enzymopathies of the skin.

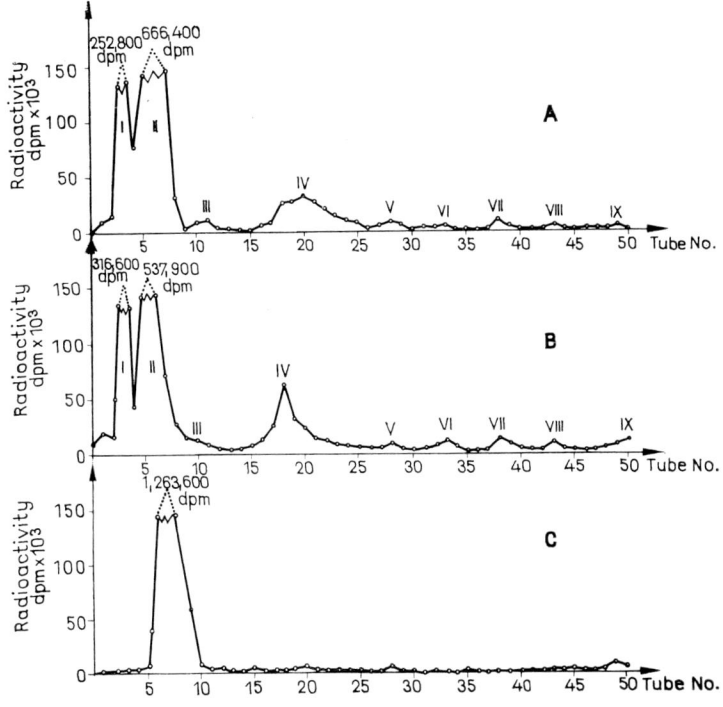

Fig. 9. Distribution of radioactivity in the eluates of the alumina column. Nos I–IX represent peaks of radioactive steroids with increasing polarity. Curve A: normal female abdominal skin; curve B: hirsute female abdominal skin; curve C: [4–^{14}C] androst-4-ene-3,17-dione substrate

REFERENCES

CAWADIAS, A. P. (1947): *Clinical Endocrinology and Constitutional Medicine.* Frederick Muller, London.
GALLEGOS, A. J. and BERLINER, D. L. (1967): *J. clin. Endocr.* **27**, 1214.
FAREDIN, I., WEBB, J. L. and JULESZ, M. (1966): In: *IInd International Congress on Hormonal Steroids.* Excerpta med. Int. Congr. Series **111**, 278.
FAREDIN, I., FAZEKAS, Á. G., TÓTH, I., KÓKAI, K. and JULESZ, M. (1967a): *Europ. J. Steroids* **2**, 223.
FAREDIN, I., WEBB, J. L. and JULESZ, M. (1967b): *Acta med. Acad. Sci. hung.* **23**, 167.
JULESZ, J. (1969): *Acta med. Acad. Sci. hung.* **26**, 375.
JULESZ, M. (1968): *Acta med. Acad. Sci. hung.* **25**, 273.
JULESZ, M. and HORVÁTH, É. (1965): In: *Deutsche Gesellschaft für klinische Medizin. 7. Wissenschaftliche Tagung*, Kühlungsborn, 21—23 Oktober 1965. p. 27.
JULESZ, M., FAREDIN, I. and TÓTH, I. (1966a): *Acta med. Acad. Sci. hung.* **22**, 25.
JULESZ, M., FAREDIN, I. and TÓTH, I. (1966b): *Acta med. Acad. Sci. hung.* **22**, 49.
JULESZ, M., FAREDIN, I. and TÓTH, I. (1971): *Steroids in Human Skin.* Akadémiai Kiadó, Budapest.
SARFATY, G. A. and LIPSETT, H. B. (1966): *Analyt. Biochem.* **15**, 184.
TÓTH, I., FAREDIN, I. and JULESZ, M. (1966): *Acta med. Acad. Sci. hung.* **22**, 35.
ZLATKIS, A., ZAK, B. and BOYLE, A. J. (1953): *J. Lab. clin. Med.* **41**, 486.

SECRETION OF LH AND FSH DURING SLEEP IN MAN*

R. T. RUBIN, A. KALES and W. ODELL

Department of Psychiatry
Milton S. Hershey Medical Center
Hershey, Penn.
and
Department of Medicine
Harbor General Hospital
Torrance, Cal., U.S.A.

Increased secretion of ACTH during sleep occurs in the early morning hours, at a time when REM sleep is maximal (Weitzman et al. 1966, Mandell et al. 1966, Rubin et al. 1969, Roffwarg et al. 1970). Increased secretion of growth hormone, on the other hand, occurs primarily in the first few hours after sleep onset and is closely related to slow-wave (stage 3–4) sleep (Takahashi et al. 1968, Honda et al. 1969, Parker et al. 1969, Sassin et al. 1969a, Mace et al. 1970). The release of ACTH can be dissociated from REM sleep by acute sleep–wake reversal (Weitzman et al. 1968), but growth hormone release follows intimately the time of onset of slow-wave sleep (Sassin et al. 1969b, Karacan et al. 1970) and is not alterable by manipulations which affect growth hormone during waking hours (Vanderlaan et al. 1970, Parker and Rossman 1971, Zir et al. 1971). The possibility that related neural mechanisms control both sleep patterns and the secretion of some anterior pituitary hormones is enhanced by evidence that biogenic amines have neurotransmitter roles both in sleep (Jouvet 1968) and in the secretion by the hypothalamus of pituitary hormone releasing and inhibiting factors (Wurtman 1971). The investigation of other pituitary hormones during sleep is thus warranted, and we report herein a study of luteinizing hormone (LH, ICSH) and follicle-stimulating hormone (FSH) release during sleep in normal young men.

Patterns of LH and FSH release in normal men have not been extensively investigated. Serum LH and FSH levels measured every two hours for one day in ten subjects were quite stable (Swerdloff and Odell 1968); other studies, however, have reported a circadian rhythm of serum FSH in men, with highest values occurring in the early morning hours (Faiman and Ryan 1967, Saxena et al. 1968). A periodicity of plasma LH levels was observed during sleep in three men, although there was no obvious relation to sleep stages (Kapen et al. 1970). Peaks of plasma testosterone, on the other hand, were found in conjunction with episodes of REM sleep in five male subjects (Evans et al. 1971).

We studied sixteen healthy male volunteers, ages 21–30, on no drugs or medications, for four consecutive nights in the sleep laboratory. Men were chosen in

---

* Report 71–50, Bureau of Medicine and Surgery, Navy Department. Supported in part by the Office of Naval Research Contract N00014–69–A–0200–4030. The opinions expressed herein are the private ones of the authors and are not necessarily those of the Department of the Navy.

order to obviate the cyclic influence of the female hypothalamus on gonadotropins. They were allowed normal meals and activity during the day. Continuous electrophysiologic (electroencephalographic, electrooculographic, and electromyographic) recordings were made each night during the hours of sleep (11:00 p.m.–7:00 a.m.). On the first night only electrophysiologic recordings were made; on the second night an antecubital venous catheter was placed but no blood was taken; on the third and fourth nights blood was sampled from an adjoining room through a ten-foot long tubing connected to the indwelling venous catheter (Vankirk and Sassin 1969, Rubin et al. 1971). The first eight subjects were sampled every thirty minutes from 11:00 p.m. to 7:00 a.m.; the second eight subjects were sampled every ten minutes between 11:00 p.m. and 1:00 a.m. and between 5:00 a.m. and 6:00 a.m. Total blood withdrawal was kept below 200 ml each night. The plasma was immediately separated and frozen until radioimmunoassay for LH and FSH (Odell et al. 1967a, b, 1968).* All samples were run in duplicate and all samples from each subject were run in the same assay. Mean intra-assay variability was 5 per cent; mean inter-assay variability was 20 per cent.

Each thirty-second epoch of EEG recording was scored as awake; stages 1, 2, 3, 4; or REM by established criteria (Rechtschaffen and Kales 1968). Compared to the subsequent three nights, the first adaptation night showed the usual greater sleep latency and lower REM time and REM % (Agnew et al. 1966, Mendels and Hawkins 1967). The only significant difference between the first two adaptation nights and the two blood-draw nights was an increased wake time after sleep onset** during the blood-draw nights, related to several occasions when subjects rolled over on the catheter while asleep and had to be momentarily awakened and untangled. There were no significant differences in sleep parameters between the two consecutive blood-draw nights.

Both LH and FSH showed patterns of nocturnal secretion that were neither similar across subjects nor constant between the two blood-draw nights for the same subject. There were episodic but unrelated peaks of both hormones throughout most nights (Figs 1 and 2).

The rhythmicity of these changes in LH and FSH was tested by fitting sine curves of 45 min, 60 min, 75 min, 90 min, 2 hours, 4 hours, 8 hours, and 24 hours for each subject.*** These analyses indicated that there was no consistent ultradian or circadian pattern across subjects for either hormone. The analysis of hormone levels by sleep stage therefore was performed without correcting the hormone data for any rhythm effects.

Generally, intersubject differences in hormone levels were great (Table 1), and differences between sleep stages averaged across subjects were small. Because there were no stage 1 data for four of the 16 subjects, this stage was omitted

---

* Antisera with marked increase in affinity of binding, and therefore sensitivity, for hormone measurement were developed and utilized in this study. Each antiserum was shown to be specific by immunologic studies and by bioassay–immunoassay correlations. These data are not presented, but studies were performed in the same fashion as previously reported.

** Time of sleep onset is marked by two continuous minutes of stage 1 or one continuous minute of stage 2 sleep.

*** Computer program by C. Nute, Navy Medical Neuropsychiatric Research Unit, San Diego, California, 92152. Dr. Ardie Lubin, of the Unit, provided helpful statistical consultation. Statistical methodology will be detailed in a subsequent report.

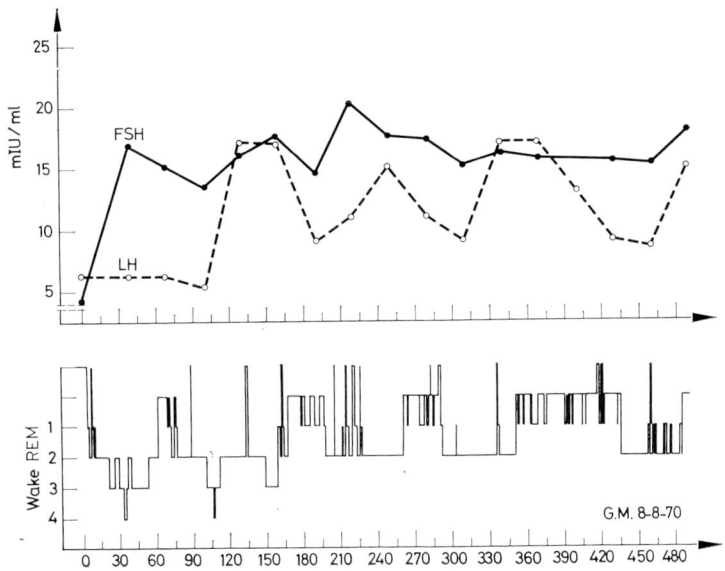

Fig. 1. Subject G. M. sampled every 30 min

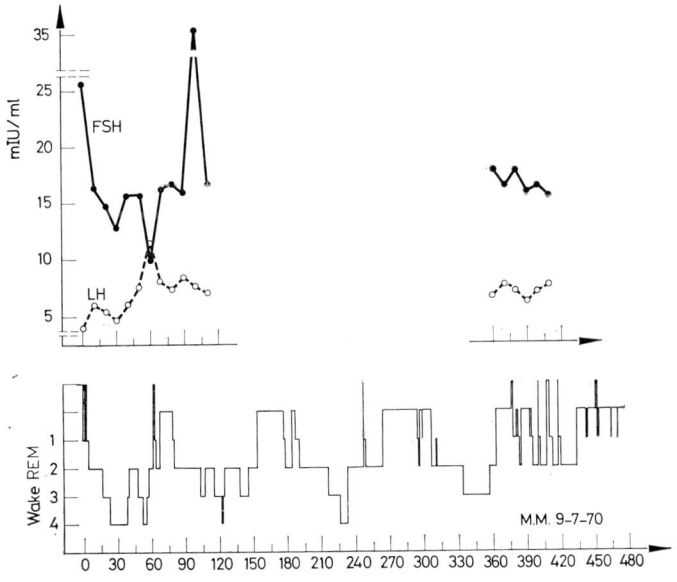

Fig. 2. Subject M.M. sampled every 10 min

in the sleep analyses. Because stages 3 and 4 had very few data points, these stages were combined in the analyses. Kendall's rank-order coefficient of concordance (Kendall 1948) comparing gonadotropin levels during awake, stage 2, stages 3 + 4, and REM across the 16 subjects was low but statistically significant for both LH (W = 0.24) and FSH (W = 0.19). By successive comparison of the individual sleep stages and combination of those that were not significantly different, the overall significance for LH was found to reside in a difference between REM sleep and all other sleep stages combined; LH was 14 per cent higher during REM sleep compared to the other sleep stages (Table 1). The significance for FSH, on the other hand, was not clearly discernible by successive comparison and combination of the individual sleep stages; FSH was not significantly increased during REM sleep (Table 1).

The results of this study suggest that the secretion of gonadotropins during sleep in normal men is pulsatile rather than periodic (Kapen et al. 1970) and varies considerably both from subject to subject and from night to night within the same subject. The discontinuous and arrhythmic nature of gonadotropin

TABLE 1

Overall mean LH and FSH levels for each subject, and % change during REM sleep compared to other sleep stages combined*

Subject	LH (mIU/ml)	% change in LH during REM sleep	FSH (mIU/ml)	% change in FSH during REM sleep
1	8.8	+14	10.3	(−6)
2	11.0	+4	12.1	(−20)
3	13.2	(−14)	16.3	+20
4	11.0	+4	15.6	+9
5	6.6	(−2)	16.0	(−11)
6	7.8	+9	5.7	(−5)
7	4.9	(−9)	6.3	+3
8	8.6	+42	12.0	(−4)
9	3.5	+90	8.4	0
10	8.0	+6	8.2	(−8)
11	9.4	+12	16.7	+7
12	7.3	+11	3.9	(−33)
13	13.0	+23	17.7	(−2)
14	15.7	+19	9.8	+1
15	24.7	+3	9.4	(−2)
16	6.5	+5	8.7	+1
Average		+14		−1

* The first eight subjects were measured at a longer time interval than the second eight subjects.

release is consistent with the pattern of release of other anterior pituitary hormones in man (Hellman et al. 1970). The modest but statistically significant increase in LH during REM sleep is of interest for several reasons. First, norepinephrine as a central neurotransmitter has been implicated both in REM sleep (Jouvet 1968) and in the secretion of LH (Wurtman 1971). Second, peak secretion of LH recently has been shown to occur during paradoxical (REM) sleep in unanesthetized, unrestrained female rats at all times of the estrous cycle (Clemens et al. 1971). Third, REM sleep-associated increases in testosterone, the release of which is stimulated by LH, were reported recently in male subjects (Evans et al. 1971). And fourth, penile erections occur during REM sleep (Oswald 1962, Fisher et al. 1965).

Of major interest is the fact that the fluctuations in both LH and FSH are small compared to the large changes in ACTH and growth hormone which occur during sleep. Recent studies of reproductive physiology using sensitive radio-immunoassay techniques indicate that major physiologic events may be associated with only small changes in LH and FSH concentrations (Odell and Moxer 1971). Thus, the modest increases in LH found during REM sleep may have important, but as yet unknown, physiologic significance. However, it also is possible that these changes reflect only the modulation of control systems within the brain and are without importance to gonadal function.

SUMMARY

Release of LH and FSH during sleep in adult men occurs in unrelated, random, arrhythmic peaks, with no consistency from night to night in the same subject. LH appears to be modestly but significantly increased (14 per cent) during REM sleep compared to non-REM sleep. FSH release is not clearly related to sleep stages.

REFERENCES

AGNEW, H. W., WEBB, W. B. and WILLIAMS, R. L. (1966): *Psychophysiol.* **2**, 263.
CLEMENS, J. A., SHAAR, C. J. and TANDY, W. A. (1971): *Endocrinology* **88**, A-72.
EVANS, J. I., MACLEAN, A. W. and ISMAIL, A. A. A. (1971): *Nature (Lond.)* **229**, 261.
FAIMAN, C. and RYAN, R. J. (1967): *Nature (Lond.)* **215**, 857.
FISHER, C., GROSS, J. and ZUCH, J. (1965): *Arch. gen. Psychiat.* **12**, 29.
HELLMAN, L., NAKADA, F. and CURTI, J. (1970): *J. clin. Endocr.* **30**, 411.
HONDA, Y., TAKAHASHI, K. and TAKAHASHI, S. (1969): *J. clin. Endocr.* **29**, 20.
JOUVET, M. (1968): *Science* **163**, 32.
KAPEN, S., BOYAR, R. and HELLMAN, L. (1970): *Psychophysiol.* **7**, 337.
KARACAN, I., WILLIAMS, R. L. and ROSENBLOOM, A. L. (1970): *Psychophysiol.* **7**, 324.
KENDALL, M. G. (1948): *Rank Correlation Methods*. Griffin, London.
MACE, J. W., GOTLIN, R. W. and SASSIN, J. F. (1970): *J. clin. Endocr.* **31**, 225.
MANDELL, M. P., MANDELL, A. J. and RUBIN, R. T. (1966): *Life Sci.* **5**, 583.
MENDELS, J. and HAWKINS, D. R. (1967): *Electroenceph. clin. Neurophysiol.* **22**, 556.
ODELL, W. D. and MOXER, D. L. (1971): *Physiology of Reproduction*. Mosby, St. Louis.
ODELL, W. D., ROSS, G. T. and RAYFORD, P. L. (1967a): *J. clin. Invest.* **46**, 248.
ODELL, W. D., RAYFORD, P. L. and ROSS, G. T. (1967b): *J. Lab. clin. Med.* **70**, 973.
ODELL, W. D., PARLOW, A. F. and CARGILLE, C. M. (1968): *J. clin. Invest.* **47**, 2551.
OSWALD, I. (1962): *Sleep and Waking*. Elsevier, Amsterdam.
PARKER, D. C. and ROSSMAN, L. G. (1971): *J. clin. Endocr.* **32**, 65.

Parker, D. C., Sassin, J. F. and Mace, J. W. (1969): *J. clin. Endocr.* **29,** 871.
Rechtschaffen, A. and Kales, A. (Eds) (1968): *A Manual of Standardized Terminology, Techniques and Scoring System for Sleep Stages of Human Subjects.* Public Health Service, U.S. Government Printing Office, Washington, D.C.
Roffwarg, H. P., Sachar, E. J. and Finkelstein, J. (1970): *Psychophysiol.* **7,** 323.
Rubin, R. T., Kales, A. and Clark, B. R. (1969): *Life Sci.* **8,** 959.
Rubin, R. T., Zir, L. M. and Smith, R. A. (1971): *Amer. J. EEG Technol.* **11,** 17.
Sassin, J. F., Parker, D. C. and Mace, J. W. (1969a): *Science* **165,** 513.
Sassin, J. F., Parker, D. C. and Johnson, L. C. (1969b): *Life Sci.* **8,** 1299.
Saxena, B. B., Demura, H. and Gandy, H. M. (1968): *J. clin. Endocr.* **28,** 519.
Swerdloff, R. S. and Odell, W. D. (1968): In: *Gonadotropins.* Ed. by E. Rosemberg. Geron-X, Los Altos, Cal. pp. 155–166.
Takahashi, Y., Kipnis, D. M. and Daughaday, W. H. (1968): *J. clin. Invest.* **47,** 2079.
Vanderlaan, W. P., Parker, D. C. and Rossman, L. G. (1970): *Metabolism* **19,** 891.
Vankirk, K. and Sassin, J. F. (1969): *Amer. J. EEG Technol.* **9,** 143.
Weitzman, E. D., Schaumberg, H. and Fishbein, W. (1966): *J. clin. Endocr.* **26,** 121.
Weitzman, E. D., Goldmacher, D. and Kripke, D. (1968): *Trans. Amer. neurol. Ass.* **93,** 153.
Wurtman, R. W. (1971): *Neurosci. Res. Prog. Bull.* **9,** 172.
Zir, L. M., Smith, R. A. and Parker, D. C. (1971): *J. clin. Endocr.* **32,** 662.

BASAL PITUITARY-GONADAL FUNCTION IN IMPOTENCY EVALUATED BY BLOOD TESTOSTERONE AND LH ASSAYS

J. J. LEGROS*, M. PALEM, J. SERVAIS, M. MARGOULIES and P. FRANCHIMONT

Institut de Médecine
Département de Clinique et de Pathologie Médicales
Université de Liège
Liège, Belgique

INTRODUCTION

Psychogenic impotency is a frequent disease whose neuroendocrine and particularly androgenic component is not perfectly understood. It is known that in man late castration or testicular organic disease does not necessarily alter the sexual potency; this agrees well with the common clinical observations of the poor efficiency of exogenous testosterone in the treatment of "impotentia coeundi". Nevertheless, a net decrease of urinary testosterone excretion has been noticed by Ismail et al. (1970) in a group of 28 impotent patients; in that study, individual values were very widespread. This work has also shown a lack of responsiveness of testes to exogenous HCG in 4 cases tested; however, to our knowledge, no sensitive LH assay has been realized until now, so that the central response to that peripheric insufficiency is not known.

Furthermore, if androgens are not necessarily implicated in the coitus, their deficiency could lead to psychological troubles which could be grafted on the proper disturbances of impotency and so could mask the psychopathogenesis of this disease.

Therefore, in this work, we have approached the study of the neuroendocrine gonadal function in this disorder in an attempt to define more exactly the dysfunction existing at that level and we hope that some of these data could later orientate the treatment in a more specific way.

MATERIAL AND METHODS

PATIENTS

Eighty-three men aged 20 to 60 were examined, the criteria for organic normality have been described elsewhere (Legros et al. 1971); all or only some of the assays were carried out in each case. Potency disturbances were primary or secondary; neither the length of the affection nor the different psychological troubles presented were taken into account in this study.

* Research Fellow. F.N.R.S.

HORMONAL ASSAYS

Fasting blood samples were collected between 11 a.m. and 4 p.m.; urinary collections were made for 24 hours preceding the day of the clinical examination.

1. *17-ketosteroids*

Performed on urine, adapted from Henry and Thevenet (1953).
Normal values are 15 ± 3 mg/24 hrs.

2. *17-hydroxycorticosteroids*

Performed on urine, according to Silber and Porter's method as modified by Scholler et al. (1957).
Normal values are 2.8 ± 1.2 mg/24 hrs.

3. *DHEA*

Performed on urine, according to Jayle et al. (1962).
Normal values are 1.5 ± 0.5 mg/24 hrs.

4. *LH*

Performed on serum by radioimmunoassay (Franchimont 1966).
Normal values are 13.14 ± 9.11 mIU/ml.

5. *Testosterone*

Performed on plasma by gas chromatography (GLC) (Palem et al. 1970), modified by the use of testosterone under the form of heptafluorobutyrate (Palem et al. 1971) sensitivity using the assay is 400 pg.
Normal values (25 men aged 18 to 22): 740 ± 230 ng/100 ml.

RESULTS

The results are presented in Table 1; patients are divided into two groups according to age (Group I between 20 to 39 years, Group II between 40 to 60 years).

TABLE 1

Age years	17-ketosteroids mg/24 h	17-hydroxy-corticosteroids mg/24 h	DHEA mg/24 h	LH mUI/ml	Testosterone ng/100 ml
20 → 39 Average age = 33.03 No. of cases = 44	12.94*±4.79** n = 34	4.25*±1.67** n = 35	1.69*±1.79** n = 33	17.45*± ±18.66** n = 38	370.1*± ±293** n = 37
40 → 60 Average age = 47.8 No. of cases = 40	10.57*±4.79** n = 37	4.10*±1.92** n = 35	1.18*±1** n = 33	17.79*± ±17.30** n = 34	326.5*± ±288.1** n = 31

* Mean value.
** S.D. = standard deviation.

DISCUSSION

There is in impotency a moderate deficiency of androgenic function as appreciated by the mean testosterone blood level; this finding confirms the results of Ismail et al. (1970), and of our team (Legros 1970).

Mean LH blood level is only slightly higher than normal mean value; this confirms to a certain extent the results of Ismail et al. (1970) concerning peripheral insufficiency and could be reflecting the conservation of testosterone LH feedback as it has been previously described in Klinefelter's disease (Franchimont 1968, Franchimont and Legros 1970). However, the correlation between testosterone and LH blood levels is weak in the first group ($r = 0.31$, d.d.l. $= 30$, $0.05 < p < 0.10$), while it does not exist in the second one ($r = 0.14$, d.d.l. $= 25$, $p < 0.10$). The mean excretion of 17-keto and DHEA is in agreement with the age of the patients and shows a decrease in the older group.

The origin of the slight decrease in androgenic functions is not yet clearly understood: it could be primary and so participate in the pathogenesis of the disease, or secondary due to the absence of sexual intercourses since it is known that coitus leads to a constant increase in testosterone excretion (Ismail and Harkness 1967).

In all cases, the great scatter of the individual testosterone and LH values is noteworthy and leads us to postulate that there is more than one single group of neuroendocrine disorder in impotency.

CONCLUSIONS

1. Mean testosterone blood level is decreased while LH blood level is slightly elevated in impotency, there remains a weak correlation between those two hormones in the younger but not in the older group.

2. Individual values are very divergent.

3. It is not yet possible to assume whether the described disturbances are primary or secondary to psychogenic impotency.

REFERENCES

FRANCHIMONT, P. (1968): In: *Protein and Polypeptide Hormones*. Ed. by M. Margoulies. Excerpta Medica, Amsterdam. Part I. p. 99.
FRANCHIMONT, P. and LEGROS, J. J. (1970): In: *The Hypothalamus*. Ed. by L. Martini, M. Motta and F. Fraschini Academic Press, New York. p. 365.
HENRY, R. and THEVENET, M. (1953): *Ann. Endocr. (Paris)* **14**, 628.
ISMAIL, A. A. A. and HARKNESS, R. A. (1967): *Acta endocr. (Kbh.)* **56**, 469.
ISMAIL, A. A. A., DAVIDSON, D. W., LORAINE, J. A., CULLEN, D. R., IRVINE, W. J., COOPER, A. J. and SMITH, C. G. (1970): In: *Reproduction Endocrinology*. Ed. by J. Irvine. Livingstone, Edinburgh. p. 138.
JAYLE, M. F., MALASSIS, D. and SCHOLLER, R. (1962): In: *Analyses des stéroïdes hormonaux*. Tome II. *Méthodes de dosages*. Ed. by M. F. Jayle. Masson, Paris. p. 37.
LEGROS, J. J. (1970): *Feuillets Psychiatriques de Liège* **3/4**, 530.
LEGROS, J. J. and FRANCHIMONT, P. (1971): In: *Proceedings of the Symposium on Gonadotrophins in Endocrine Disorders of Human Reproduction*. Smokoveck, Czechoslovakia. (In press).
PALEM, M., MAQUINAY, A., MARGOULIES, M. and CONINX, P. (1969): *Rev. franç. Étud. clin. biol.* **14**, 96.
PALEM, M., MAQUINAY, A. and MARGOULIES, M. (1971): (In press).
SCHOLLER, R., BUSIGNY, M. and JAYLE, M. F. (1957): *Arch. Soc. franç. Biol. med.* **2**, 47.